Surgical Techniques of Focused Ultrasound Ablation in Benign Uterine Diseases

Yonghua Xu • Lixia Yang • Felix Wong
Editors

Surgical Techniques of Focused Ultrasound Ablation in Benign Uterine Diseases

SSTP

Springer

Editors
Yonghua Xu
Imaging and Interventional Radiology
Xuhui Hospital of Fudan University/Shanghai
Xuhui Central Hospital
Shanghai, China

Lixia Yang
Imaging and Interventional Radiology
Xuhui Hospital of Fudan University/Shanghai
Xuhui Central Hospital
Shanghai, China

Felix Wong
Obstetrics and Gynaecology
Liverpool Hospital,
The University of New South Wales
Sydney, Australia

ISBN 978-981-19-7179-2 ISBN 978-981-19-7180-8 (eBook)
https://doi.org/10.1007/978-981-19-7180-8

Jointly published with Shanghai Scientific and Technical Publishers
The print edition is not for sale in China (Mainland). Customers from China (Mainland) please order the print book from: Shanghai Scientific and Technical Publishers.

This Springer imprint is published by the registered company Springer Nature Singapore Pte Ltd.
The registered company address is: 152 Beach Road, #21-01/04 Gateway East, Singapore 189721, Singapore

Preface

From year 2005, we realised that the focused ultrasound ablation treatment for benign gynaecological diseases is very promising. It is a new surgical modality that enables us to perform non-invasive and virtual surgery. In January 2021, we published a Chinese book, which detailed the practical applications of high intensity focused ultrasound (HIFU) ablation, especially in difficult HIFU ablation cases and complications that our team had encountered.

The Chinese book used numerous illustrative case series to illustrate how to apply HIFU ablation in various uterine pathologies. It contained more than 1000 MRI pictures illustrating many uterine pathological diagnoses and treatment results. As the focused ultrasound ablation is a non-invasive surgery without pathology confirmation, we usually rely on MRI diagnoses. The book's detailed MRI illustration of fibroids and adenomyosis provided the prerequisite information on how to interpret and better understand the MRI findings, assess its suitability for HIFU treatment, and their responses to HIFU ablation, and their interpretation of the treatment results.

During the past 20 years, the HIFU ablation for treating benign gynaecological diseases has been rapidly developed in China. Improved clinical training and advanced treatment with new safety protocols for the HIFU ablation have expanded the safety margin and improved the effectiveness of HIFU ablation. Currently, we wrote this English version of our book. Hopefully, we can deliver more information about this new HIFU technology worldwide, especially in English-speaking countries.

This English version of our book is especially suitable for overseas doctors learning HIFU ablation treatment. Based on the vast HIFU experiences in China, this book is of great value in guiding doctors to select suitable patients for HIFU, assess the suitability of treatment, and avoid complications related to HIFU treatment. Those gynaecologists who want to use a non-invasive approach to help their patients should read this book.

The English literature on Focused Ultrasound Surgery did not always provide detailed information on the techniques and problems in treating uterine fibroids and adenomyosis. This book contains numerous case studies with detailed information on MRI assessment and HIFU treatment that serves and helps how to tackle difficult ultrasound ablation cases.

In this book, the treatments of the huge fibroids with a size of 19.8 cm and multiple fibroids over one hundred were impressive. HIFU does not mean providing the best treatment options available. However, it creates a new direction where non-invasive ablation treatment can relieve the symptoms of large fibroid or numerous fibroids while preserving the uterus.

We admit that there are a few limitations to the book. Not many patients had long-term follow-ups. Despite nearly all ablation treatments being successful and safe, there were recurrences of fibroids and adenomyosis in some patients on the follow-up MRI scans, even though they might not have symptoms. This book comprises only case reports, with no statistical results available for the above HIFU treatment. Besides, it is to share our experience from our case reports on how to assess, evaluate, and achieve a complete ablation. Lastly, this book illustrates HIFU treatment from only one hospital centre; therefore, the treatment methods, duration, power, and complications might be biased towards one's own practice. Hopefully, our book will raise awareness of the feasibility of HIFU treatment and the potential complications of this non-invasive treatment.

This non-invasive HIFU procedure can offer an alternative therapy to surgical treatment even though the limitation of treatment will depend on various factors. Compared to traditional gynaecological surgeries, the thermal ablation treatments for fibroids and adenomyosis using HIFU technology, microwave, and radiofrequency have much fewer complications, especially life-threatening haemorrhage, infection, and organ injuries. Therefore, non-invasive and virtual surgery using HIFU ablation should become a common surgery of the future.

Shanghai, China Yonghua Xu
Shanghai, China Lixia Yang
Sydney, Australia Felix Wong

Contents

About the Editors

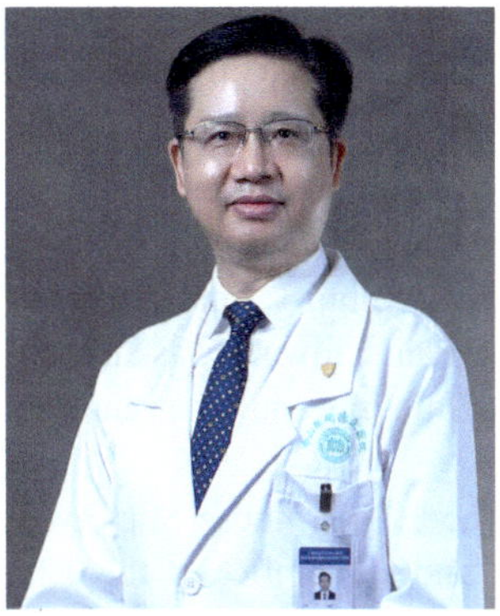

Yonghua Xu, MD PhD Yonghua Xu MD PhD, Chairman and Professor, Department of Imaging and Interventional Radiology, Zhongshan-Xuhui Hospital of Fudan University, Shanghai, China.

Dr. Xu received his medical degree at Central South University Xiangya Medical School in 1991. He completed resident training in 1994 and became an attending and consulting radiologist at Shanghai No. 8 Peoples' Hospital from 1994 to 2002. Dr. Xu had got interventional fellowship training at the Department of Radiology of Indiana University School of Medicine from 2002 to 2005 and worked as a clinical research fellow at Imaging Department of Massachusetts General Hospital and Harvard Medical School until 2007, then joined in Zhongshan-Xuhui Hospital of Fudan University as the Chairman of the Department of Imaging and Interventional Radiology and the Director of the Biomedicine Imaging Technology Laboratory. He also got PhD degree in clinical oncology at Chongqing Medical University in 2015.

Dr. Xu, a pioneer in the use of MR-guided HIFU ablation for the treatment of uterine fibroids in China, broadens the ultrasound-guided HIFU clinical applications for the treatment of all types of fibroids, adenomyosis, hepatic cancer and metastasis, pancreatic cancer, breast cancer, adrenal and renal tumours, aggressive fibromatosis, and some abdominal solid tumours. He accomplished the world's first HIFU ablation telesurgery through the 5G network and led his group to join the multicentre clinical trials funded by the National Key Technology Research and Development Program of China and has received the state awards for researches from the government and the teaching awards from Fudan University.

Dr. Xu is a board member of the International Society of Mini- and Non-invasive Medicine, the associate chairman of the ultrasonic therapy and bioeffect committee of Chinese Association of Ultrasound in Medicine and Engineering, the fellow of the mini- and non-invasive medicine committee of Chinese Medical Doctor Association and the permanent member of the ultrasound ablation committee of China Anti-Cancer Association, and he is currently the editorial board member of Journal of Interventional Radiology (China) and Chinese Journal of Ultrasound in Medicine. He was a member of the RSNA, European Society of Radiology, and the Society of Interventional Radiology.

Dr. Xu has published over 100 publications and edited five books, and given more than 100 invited lectures in the field of radiology and image-guided HIFU ablation both domestically and internationally.

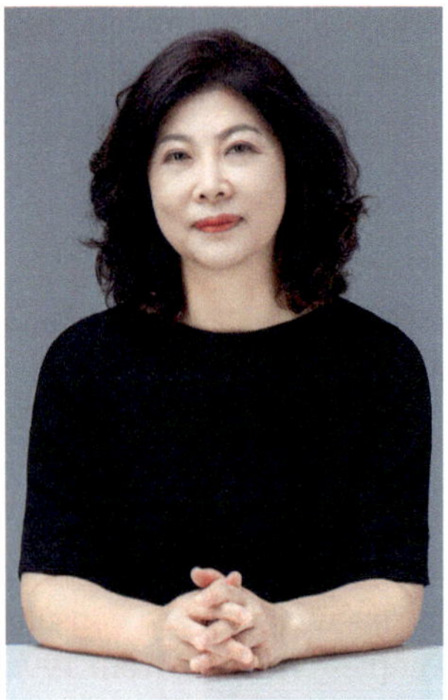

Lixia Yang, MD, PhD Lixia Yang, MD, PhD, Chief Physicians and Associate Professor, Department of Imaging and Interventional Radiology, Zhongshan-Xuhui Hospital of Fudan University, Shanghai, China.

Dr. Yang received her medical degree at Shihezhi Medical College in 1995 and got PhD degree in Medical Imaging at Xinjiang Medical University in 2008. She completed resident training in 2003 and became attending and consulting radiologist in the first affiliated hospital of Xinjiang Medical University from 2003 to 2008. Dr. Yang had completed the fellowship training at the department of radiology of Shanghai Ruijing Hospital and then joined in Shanghai Xuhui Central Hospital and Zhongshan-Xuhui Hospital of Fudan University as an associate professor and chief physician of Imaging and Interventional Radiology.

Dr. Yang was the secretary of the 12th Chinese Society of Magnetic Resonance in Medicine and a member of the 12th Youth Committee of Chinese Society Radiology (CSR), RSNA, and SFN. She is the editorial board member of Chinese Journal of Magnetic Resonance Imaging.

Dr. Yang is an experienced clinician in HIFU ablation treatment of uterine fibroids. She is one of the doctors firstly using 5G networks to provide a remote HIFU ablation surgery in the world. She is good at the tumour diagnosis by MRI, especially in evaluation before and after treatment related to the focused ultrasound ablation surgery. Dr. Yang's research team has conducted several clinical trials to evaluate the effectiveness of both ultrasound ablation and surgery operation for the treatment of uterine fibroids. She participated in more than 30 clinical trials of imaging requirement including the MR-guided focused ultrasound clinical trial.

Dr. Yang has co-authored over 40 peer-reviewed academic articles and six books. She presided and participated in over ten research projects funded by NSFC and the provincial government. She has received many honours and awards for excellent research and teaching in the levels of the government and Fudan University.

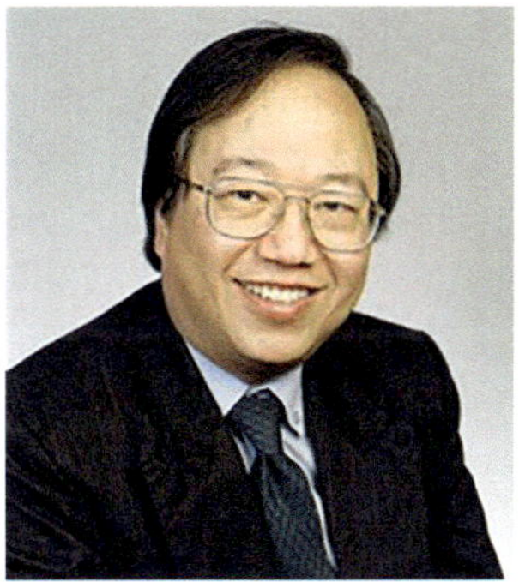

Felix Wong Professor Felix Wong is a (retired) Professor of the University of New South Wales. He graduated from the University of Hong Kong in 1976 and was appointed as the foundation Professor of the University of New South Wales at Liverpool Hospital in 1991.

Professor Wong is renowned for his contribution to medical education in Asia Pacific Countries. In the last 30 years, he had also been invited as a guest speaker and/or as an organising committee member in up to many national and international endoscopy and O&G workshops. He received ten visiting professorships from other universities and 10 honorary consultant positions from Maternal and Child Health Hospitals, China.

For his contribution to his speciality area, he had received many awards, including a Guangdong Friendship Award 2003 and an Endoscopists Award 2005 for his significant contribution to the field of endoscopy in China and a medical ambassador from the Gynecological Endoscopy Group of the Chinese Medical Association. He is currently the Vice President of the World Association of Chinese Obstetricians and Gynecologists and the Foundation Chairman of the Focused Ultrasound Surgery Association (FUSA) in Hong Kong.

In 2006, he was honoured by a Ho Chi Minh City Badge Award by The People's Committee of Ho Chi Minh City to recognise his continuous contribution to strengthening friendly relationships with HCMC people. In 2009, he received the Endos Award in Medical Science and Technology, China, for his excellent achievement in endoscopic surgery. He was honoured with Lifetime Achievement Award by Asia-Pacific Association for Gynecologic Endoscopy and Minimally Invasive Therapy (APAGE) in 2017 and the Outstanding Contribution Award by the European Society for Gynaecological Endoscopy (ESGE) in 2018.

Professor Wong has published 14 books and more than 230 papers in local and international journals.

1 Principles and Procedure of Focused Ultrasound Ablation Surgery

Yonghua Xu, Felix Wong, and Lixia Yang

Abstract

The principle, therapeutic strategy, and sonication process of ultrasound-guided and magnetic resonance-guided focused ultrasound ablation in the treatment of uterine benign diseases are described in detail. The sonication processes are monitored with sonographic imaging using ultrasound-guided method, and with real-time temperature mapping using MR-guided method for therapeutic safety and efficacy. After the treatment, the contrast-enhanced MRI is performed for assessing ablative effects with non-perfused volume. The efficacy, sonication energy efficiency, treatment time, and safety of ultrasound-guided high-intensity focused ultrasound (USgHIFU) are compared with those of magnetic resonance-guided high-intensity focused ultrasound (MRgHIFU) for the complete ablation of uterine fibroids. Their advantages and disadvantages are discussed.

Telemedicine and telesurgery have transformed healthcare delivery so that services can be provided in clinics or sites outside acute hospitals. The focused ultrasound ablation surgery is one of the latest developments, which enables doctors to operate on a computer console under direct ultrasound monitoring. Coupled with the rapid development of 5G communication technology in China, the world's first focused ultrasound ablation telesurgery through the 5G-backed network was performed in Shanghai, China. The digital technology development and limitations of HIFU in the future are highlighted.

Keywords

Ultrasound · MRI · Temperature mapping · High-intensity focused ultrasound · Ablation · Contrast-enhanced MRI · Efficacy · Safety · Telesurgery

Tumor ablation is to cause coagulative necrosis inside tumors by physical or chemical approaches. The ablation procedures as determined by the Radiological Society of North America (RSNA) in 1997 include chemical ablation, thermal ablation, and cryoablation. Focused ultrasound ablation surgery (FUAS) or high-intensity focused ultrasound (HIFU) is one of the thermal ablation procedures; however, it does not require the insertion of an applicator into a target tissue, which is different from other ablation therapies. Focused ultrasound waves, an extracorporeal source, can penetrate the human body and act on the target focal region to be treated by its biophysical effects to achieve the instantaneous coagulative necrosis of the tissue. In contrast, the tissues and organs on the "path" of ultrasound outside the treatment area are not or less damaged, for which the "thermal ablation" of the tissue is achieved. This emerging technique for local treatment of tumors perfectly reflects the concept of "treatment that is to minimize harm to patients." However, a successful ablation procedure depends on the precise positioning of the target region and the real-time treatment effect monitoring feedback and assessment. In order to ensure the safety and effectiveness of focused ultrasound ablation in clinical application, image guidance and monitoring techniques for treatment are essential. Currently, either ultrasound or magnetic resonance imaging guidance, offering integrated therapy planning, real-time control, and evaluation, has been commonly applied in routine clinical treatment, thus ensuring focused ultrasound ablation treatment safety and efficacy.

Y. Xu (✉) · L. Yang
Zhongshan-Xuhui Hospital, Fudan University, Shanghai, China

F. Wong
The University of New South Wales, Sydney, NSW, Australia

Y. Xu et al. (eds.), *Surgical Techniques of Focused Ultrasound Ablation in Benign Uterine Diseases*,
https://doi.org/10.1007/978-981-19-7180-8_1

1.1 Ultrasound Guided Focused Ultrasound Therapy

1.1.1 Principles of Treatment

Sonographically guided high-intensity focused ultrasound (HIFU) ablation therapy is a non-invasive thermal ablation procedure delivering the ultrasonic energy of 1 w/cm^2 emitted from the transducer to form highly concentrated energy around 5000 to 10,000 w/cm^2 at the focal region of the target area. It can generate an instantaneous high temperature (60–100 °C) in the focal region for more than 1 s, resulting in irreversible coagulative necrosis, which is the ablation by the thermal effect and acoustic cavitation of the ultrasonic focusing energy in the target tissue (Fig. 1.1a) [1–3]. The basic mode of "removal" of tumors with HIFU is to use a small biological focal region (BFR) movement to increase the volume for thermal ablation and employ a point-line-plane-stereo combination strategy to finally achieve the three-dimensional "conformal resection" with sharp margins between treated and healthy tissue (Fig. 1.1b) [4].

1.1.2 Treatment Procedure

1.1.2.1 Treatment Equipment

The focused ultrasound tumor treatment system is made up of six parts: an ultrasonic energy delivery system, treatment bed system, motion system, control system, water circulation system, and power supply system.

JC 200 focused ultrasound tumor treatment systems are comprehensive focused ultrasound tumor treatment systems following the JC focused ultrasound tumor treatment systems (Fig. 1.2a). Compared with the JC system, it has several sub-models to meet the therapeutic needs of different specialties.

There are currently five sub-models in the JC 200 series: JC 200A (for the treatment of liver tumors and soft tissue tumors); JC 200B (for the treatment of breast cancer, breast fibroadenoma, and soft tissue tumors); JC 200C (for the treatment of bone tumors and soft tissue tumors); JC 200D and JC 200D1 (for the treatment of uterine fibroids and soft tissue tumors).

JC300 focused ultrasound tumor treatment system is a new comprehensive system that integrates the artificial intelligent treatment plan system (TPS), 3D image processing software, telemedicine conduct-sharing for diagnosis and treatment plan (Fig. 1.2b), and this system has a one-stop station with an accurate fully digital mode. It is characterized by small focus, high sound intensity, and small side flaps. Thus it is indicated for solid tumors such as liver tumors, bone tumors, breast tumors, uterine fibroids, and soft tissue tumors.

1.1.2.2 Treatment Process

At present, there are three types of ultrasound-guided techniques for FUAS of tumors or lesions in clinical practice: ultrasound sonography, color Doppler ultrasound imaging, and contrast-enhanced ultrasound (CEUS). Although the ultrasound image can show the tomographic structure of the

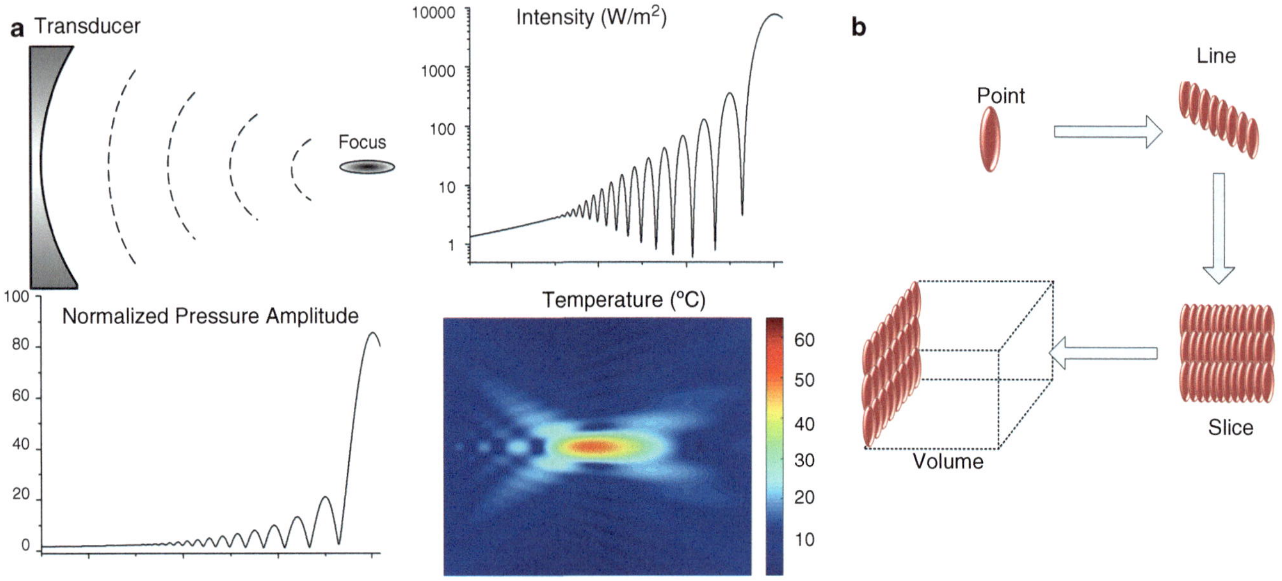

Fig. 1.1 Principles of high-intensity focused ultrasound ablation therapy. (**a**) The ultrasonic energy of 1 w/cm^2 emitted from the transducer can be delivered to the focal region by 5000–10,000 w/cm^2 (Provided by Prof. Dong Zhang); (**b**) The basic mode of "removal" of tumors with HIFU

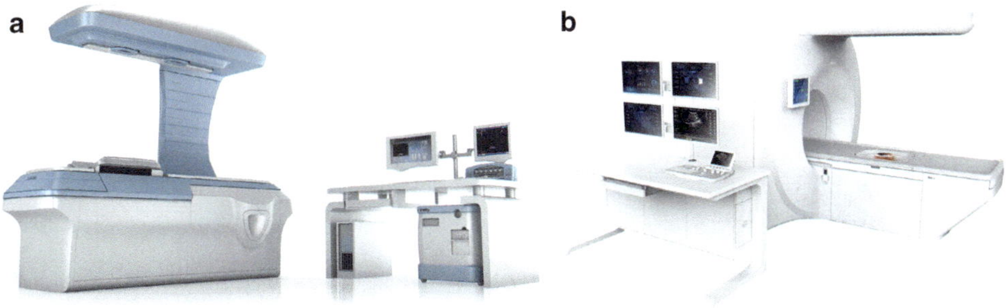

Fig. 1.2 Focused ultrasound tumor treatment systems. (**a**) JC 200; (**b**) JC 300

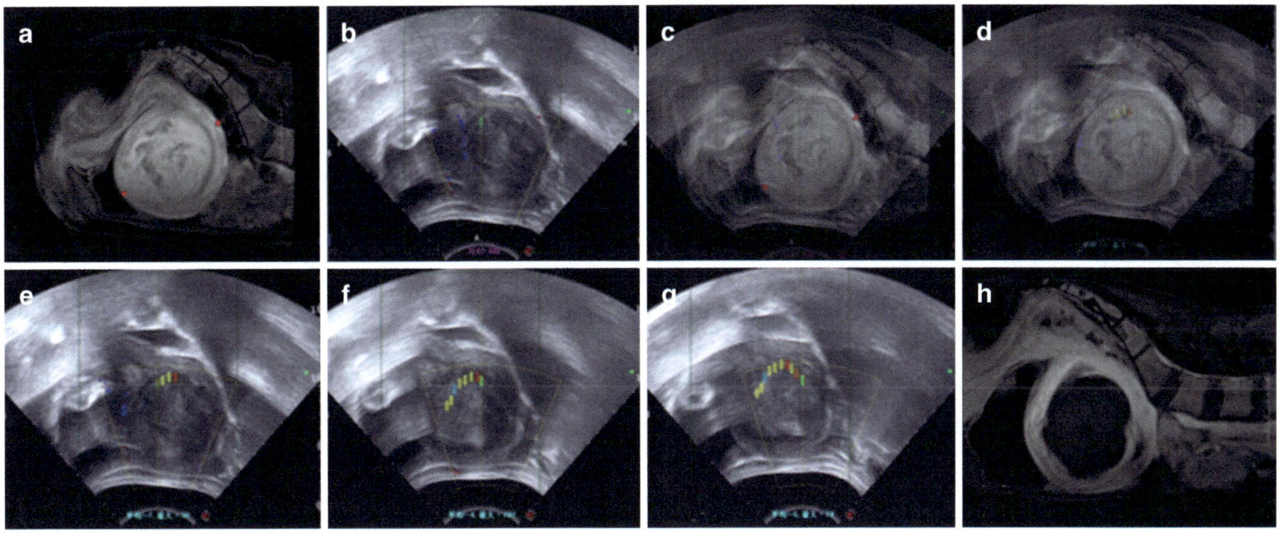

Fig. 1.3 Image fusion system: Registration and fusion of ultrasound images and MRI images for treatment positioning by the volumetric ablation strategy. (**a**) Contrast-enhanced MRI before treatment: The largest sagittal plane of uterine fibroids; (**b**) The largest sagittal plane of fibroids by ultrasound before treatment; (**c**) MRI and ultrasound fusion images of A and B based on the TPS; (**d–g**). Along with the deep and rear layers of fibroids, the sonication points were deployed in the focal region at an interval of 5 mm, and then a point-by-point treatment mode was performed. The enhanced ultrasound echo of the internal fibroids occurred during treatment and eventually covered the entire fibroid; (**h**) After treatment, the contrast-enhanced MRI scan showed that the fibroid was completely non-perfused

tissue and its surroundings, it has more noise, and the image quality is easily affected by many factors. The three-dimensional virtual navigation system performs the registration and fusion of the monitored ultrasound image and MRI T2WI fat saturation images or T1WI contrast-enhanced images for the planned positioning of fibroids before treatment to achieve computer-assisted virtual positioning and navigation during tumor or lesion treatment (Fig. 1.3). The real-time imaging with ultrasound images and the high-resolution imaging with MRI images are perfectly integrated. Although the resolution of the ultrasound image itself is relatively low, the tissues subjected to coagulative necrosis after focused ultrasound ablation are well displayed, showing the echo enhancement area (Fig. 1.4). Color Doppler ultrasound can show the blood flow in and around the tumor or lesion well (Fig. 1.5). CEUS is used to observe changes in the blood perfusion in tumors or lesions before and after treatment and evaluate the therapeutic effects of focused ultrasound ablation (Fig. 1.6).

USgHIFU is a safe, effective, and patient-friendly therapeutic option for uterine fibroids, which reduces overall healthcare costs with few adverse events, shorter hospital stay, and quicker postoperative recovery to normal activities like work, tours, and suitable sports.

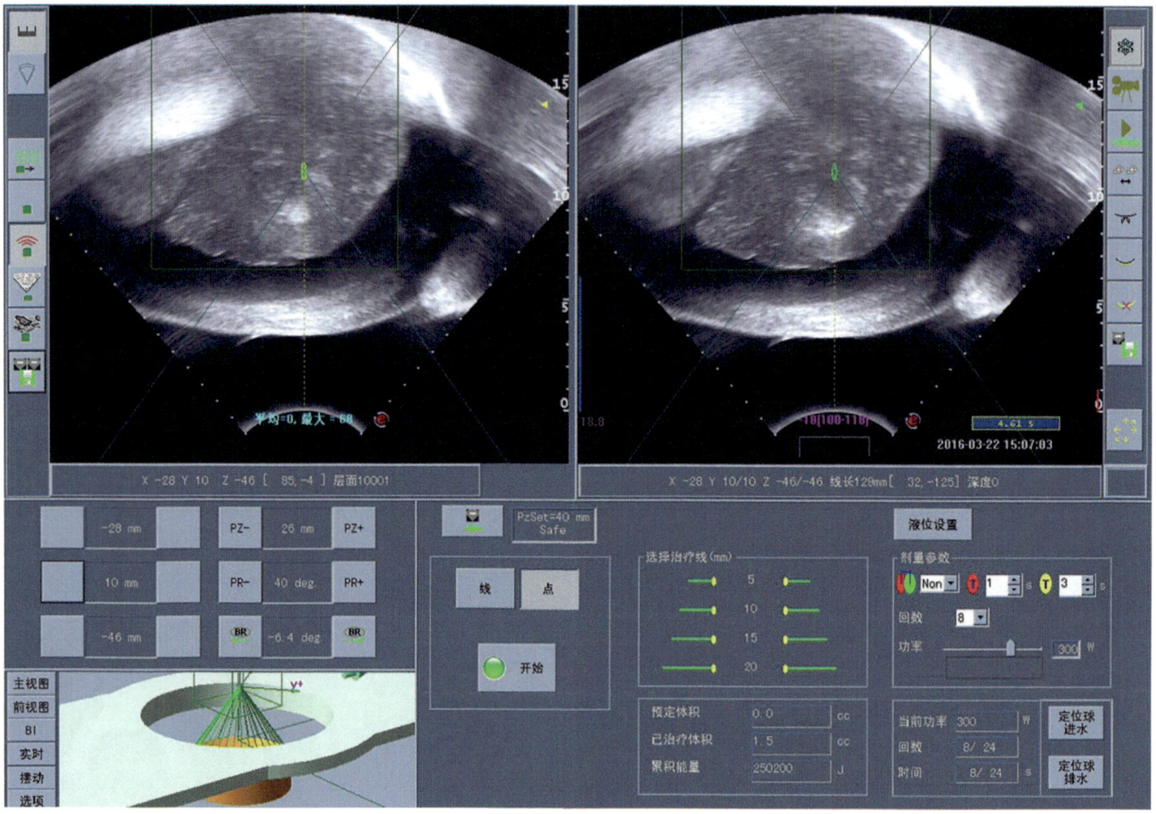

Fig. 1.4 Real-time ultrasound image during focused ultrasound ablation procedure. The internal fibroid showed grayscale changes from low echo to high echo during treatment

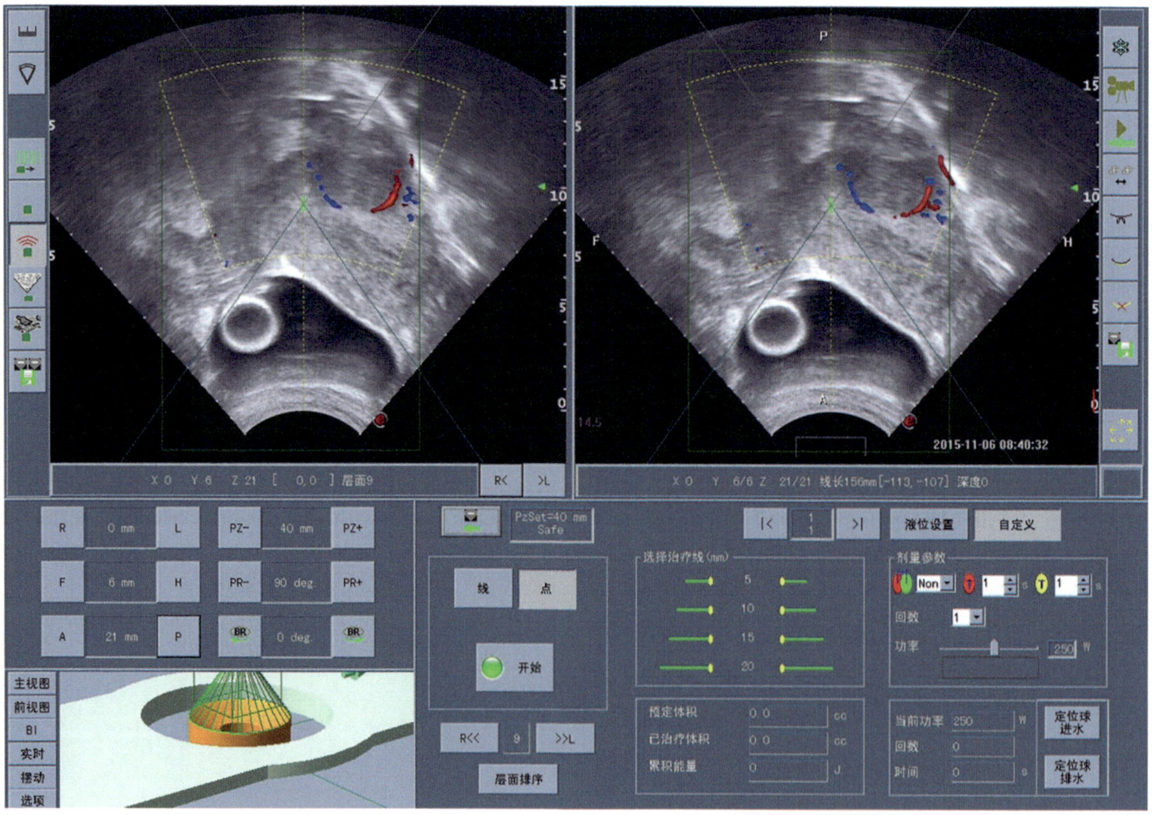

Fig. 1.5 Color Doppler ultrasound image showed the blood supplied vessels were dispersed around the margin of the fibroid

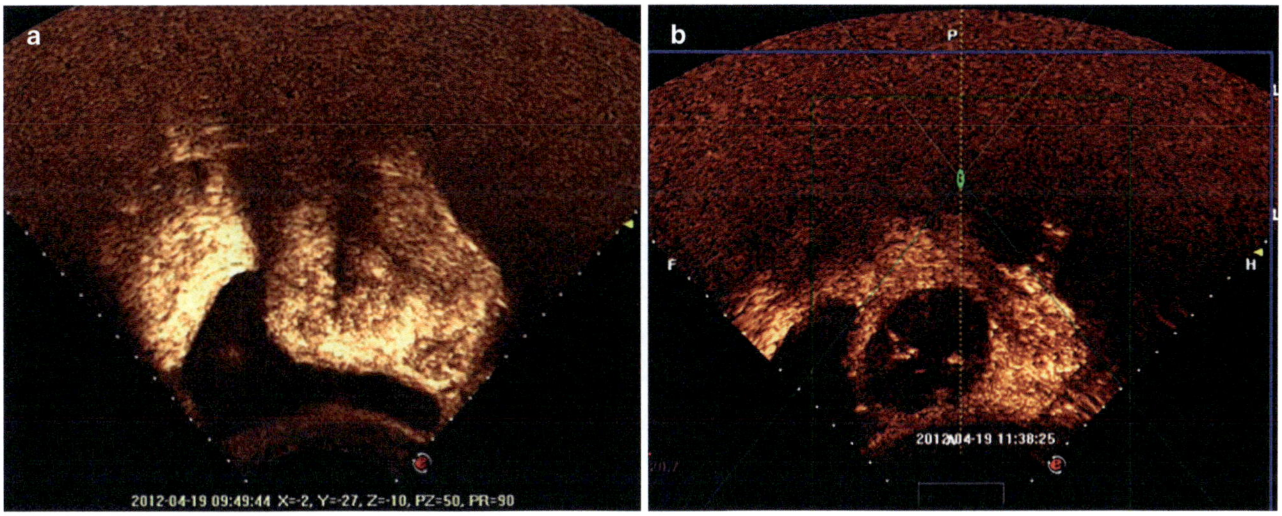

Fig. 1.6 CEUS images showed the blood perfusion in fibroid before treatment (**a**) and the ablated fibroid with non-perfusion (coagulative necrosis) after treatment (**b**)

1.2 Magnetic Resonance Guided Focused Ultrasound Therapy

1.2.1 Principles of Treatment

The temperature below 55 °C within 4 s can only cause the degeneration rather than necrosis of tumor cells. When the instantaneous temperature at the treatment area reaches 60 °C or above and lasts for 1 s or more, the positive effect of tumor necrosis can be achieved. Magnetic resonance thermometry technology can obtain a spatial distribution map of temperatures by quantifying temperature-related parameters [5]. The temperature mapping through the special sequence of MRI, Proton Resonance Frequency Shift (PRFS), can provide real-time temperature monitoring at the speed of 1 frame per second for focused ultrasound ablation treatment, which not only helps to ensure the coagulative necrosis of the target tissue (≥60 °C) but also prevents the damage to normal surrounding tissues due to overheating, especially the cavitation resulting in unpredictable damage (Fig. 1.7) [5, 6].

MRI-guided high-intensity focused ultrasound (MRgHIFU) treatment is generally provided with an ultrasound release power of 200–400 W (Fig. 1.8), which is adjusted according to the size of the irradiation area and feedback of temperature for fibroids to be treated while taking into account the patient's tolerance and reaction. Once the temperature in the targeted volume elevates at the threshold of 60 °C and above, it means that the exact thermal ablation effects are obtained. The operator can move to the next targeted focus. Therefore, the released acoustic energy would be manipulated to ensure the treatment efficacy and safety based on the detected temperature of the treated region and its surrounding area [7].

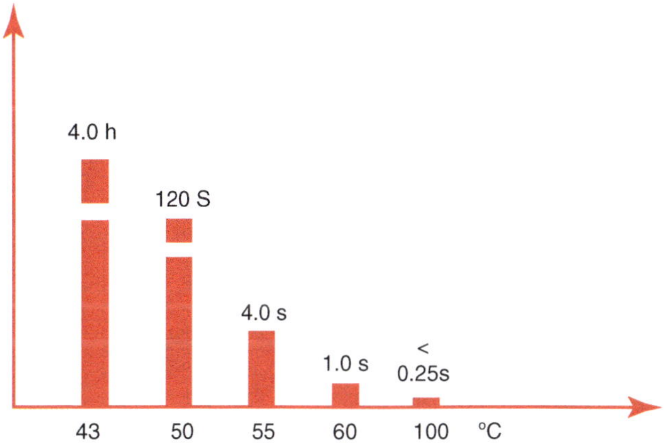

Fig. 1.7 The correlation between thermal temperature and time for killing cells

1.2.2 Treatment Procedure

1.2.2.1 Treatment Equipment

The MRgHIFU tumor treatment system is a combination of 1.5 T MRI and JM 2.5C high-intensity focused ultrasound tumor treatment system. MRI guides HIFU treatment in this system and provides real-time temperature monitoring (Fig. 1.9).

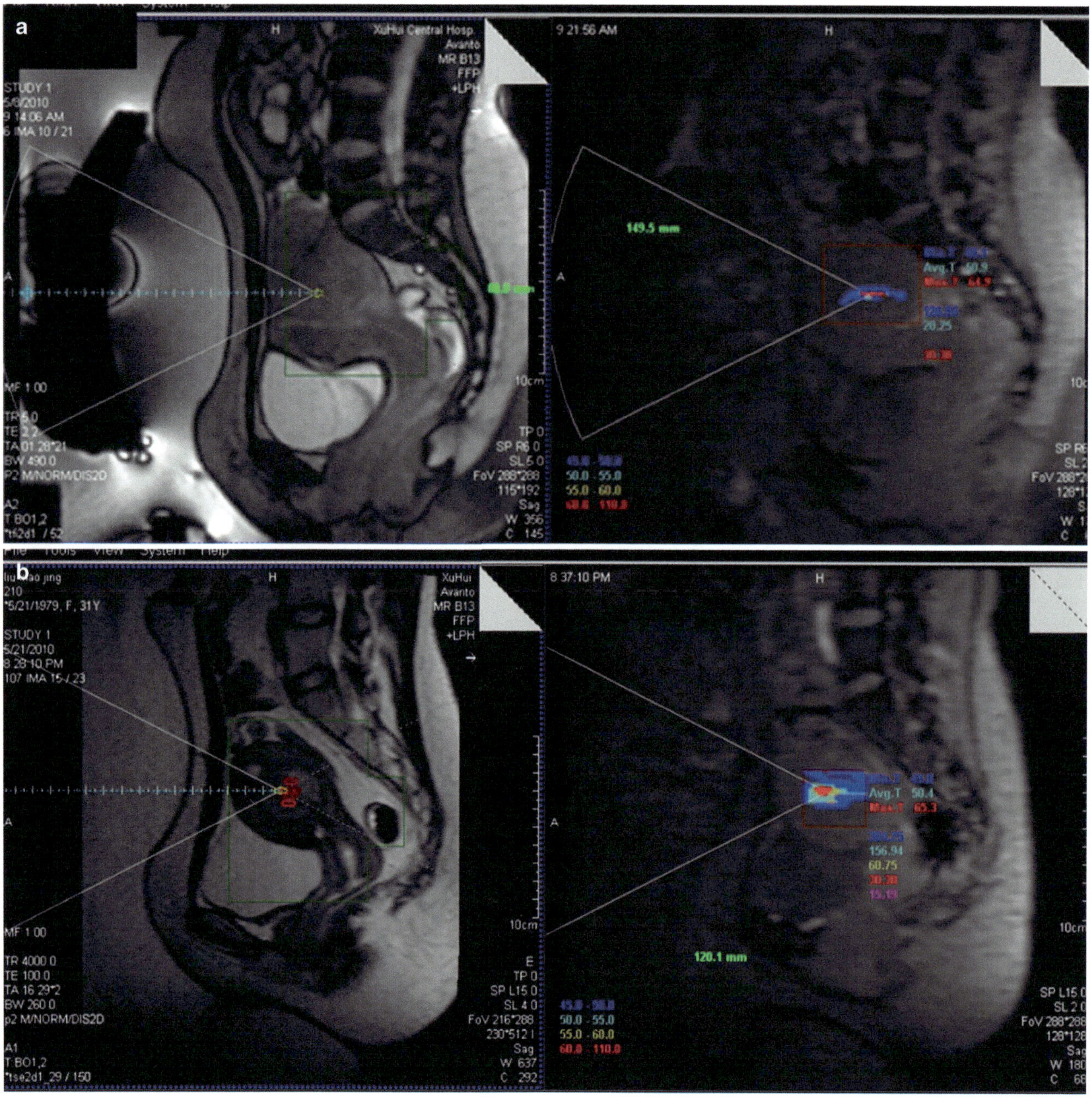

Fig. 1.8 MRI temperature monitoring the changes in temperature at the focal regions for different acoustic powers during MRgHIFU treatment of uterine fibroids. (**a**) 200 W; (**b**) 250 W; (**c**) 300 W; (**d**) 400 W. (The left figures: T2WI sagittal view for planning and positioning; the right figures: MR-thermometry mapping for the respective anatomical images)

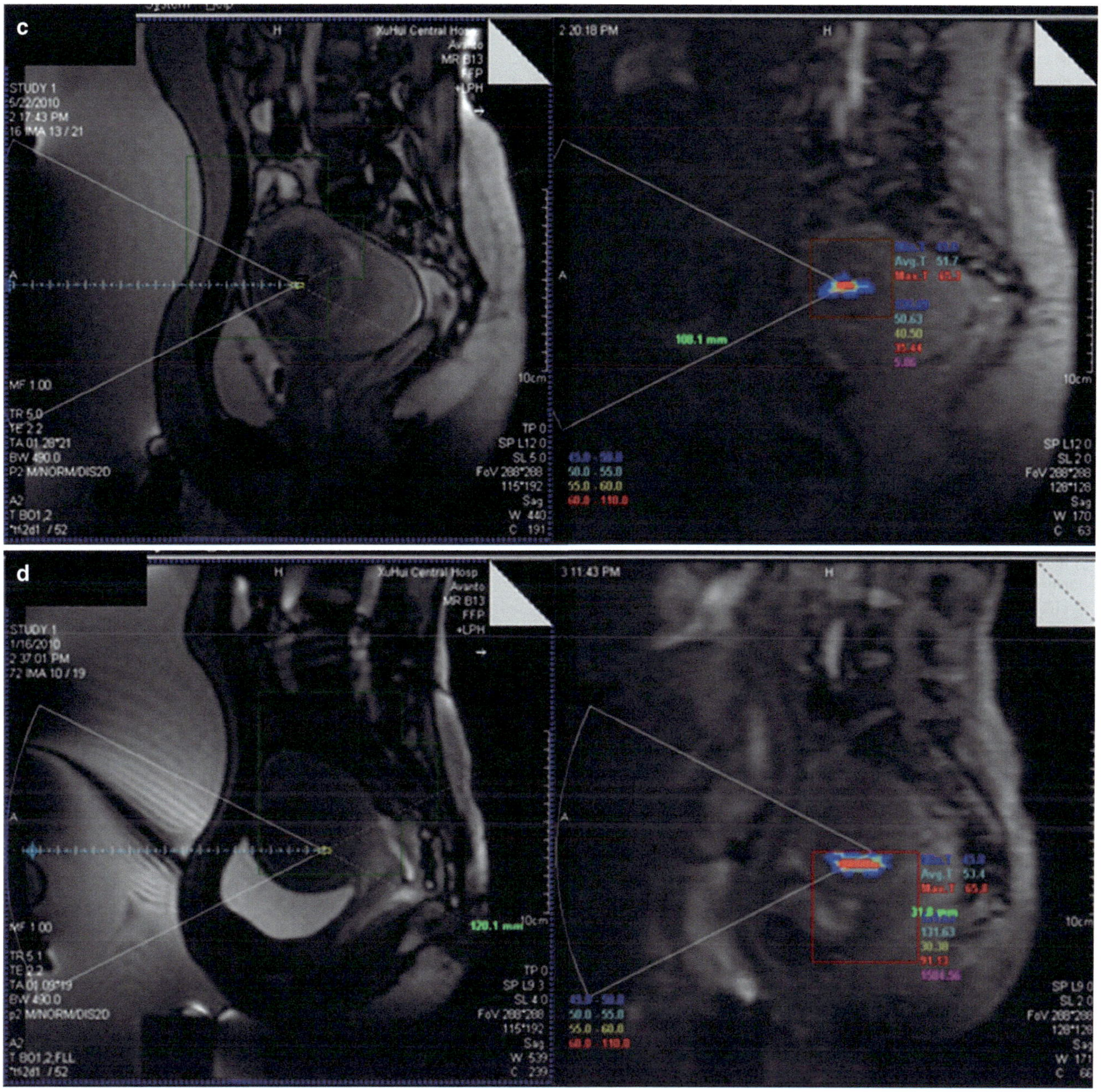

Fig. 1.8 (continued)

1.2.2.2 MRgHIFU Procedure

The patient lies prone on the HIFU treatment bed, with the inferior abdominal wall in a degassed water tank. The degassed water balloon is placed between the abdominal wall and the transducer (Fig. 1.10). Before focused ultrasound ablation treatment, the coronal, sagittal, and axial anatomical structure images are acquired through MRI scanning to formulate a treatment plan. The MR imaging of the proton resonance frequency shift (PRFS) sequence is employed for monitoring therapeutic temperature changes. The physical focus is adjusted to match the biological focus with the temperature mapping for the focal region calibration. Thus, focused ultrasound ablation of uterine fibroids can be initiated according to the treatment plan system. During MRgHIFU treatment, the intensities of the temperature elevation in the target and surrounding areas are observed with real-time MR thermometry (Fig. 1.11) while the patient holds an emergency stop but-

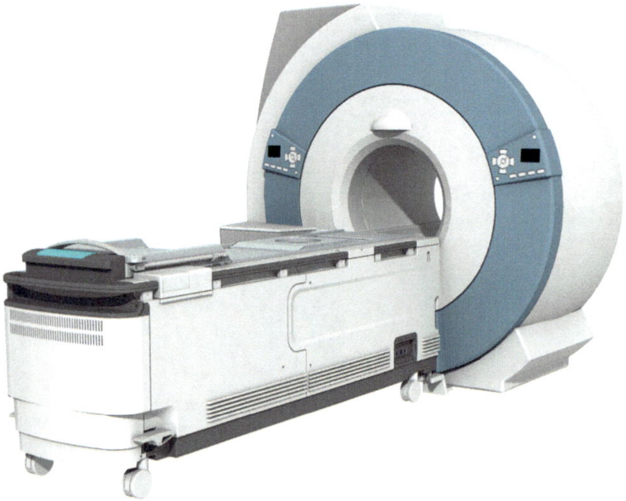

Fig. 1.9 JM 2.5C MRgHIFU tumor treatment system with integrated MRI and high-intensity focused ultrasound therapy unit

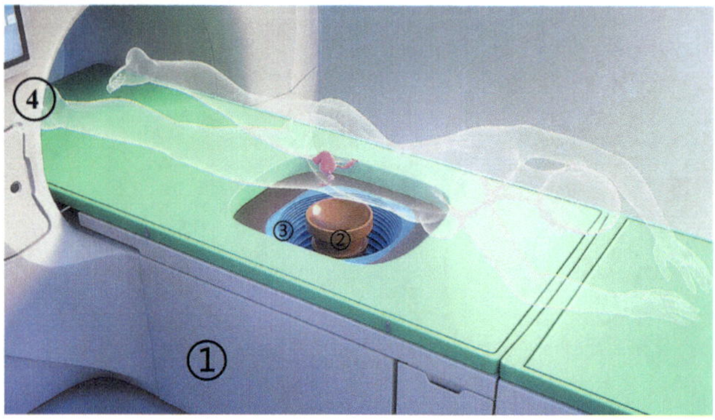

Fig. 1.10 A schematic diagram of the MRIgHIFU procedure in the treatment of uterine fibroids (1. treatment bed, 2. transducer, 3. water tank, 4. MRI)

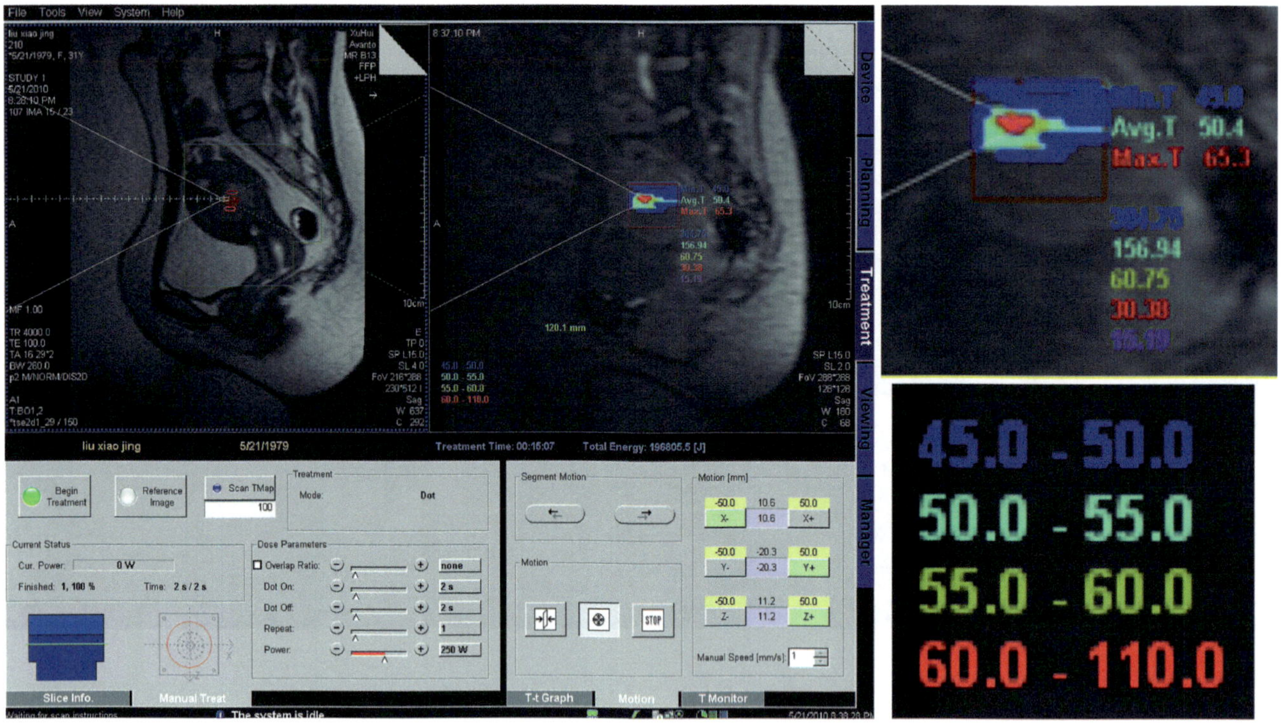

Fig. 1.11 MRgHIFU procedure with temperature feedback to control acoustic energy and powers. MRI sagittal T2WI showed the location of the fibroids with the targeted focal regions based on the treatment plan (left); at the same slice, the real-time temperature mapping showed the temperature rise of the target focus and its surrounding area with the maximum temperature of 65.3 °C at the focal region (right). Note: The red and yellow in the temperature map represent ≥60 and 55–60 °C, respectively. Sonication with an acoustic power of 300 W produced the area of the focal region in red by 35.44 mm^2 (horizontal shaft 4 mm, long shaft 11–12 mm)

ton in her hand (Fig. 1.12). Once the temperature at the treatment site rises to or over the threshold value of 60 °C, the sonication would be stopped since the dose of acoustic energy deposits sufficiently in the target to cause coagulative necrosis. If unbearable discomfort or pain, the abdominal skin hot, or the lower limb numb occurs, the emergency stop button can be pressed by the subjective to cease the treatment [8, 9].

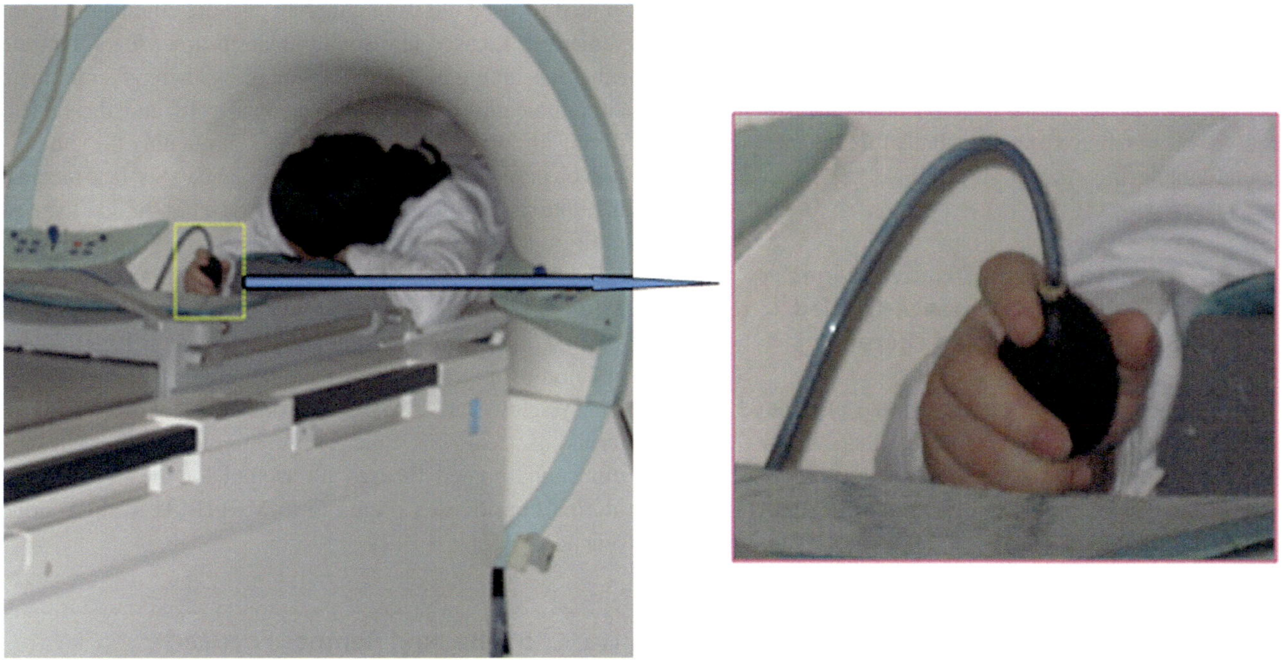

Fig. 1.12 The stop button of MRI-guided focused ultrasound tumor treatment system was held by the patient for any emergency

1.3 Comparison of Two Guidance Modalities for Focused Ultrasound Therapy

In 2002, the first clinical study of ultrasound-guided high-intensity focused ultrasound ablation in the treatment of uterine fibroids was reported in China [10]. In 2004, the U.S. FDA approved the clinical application of MRI-guided focused ultrasound to treat uterine fibroids. At present, the mainly available technologies for non-invasive image-guided focused ultrasound ablation therapy employ either MRI or ultrasound for lesion targeting and efficacy evaluation. In ultrasound-guided HIFU treatment systems, real-time ultrasonography is used to monitor the echo changes in the treatment or the feedback for manipulating sonication to achieve safe and effective thermal ablation of the target tissue [11, 12]. During the MRgHIFU procedure, the temperature change at the treatment area is monitored in real time with the temperature mapping sequence. Then the ultrasonic power and sonication energy are released based on them. When the temperature at the focal region is up to 60 °C or above, the coagulative necrosis of the tissue subjected to thermal ablation can be determined, and the sonication will be stopped immediately. Thus, the therapeutic ultrasound energy is effective but not excessive, thereby ensuring the safety and effectiveness of the treatment [13]. The advantages and disadvantages of the two guidance modalities for focused ultrasound therapy and how to choose them in the clinical application are discussed as follows.

1.3.1 Advantages and Disadvantages of Ultrasound-Guided Focused Ultrasound Ablation

After the registration and fusion of ultrasound-magnetic resonance images with the pre-treatment MRI image according to the treatment plan, the USg-HIFU system uses ultrasound to define the targeted fibroid(s) accurately and guide the procedure in real time. The echogenicity changes in the therapeutic area were monitored as feedback to determine the release of acoustic energy for achieving a safe and effective thermal ablation. There is no consensus that USgHIFU is accurately effective and safe for the ablation of uterine fibroids since the other commercially available focused ultrasound diathermy systems can only be used as adjuvant therapy. Different from their lower treatment temperatures that cannot achieve the effect of coagulative necrosis at the target tissue, the USgHIFU system has addressed the two concerning issues: (1) Gray-scale changes of ultrasonic echogenicity at the targeted area can predict the effectiveness of the ablation; (2) the suitable sonication energy is released based on the contrast-enhanced ultrasound during the procedure for avoiding excessive therapy while allowing supplementary sonication to ablate a residual portion of fibroid. And it has the following advantages: (1) guidance and feedback with real-time imaging; (2) convenient operation with shorter treatment time; (3) the treatment indications are broader. However, there are also the following disadvantages: (1) The resolution of ultrasound images is relatively low, which needs to be solved by fusion of ultrasound-magnetic resonance images, but there are still difficulties in image recognition for non-professional or untrained doctors; (2) the imaging technique of temperature measurement has not yet been achieved for the clinical treatment with ultrasound monitoring.

1.3.2 Advantages and Disadvantages of Magnetic Resonance-Guided Focused Ultrasound Therapy

The magnetic resonance-guided focused ultrasound has the advantage of real-time thermometry that allows measurement and adjustment of the deposited energy during the treatment. There are currently three MRgHIFU devices approved by the China Food and Drug Administration (CFDA) and FDA in many countries: ExAblate 2000 MR-guided focused ultrasound (MRgFUS) from InSightec (Haifa, Israel), JM2.5C MRgHIFU from Chongqing Haifu (Chongqing, China), and Sonalleve MR-HIFU from Profound Medical (Mississauga, Canada). All of them have been available in the clinical treatment of uterine fibroids.

The advantages of magnetic resonance-guided focused ultrasound therapy are as follows: (1) The temperature elevation at the focal region (targeted lesion) is monitored through the real-time MR imaging of thermal measurement sequence, and the effect of ablation treatment is evaluated, while the surroundings of the focal region are observed simultaneously for ensuring the treatment safety; (2) the image resolution of soft tissues guided by MRI is better than that by ultrasound, and the image slices obtained for treatment plan are easily standardized. However, the following disadvantages of this guidance modality restrict its wide clinical application: (1) the overall cost-effectiveness is poor since both the magnetic resonance imaging system and the focused ultrasound treatment system matched with the magnet have high costs, and the slow process of MR imaging and cumbersome operating procedures make the treatment time-consuming; (2) the patient in the treatment room is inconvenient to communicate with the operator(s) in the control room for the feedback during treatment; (3) the environmental requirement for the MRI room is relatively high, and the metallic implants in the body are strictly contraindicated. Conventionally intraoperative monitoring and rescue equipment are difficult to be deployed for patient safety.

In summary, both ultrasound and magnetic resonance-guided modalities provide new non-invasive treatment modes with their own advantages and disadvantages. Their treatment safety, reliability, and effectiveness have been widely recognized in clinical practice. The ultrasound-guided focused ultrasound therapy is more efficient and convenient in focused ultrasound ablation procedures than the time-consuming MRgHIFU procedures; there is an intimate communication between the medical staff and the patient during ultrasound-guided treatment, eliminating the patient's nervousness to improve her compliance. So far, medical institutions worldwide have used ultrasound-guided focused ultrasound ablation to treat more than 120,000 cases of uterine fibroids, which far exceeds about 20,000 cases of MRgHIFU ablation. Our results of a comparative study showed that ultrasound-guided HIFU and MRgHIFU for ablation of uterine fibroids have the equivalent energy efficiency. However, USgHIFU is superior to MRgHIFU in terms of treatment time [11]. This might be why the ultrasound-guided focused ultrasound for the treatment of uterine fibroids was preferred to MRgHIFU in the routine practice.

1.4 5G-Backed Remote Focused Ultrasound Therapy and Future "Digital Medicine"

The internet-based remote medical diagnosis and treatment emerging in the twenty-first century have greatly subverted the past clinical service process. As far as the vast majority of patients are concerned, they have not yet fully adapted to the new medical pattern. The development and application of Internet-based healthcare services also pose a challenge to the physicians' current scenarios of diagnosis and treatment practical application. Traditional on-site medical environments and patients' habits of hospital visits have also slowed down the development of Internet-based healthcare services to a certain extent. The abrupt COVID-19 pandemic in 2020 brought about tremendous changes in the medical field. The SARS-CoV-2 virus infected hundreds of millions of people and affected the lifestyles of medical staff and patients around the world. The COVID-19 epidemic has prompted medical personnel and patients to realize the importance of telemedicine. Medical institutions at all levels have also increased their deployment and investment in telemedicine. Telemedicine can be defined as the provision of healthcare services, including disease prevention, diagnosis, and treatment using information and communication technologies, such as video conferencing, electronic communication, and telephone. The rapid development of new communication technologies has made network transmission faster, and two-way communication has almost no time delay, which provides a basic guarantee for doctors to provide safe, effective, and satisfactory medical services to patients. Furthermore, unlike traditional "on-site" medical practice, telemedicine and remote surgical procedures enable physicians to provide services to patients in other clinics or places outside the hospital.

High-intensity focused ultrasound (HIFU) therapy is now increasingly applied in the clinical treatment of uterine fibroids, adenomyosis, and other solid tumors. This targeted thermal ablation technique requires only sedation and analgesia during treatment. Almost all patients can tolerate the whole treatment process with clear consciousness. The treatment process usually only requires 1–3 h. After the ablation treatment, the patients can return to work after a rest of a few hours or within 1–2 days generally. The focused ultrasound ablation is a non-invasive therapy that disrupts the traditional concepts of scalpel cutting and puncture needle ablation. It is a target thermal ablation treatment technique without incision, bleeding, or scar. So far, it has been used to treat malignant tumors such as liver cancer, pancreatic cancer, kidney cancer, breast cancer, prostate cancer, and benign tumors such as uterine fibroids. However, compared with other disciplines and techniques, there is a lack of focused ultrasound ablation surgery experts with rich clinical experience and proficient skills, limiting the development and clinical application of the focused ultrasound ablation technique. Since the outbreak of the COVID-19 in early 2020, the measures of strict home isolation and preventing epidemic control requirements have made it difficult for many patients to leave the local area to seek healthcare services from experts or big hospitals in other places.

With the expansion of internet-based healthcare services, wireless communication has evolved from the voice-based 2G to the data-based 3G and 4G and currently entering the 5G era. The 5G communication had the characteristics of low latency and large bandwidth superior to 4G networks. Its capability meets the core requirements of mobile health and telemedicine, which makes access and provision of medical services no longer restricted by time and space. HIFU treatment system is a highly digitalized medical device with "innate advantages" combined with 5G. It can realize wireless telemedicine applications based on video and remote force feedback technology. The focused ultrasound treatment equipment uses 5G-backed remote ultrasound images for real-time guidance; the physician can remotely control the therapeutic probe to treat the patient through the computer interface. The physician and the patient do not meet each other face-to-face during the whole process. The communication between the console and the treatment bed is controlled by a high-speed cable, which is superior to surgical robots and minimally invasive surgical robots for remote operation in many aspects. The HIFU operators can perform remote focused ultrasound surgery through a high-speed 5G network with large broadband and low latency (ith ms).

At 14:00 pm on October 14, 2019, the world's first 5G remote focused ultrasound surgery was performed successfully by Dr. Xu and Dr. Yang from the Department of Imaging and Interventional Radiology, Fudan University Zhongshan-Xuhui Hospital in Shanghai. The experts actually presented at the Shanghai International Medical Center located east of Huangpu River (Fig. 1.13a). The operation signal is transmitted in real time through a 5G-backed network. They could perform the focused ultrasound ablation procedure in the Ultrasound Treatment Center of Xuhui Central Hospital at the west of the Huangpu River (Fig. 1.13b), which is 30 kilometers away. A 39-year-old patient with multiple uterine fibroids underwent remote focused ultrasound ablation surgery (Fig. 1.14). Witnessed by many news media, the entire surgery lasted 52 minutes without any signal lag or delay.

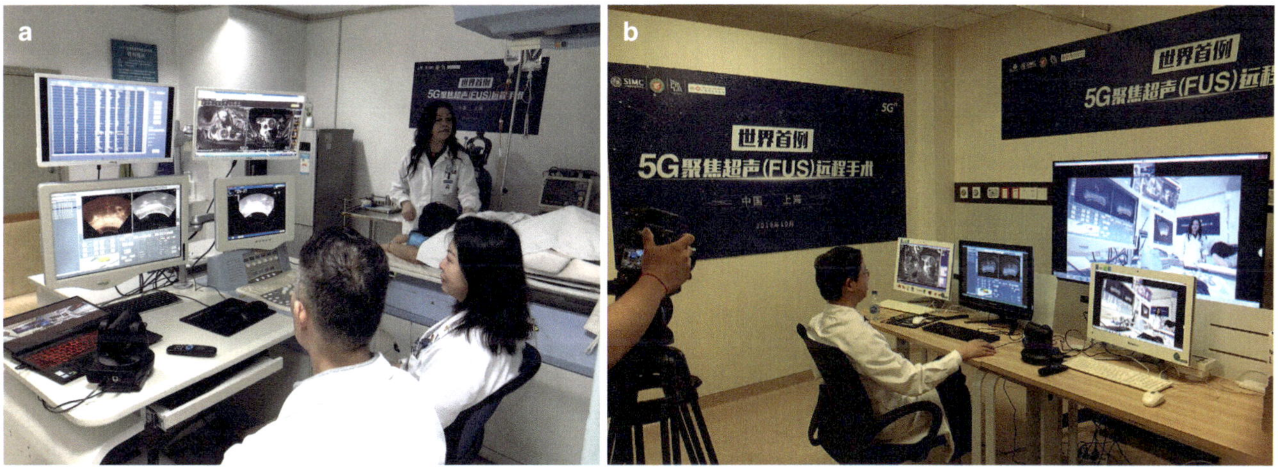

Fig. 1.13 The scenes of the first 5G-backed remote focused ultrasound surgery (FUS). (**a**) Shanghai International Medical Center (East Shanghai), the 5G-based operation site of remote FUS; (**b**) the Ultrasound Treatment Center of Xuhui Central Hospital (West Shanghai), where the focused ultrasound surgery was performed remotely

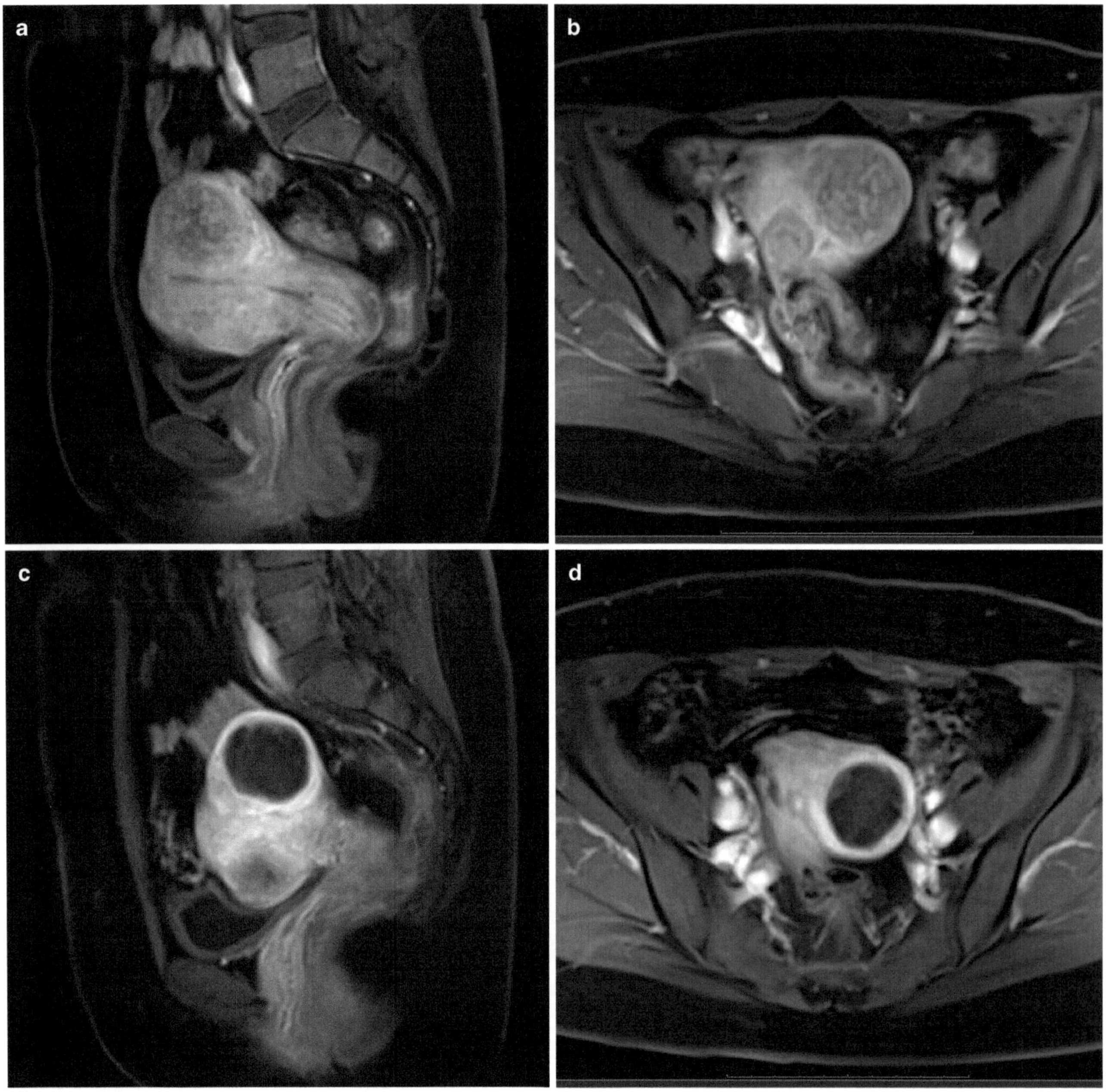

Fig. 1.14 The uterine intramural fibroids before and after remote FUS more than 95% non-perfused volume of fibroid after remote FUS. (**a**) T1WI_FS + C sagittal before treatment; (**b**) T1WI_FS + C axial before treatment; (**c**) T1WI_FS + C sagittal after treatment; (**d**) T1WI_FS + C axial after treatment

Both uterine intramural fibroids and subserosal fibroids of the patient were precisely ablated even without damage to the tumor membranes (Fig. 1.15) [14].

The application and promotion of 5G-backed remote surgery will undoubtedly accelerate the development of internet-based healthcare services. The real-world application of digital healthcare services in the future will allow experts to carry out diagnoses and treatment in their own offices without the need to travel to other places. This greatly reduces their time spent traveling and thus improves the efficiency of medical practices. Furthermore, the advanced medical services from medical staff in the regional hospitals will be continuously improved. In terms of patients, they can also receive treatment from the top experts without leaving their home hospital. These undoubtedly build an invisible bridge and break the space restriction between the physician and the patient. Patients in remote areas can also obtain high-quality medical resources, especially to improve their healthcare services and greatly save their medical costs (including travel, accommodation expenses, etc.). Meanwhile, all pub-

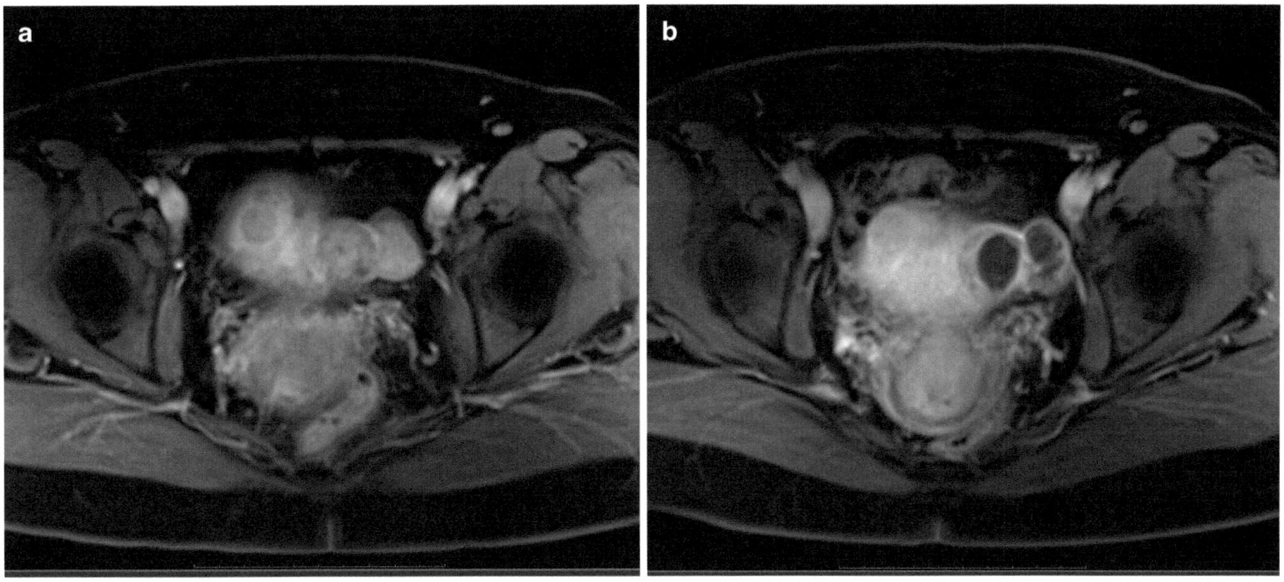

Fig. 1.15 The uterine subserosal fibroids before and after remote FUS. (**a**) T1WI_FS + C axial before treatment; (**b**) T1WI_FS + C axial after treatment(ablated fibroid without damaging the tumor membranes)

lic medical facilities and institutes can be fully utilized to cope with the COVID-19 crisis and to minimize the risks of cross-infections of this very infectious disease since the hundreds to thousands of patients requiring medical consultations and subsequent surgeries would not be allowed to get into doctors' clinics and hospitals in this pandemic period.

References

1. Li SJ, Xu J, Lian XW, et al. Principle of high intensity focused ultrasound (HIFU) and its utilization on the treatment of carcinomas. Pract J Cardiac Cereb Pneumal Vasc Dis. 2009;17(6):532–3.
2. Haar GT, Coussios C. High intensity focused ultrasound: past, present and future. Int J Hyperth. 2007;23(2):85–7.
3. Miller DL, Smith NB, Bailey MR, et al. Overview of therapeutic ultrasound applications and safety considerations. J Ultrasound Med. 2012;31(4):623–34.
4. Li FQ, Wang ZB, Du YH, et al. Study on therapeutic dosimetry of HIFU ablation tissue. J Biomed Eng. 2006;23(4):839–43.
5. McDannold NJ, King RL, Jolesz FA, et al. Usefulness of MR imaging-derived thermometry and dosimetry in determining the threshold for tissue damage induced by thermal surgery in rabbits. Radiology. 2000;216(2):517–23.
6. Jolesz FA, Hynynen K, McDannold N, et al. MR imaging-controlled focused ultrasound ablation: a noninvasive image-guided surgery. Magn Reson Imaging Clin N Am. 2005;13(3):545–60.
7. Rabinovici J, David M, Fukunishi H, et al. Pregnancy outcome after magnetic resonance-guided focused ultrasound surgery (MRgFUS) for conservative treatment of uterine fibroids. Fertil Steril. 2010;93(1):199–209.
8. Xu YH, Fu ZX, Yang LX, et al. Feasibility, safety, and efficacy of accurate uterine fibroid ablation using magnetic resonance imaging-guided high-intensity focused ultrasound with shot sonication. Ultrasound Med. 2015;34:2293–303.
9. Wang Y, Wang ZB, Xu YH. Efficacy, efficiency, and safety of magnetic resonance-guided high intensity focused ultrasound for ablation of uterine fibroids: comparison with ultrasound-guided method. Korean J Radiol. 2018;19(4):724–32.
10. Wang W, Liu WY, Zhou JM, et al. Treatment of symptomatic uterine leiomyomata with high intensity focused ultrasound: a preliminary clinical study [J]. Chin J Ultrasonogr. 2002;11(3):161–3.
11. Fu ZX, Wang Y, Xu YH. Comparative study between MRI guided and US guided high intensity focused ultrasound for complete ablation of uterine fibroids. Chinese Comput Med Imaging. 2016;22:468–72.
12. Zhang L, Chen WZ, Liu YJ, et al. Feasibility of magnetic resonance imaging-guided high intensity focused ultrasound therapy for ablating uterine fibroids in patients with bowel lies anterior to uterus. Eur J Radiol. 2010;73(2):396–403.
13. Froeling V, Meckelburg K, Schreiter NF, et al. Outcome of uterine artery embolization versus MRguided high-intensity focused ultrasound treatment for uterine fibroids: long-term results. Eur J Radiol. 2013;82(12):2265–9.
14. Wong WSF, Zhang L, Xu Y. High intensity focused ultrasound (HIFU) telesurgery play a role in "digital healthcare"-the first 5G-backed HIFU ablation procedures. Clin Surg. 2021;6:3199.

Imaging Diagnosis of Uterine Fibroids

2

Lixia Yang, Felix Wong, Yu Cheng, Qing Song Yang, Zhongxiang Fu, and Liqun Sun

Abstract

The aim of this chapter is to overview the normal anatomy of the uterus and the diagnosis and classification of uterine fibroid by MRI, CT, and ultrasonography. All types of fibroids are modified per focused ultrasound ablation procedure, and the MR imaging with different sequences of each type is given, especially for broad ligament fibroid and adenomyomatosis, emphasizing the differential diagnosis between the benign uterine diseases (endometrial polyps, fibroids, adenomyosis, etc.) and the malignant uterine diseases (cervical carcinoma, endometrial carcinoma, and uterine sarcoma). The ultrasound and CT findings of uterine fibroids and their special types with differential diagnoses are described.

Keywords

Ultrasonography · CT · MRI · Uterine fibroid · Diagnosis Classification

The treatment option, efficacy evaluation, and differential diagnosis of uterine fibroids should fully rely on imaging techniques to provide relevant information. Currently, the most commonly used clinical imaging techniques include magnetic resonance imaging (MRI), computed tomography (CT), and ultrasound. Ultrasound is the first choice for routine examinations. For those with contraindications to MRI or those with degeneration and calcification of uterine fibroids, CT examination can be used. MRI is popular clinically because of its higher soft tissue resolution and tissue contrast, especially in selecting treatment options for uterine fibroids, evaluation before and after treatment, and follow-up. This chapter mainly introduces the application of MRI, CT, and ultrasound in the diagnosis of uterine fibroids, with an emphasis on the diagnostic value of MRI.

2.1 MRI Diagnosis of Uterine Fibroids

The uterus is a female reproductive organ, and sagittal MR Imaging of a normal adult uterus can clearly show its gross morphology and anatomical characteristics. The uterus can be divided into the uterus body and the cervix. The shape is generally inverted fusiform, wide at the fundus and narrow at the cervix. The uterus is located in the center of the pelvic cavity, with the bladder in front and below, the rectum in the rear, the small intestine in front and above, and the symphysis pubis in the bottom.

2.1.1 MRI Findings of a Normal Uterus

2.1.1.1 Uterine Body

The uterine body is mainly composed of three layers of tissue: endometrium (mucosa), muscularis, and adventitia (serosa) from inside to outside. Due to a certain amount of viscous fluid in the uterine cavity on MRI, slightly higher signal intensity was present on T1WI (Fig. 2.1a), and significantly higher signal intensity was present on T2WI (Fig. 2.1b, c). The uterine body usually shows uniform hypointensity on T1WI (Fig. 2.1d); different signals on T2WI can present delamination, the innermost lining layer for slightly high signal, next to the lining base of the low signal of the belt

L. Yang (✉) · Y. Cheng · Z. Fu
Zhongshan-Xuhui Hospital, Fudan University, Shanghai, China

F. Wong
The University of New South Wales, Sydney, NSW, Australia

Q. S. Yang
Department of Interventional Radiology, Changhai Hospital, Naval Medical University, Shanghai, China

L. Sun
Department of Ultrasound, International Peace Maternity & Child Health Hospital, School of Medicine, Shanghai Jiao Tong University, Shanghai, China

Y. Xu et al. (eds.), *Surgical Techniques of Focused Ultrasound Ablation in Benign Uterine Diseases*,
https://doi.org/10.1007/978-981-19-7180-8_2

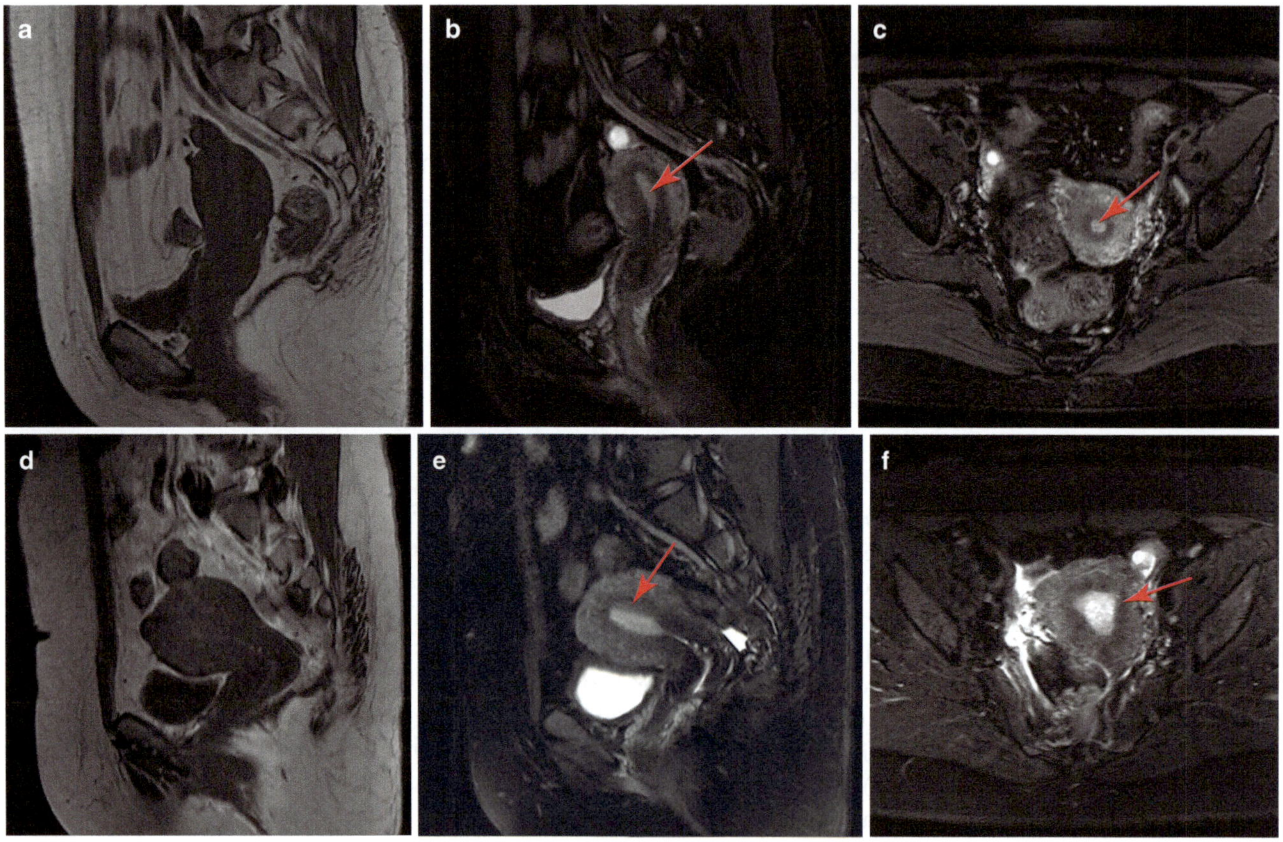

Fig. 2.1 Normal uterine body. (**a**) T1WI sagittal; (**b**) T2WI_FS sagittal; (**c**) T2WI_FS axial; (**d**) T1WI sagittal; (**e**) T2WI_FS sagittal; (**f**) T2WI_FS axial

(Junctional Zone, JZ), on the outside of the high signal of uterine muscle layer (Fig. 2.1e, f, arrow showing low-signal junction zone).

2.1.1.2 Uterine Isthmus

The isthmus is located at the narrow part of the junction between the end of the uterine body and the uterine cervix. It is the most common site for cesarean section in women (Fig. 2.2a, arrow shows the isthmus incision). The isthmus was not obvious on T1WI (Fig. 2.2b), and the sagittal view on T2WI clearly showed hypointensity in the isthmus (Fig. 2.2c).

2.1.1.3 Uterine Cervix

The cervix of the uterus is located at the entrance of the uterine body. T2WI can clearly show the uterus against the mucus in the cervical canal. The structure and stratification of the cervix are as follows, the innermost layer being the mucosal layer with a slightly higher signal. In the middle is the cervical fibrous matrix layer with a relatively low signal, which is continuous with the isthmus of the uterine body. The outermost layer is the isometric signal muscular layer, which is continuous with the muscular layer of the uterine body (Fig. 2.3a, b, arrow shows the mucosal layer with a slightly higher signal). Some of the most common cysts in the cervical region of the uterus, such as the Nabothian cyst, showed high signal intensity on T2WI (Fig. 2.3c).

2.1.1.4 Uterine Ligament

The uterine ligament is an important part of the uterine appendage to maintain the normal position and shape of the uterus. It mainly consists of four pairs of ligaments: the main uterine ligament, the broad uterine ligament, the round uterine ligament, and the uterosacral ligament. The uterine ligaments showed isointense signal intensity on T1WI (Fig. 2.4a, e) and medium-high signal intensity on T2WI axial and coronal (Fig. 2.4b–d, f). The boundaries between the ligaments were not clearly displayed.

2.1.1.5 Uterus and Ovaries

The ovaries on both sides of the uterus usually show moderate to high signal intensity on T2WI, and the ovarian follicles show higher signal intensity (Fig. 2.5a, b). The common ovarian cysts showed significantly high signal intensity on T2WI (Fig. 2.5c) and low signal intensity on T1WI (Fig. 2.5d). In contrast, chocolate cysts showed mixed signal

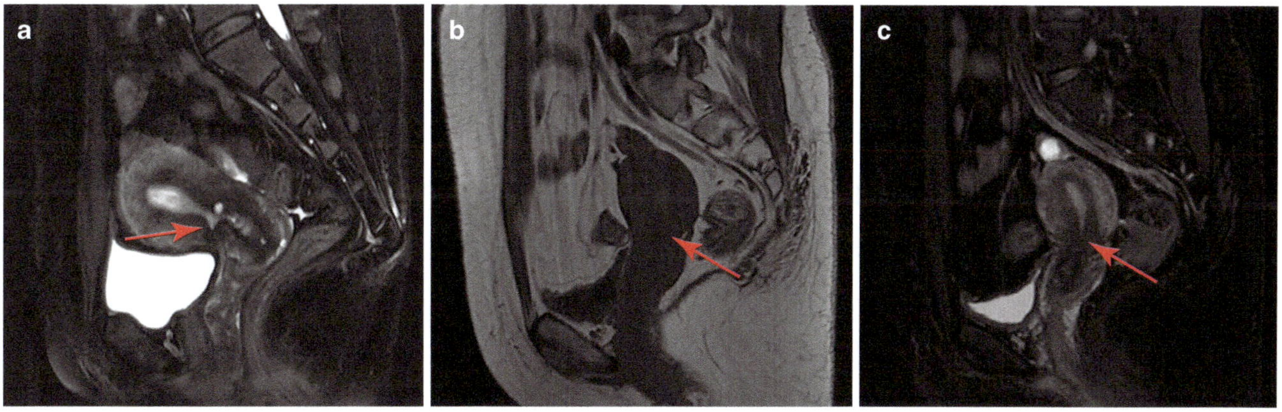

Fig. 2.2 Normal uterine isthmus. (**a**) T2WI_FS sagittal; (**b**) T1WI sagittal; (**c**) T2WI_FS sagittal

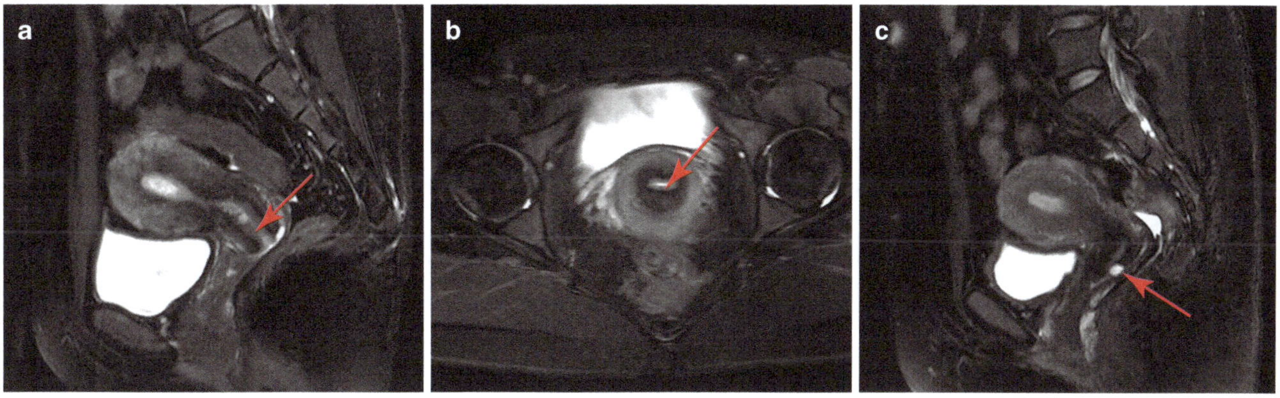

Fig. 2.3 Normal uterine neck. (**a**) T2WI_FS sagittal; (**b**) T2WI_FS axial; (**c**) T2WI_FS sagittal

intensity on T2WI (Fig. 2.5e) and significantly high signal intensity on T1WI (Fig. 2.5f).

2.1.1.6 Uterine Functional Imaging

Diffusion weighted imaging (DWI) is one of the most commonly used sequences in uterine MRI functional imaging. It is highly sensitive to malignant uterine tumors and usually uses axial imaging. For uterine DWI functional imaging, a single b value or multiple b values can be selected to reconstruct the apparent diffusion coefficient (ADC) of quantitative parameters to improve the sensitivity of lesion detection and further quantitative analysis of lesions. Low b values range from 0 to 100 s/mm^2 (Fig. 2.6a), while high b values are usually greater than 500 s/mm^2 (Fig. 2.6b). Both DWI and ADC images can roughly show the three-layered structure of the uterine body (Fig. 2.6c).

2.1.1.7 Uterine T1WI Dynamic Enhanced Imaging

In dynamic uterine contrast-enhanced MRI, the blood supply to different parts of the uterine body was different after the injection of Gadopentetic acid (Gd-DTPA) contrast agent in venous mass. In T1WI contrast-enhanced imaging, the myometrium rich in blood supply was enhanced first, and the enhancement performance varied with time. Early enhancement usually starts from the outer layer and sometimes from the inner layer, followed by uniform enhancement of the entire muscular layer (Fig. 2.7).

2.1.2 Classifications and Types of Uterine Fibroids

Uterine leiomyoma, also known as uterine fibroid, is a benign tumor comprising uterine smooth muscle and fibrous connective tissue. It is the most common gynecological tumor. The classifications of uterine fibroids and subtypes method can be divided into uterine body fibroids and cervical fibroids by their growing location; the former accounts for about 90%, and the latter accounts for about 10%. The relationship between myoma and uterine wall can be divided into four kinds: intramural myoma, submucosal myoma, subserosal myoma, and broad ligament myoma. The classification of uterine fibroids widely adopts the classification standard of the International Federation of Gynecology and Obstetrics (FIGO) [1]. FIGO divides uterine fibroids into nine types, represented by Arabic numerals 0 ~ 8 or Greek I ~ VIII

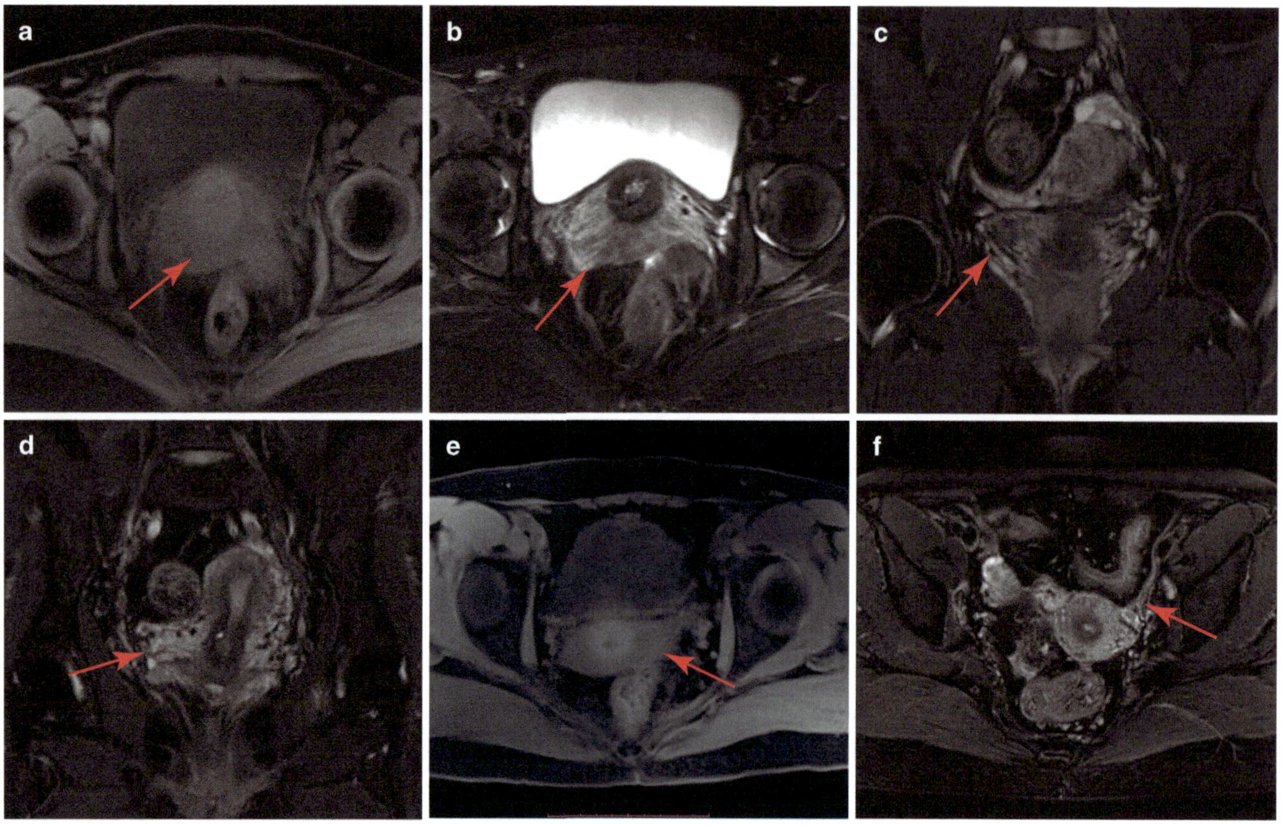

Fig. 2.4 Normal uterine ligaments. (**a**) T1WI_FS axial; (**b**) T2WI_FS axial; (**c**, **d**) T2WI_FS coronal; (**e**) T1WI_FS axial; (**f**) T2WI_FS axial

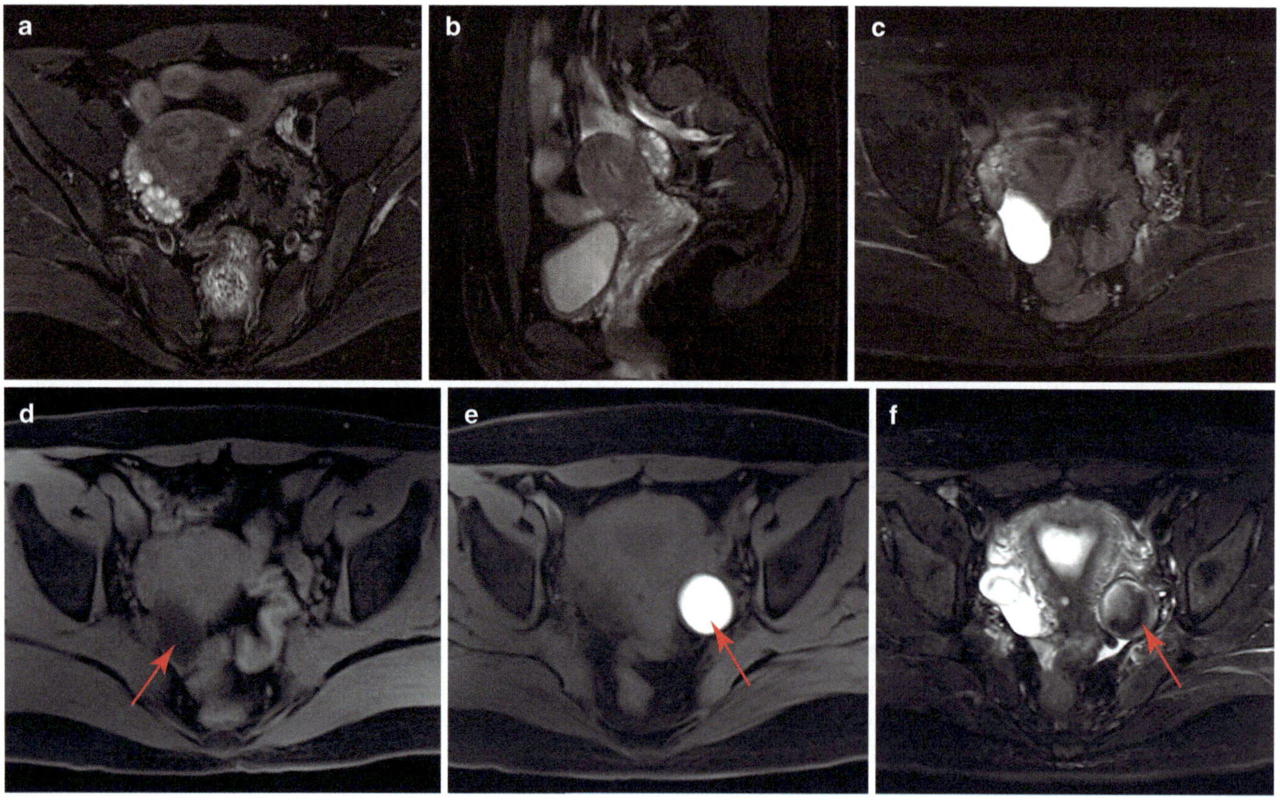

Fig. 2.5 Normal uterine ovary. (**a**) T2WI_FS axial; (**b**) T2WI_FS sagittal; (**c**) T2WI_FS axial; (**d**) T1WI_FS axial; (**e**) T2WI_FS axial; (**f**) T1WI_FS axial

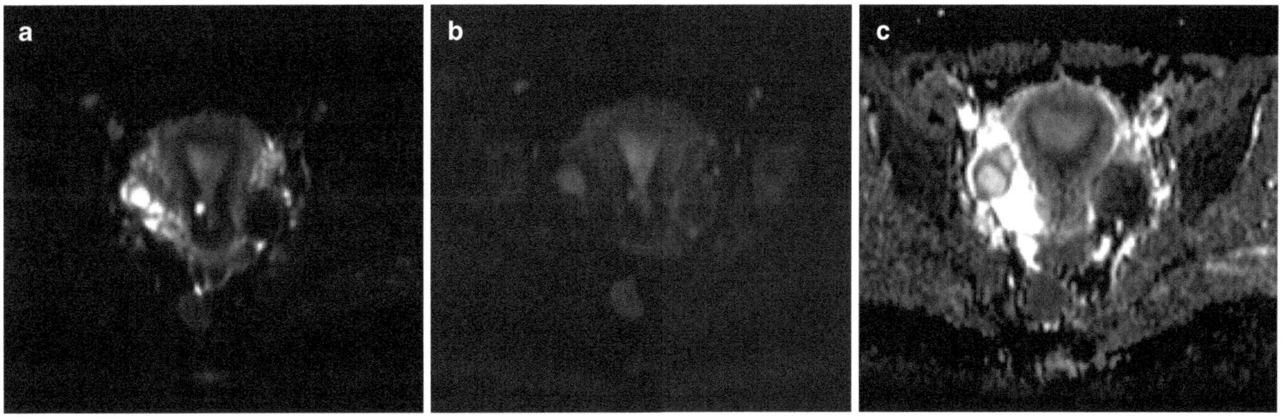

Fig. 2.6 Functional imaging of normal uterine DWI. (**a**) DWI axial (b = 50 s/mm^2); (**b**) DWI axial (b = 800 s/mm^2); (**c**) ADC axial

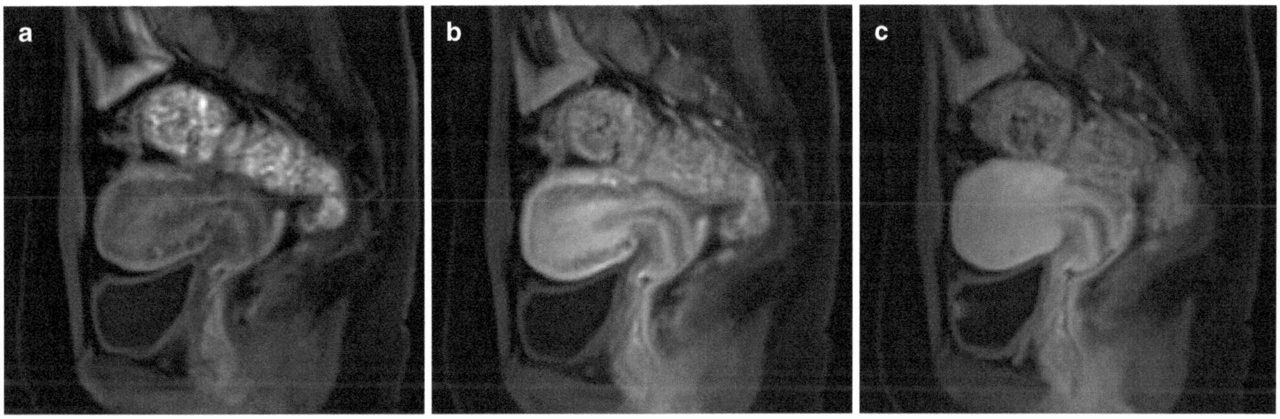

Fig. 2.7 Dynamic enhancement of T1WI in normal uterine. (**a**). T1WI_FS + C ultra-early sagittal; (**b**) T1WI_FS + C early sagittal; (**c**) T1WI_FS + C late sagittal

(Fig. 2.8): Type 0: pedunculated submucosal myoma; Type I: submucous myoma, expansion to muscular layer less than 50%; Type II: submucous myoma, expansion to muscular layer at least 50%; Type III: intramural myoma, close to the endometrial cavity but distant from uterine serosa 5 mm or more; Type IV: intramural myoma, near the uterine serosa layer, and the myoma protrudes to the serous layer <50%; Type V: intramural myoma (hybrid), the myoma occupies the whole myometrial layer; Type VI: myoma protrudes through the uterine serosa; Type VII: myoma lies entirely over the uterine serosa with a pedicle; Type VIII: special types of myoma in other parts of the uterus (the cervix, uterine horn, and broad ligament).

FIGO classification of uterine fibroids focuses on indicating the location of fibroids and the relationship with endometrium. The smaller the number, the closer the fibroids are to the endometrium; the larger the number, the closer the fibroids are to the serous membrane of the uterus.

2.1.2.1 Submucosal Uterine Fibroids (Type 0 to II)

Submucous myoma accounts for about 10% of the total number of fibroids, which grows into the uterine cavity through a protrusion process, with the endometrium covering the surface of the protruded fibroid. According to FIGO classification criteria, submucosal uterine fibroids can be classified into the following three types: (1) Type 0: pedunculated submucosal fibroids. The fibroid is completely located in the uterine cavity, connected to the endometrium through a pedicle on one side, and the fibroid does not extend to the muscular layer (Fig. 2.9). (2) Type I: this submucous fibroid does not have a pedicle, it expands to the muscular layer of 50% or less, and the angle between the fibroid and the uterine muscular wall forms an acute angle (Fig. 2.10). (3) Type II: this submucous fibroid expands to the muscular layer >50%, and the angle between the fibroid and the uterine muscular wall forms an obtuse angle (Fig. 2.11).

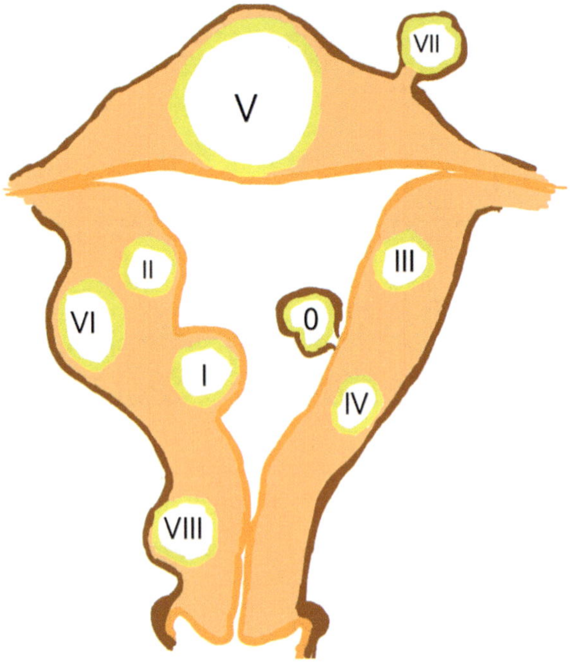

Fig. 2.8 Location typing of uterine fibroids. Classification Schematic Diagram [2]

MRI Findings

Submucosal fibroids are usually homogeneous and hypointense signals on conventional T1WI imaging. Due to the difference in the intrauterine fluid signal, the contrast can be improved, and the boundary of fibroids can be displayed to a certain extent (Figs. 2.9d and 2.10a). Compared with T1WI imaging, T2WI can significantly observe the morphology and characteristics of submucosal fibroids. Most of the submucosal fibroids are single but occasionally multiple (Fig. 2.10b), usually round in appearance. Due to the significant contrast provided by intrauterine fluid, the boundary and pedicle of a submucosal fibroid can be clearly shown (Fig. 2.9k).

Fibroids can grow in various locations of the uterine body, such as the anterior wall (Fig. 2.10d), the posterior wall (Fig. 2.11h), the lateral wall, or the fundus (Fig.2.10j). The size of submucosal fibroids varies; when the fibroid is small, it basically does not affect the normal uterine form (Fig. 2.9a). On the contrary, when the fibroid is bigger, it often grows into the uterine cavity, leading to uterine enlargement (Fig. 2.10d). Due to the gravity, a part of the larger submucosal fibroid can gradually push downward to the nearby internal cervical opening, and the opening of the cervix may become narrow or blocked (Fig. 2.11h). Submucosal fibroids increase the endometrial surface and occupy space in the uterine cavity, affecting the menstrual blood flow. Therefore, it may cause abnormal uterine body contraction, producing dysmenorrhea, and accompanied by an increased menstrual flow and period disorders.

The submucosal fibroids usually present a relatively uniform low intense signal on T2WI (Fig. 2.9j), and a few may present isointense signals (Fig. 2.10d), high intense signals (Fig. 2.11a), or mixed signals (Fig. 2.10k) relative to that of the uterine muscle. When fibroids grow larger, a certain degree of degeneration and necrosis can be observed, resulting in uneven signals inside the fibroids.

DWI functional imaging is not sensitive to the diagnosis of fibroids, and fibroids usually present relatively uniform low intense signals (Fig. 2.9l), while a few present isointense signals (Fig. 2.10l). Because intrauterine fluid presents slightly hyperintense signals, the boundary of submucosal fibroids can be shown to a certain extent.

Contrast-enhanced T1WI usually shows fibroid is a relatively homogeneous high signal, a few for the inhomogeneous signal with unobvious boundary (Fig. 2.11c). Because of the difference in blood flow to the submucosal fibroids and the uterine muscle layer, sometimes fibroids can be observed with overall T1W1 signals appearing slightly lower (Fig. 2.11i) or slightly higher than that of the uterine muscle layer. Degenerative necrosis with no perfusion in the fibroid may show an area of low intense signals (Fig. 2.10n).

Differential Diagnosis

- **Endometrial polyp**: Endometrial polyp (EP) is a benign tumor projecting from the endometrial surface composed of endometrial glands and fibrotic endometrial stroma containing thick-walled blood vessels. On T2WI images, EP can show endometrial defect or bulge with isointense signals or slightly hypointense signals (Fig. 2.12b), which is not easy to distinguish from type 0 submucosal fibroid, especially type 0 submucosal fibroid tends to form pedicle and grows like a foreign body in the uterine cavity. Therefore, the differentiation between EP and type 0 submucosal fibroids is more difficult and often requires clinical and pathological confirmation.
- **Endometrial carcinoma**: Endometrial carcinoma (EC) is one of the most common malignancies of the female reproductive system. It usually occurs in older women. On T2WI images, EC usually shows isointense signals or slightly hyperintense signals and irregular lesions in local endometrial or intrauterine areas (Fig. 2.13a, b, g). Conventional MRI T1WI was difficult to identify accurately (Fig. 2.13e). DWI functional imaging showed that endometrial carcinoma presented high intense signals at a high b value (Fig. 2.13c), while ADC showed slightly low signals (Fig. 2.13d). The early stage of dynamic contrast-enhancement T1WI showed that the endometrial enhancement zone surface was irregular, with a certain degree of destruction (Fig. 2.13f, h, i).
- **Adenomyoma**: Adenomyoma (AM) is one of types of adenomyosis in which ectopic infiltration of the endometrium and basal stroma into the myometrium. It may be located in

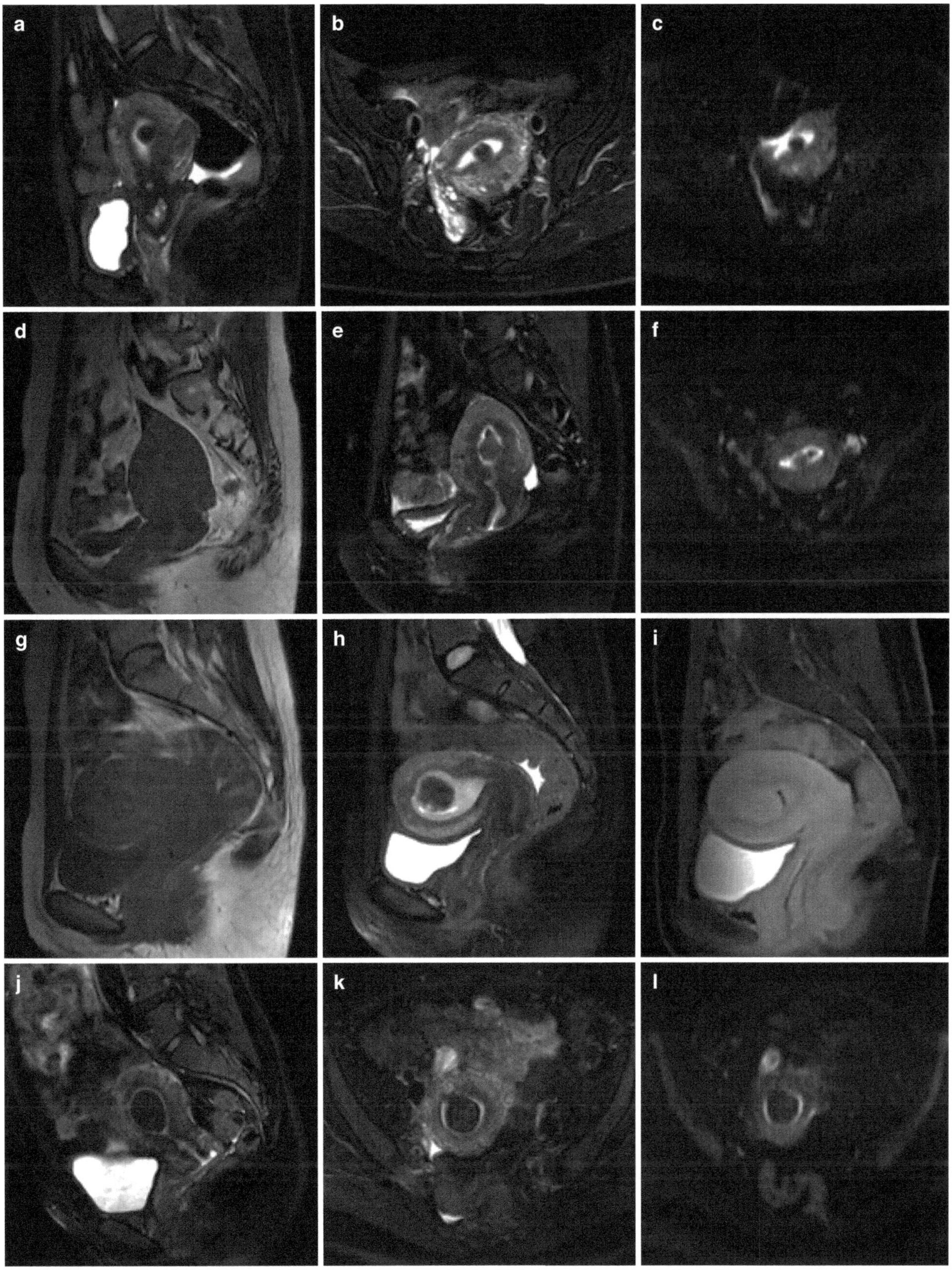

Fig. 2.9 Submucosal uterine fibroids (Type 0). (**a**) T2WI_FS Sagittal; (**b**) T2WI_FS axial; (**c**) DWI axial (b = 800 s/mm^2); (**d**) T1WI sagittal; (**e**) T2WI_FS sagittal; (**f**) DWI axial (b = 800 s/mm^2); (**g**) T1WI sagittal; (**h**). T2WI_FS sagittal; (**i**). T1WI_FS + C sagittal; (**j**) T2WI_FS Sagittal; (**k**) T2WI_FS axial; (**l**) DWI axial (b = 800 s/mm^2); (**m**) T2WI_FS sagittal; (**n**) T1WI_FS axial; (**o**) DWI axial (b = 800 s/mm^2); (**p**) T1WI_FS + C axial; (**q**) T1WI_FS + C sagittal; (**r**) T1WI_FS + C coronal

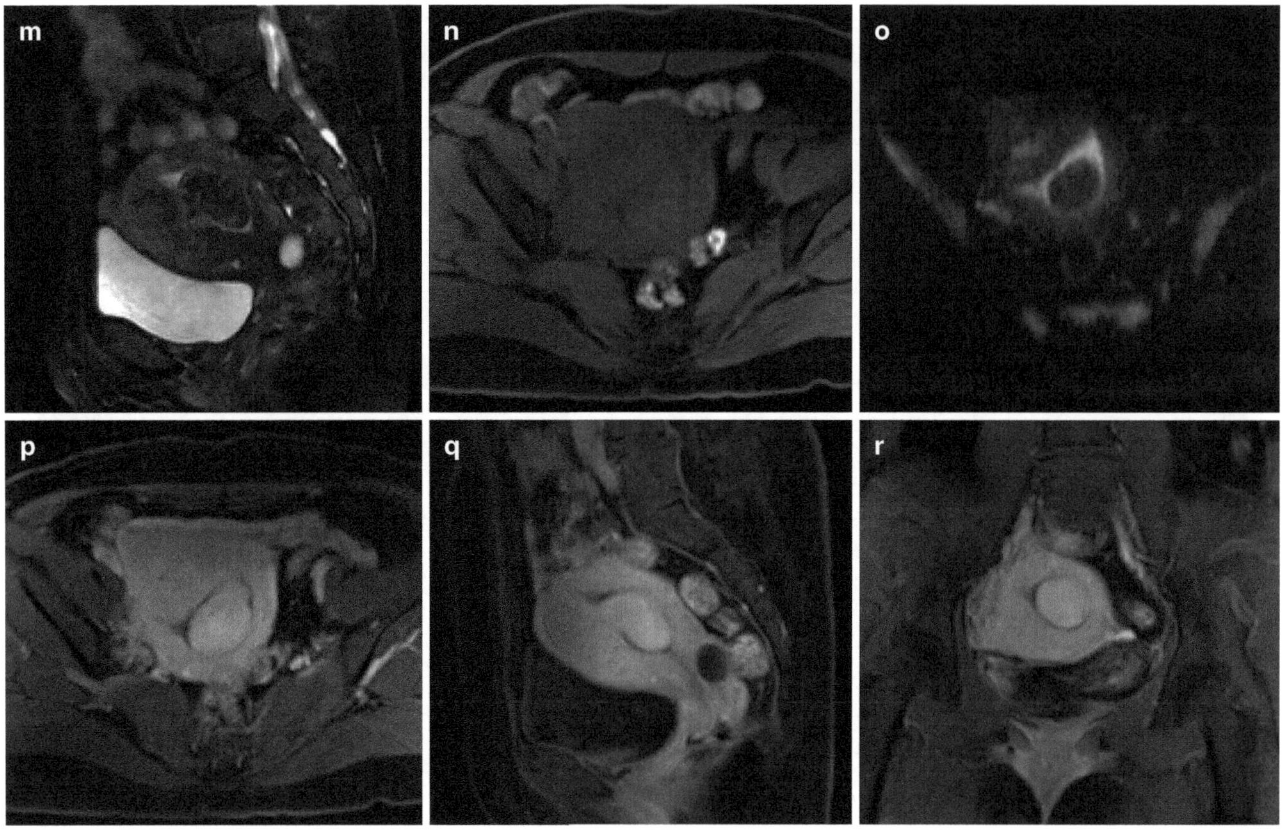

Fig. 2.9 (continued)

the uterine muscular layer to form a circumscribed nodular aggregate of benign endometrial glands surrounded by endometrial stroma with leiomyomatous smooth muscle. However, unlike fibroids, adenomyoma has no pseudocapsule and no obvious boundary from the surrounding muscular layer, so removing it from the muscular layer is difficult. Uterine adenomyoma needs to distinguish from the type II submucosal uterine fibroid. A normal uterine endometrial-myometrial junction (EMJ) thickness is less than 6 mm on T2WI. Adenomyoma is of an intramural mass with isointense signal on T1WI and hypointense signal similar to the EMJ on T2WI, mostly in the posterior wall of the uterus. Often within the tumor, it may sometimes be accompanied by dot-like high intense signals and has similar enhancement as EMJ but no enhanced blood vessels around it. Patients are often characterized by pain during menstruation (Fig. 2.14).

2.1.2.2 Intramural Uterine Fibroids (Type III, IV)

The intramural fibroid is one of the most common types of uterine leiomyoma, which grows in the myometrium and is surrounded by normal myometrial tissue. According to FIGO classification criteria, intramural uterine fibroids can be divided into two main types. (1) The intramural fibroid has its inner border in contact with the endometrium (type III): the fibroid grows close to the uterine cavity, but its outer border is 5 mm or more from the uterine serosal layer (Fig. 2.15). (2) The intramural fibroid has its outer border in contact with the serosa (type IV): the fibroid grows in the myometrium, but its location is close to the uterine serosal layer, and the fibroid protrudes over the serosal layer <50% (Fig. 2.16).

MRI Findings

Conventional T1WI plain scan of fibroids usually presents uniform isointense low signals with unclear boundaries. Some fibroids may present lower signals than the muscular layer, which can show the boundary of fibroids to some extent (Fig 2.15d). Compared with a plain T1WI scan, conventional T2WI can clearly observe the morphology and characteristics of the fibroid. Uterine fibroids are usually multiple in the uterine muscular wall, and there could be two or more intramural fibroids (Fig. 2.15i).

Most fibroids are usually round in shape; a few are irregularly shaped (Fig. 2.15a). Most have a pseudocapsule and show relatively clear boundaries. Fibroids can grow anywhere in the uterine body, such as the anterior wall (Fig. 2.16b), the posterior wall (Fig. 2.16n), the lateral wall, or the fundus of the uterus (Fig. 2.15i). When uterine fibroids are small, they do not change the form of the uterus (Fig. 2.16m). Type III intramural fibroid is in contact with endometrium. When the fibroid grows to a larger size, the endometrium can show a certain degree of compression. The EMJ can be observed with low signals on T2WI and slightly

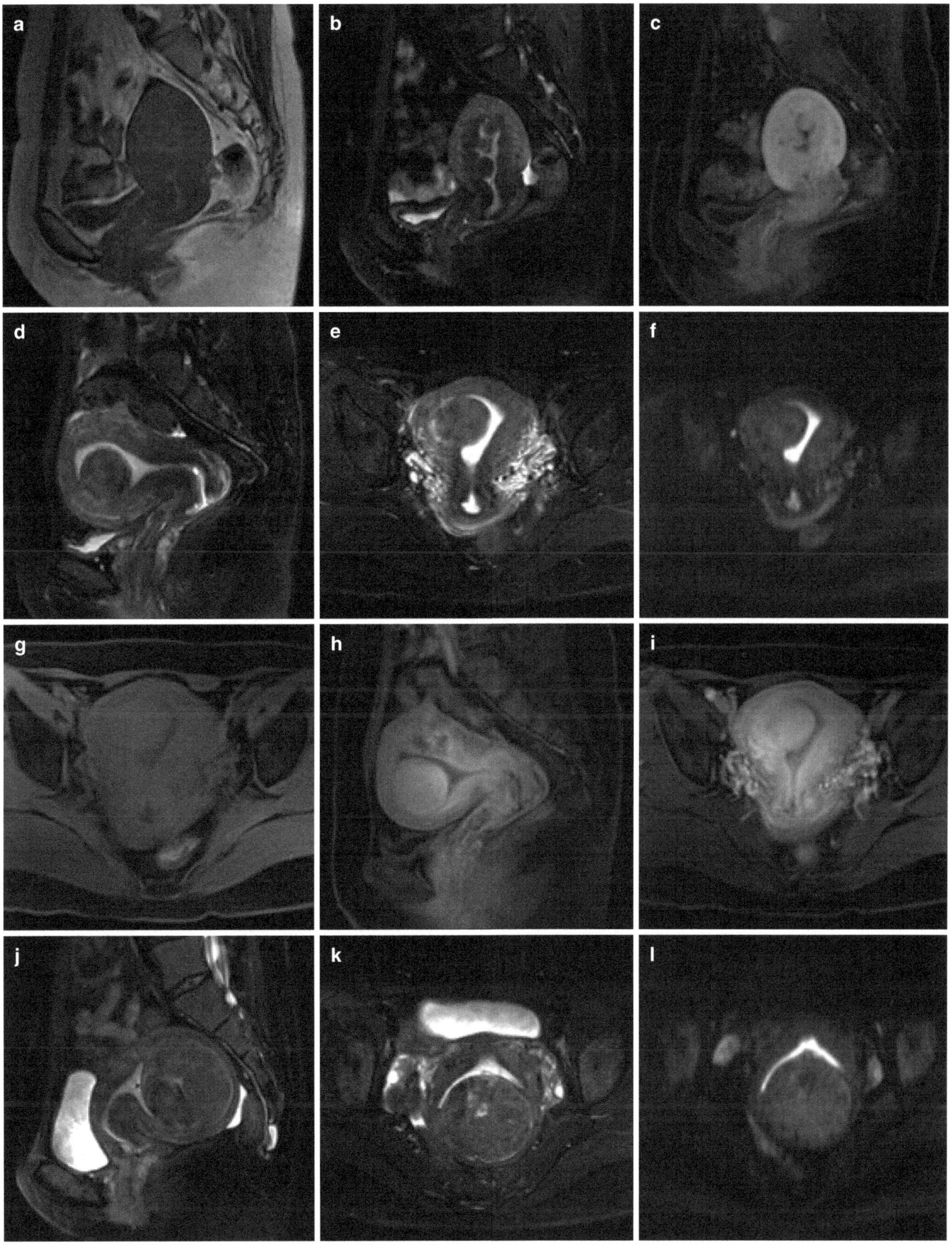

Fig. 2.10 Submucosal uterine fibroids (Type I). (**a**) T1WI sagittal; (**b**) T2WI_FS sagittal; (**c**) T1WI_FS + C sagittal; (**d**) T2WI_FS sagittal; (**e**) T2WI_FS axial; (**f**) DWI axial (B = 800 s/mm^2); (**g**) T1WI_FS axial; (**h**) T1WI _FS + C sagittal; (**i**) T1WI_FS + C axial; (**j**) T2WI_FS sagittal; (**k**) T2WI_FS axial; (**l**) DWI axial (b = 800 s/mm^2); (**m**) T1WI_FS axial; (**n**) T1WI_FS + C sagittal; (**o**) T1WI_FS + C axial

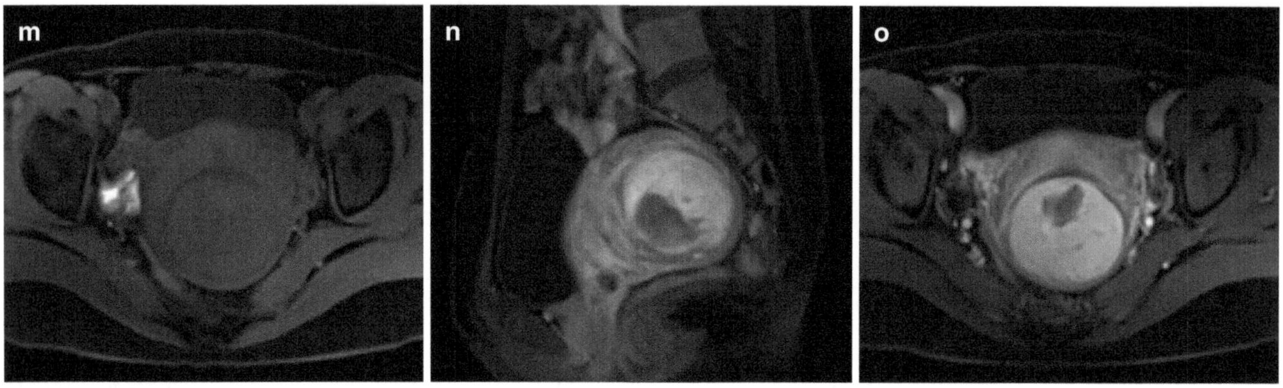

Fig. 2.10 (continued)

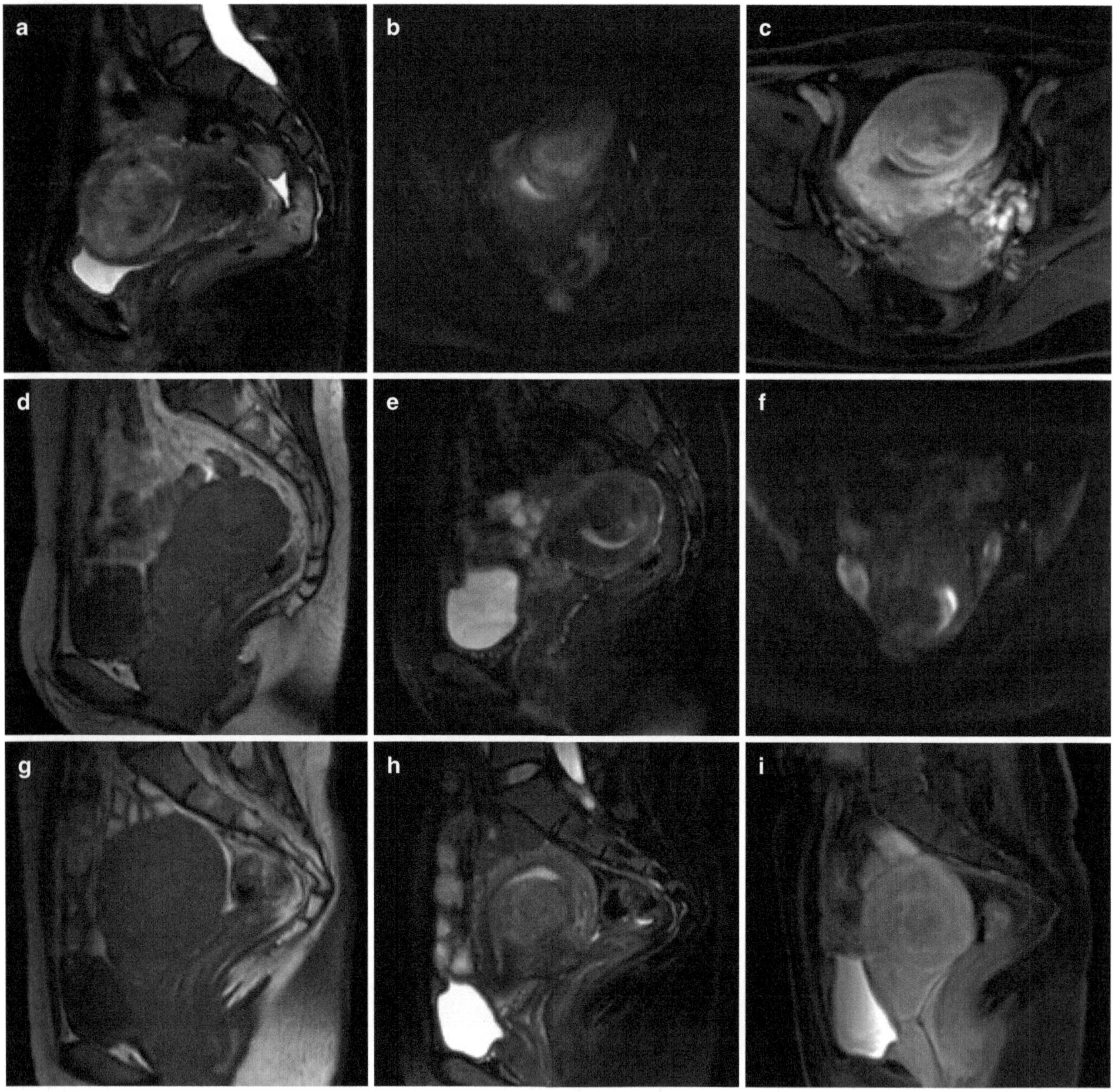

Fig. 2.11 Submucosal uterine fibroids (Type II). (**a**) T2WI_FS sagittal; (**b**) DWI axial (b = 800 s/mm^2); (**c**) T1WI_FS + C axial; (**d**) T1WI sagittal; (**e**) T2WI_FS sagittal; (**f**) DWI axial (b = 800 s/mm^2); (**g**) T1WI sagittal; (**h**) T2WI_FS sagittal; (**i**) T1WI_FS + C sagittal

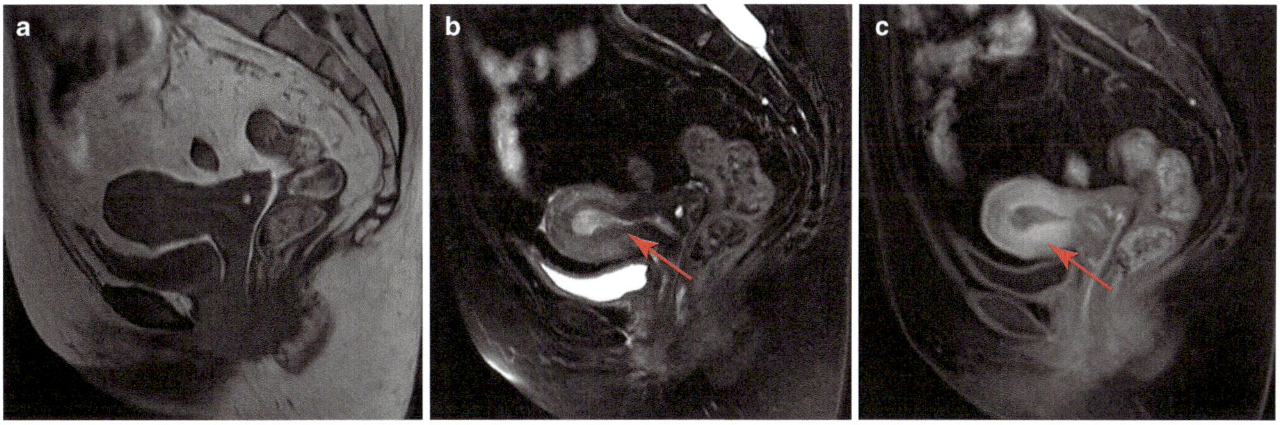

Fig. 2.12 Endometrial polyps. (**a**) T1WI sagittal; (**b**) T2WI_FS sagittal; (**c**) T1WI_FS + C sagittal

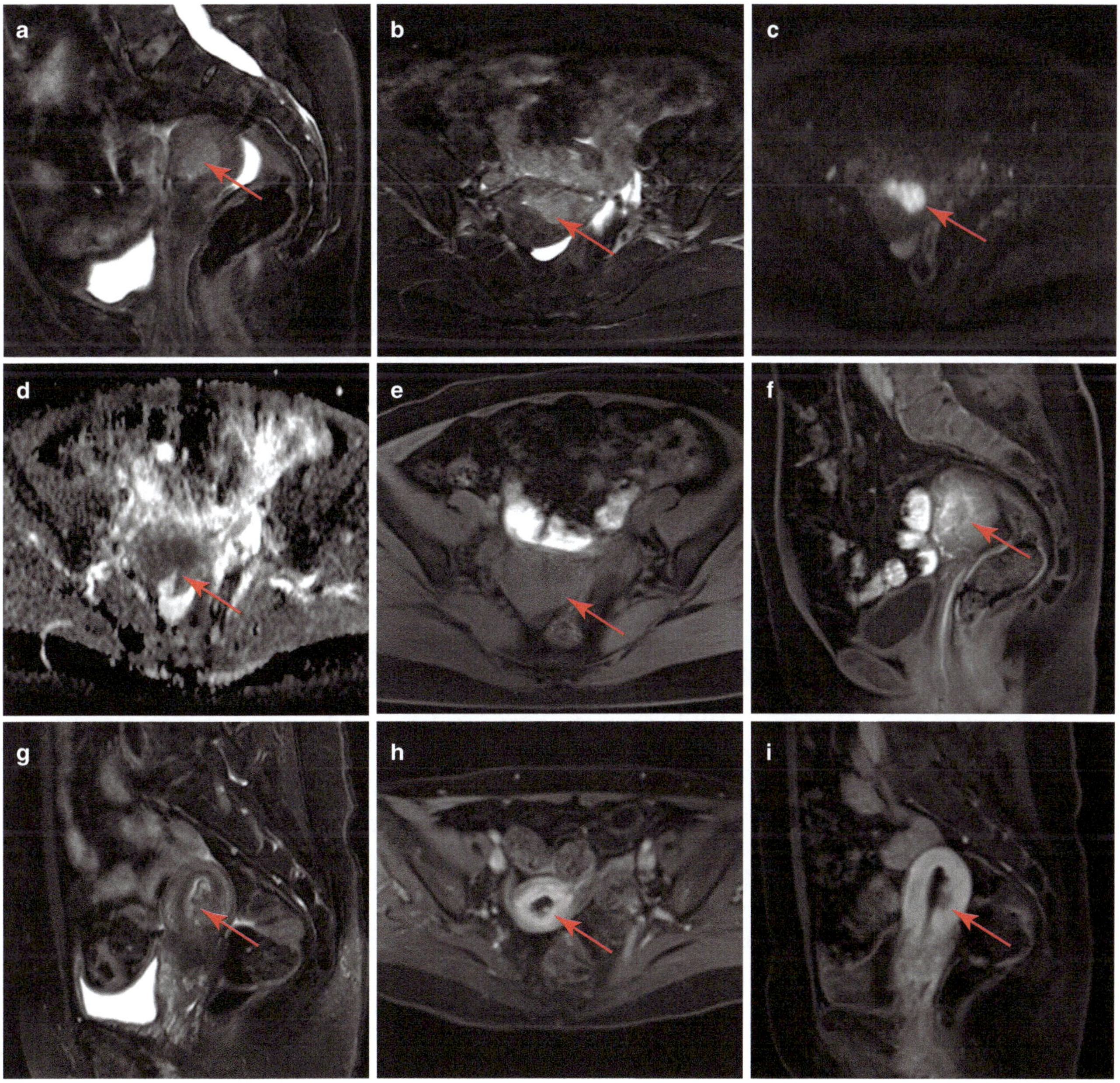

Fig. 2.13 Endometrial carcinoma. (**a**) T2WI_FS sagittal; (**b**) T2WI_FS axial; (**c**) DWI axial (b = 800 s/mm^2); (**d**) ADC axial; (**e**) T1WI_FS axial; (**f**) T1WI_FS + C sagittal; (**g**) T2WI_FS sagittal; (**h**) T1WI_FS + C axial; (**i**) T1WI _FS + C sagittal

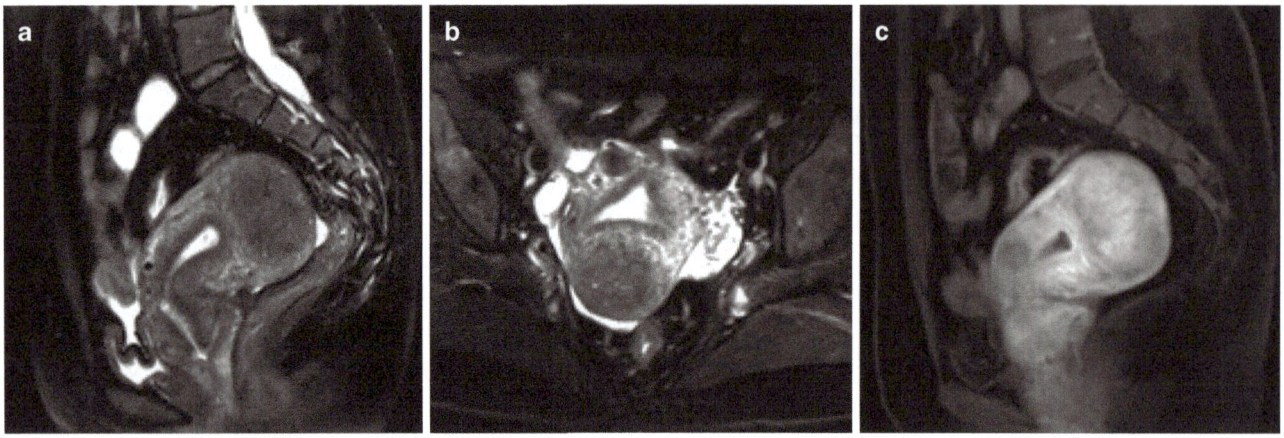

Fig. 2.14 Adenomyoma. (**a**) T2WI_FS sagittal; (**b**) T2WI_FS axial; (**c**) T1WI_FS + C sagittal

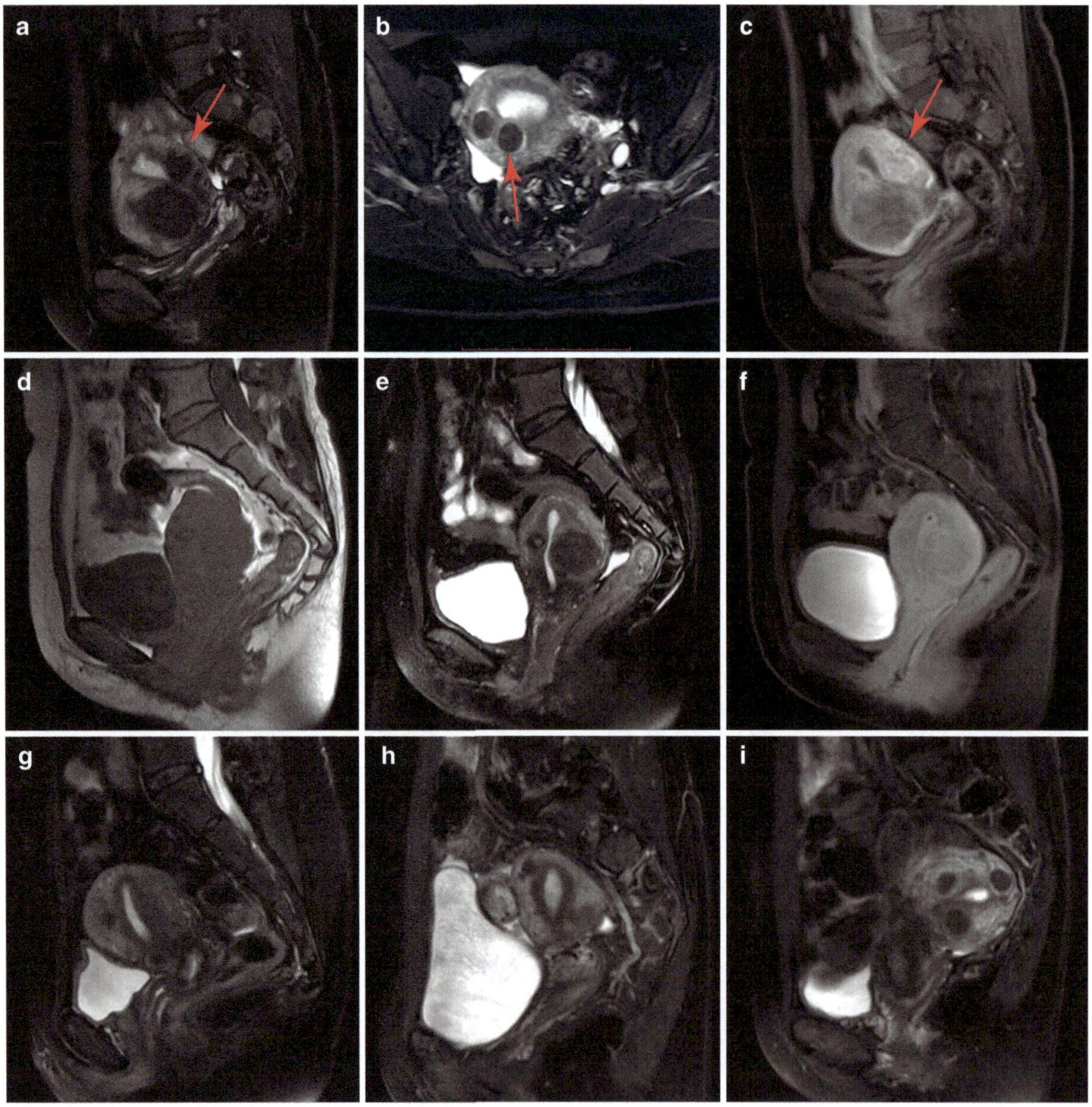

Fig. 2.15 Intramural uterine fibroids (Type III). (**a**) T2WI_FS sagittal; (**b**) T2WI_FS axial; (**c**) T1WI_FS + C sagittal; (**d**) T1WI sagittal; (**e**) T2WI_FS sagittal; (**f**) T1WI_FS + C sagittal; (**g–i**) T2WI_FS sagittal

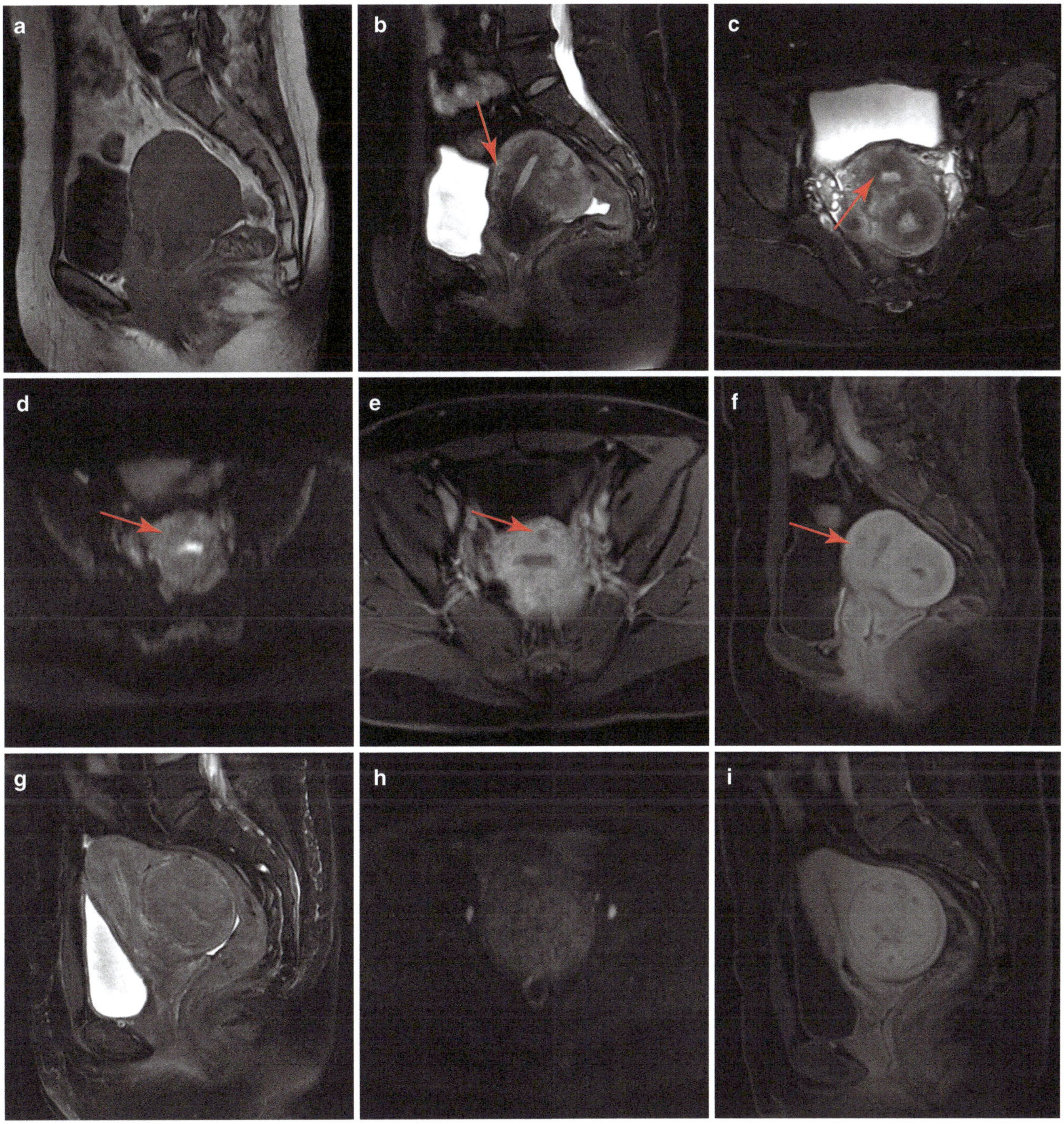

Fig. 2.16 Intramural uterine fibroids (Type IV). (**a**) T1WI sagittal; (**b**) T2WI_FS sagittal; (**c**) T2WI_FS axial; (**d**) DWI axial (b = 800 s/mm^2); (**e**) T1WI_FS + C axial; (**f**) T1WI_FS + C sagittal; (**g**) T2WI_FS sagittal; (**h**) DWI axial (b = 800 s/mm^2); (**i**) T1WI_FS+ C sagittal; (**j**) T1WI sagittal; (**k**) T2WI_FS sagittal; (**l**) T1WI_FS + C sagittal; (**m–o**).T2WI_FS sagittal

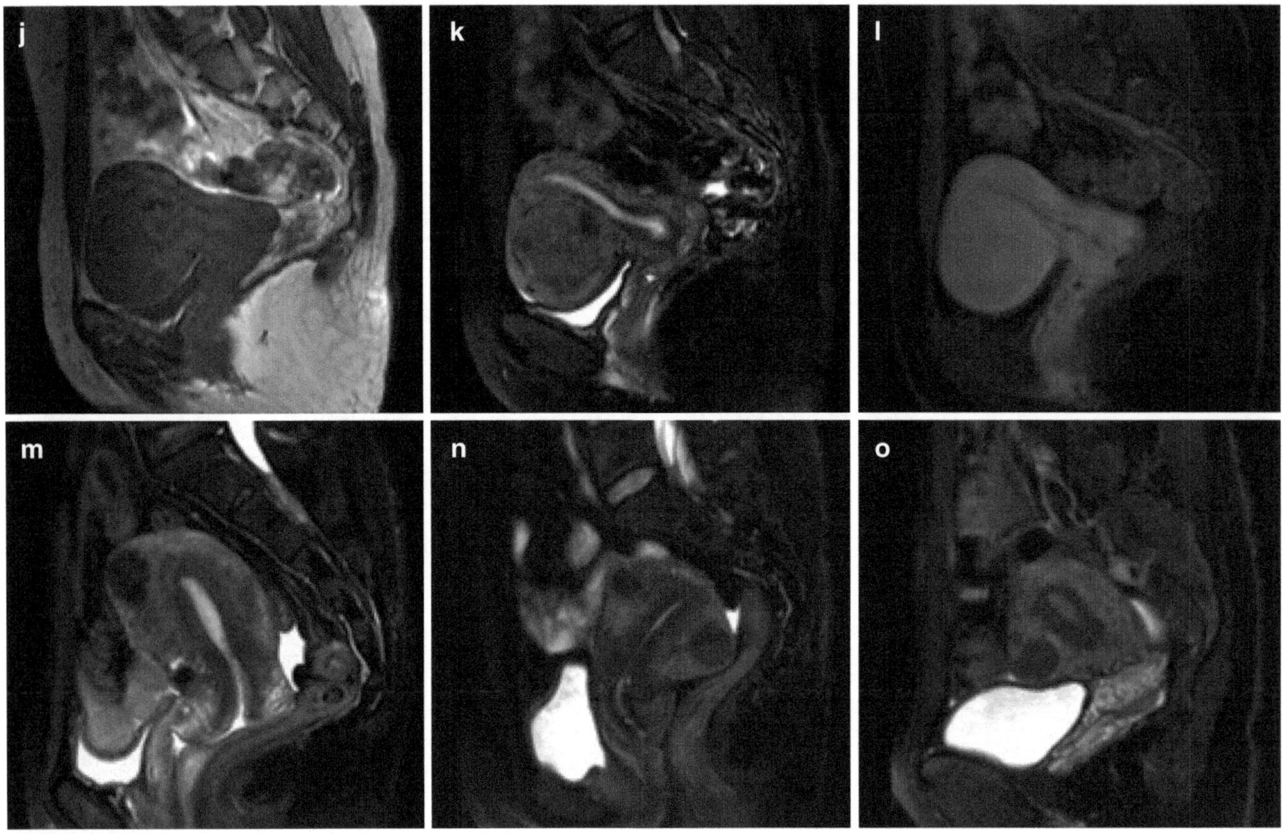

Fig. 2.16 (continued)

protruding into the uterine cavity (Fig. 2.15a, e). When Type IV intramural fibroid grows to a certain size, it can obviously protrude over the uterine serosal layer, but the fibroid part is usually not more than 50% (Fig. 2.16m–o). Only intramural fibroids alone usually have little influence on patients, but if combined with other types of fibroids, the patients' clinical symptoms are obvious.

Intramural fibroids usually show relatively uniform low isointense signals on T2WI. DWI functional imaging is not significantly sensitive to intramural fibroids and usually presents relatively uniform low isointense signals (Fig. 2.16h). Due to the relatively low resolution of DWI and the presence of some magnetic sensitive artifacts, it is difficult to identify some small intramuscular uterine fibroids on DWI imaging (Fig. 2.16d).

Contrast-enhanced T1WI usually shows that intramural fibroids present relatively uniform low isointense signals with unclear boundaries. They may present slightly lower signals (Fig. 2.16e) or slightly higher signals relative to the uterine muscular layer (Fig. 2.15c) due to the difference in blood supply between the fibroids and the muscular layer.

Differential Diagnosis

Submucous fibroid type II and intramural fibroid type III have direct contact with the endometrium in common. Submucosal fibroid (type II) shows fibroid extension to the myometrium, with its part in the muscular layer >50%; intramural uterine fibroid (type III) is an intramural myoma with close contact to the endometrium. Significant differences between the two types can be observed on MRI T2WI. For the intramural fibroid, the low signals of the endometrial myometrium junction can be seen compressed and protruding into the uterine cavity. At the same time, the submucosal fibroid will have the endometrial myometrium junction protruding into the uterine myometrial layer, which is not difficult to distinguish on conventional MRI imaging.

2.1.2.3 The Intramural Uterine Fibroid (Type V)

According to the FIGO classification, intramural uterine fibroids (type V) can run through all the myometrial layers and are connected to the endometrium and the serosa. Still, the part of fibroids in either the endometrial or the serosal layers should not be more than 50%. Type V intramural uterine fibroid is the most common type of intramural uterine fibroid. It can cause uterine deformities in both the endometrium and the serosa; therefore, the clinical symptoms are similar to the superadditional symptoms due to both endometrial and serosal abnormalities.

MRI Findings

Conventional MRI of type V fibroid usually shows uniform and low isointense on T1WI, and the boundary of the fibroid can be shown by comparing the pelvic fat with the intrauterine fluid (Fig. 2.17a). Routine T2WI can observe the morphology and characteristics of intramural fibroids. They are usually single, round, and with pseudocapsules. One side of the fibroid protrudes into the uterine cavity, the other side protrudes into the pelvis, and the boundary on both sides is relatively clear.

Intramural fibroids are usually large and cause some distortion of the uterine body. When the fibroid is small, the effect on the normal uterine body is small (Fig. 2.17g). The fibroids can locate anywhere in the uterine body. A fibroid in the anterior uterine wall can compress the bladder (Fig. 2.17b), in the posterior wall can compress the rectum (Fig. 2.17k), and the lateral wall can push against the uterine appendages (Fig. 2.17d). The fundal fibroid pushes against the neighboring bowels (Fig. 2.17p).

T2WI images showed different fibroid signals, including low signals (Fig. 2.17b), isosignals (Fig. 2.17d), high signals (Fig. 2.17p), or mixed signals (Fig. 2.17k).

DWI functional imaging is insensitive to the diagnosis of fibroids and usually presents a relatively uniform low signal (Fig. 2.17e). In contrast, a few fibroids may present isosignals (Fig. 2.17h) or slightly high signals (Fig. 2.17q).

Contrast-enhanced T1WI usually shows hyperintensity of fibroids. Due to the difference in blood supply between fibroids and uterine myometrium, fibroids may show slightly higher or lower intensity signals relative to the muscle layer (Fig. 2.17c). In contrast, larger fibroids may have cystic

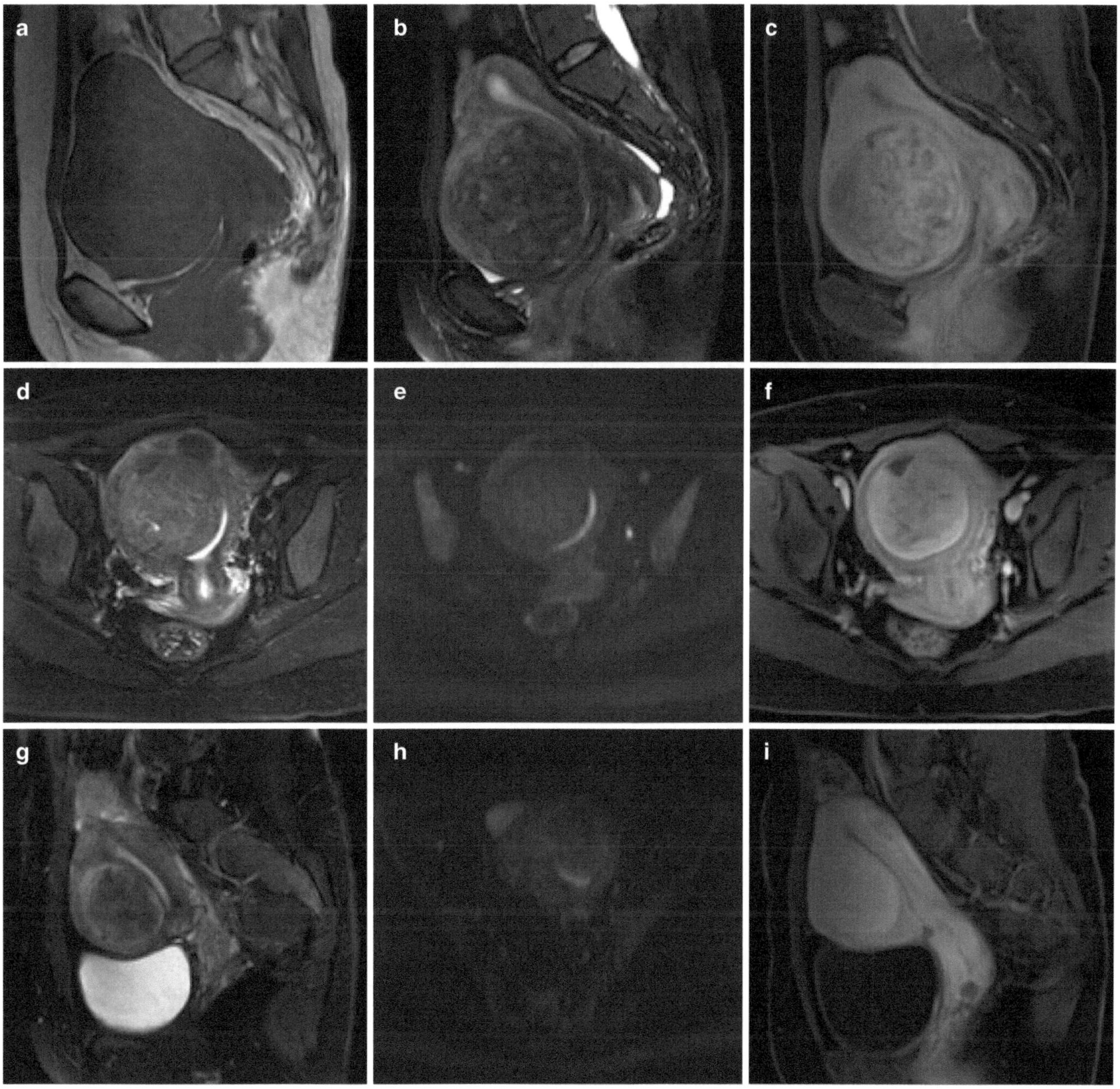

Fig. 2.17 Uterine fibroids (Type V). (**a**) T1WI sagittal; (**b**) T2WI_FS sagittal; (**c**) T1WI_FS + C sagittal; (**d**) T2WI_FS axial; (**e**) DWI axial (b = 800 S /mm^2); (**f**) T1WI_FS + C axial; (**g**) T2WI_FS sagittal; (**h**) DWI axial (b = 800 s/mm^2); (**i**) T1WI_FS + C sagittal; (**j**) T1WI sagittal; (**k**) T2WI_FS sagittal; (**l**) DWI axial (b = 800 s/mm^2); (**m**) T1WI_FS + C sagittal; (**n**) T1WI_FS + C axial; (**o**) T1WI_FS + C coronal; (**p**) T2WI_FS sagittal; (**q**) DWI axial (b = 800 s/mm^2); (**r**) T1WI_FS + C sagittal

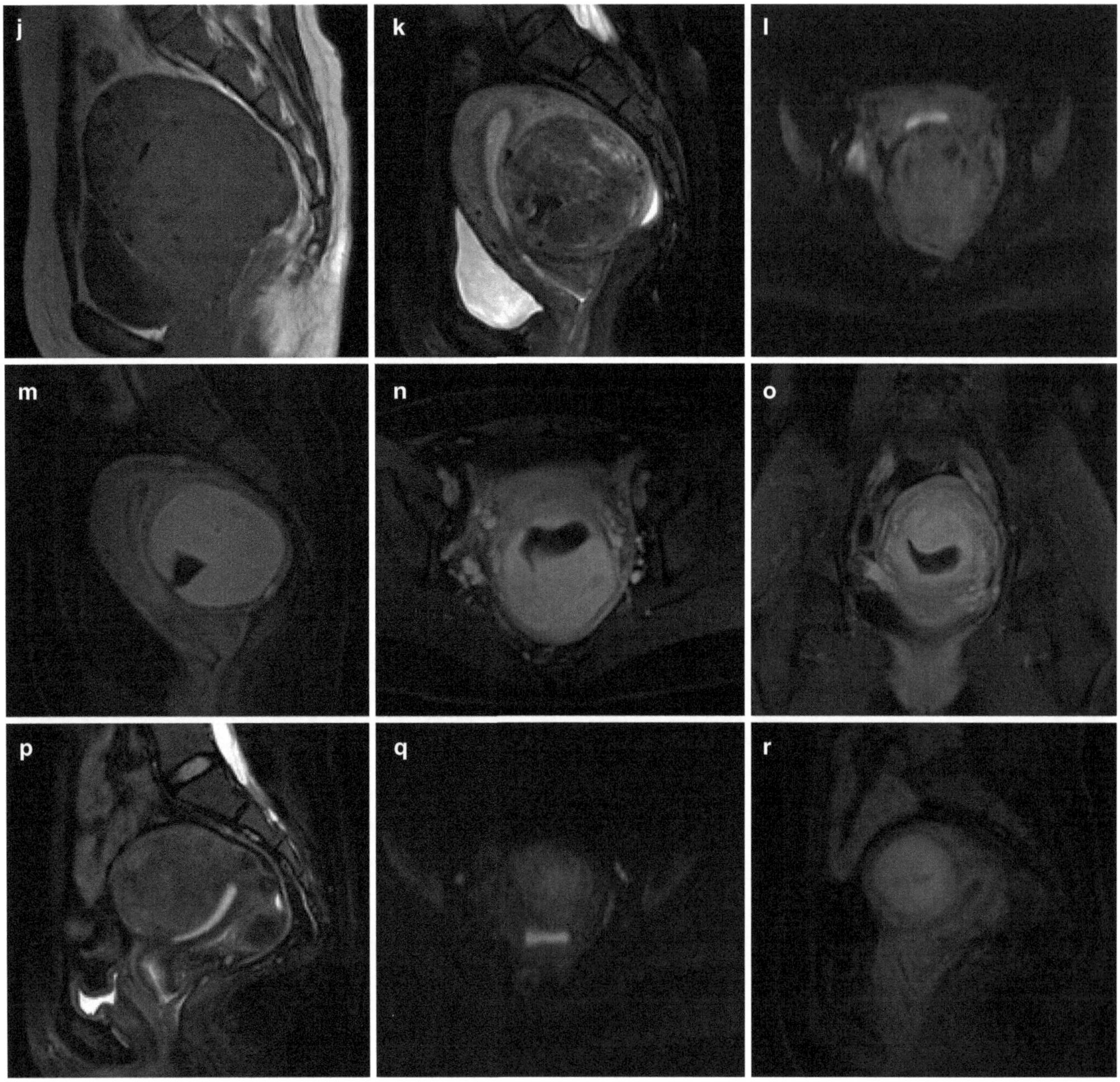

Fig. 2.17 (continued)

necrosis and calcification, showing a low-intensity non-perfusion area (Fig. 2.17n).

2.1.2.4 Subserosal Hysteromyoma (Type VI, VII)

Subserosal fibroid accounts for 20–30% of uterine fibroids, which refers to the intramural fibroids close to the serous layer of the uterus. It squeezes out of the outer serosal layer of the uterus, and the uterine serosa covers its surface. According to the FIGO classification, subserosal fibroids were divided into two types. (1) Type VI: the fibroid protrudes out of the uterine serosa, with its side covered by the serous membrane. Its part also pushes into the pelvic cavity (Fig. 2.18). (2) Type VII: the fibroid is completely in the serosal layer. The fibroid is almost entirely wrapped around by the serous membrane. Some fibroid parts may connect to the uterus by a pedicle or serous membrane, and it generally does not affect the normal uterine body (Fig. 2.19).

MRI Findings

Conventional MRI shows fibroids have homogeneously low signals on T1WI. The subserosal fibroid is usually of low signals due to the fat in the pelvis providing significant contrast. Thus, it can clearly display the border side of the subserosal fibroid (Fig. 2.18a). The type VII subserosal fibroid can display the connected pedicle (Fig. 2.19d). Contrary to the plain T1WI scan, conventional T2WI could clearly reveal

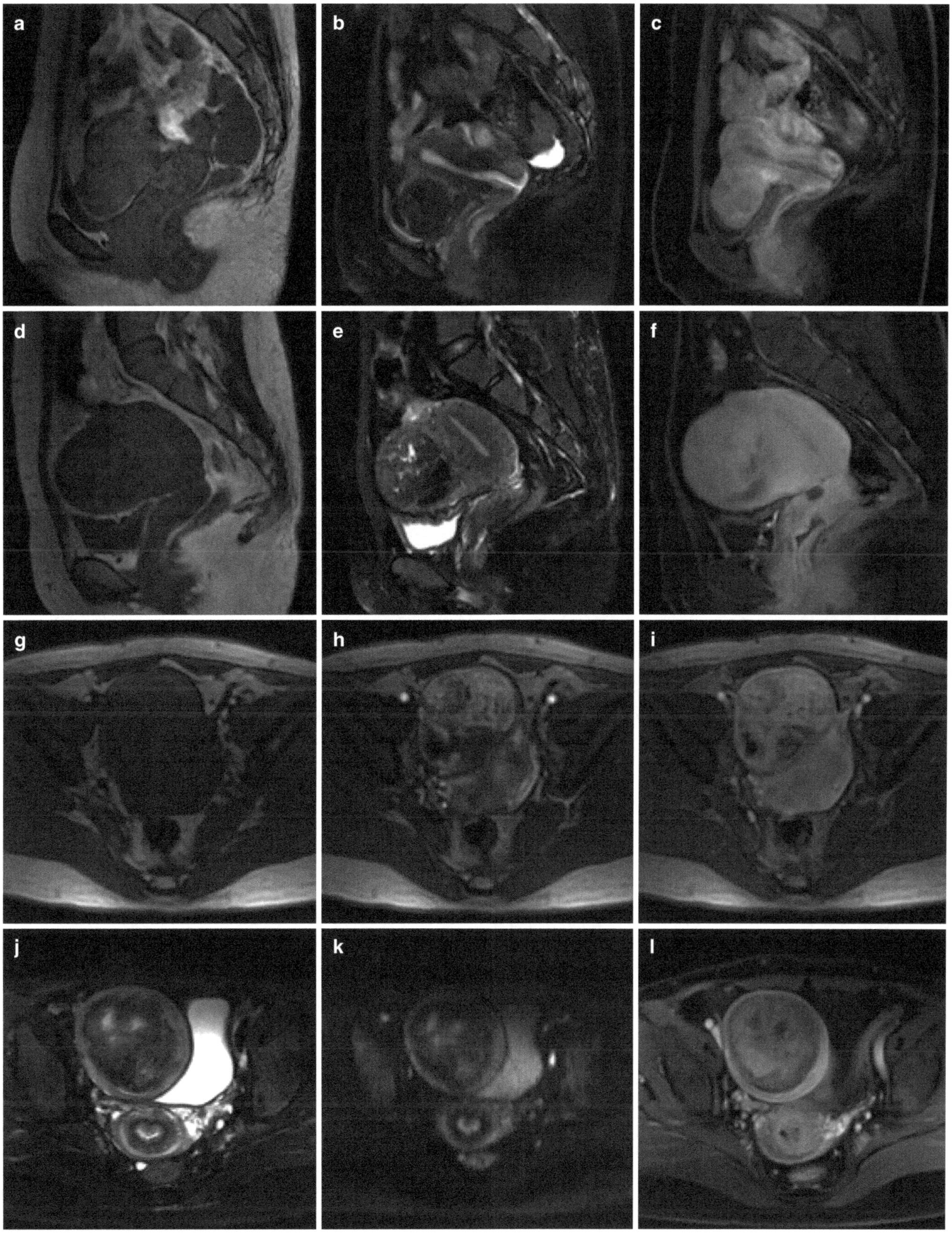

Fig. 2.18 Subserosal hysteromyoma (Type VI). (**a**) T1WI sagittal; (**b**) T2WI_FS sagittal; (**c**) T1WI_FS + C sagittal; (**d**) T1WI sagittal; (**e**) T2WI_FS sagittal; (**f**) T1WI_FS + C sagittal; (**g**) T1WI_Dynamic axial; (**h**, **i**) T1WI_Dynamic +C axial; (**j**) T2WI_FS axial; (**k**) DWI axial (b = 800 s/mm^2); (**l**) T1WI_FS + C axial; (**m–o**) T2WI_FS sagittal

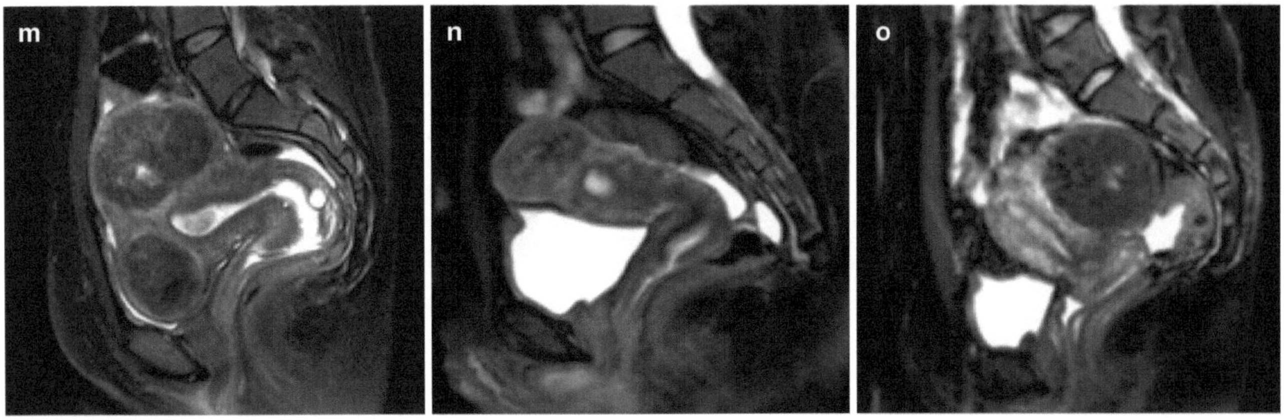

Fig. 2.18 (continued)

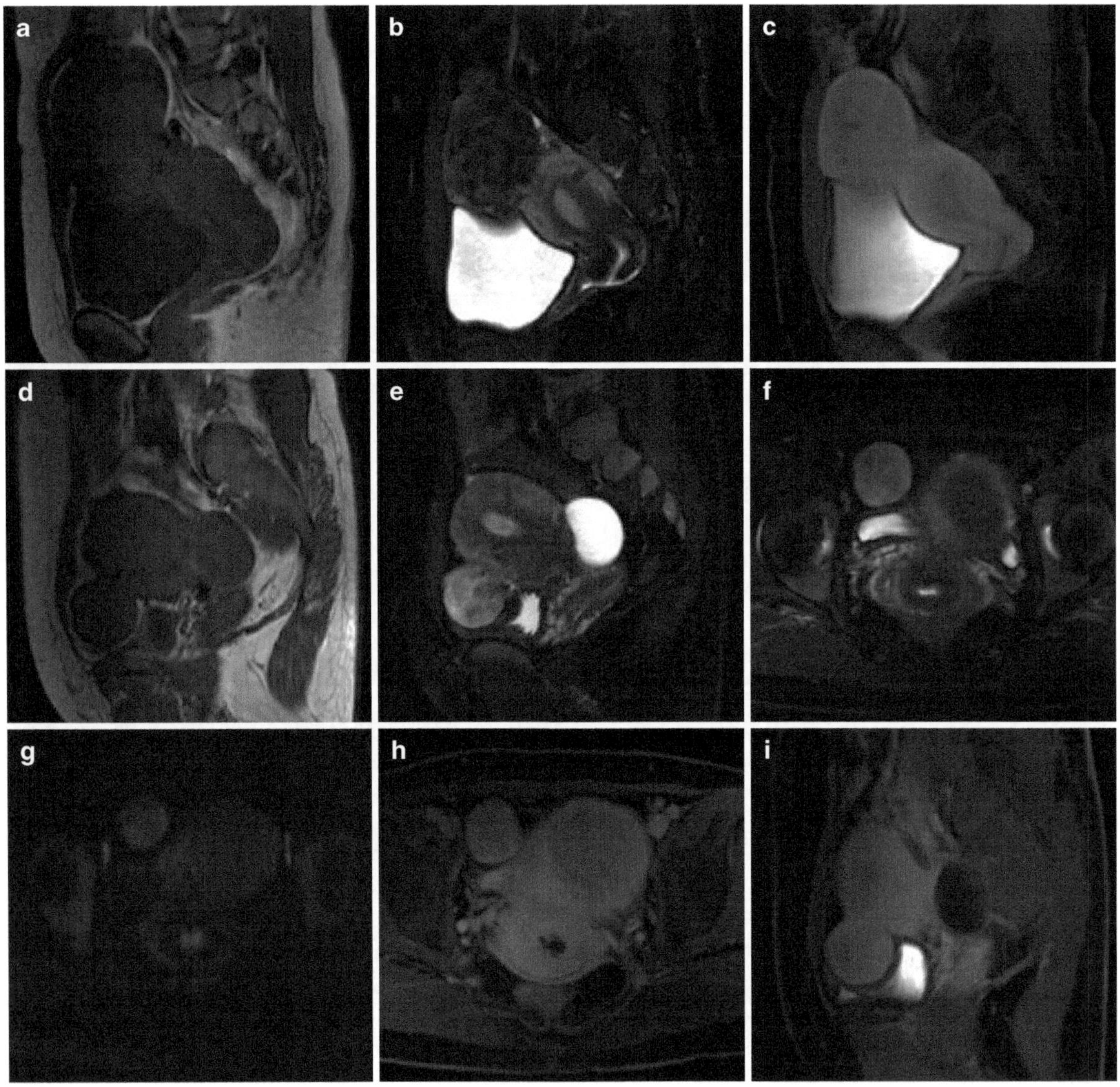

Fig. 2.19 Subserosal fibroid (Type VII). (**a**) T1WI sagittal; (**b**) T2WI_FS sagittal; (**c**) T1WI_FS + C sagittal; (**d**) T1WI sagittal; (**e**) T2WI_FS sagittal; (**f**) T2WI_FS axial; (**g**) DWI axial (b = 800 s/mm^2); (**h**) T1WI_FS + C axial; (**i**) T1WI_FS + C sagittal; (**j**) T1WI sagittal; (**k**) T2WI_FS sagittal; (**l**) T2WI_FS axial; (**m**) T1WI_FS + C axial; (**n**) T1WI_FS + C sagittal; (**o**) T1WI_FS + C coronal

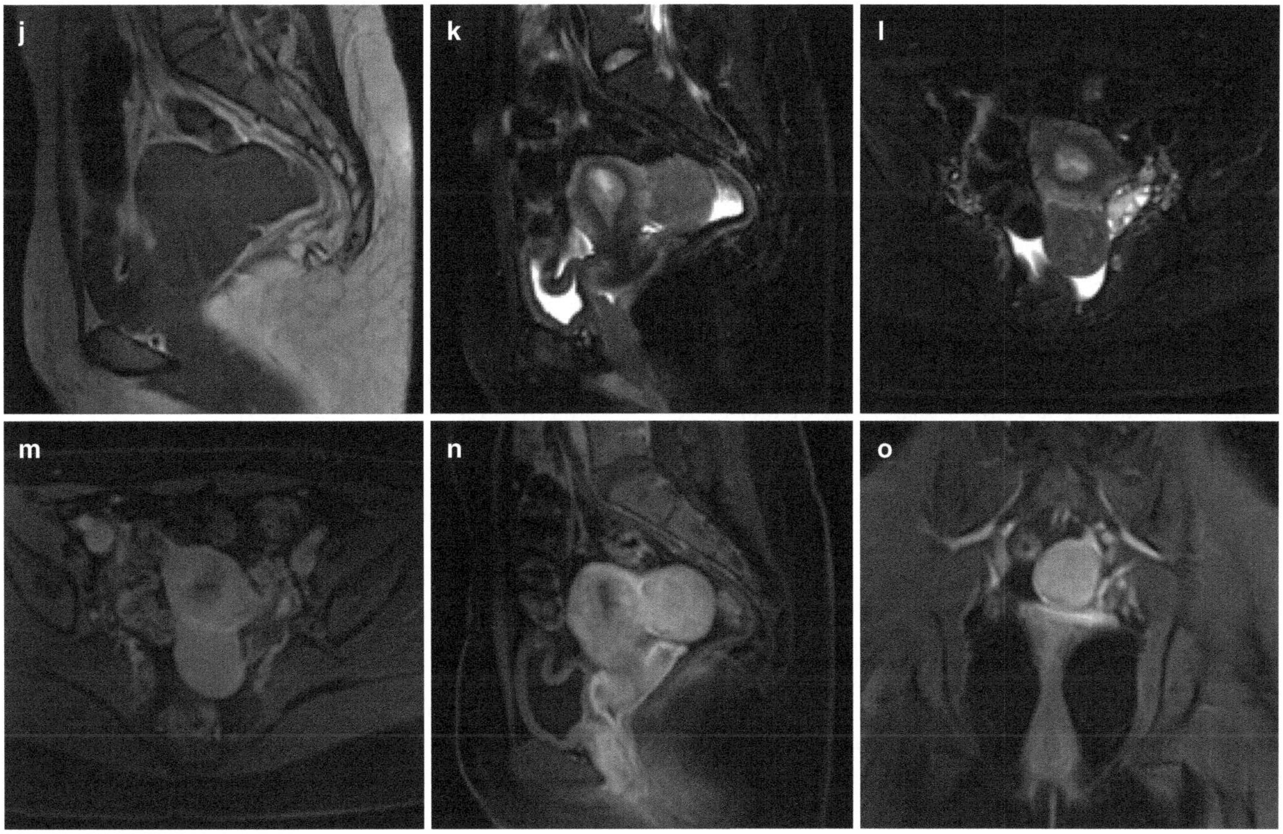

Fig. 2.19 (continued)

the morphology and characteristics of fibroids. The subserosal fibroid is usually solitary, but occasionally two or more subserosal fibroids can occur (Fig. 2.18m).

The fibroids usually appear quasi-round, and most have a pseudocapsule, showing relatively well-defined boundaries. Type VII subserosal fibroid has little influence on the normal uterine morphology. The fibroid can grow in any position of the uterine body. A subserosal fibroid in the anterior wall can compress the bladder (Fig. 2.18a–i), and in the posterior wall, it can compress the rectum (Fig. 2.18o). At the lateral wall, it can push toward the uterine body adnexa (Fig. 2.18g–i). A fundal fibroid may push against the surrounding bowels (Fig. 2.19b). Patients generally have no obvious symptoms because subserosal fibroids do not affect the endometrium. However, a pedunculated subserosal fibroid in the pelvic cavity is in a semi-free state. Sometimes acute or chronic torsion of the fibroid can produce abdominal pain.

The subserosal fibroid showed mixed signals on T2WI, usually showing relatively uniform low signals, with some showing isointense signals (Fig. 2.18n), hyperintense signals (Fig. 2.19e), or mixed signals (Fig. 2.18e, j). Cystic necrosis may occur when these fibroids grow larger (Fig. 2.18j, o).

DWI functional imaging is insensitive to the diagnosis of subserosal uterine fibroids. Usually, they present relatively uniform low intense signals, with a few presenting isointense signals or slightly high intense signals (Fig. 2.19g).

Usually, T1WI contrast-enhanced imaging of these fibroids revealed relatively uniform high signals (Fig. 2.19c, n, o). The fibroid side in contact with the muscular layer is not obvious. Because of differences in the blood flow to the fibroid and the muscle layer, the fibroid can present slightly low signals than the muscular layer (Fig. 2.19h) or slightly high signals. As a subserosal fibroid can undergo cystic degeneration with necrosis, it can show a low signal with no perfusion zone (Fig. 2.18l). T1WI dynamic contrast-enhanced imaging can demonstrate the progressive enhancement of fibroids (Fig. 2.18g–i).

Differential Diagnosis

- **Broad ligament fibroid:** It refers to fibroids that grow within the region of the broad ligament. When a subserosal fibroid grows in the broad ligament region, the differentiation between the two can be relatively difficult and usually requires surgical diagnosis.

- **Chocolate cyst of the ovary**: The chocolate cyst of the ovary is an ectopic lesion with endometriosis in the ovarian region, usually on one side of the ovary. Conventional T2WI presents both high and low mixed signals or high isointense signals (Fig. 2.20a, b). The T1WI plain scan shows significantly high signals. The lesion is usually round with relatively clear boundaries (Fig. 2.20c). T1WI contrast-enhanced images show no significant change in the chocolate cysts compared with plain T1WI, and there is a non-perfusion capsule.
- **Uterine sarcoma:** Uterine sarcoma is a relatively rare uterine malignancy, of which leiomyosarcoma is the most common. The conventional T1WI of uterine sarcoma will show moderately low intense signals, with the common necrotic cystic degeneration showing even lower intense signals. A few sarcomas may show high intense signals with varying degrees of bleeding (Fig. 2.21d). T2WI fat-saturation imaging shows that the overall signal intensity of the sarcoma is higher than that of the myometrium, with hyperintense signals for necrotic cystic degeneration or hemorrhage within the sarcoma. Low intense signals for calcification occur in a few sarcomas (Fig. 2.21a, b). DWI imaging is sensitive to the diagnosis of sarcoma and presents a significantly high intense signal (Fig. 2.21c). The contrast-enhanced T1WI shows heterogenous enhancement of uterine sarcoma (Fig. 2.21e, f). Therefore, uterine sarcomas are not difficult to identify by MRI.
- **Intramural uterine fibroids (Type IV, V):** When a fibroid grows to a certain size, it protrudes out of the serosal layer; there is a need to distinguish between subserosal fibroid (type VI) and intramural fibroids (type IV and type V). The intramural fibroid (type IV) grows intramurally, with its growth always in the myometrium and its border totally surrounded by the myometrium (Fig. 2.22a). When the fibroid grows significantly in the uterine muscular layer, usually there is no normal myometrium between the fibroid and the normal myometrium, without obvious compression of the endometrium. The protruded part of the fibroid is generally no more than 50% (Fig. 2.22b). The intramural uterine fibroid (type V) grows completely inside the uterine muscular layer from the endometrium to the serosal layer. The uterine endometrium and serosa can be significantly under compression by the fibroid with no normal muscular layer between them (Fig. 2.22c, d). The subserosal fibroid (type VI) is a fibroid in the muscular layer, protruding to the serosal layer. There is usually a visible normal muscular layer between the fibroid and the endometrium, and the normal myometrium seems slightly compressed (Fig. 2.22e, f).

2.1.2.5 Special Types: Cervical Fibroid (Type VIII)

Cervical fibroids in the uterus are the fibroids of the uterus that grow in the uterine cervix. Usually, the fibroids are small, grow in the anterior cervix, and their incidence is low, about 2.2–8% of the uterine fibroids.

MRI Findings

Routine T1WI plain scan is difficult to identify cervical fibroids, and they usually show low intense signals with poorly defined boundaries (Fig. 2.23a). T2WI can clearly reveal the location, morphology, and characteristics of cervical fibroids. They are usually solitary and round in appearance with clear boundaries (Fig. 2.23b, c).

Cervical fibroids vary in size. When fibroids are small, they do not affect normal uterine morphology, and patients have no obvious symptoms. When the fibroids are large, the cervical morphology may appear deformed. The lip or wall of the cervix where the fibroids are located is thickened, while the contralateral cervical site is stretched and thinned (Fig. 2.23j). Suppose the cervical fibroid grows in the posterior wall of the cervix (Fig. 2.23m). The fibroid can gradually grow into the cervical canal cavity, causing compression or blockage of the cervical opening (Fig. 2.23g).

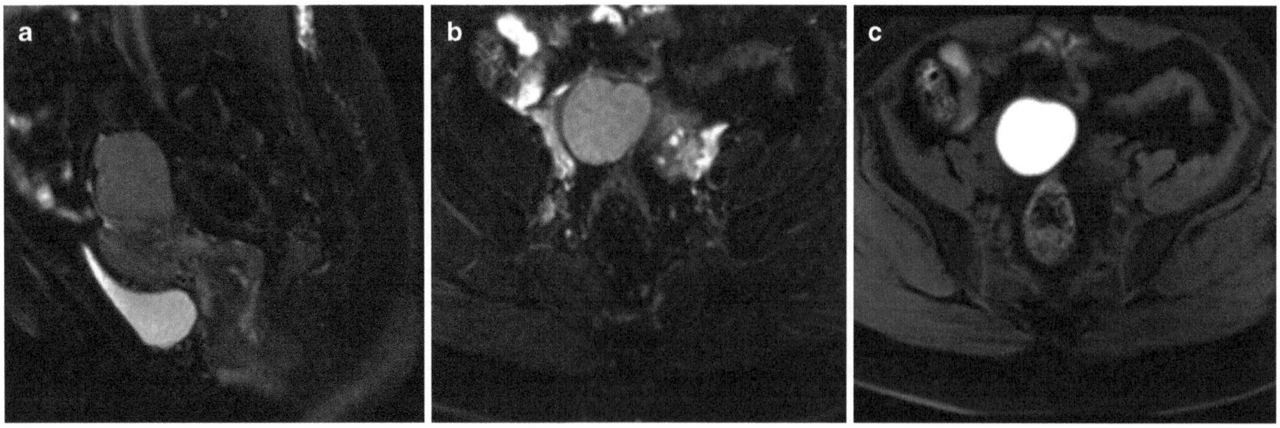

Fig. 2.20 Chocolate cyst of ovary. (**a**) T2WI_FS sagittal; (**b**) T2WI_FS axial; (**c**) T1WI_FS axial

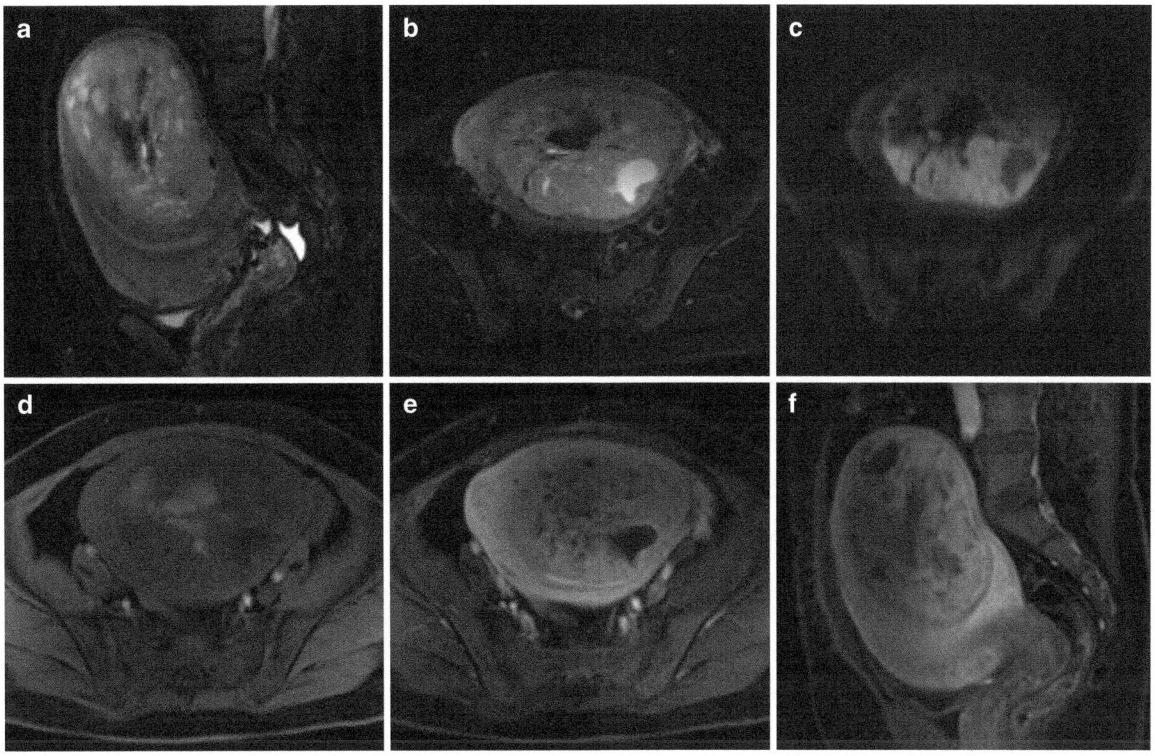

Fig. 2.21 Uterine sarcoma. (**a**) T2WI_FS sagittal; (**b**) T2WI_FS axial; (**c**) DWI axial (b = 800 s/mm^2); (**d**) T1WI_FS axial; (**e**) T1WI_FS + C axial; (**f**) T1WI_FS + C coronal

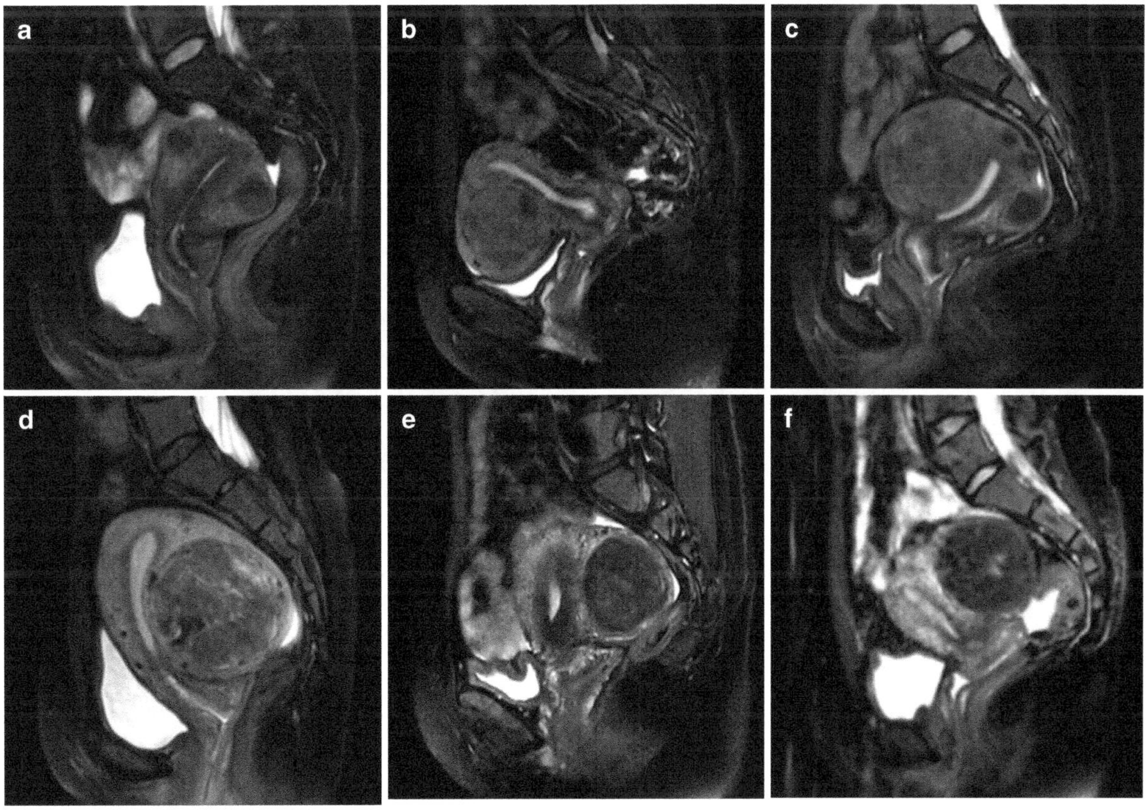

Fig. 2.22 Intramural (Type IV and V) and subserosal hysteromyoma (Type VI). (**a**–**f**) T2WI_FS sagittal

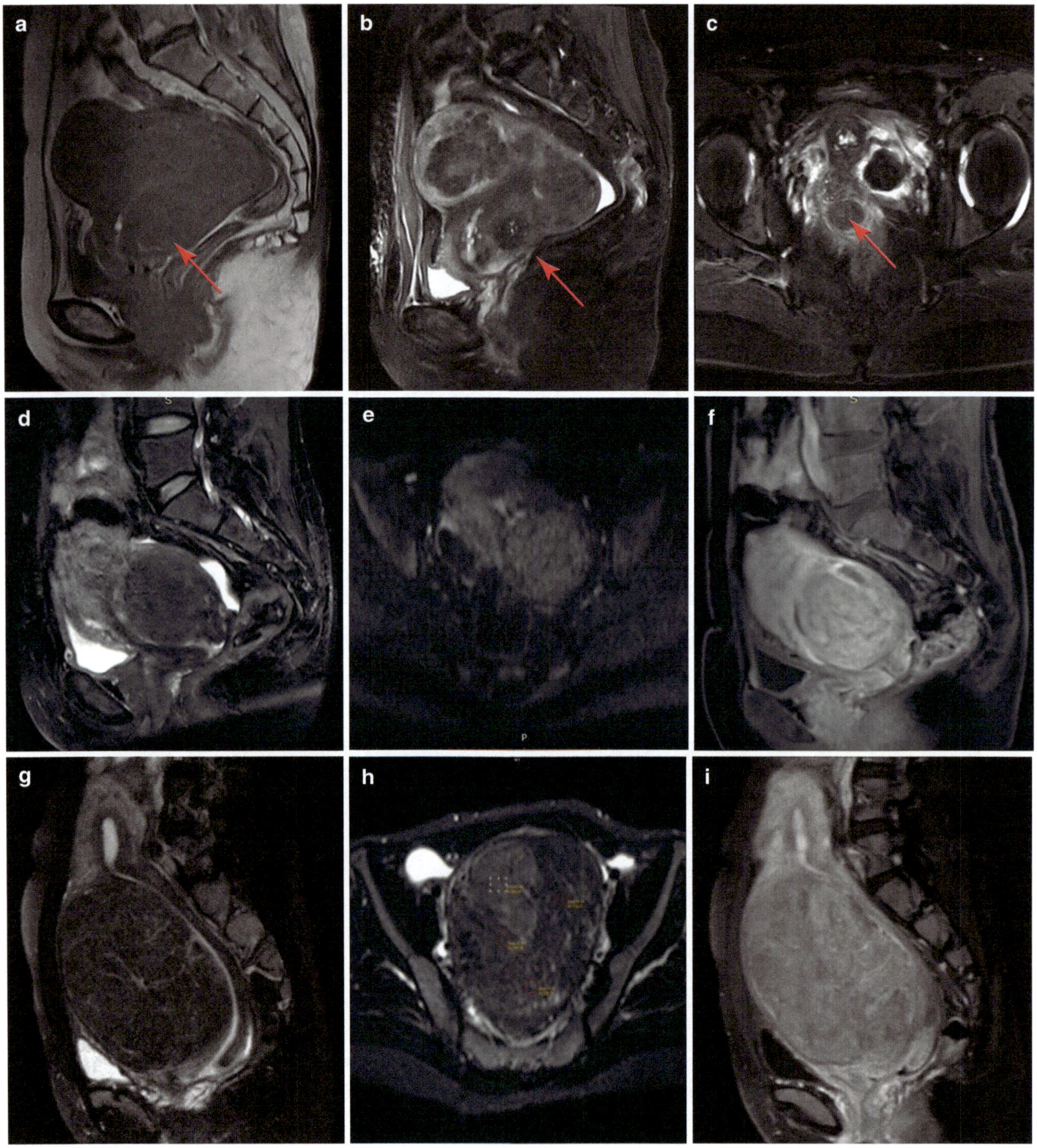

Fig. 2.23 Cervical fibroids. (**a**) T1WI sagittal; (**b**) T2WI_FS sagittal; (**c**) T2WI_FS axial; (**d**) T2WI_FS sagittal; (**e**) DWI axial (b = 800 s/mm^2); (**f**) T1WI_FS + C sagittal; (**g**) T2WI_FS sagittal; (**h**) T2WI_FS axial; (**i**) T1WI_FS + C sagittal; (**j**) T2WI_FS sagittal; (**k**) DWI axial (b = 800 s/mm^2); (**l**) T1WI_FS axial; (**m**) T2WI_FS sagittal; (**n**) DWI axial (b = 800 s/mm^2); (**o**) T1WI_FS + C sagittal

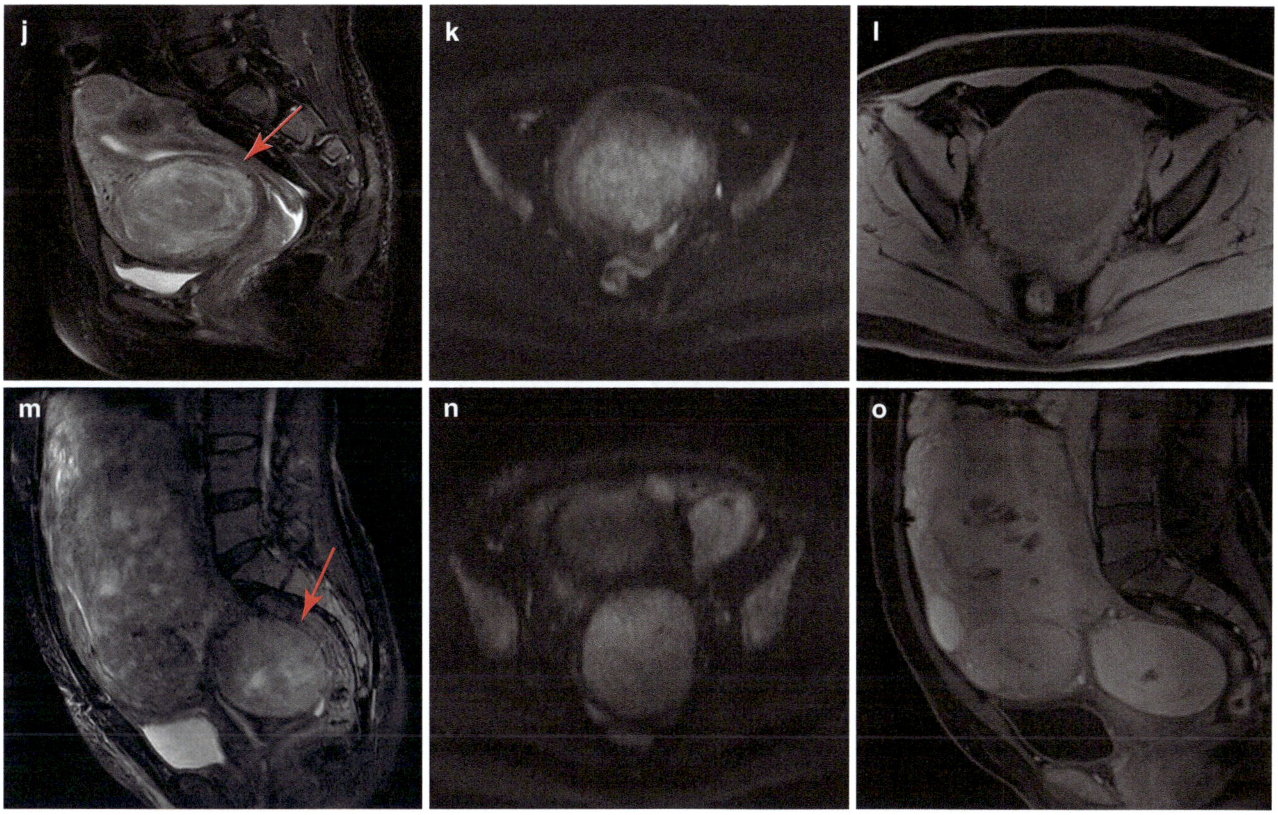

Fig. 2.23 (continued)

T2WI imaging of cervical fibroid usually presents with relatively uniform low isointense signals (Fig. 2.23d, g). Still, it can also be isointense signals, high intense signals (Fig. 2.23m), or mixed signals (Fig. 2.23j).

Due to the low-resolution and magnetic-sensitive artifacts of DWI imaging, it is sometimes difficult to find small cervical fibroids. DWI imaging is also insensitive to the diagnosis of fibroids, showing uniform and low intense signals relative to the muscular layer (Fig. 2.23e). In contrast, some cervical fibroids show isointense or slightly high intense signals (Fig. 2.23n).

Contrast-enhanced T1WI imaging shows that fibroids are usually high intense signals. Still, due to the difference in blood supply and size of cervical fibroids, fibroids can show slightly higher signals (Fig. 2.23f) or lower signals (Fig. 2.23i) than the muscular layer.

Differential Diagnosis

- **Cervical cancer:** Cervical cancer is a malignant tumor growing in the uterine cervix. It usually occurs in women of childbearing age between 30 and 60 years old. Conventional T1WI shows the low isointense or slightly high intense signals (Fig. 2.24a), while T2WI shows high or mixed signals (Fig. 2.24b, g). Cervical cancer can also be staged according to the integrity of the cervical stroma. Compared with cervical fibroids, DWI imaging has certain sensitivity to diagnose cervical cancer, usually showing high intense signals on DWI images (Fig. 2.24c, h) and low intense signals on ADC images (Fig. 2.24d, i). According to the patient's clinical history and MRI results, it is not difficult to identify the nature of the cervical lesion, and a pathological biopsy is needed to confirm the diagnosis.

2.1.2.6 Special Type: Broad Ligament Fibroids

Broad ligament fibroids account for 1.5–2% of uterine fibroids and can be divided into true and false broad ligament fibroids according to their origin. (1) True broad ligament fibroid originates from the round ligament, utero-ovarian ligament, ovary, or the surrounding tissues of uterine blood vessels. It grows between the anterior and posterior peritoneum of the broad ligament and is not connected with the uterus. Its occurrence and development had nothing to do with the uterine wall. (2) The pseudo-broad ligament fibroid (Figs. 2.25 and 2.26) arises from the uterine lateral wall of its body or cervix and grows into the anterior and posterior peritoneum of the broad ligament. They are actually subserosal fibroids. At present, it is difficult to distinguish between true and pseudo broad ligament fibroids accurately by MRI imaging, and further pathological examination is needed.

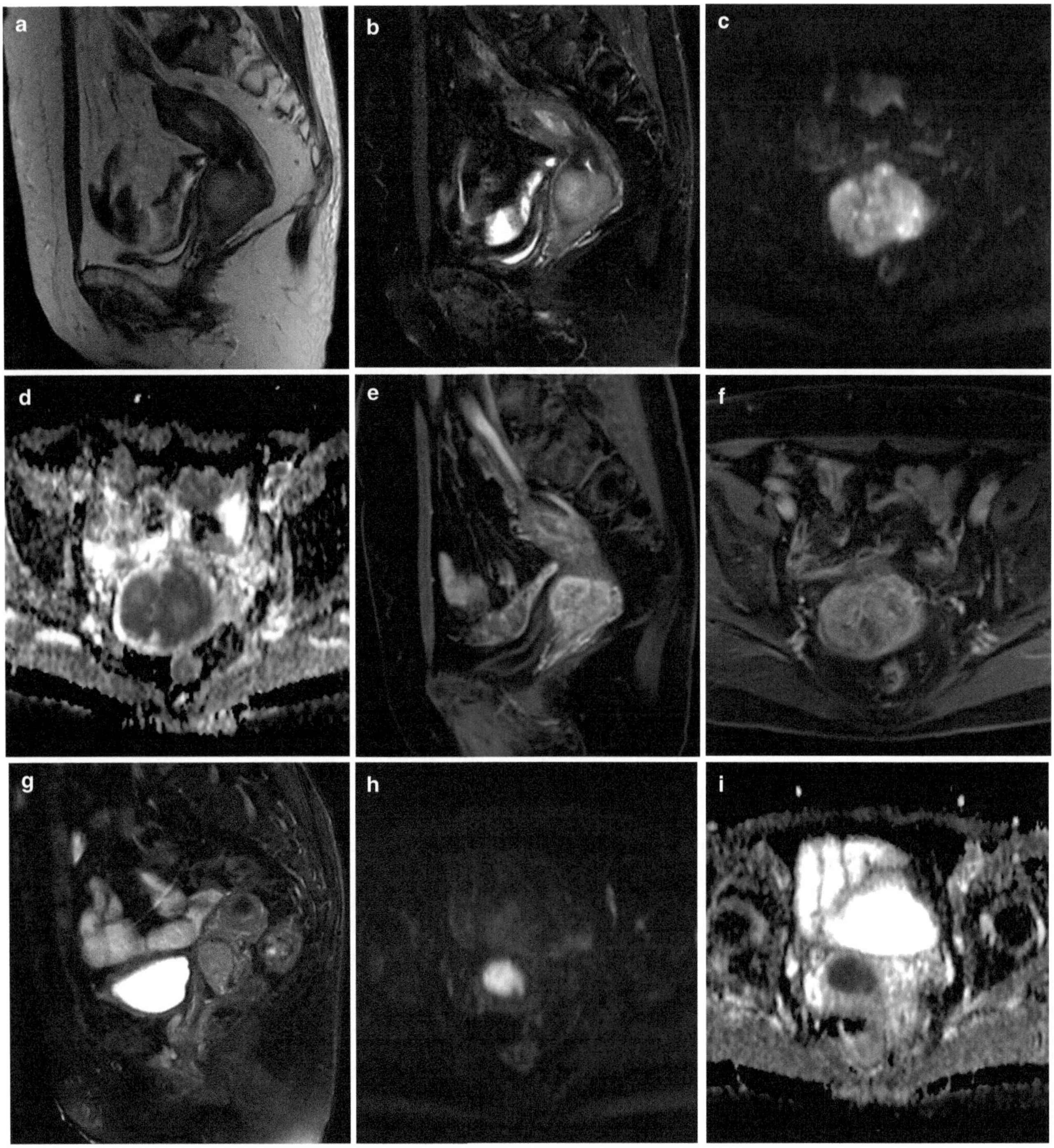

Fig. 2.24 Cervical cancer. (**a**) T1WI sagittal; (**b**) T2WI_FS sagittal; (**c**) DWI axial (b = 800 s/mm^2); (**d**) ADC axial; (**e**) T1WI_FS + C sagittal; (**f**) T1WI_FS + C axial; (**g**) T2WI_FS sagittal; (**h**) DWI axial (b = 800 s/mm^2); (**i**) ADC axial

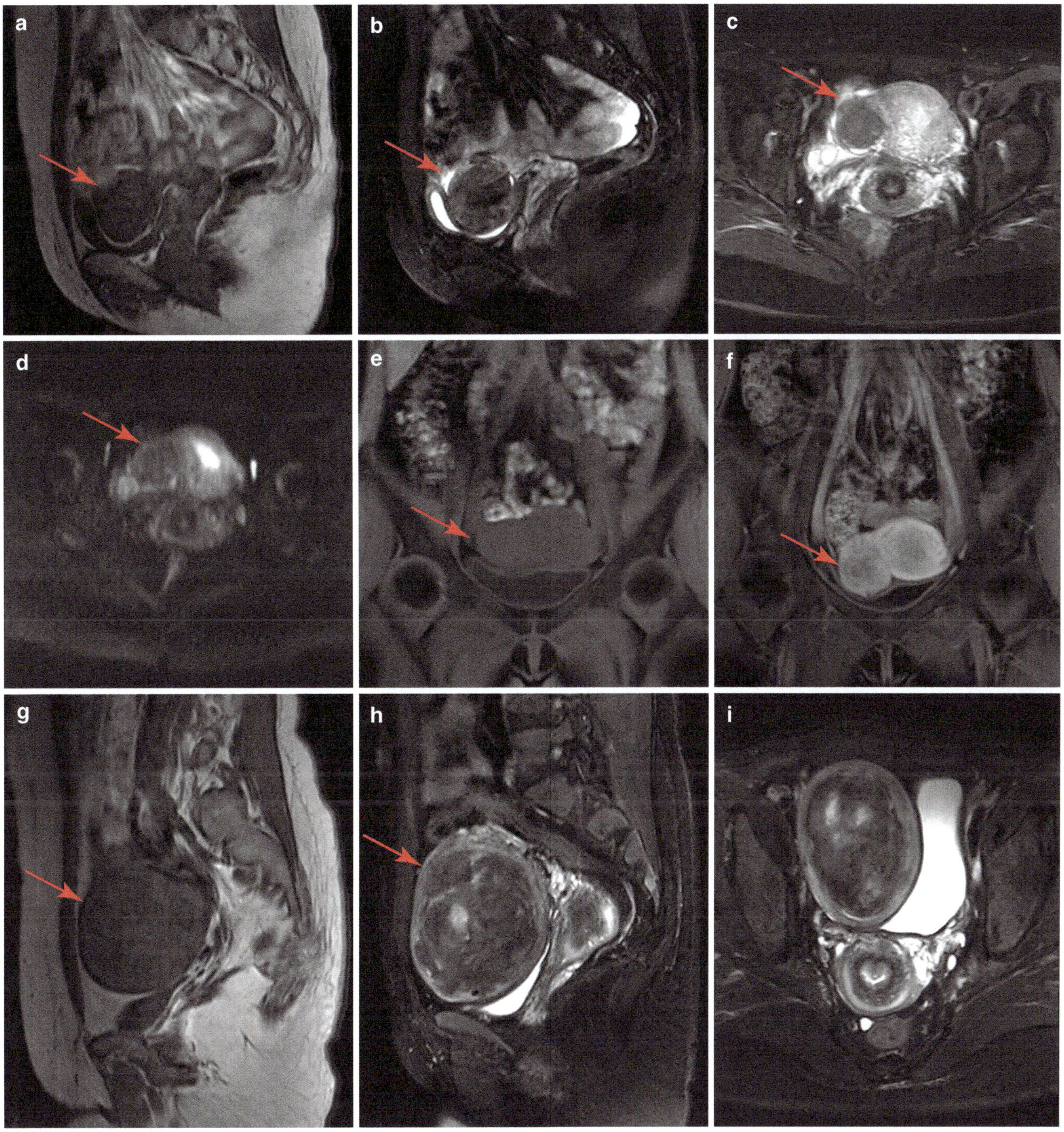

Fig. 2.25 Broad ligamentous fibroid. (**a**) T1WI sagittal; (**b**) T2WI_FS sagittal; (**c**) T2WI_FS axial; (**d**) DWI axial ($b = 800$ s/mm^2); (**e**) T1WI_FS coronal; (**f**) T1WI_FS + C coronal; (**g**) T1WI sagittal; (**h**) T2WI_FS sagittal; (**i**) T2WI_FS axial; (**j**) DWI axial ($b = 800$ s/mm^2); (**k**) T1WI_FS axial; (**l**) T1WI_FS + C coronal; (**m**) T2WI_FS sagittal; (**n**) T2WI_FS axial; (**o**) T1WI_FS + C axial

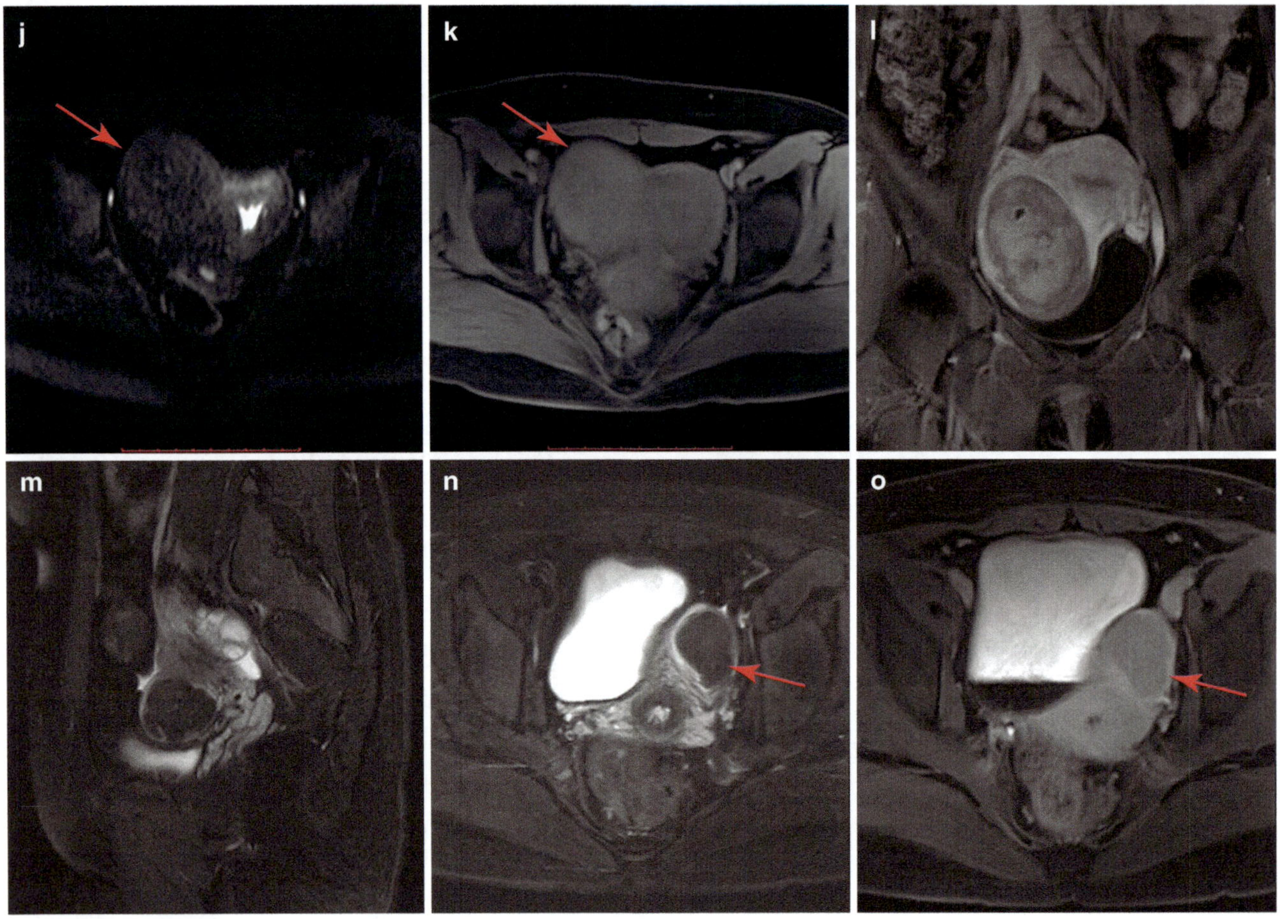

Fig. 2.25 (continued)

MRI Findings

Routine T1WI imaging shows low intense signals for the broad ligament fibroids, and the boundaries of the fibroids can be shown because they occupy the pelvic space with the pelvic fat providing the contrast (Fig. 2.25g). T2WI imaging can clearly define the morphology and characteristics of fibroids. Broad ligament fibroid is usually solitary, arising from the lateral wall of the uterus, and is round in appearance with a clear boundary. The fibroid generally does not affect the normal uterine body morphology, and the patient has no apparent clinical features (Fig. 2.25c). When the fibroid grows larger, it can compress onto the uterine wall (Fig. 2.26i) or the bladder (Fig. 2.25i).

T2WI imaging shows that broad ligament fibroids usually present with relatively uniform low isointense signals (Fig. 2.25m), but some may present isointense signals (Fig. 2.26a), high intense signals, or mixed signals (Fig. 2.26h).

DWI imaging is insensitive to the diagnosis of fibroids. Usually, it presents with uniform and isointense signals relative to the muscular layer (Fig. 2.25j), while a few fibroids present isointense or slightly hyperintense signals (Fig. 2.26j).

Contrast-enhanced T1WI imaging shows that the broad ligament fibroid usually presents a relatively uniform isointense signal, slightly lower (Fig. 2.25o), or higher signals (Fig. 2.26l) relative to the uterus due to the difference in the location and blood supply of the broad ligament fibroids.

2.1.2.7 Special Type: Multiple Uterine Fibroids

Multiple uterine fibroids account for 1.5–2% of uterine fibroids, which refer to the number of fibroids ≥3, including two or more types of fibroids—the submucosal, intramural, and subserosal fibroids.

MRI Findings

Routine T1WI imaging usually showed multiple uterine fibroids with uniform, low intense signal, unclear boundaries, deformed uterine body morphology, that makes the types not clearly identified (Fig. 2.27d). On the contrary, the morphology and characteristics of multiple uterine fibroids can be observed on T2WI. The fibroids are usually round in shape, most of them have pseudocapsule, and the boundary is relatively clear. Some fibroids can fuse together (Fig. 2.27p).

Multiple uterine fibroids can grow in any position of the uterine body, such as the anterior wall, posterior wall, lateral wall, uterine fundus, or cervix. More fibroids grow in the anterior and posterior walls of the uterus (Fig. 2.27e). When the number of fibroids is small, and their sizes are small, the effect on the normal uterine morphology is minimal. Then the patient has no obvious clinical symptoms (Fig. 2.27a). When the fibroids are many and their sizes are large, the uterine body morphology can change a lot (Fig. 2.27m), such as pushing the surrounding tissues and organs (Fig. 2.27r), intrauterine space-occupying lesions (Fig. 2.27e), cervical obstruction, or stenosis (Fig. 2.27q).

Due to certain differences in the fibroids' type, number, and size, T2WI signal characteristics of multiple uterine fibroids in the same patient can differ. Usually, many fibroids are uniformly low isointense signals on T2WI (Fig. 2.27p), while some fibroids may show isointense, high intense signals, or mixed signals (Fig. 2.27e).

DWI imaging is not sensitive to the diagnosis of multiple fibroids and usually presents with relatively uniform low isointense signals, with some showing isointense signals. These fibroids have a relatively clear boundary (Fig. 2.27g).

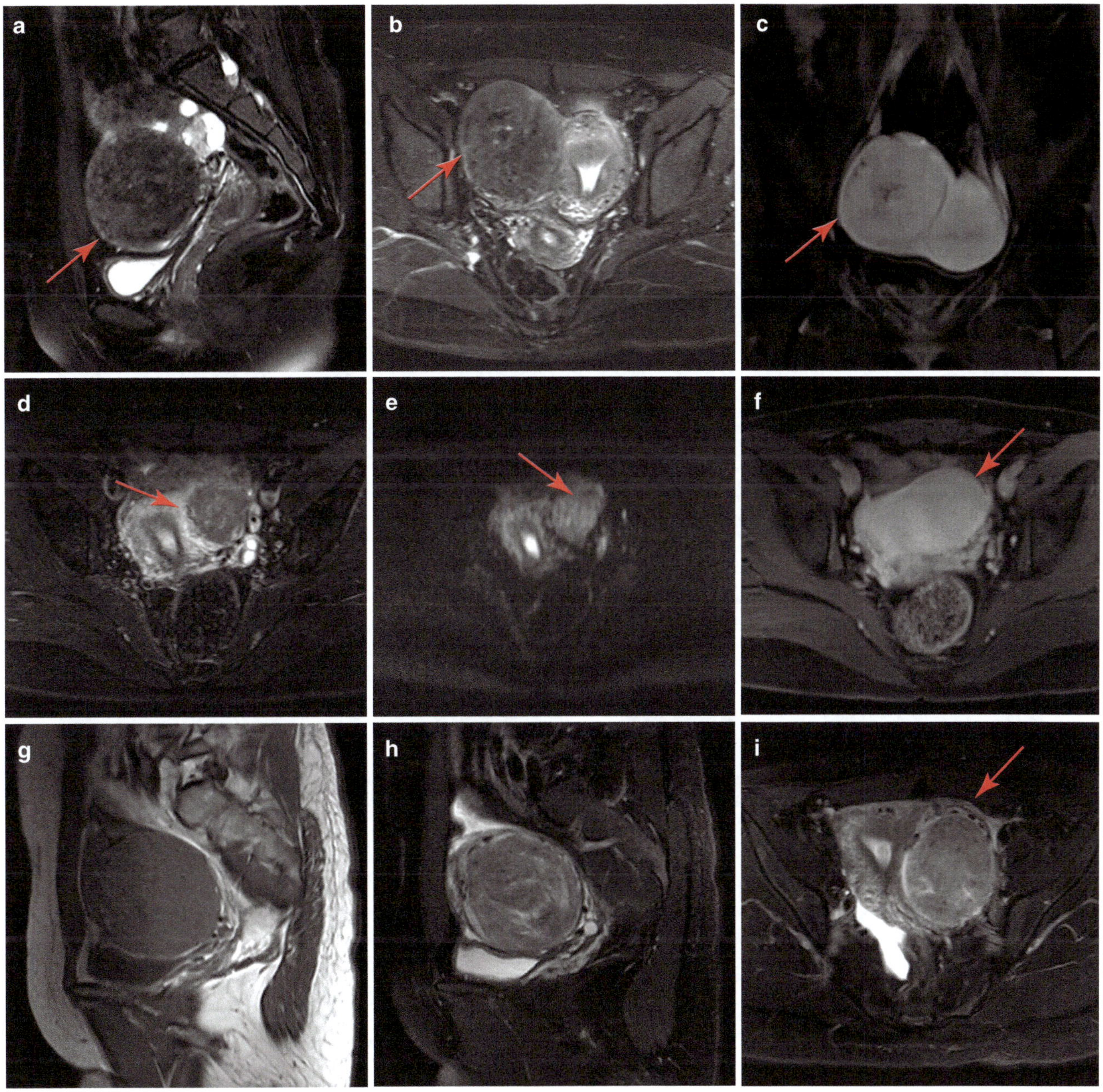

Fig. 2.26 Broad ligament fibroid. (**a**) T2WI_FS sagittal; (**b**) T2WI_FS axial; (**c**) T1WI_FS + C coronal; (**d**) T2WI_FS axial; (**e**) DWI axial (b = 800 s/mm^2); (**f**) T1WI_FS + C axial; (**g**) T1WI sagittal; (**h**) T2WI_FS sagittal; (**i**) T2WI_FS axial; (**j**) DWI axial (b = 800 s/mm^2); (**k**) T1WI_FS + C axial; (**l**) T1WI_FS + C coronal

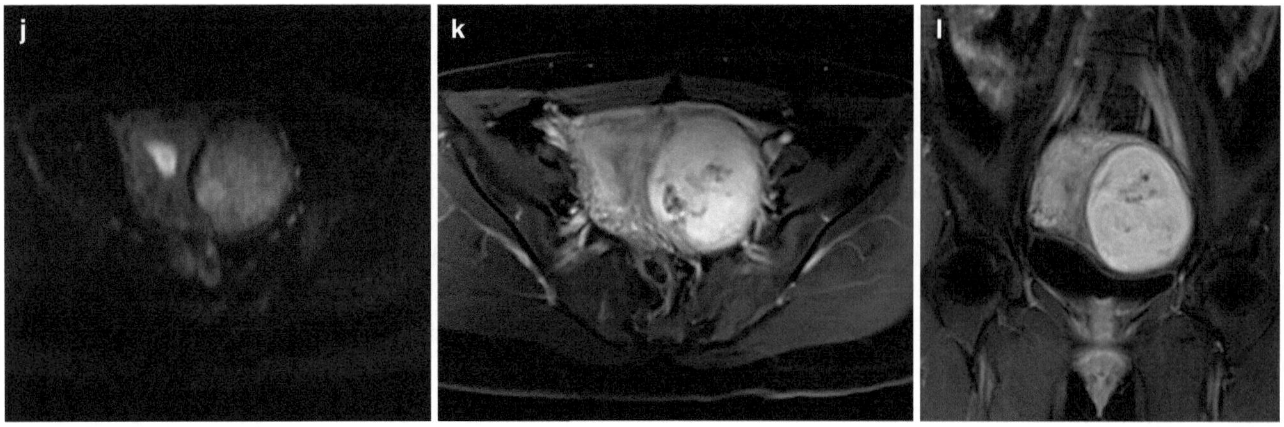

Fig. 2.26 (continued)

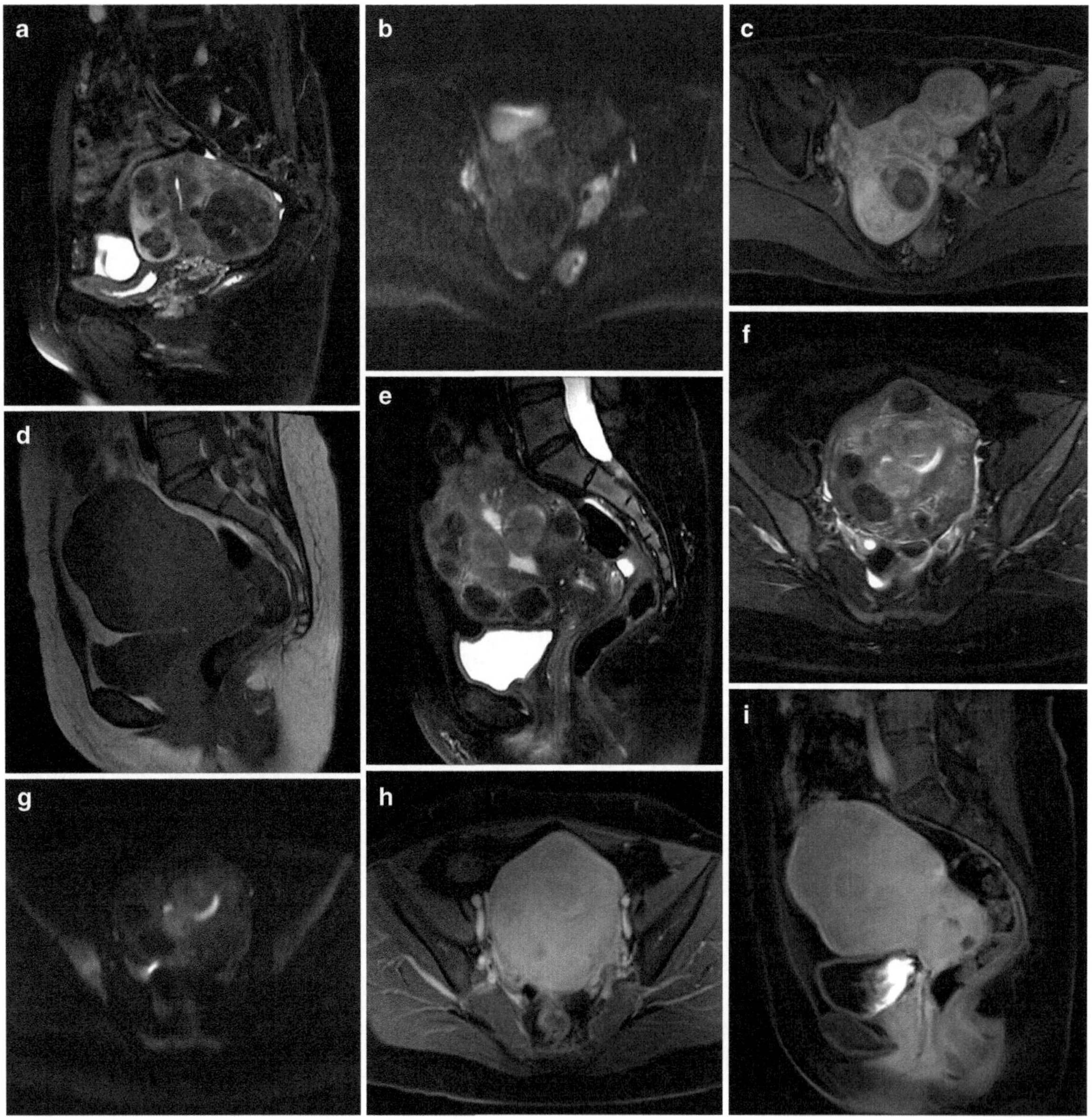

Fig. 2.27 Multiple uterine fibroids. (**a**) T2WI_FS sagittal; (**b**) DWI axial (b = 800 s/mm^2); (**c**) T1WI_FS + C axial; (**d**) T1WI sagittal; (**e**) T2WI_FS sagittal; (**f**) T2WI_FS axial; (**g**) DWI axial (b = 800 s/mm^2); (**h**) T1WI_FS + C axial; (**i**) T1WI_FS + C sagittal; (**j**) T1WI_Dynamic axial; (**k–l**) T1WI_Dynamic+C axial; (**m**) T2WI_FS sagittal; (**n**) DWI axial (b = 800 s/mm^2); (**o**) T1WI_FS + C sagittal; (**p–r**) T2WI_FS sagittal

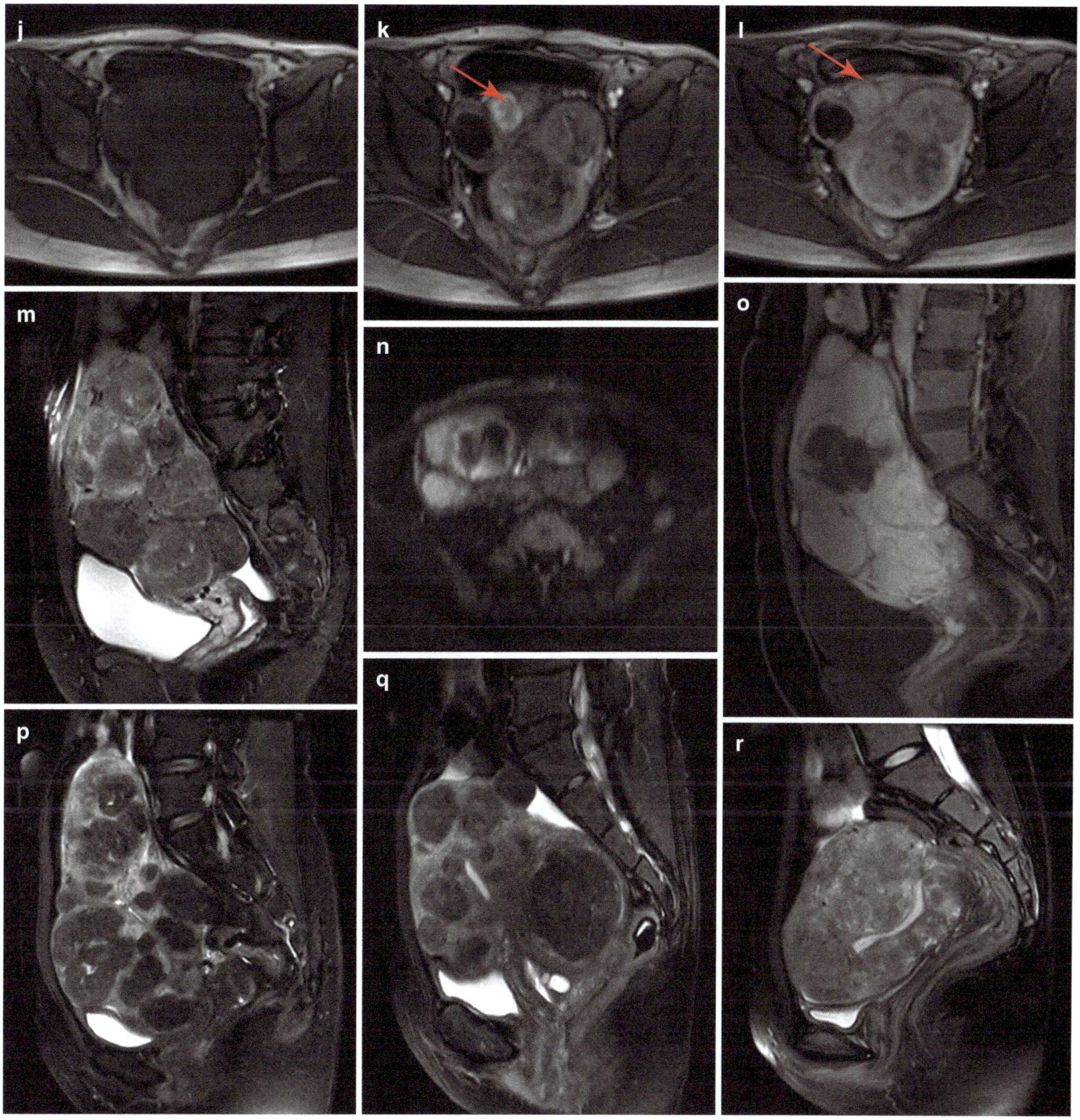

Fig. 2.27 (continued)

The contrast-enhanced T1WI imaging shows that multiple uterine fibroids usually have relatively uniform low isointense signals. Due to the location and blood supply of multiple fibroids, the inner part of the fibroids may have slightly higher (Fig. 2.27o) or slightly lower (Fig. 2.27i) signal relative to the muscular layer. The enhancement difference of different fibroids can be observed by dynamic enhancement on T1WI. For example, the fibroids with rich blood supply can be enhanced early, the smaller fibroids can be enhanced uniformly, and the larger fibroids show gradually progressive target ring-like enhancement to the center. Some fibroids may show low intense signals with areas of non-perfusion necrosis (Fig. 2.27j–l).

Differential Diagnosis

- **Uterine myomatosis** It is a diffuse growth of fibroids in the myometrium and is usually characterized by numerous, small, fused, circular nodules. Unlike multiple uterine fibroids, leiomyomatosis is a fusion of many small fibroids without obvious boundaries, and the uterine morphology presents with a symmetrical increase in size. On the other hand, multiple uterine fibroids are usually seen as multiple circular nodules with distinct boundaries. T2WI imaging shows multiple uterine fibroids with low intense signals, well-defined boundaries, and sometimes partial cystic necrosis. Uterine leiomyomatosis usually shows uniformly low intense signal, no obvious boundary, and the uterus is symmetrically enlarged and protruding into the abdominal cavity.

2.1.2.8 Special Type: Uterine Leiomyomatosis

Uterine leiomyomatosis (UL), also known as diffuse uterine leiomyomatosis (DUL), is a very rare growth mode of uterine fibroids, accounting for 0.08–1.94% of the incidence of uterine fibroids (Fig. 2.28).

MRI Findings

Routine T1WI imaging showed low isointense signals of the uterine leiomyomatosis with enlarged uterine body shape and ill-defined boundaries (Fig. 2.28a).T2WI imaging can clearly display forms and features of uterine leiomyomatosis that differ from the common multiple uterine fibroids; uterine leiomyomatosis usually shows fused leiomyoma nodules with unclear boundary, diameter < 3 cm, accumulating in the whole body of the uterus. It also causes a uniformly enlarged uterine body, diffused thickening in the muscular layer that becomes invisible. Some inner fibroids are fusiform, and occasionally some may have a pseudocapsule with well-defined boundaries (Fig. 2.28b). The clinical manifestations of the patients have no specific presentations, and patients in the early stage of the disease have no clinical symptoms. With the increase in sizes of these fibroids, some fibroids can protrude into the endometrial cavity and also gradually compress the surrounding tissues and organs in the pelvis, resulting in a series of pressure and pain symptoms.T2WI imaging shows that fibroids of different locations and sizes in the

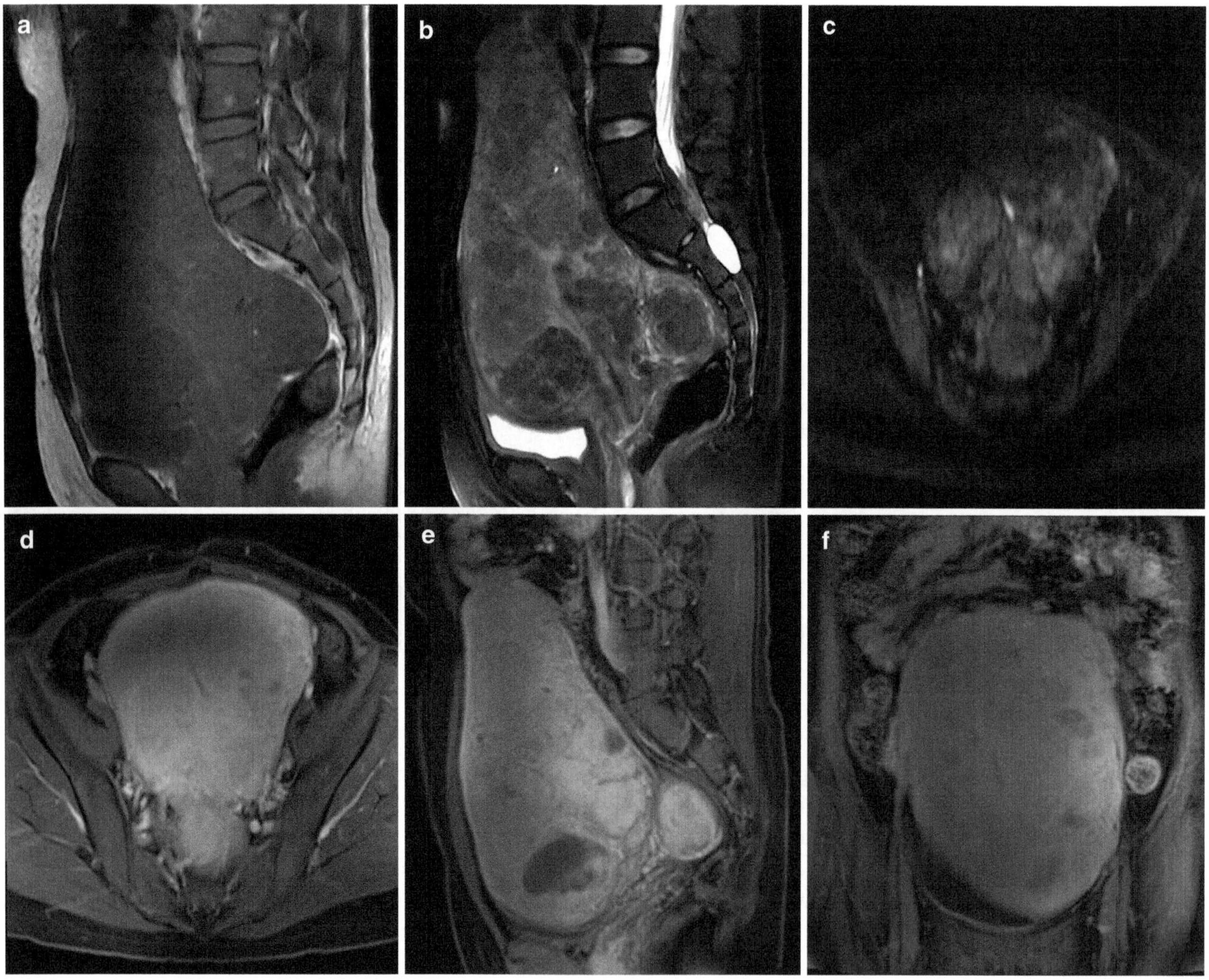

Fig. 2.28 Uterine leiomyomatosis. (**a**) T1WI sagittal; (**b**) T2WI_FS sagittal; (**c**) DWI axial (b = 800 s/mm^2); (**d**) T1WI_FS + C axial; (**e**) T1WI_FS + C sagittal; (**f**) T1WI_FS + C coronal; (**g**) T1WI sagittal; (**h**) T2WI_FS sagittal; (**i**) DWI axial (b = 800 s/mm^2); (**j**) T1WI_FS + C axial; (**k**) T1WI_FS + C sagittal; (**l**) T1WI_FS + C coronal

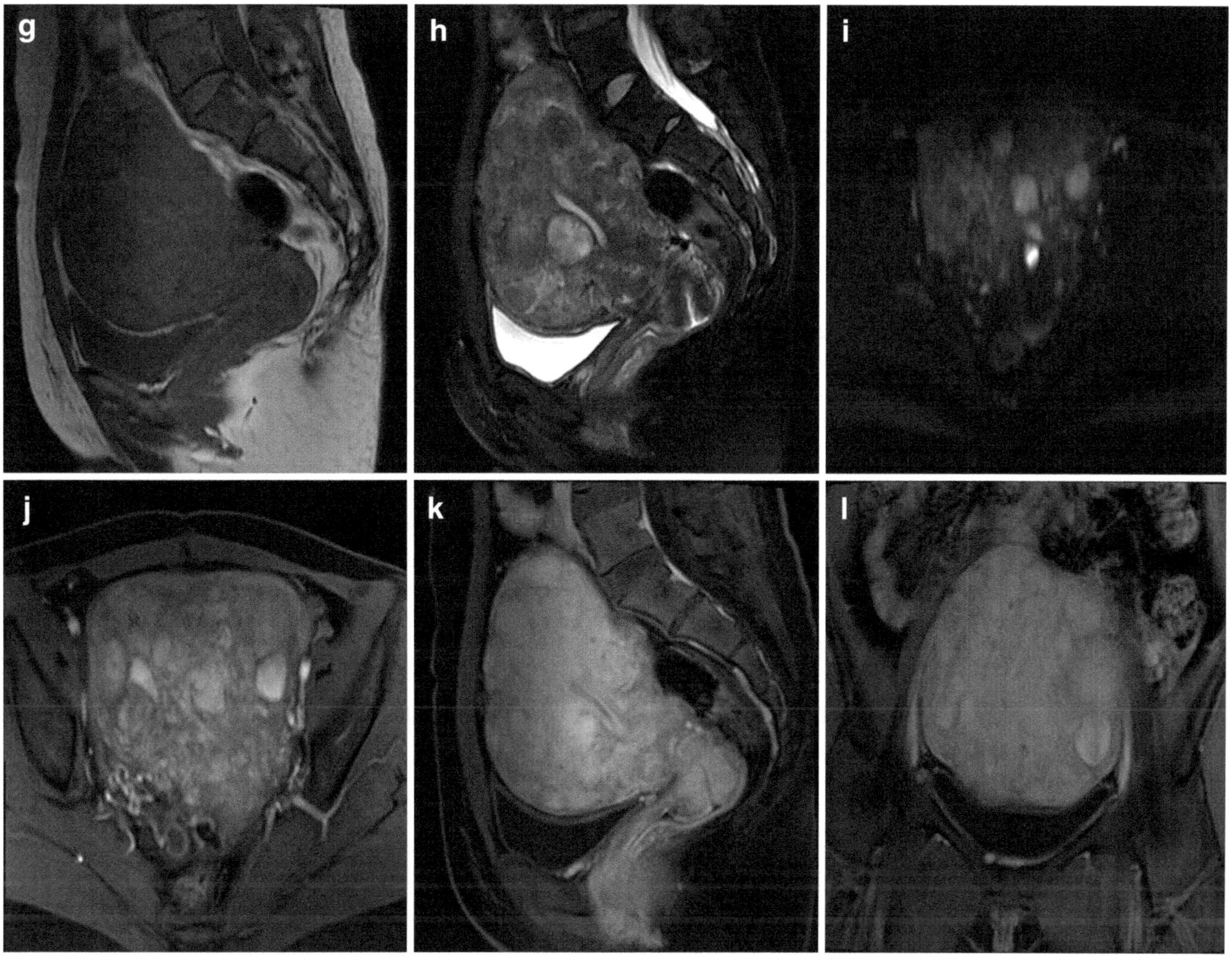

Fig. 2.28 (continued)

uterine leiomyomatosis can have certain signal differences. The fibroids are usually relatively uniform and isointense, and a few fibroids may have low intense or slightly high intense signals (Fig. 2.28h). DWI imaging has no obvious specificity for the diagnosis of uterine leiomyomatosis and usually presents as diffuse low intense or isointense signals (Fig. 2.28c, i).

As uterine leiomyomatosis has fibroids of different sizes and fused with fibroids from different locations, it shows different intensity of signals on T1WI contrast-enhanced imaging. Usually, these fibroids show diffuse high intense signals, with numerous round nodules inside the tumor (Fig. 2.28j). They seem to have a visible boundary, with some fibroids showing low intense signals with non-perfusion areas (Fig. 2.28e).

Differential Diagnosis

- **Multiple uterine fibroids:** Uterine leiomyomatosis and multiple uterine fibroids are generally not difficult to distinguish. Multiple uterine fibroids usually have multiple round-like fibroid nodules with distinct boundaries. Uterine leiomyomatosis is a fusion of small fibroids that generally do not have a clear boundary.

2.1.3 Signal Characteristics and Classification of Uterine Fibroids

FIGO classification criteria focus on the growth site of uterine fibroids and the relationship between fibroids and the endometrium, muscular layer, and serosa. Many clinical studies and practical experience on uterine fibroids have proved that the signal characteristics of uterine fibroids on T2WI imaging reflect the difficulty of focused ultrasound ablation of fibroids to a certain extent [3].

According to the signal characteristics (grayscale value) of uterine fibroids on T2WI images, the signal intensity of uterine fibroids on T2WI was compared with that of skeletal muscle (usually rectus abdominis) and normal myometrium, and uterine fibroids were roughly divided into the following five types [4, 5]: (1) T2WI low signal intensity: The signal intensity of fibroids is similar to that of skeletal muscle (Fig. 2.29). (2) T2WI isointense signal: The signal intensity of fibroids was lower than that of the myometrium but higher than that of skeletal muscle (Fig. 2.30). (3) T2WI inhomogeneous hyperintensity: Fibroids have tissue degeneration and necrosis, and there are patches or strips (>5 mm in width) of high and low signal shadows close to endometrial signal or close to skeletal muscle signal in fibroids (Fig. 2.31). (4) T2WI uniform mild hyperintensity: The fibroid signal was evenly distributed, and the intensity of the fibroid signal was equal to or slightly higher than that in the myometrium and significantly lower than that in the endometrium (Fig. 2.32). (5) Uniform and significantly high T2WI signal: The signal intensity of fibroids was significantly higher than that of the myometrium and close to or equal to that of the endometrium (Fig. 2.33).

2.1.4 Special Signal Fibroids: Red Degeneration of Uterine Fibroid

Uterine fibroid red degeneration, is one of the various forms of uterine fibroid degeneration. It usually occurs during pregnancy or postpartum, accounting for 1.9–25% of uterine fibroids, and 13.0–40.0% are related to pregnancy [6]. Uterine fibroid red degeneration is usually considered due to fibroids ischemia, necrosis, hemolysis, thrombosis, and embolism, followed by the overflows of the corresponding red hemoglobin into the myoma, producing the red coloration. Patients are usually characterized by fever-associated severe abdominal pain, mild increased WBC, and local abdominal tenderness. It is also known as the natural necrosis of fibroid. After its diagnosis, the patient generally doesn't need focused ultrasound ablation.

2.1.4.1 MRI Findings

A routine T1WI plain scan shows a slightly higher signal intensity of the red-like degenerated fibroid (Fig. 2.34d, g). The signal may be uniform or mixed and usually shows the fibroid boundary. On the contrary, T2WI imaging can clearly define the morphology and characteristics of fibroids. The red degeneration of fibroids is usually single (Fig. 2.34h), and occasionally there are ≥2 fibroids with red degeneration (Fig. 2.34a). The fibroids are round, most of them have pseudocapsule, and the boundary of fibroids can be clearly displayed.

Red degeneration fibroids can be in submucosal, intramural, or subserosal fibroids, more for intramural fibroids. The fibroid morphology varies in size and is associated with the type of fibroid caused by their morphological changes and

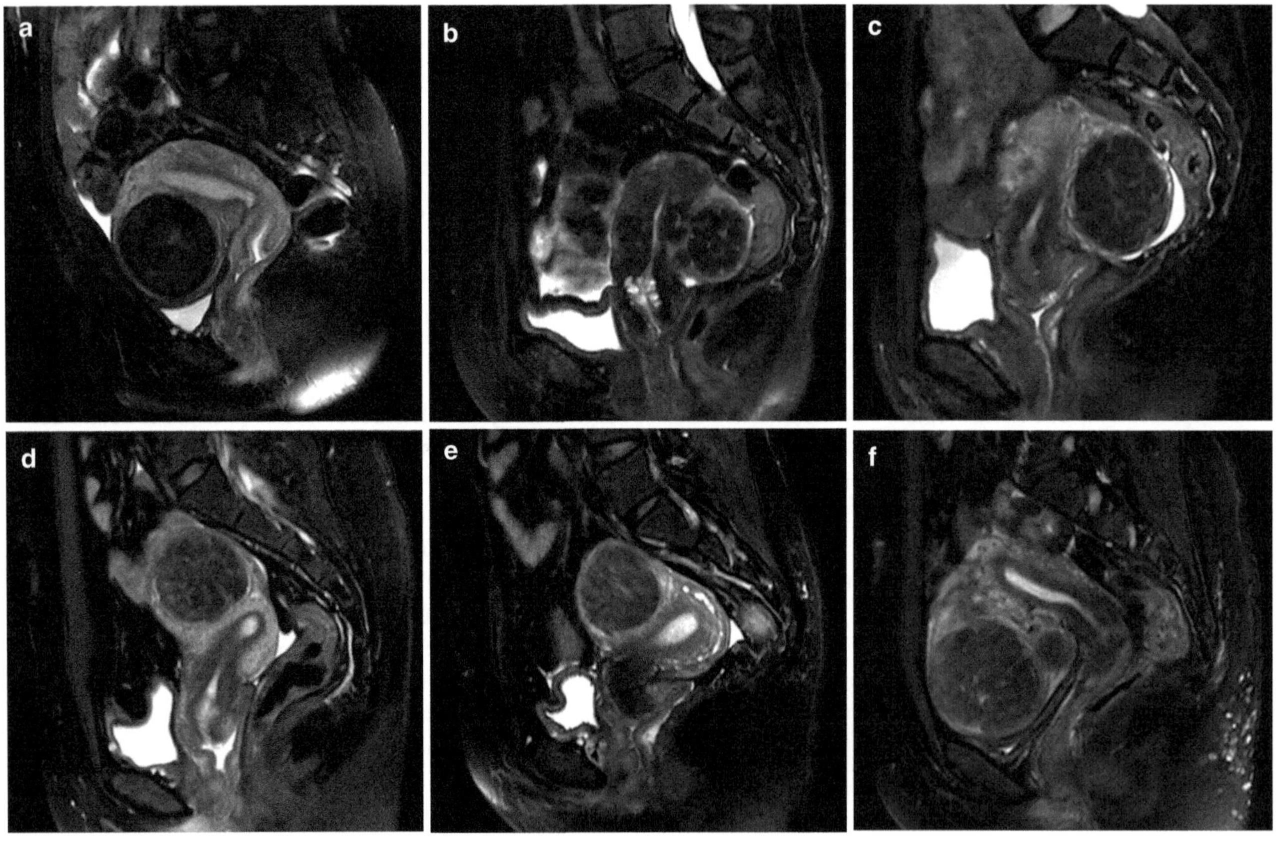

Fig. 2.29 T2WI hypointense fibroids: (**a**–**f**) T2WI_FS sagittal

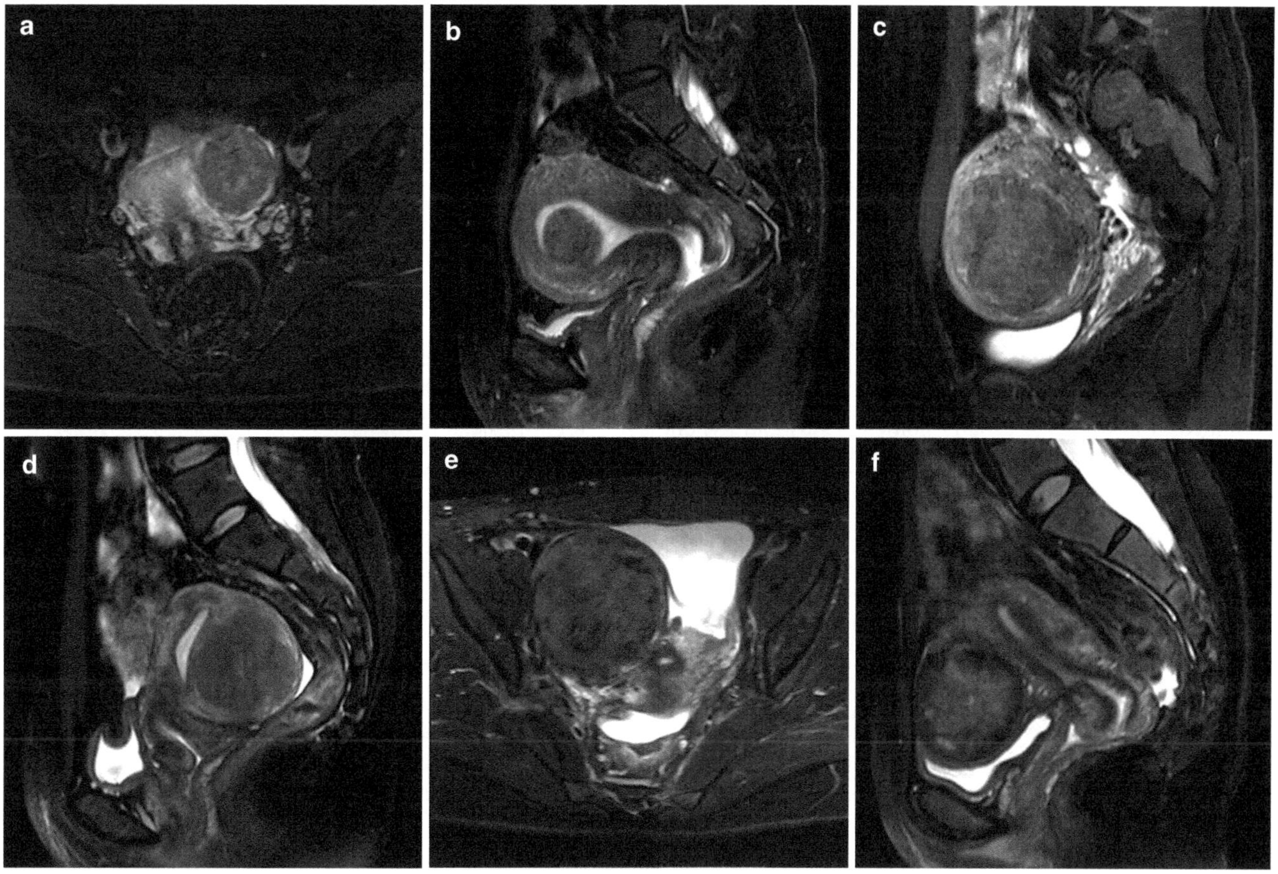

Fig. 2.30 T2WI isosignal uterine fibroids: (**a**) T2WI_FS axial, (**b–f**) T2WI_FS sagittal

symptoms. Some combined fibroids types can have red degeneration at the same time.

T2WI imaging shows that fibroid with red degeneration usually presents with mixed signals (Fig. 2.34b, h) or even slightly higher signals. Some larger fibroids may also present cystic necrosis with higher intense signals.

DWI imaging is sensitive to the diagnosis of uterine fibroids with red lesions, usually presenting slightly higher mixed signals (Fig. 2.34c, i), and a few presenting slightly higher signals with clear boundaries.

The contrast-enhanced T1WI shows uterine fibroids with red degeneration usually show uniform low intense signals (Fig. 2.34e, k). A few fibroids also have slightly blood supply signals that can be seen inside the fibroid and marginal areas. The fibroid boundary is usually clear and smooth.

2.1.4.2 Differential Diagnosis

- **Uterine fibroids**: Routine T1WI scan of fibroids usually shows uniform and low isointense signals without clear boundaries. DWI imaging usually shows low isointense signals, and The contrast-enhanced T1WI shows the presence of blood supply. The red degeneration of the fibroid is a process of natural necrosis of the fibroid, usually showing a mixed signal on T2WI and a slightly high signal on T1WI, which can show a certain boundary. The DWI imaging can have slightly higher mixed signals, the contrast-enhanced T1WI showed the fibroids have no blood supply, like the fibroids after focused ultrasound ablation. Therefore, it is generally not difficult to distinguish between T1WI plain scan and T1WI-enhanced imaging.
- **Uterine malignancy**: Uterine malignancy is usually manifested by increased intensity of signals on T1WI with a certain boundary. DWI imaging usually presents slightly high mixed signals or significantly high signals. But malignant tumors on T1WI enhancement usually present slightly high mixed signals with obvious blood supply and boundary. However, the uterine fibroids with red-like degeneration usually shows no blood supply on the contrast-enhanced T1WI, so it is not difficult to differentiate.

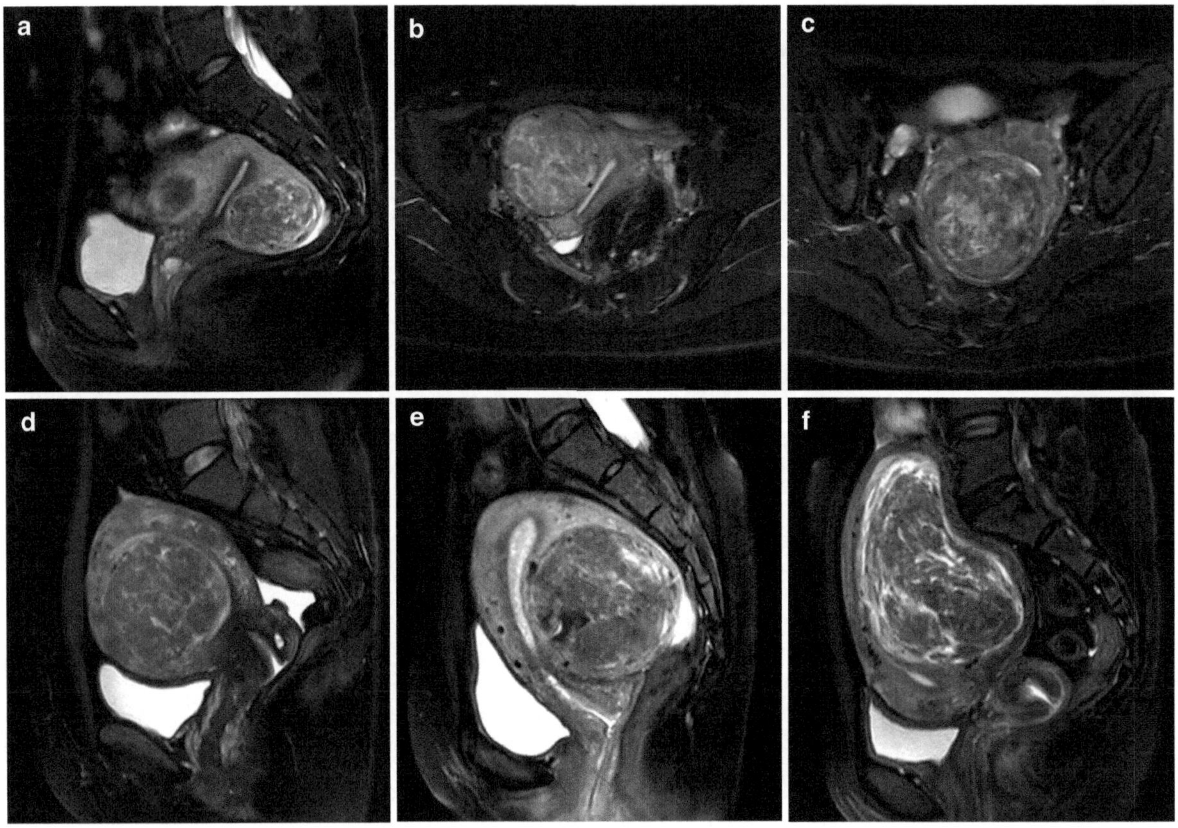

Fig. 2.31 Uterine fibroids with heterogenous hyperintensity on T2WI: (**a**) T2WI_FS sagittal, (**b**, **c**) T2WI_FS axial, (**d**–**f**) T2WI_FS sagittal

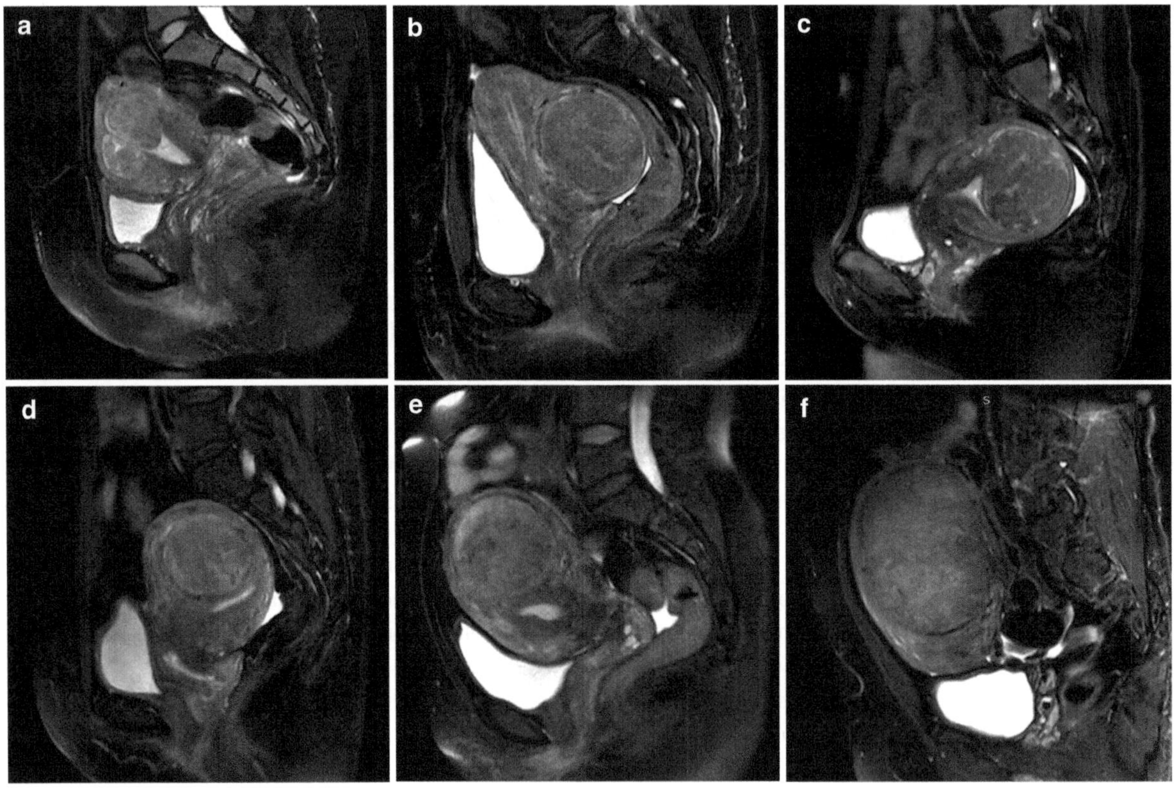

Fig. 2.32 The fibroids with slightly homogeneous hyperintensity on sagittal T2WI (**a**–**f**)

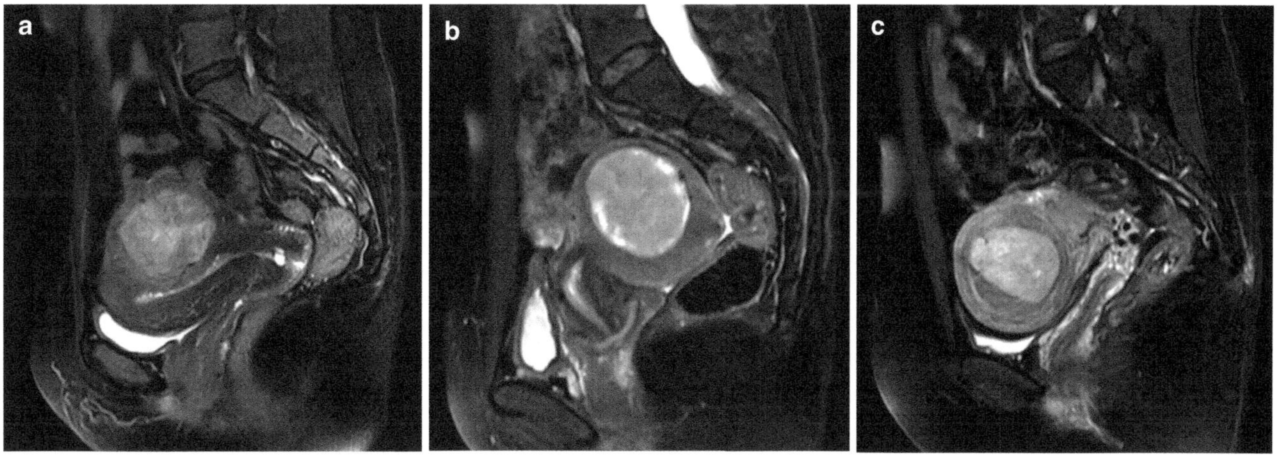

Fig. 2.33 Significant hyperintensity uterine fibroids on T2WI: (**a**–**c**) T2WI_FS sagittal

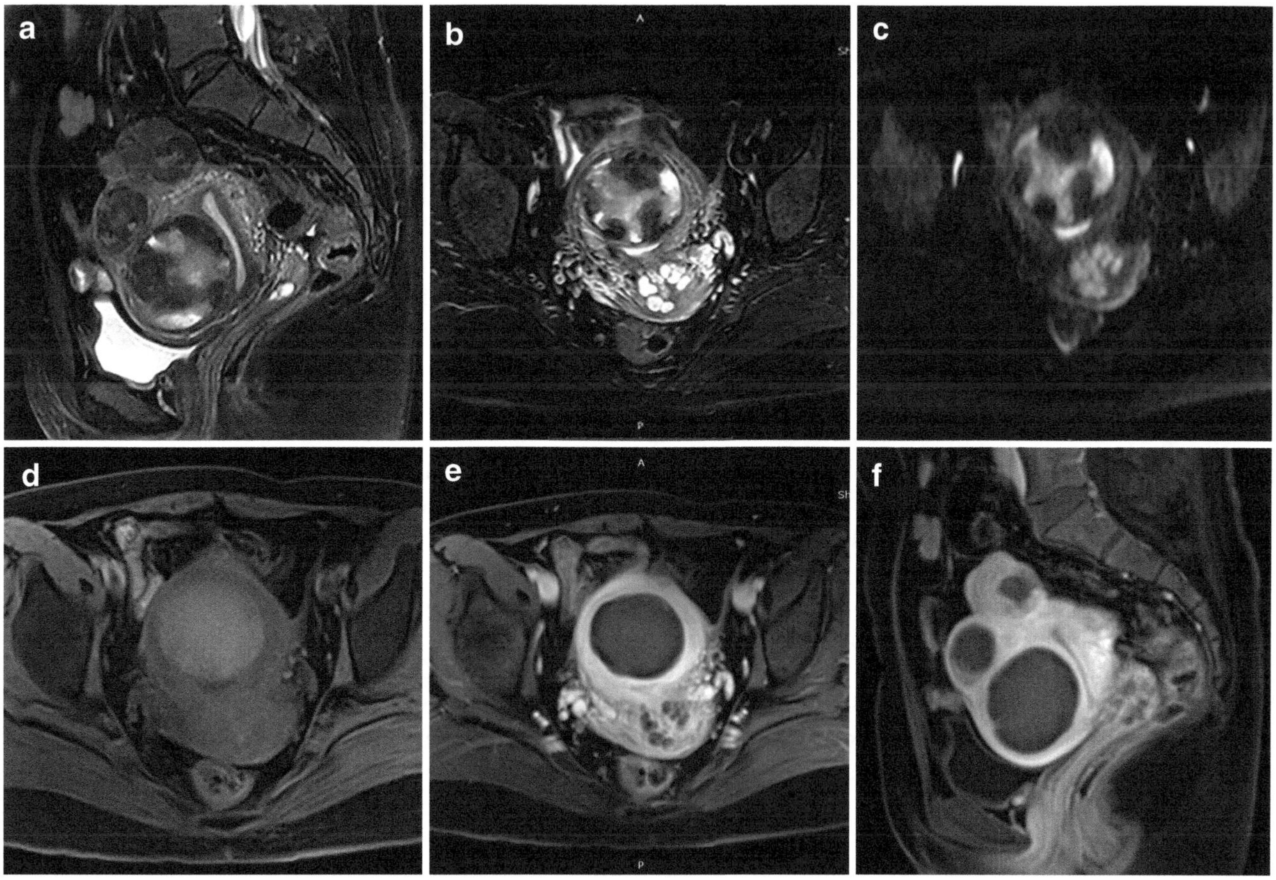

Fig. 2.34 Uterine fibroids have reddish-like degeneration. (**a**) T2WI_FS sagittal; (**b**) T2WI_FS axial; (**c**) DWI axial (b = 800 s/mm^2); (**d**) T1WI_FS axial; (**e**) T1WI_FS + C axial; (**f**) T1WI_FS + C sagittal; (**g**) T1WI sagittal; (**h**) T2WI_FS sagittal; (**i**) DWI axial (b = 800 s/mm^2); (**j**) T1WI_FS axial; (**k**) T1WI_FS + C axial; (**l**) T1WI_FS + C sagittal

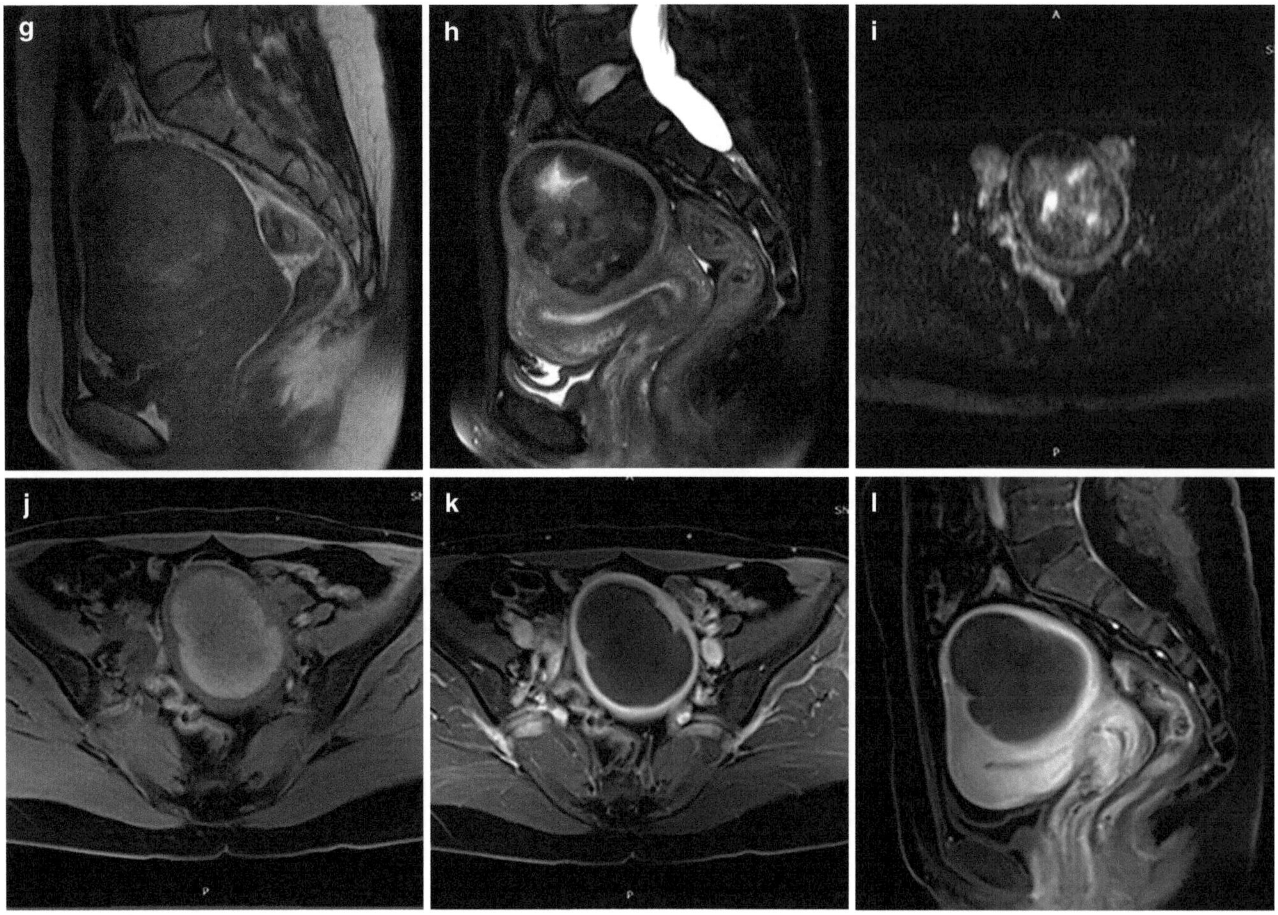

Fig. 2.34 (continued)

2.2 CT Diagnosis of Uterine Fibroids

2.2.1 CT Findings of a Normal Uterus

Due to the lack of obvious soft tissue density contrast, computed tomography (CT) is significantly inferior to magnetic resonance imaging regarding the image resolution of the normal body of the uterus. Usually, the body of the uterus presents a homogeneous signal of soft tissue density on CT imaging, and only changes in the shape and size of the body of the uterus can be observed. In most cases, the density of uterine fibroids is similar to that of normal myometrium, and thus it is difficult to distinguish its boundaries. Sometimes the pseudocapsule of the fibroids, the nourishing blood vessels of the fibroids, and the like are occasionally seen. When the fibroids appear in cystic transformation, hemorrhage, degeneration, necrosis, and so on, it can enhance the contrast of the fibroids on the CT imaging, for which the diagnostic confidence can be improved.

2.2.1.1 Body of Uterus

The plain CT scan of a normal body of the uterus shows homogeneous soft tissue density (CT value = 20–80 Hu), ill-defined three-layer structure, and uterine effusion with a slightly low density (Fig. 2.35).

2.2.1.2 Uterine Cervix

Compared with the MRI of a normal uterus, the cervix and isthmus of the normal uterus show the same soft tissue signal density as that of the body of the uterus on the plain CT scan, which is difficult to distinguish accurately (Fig. 2.36).

2.2.1.3 Ovary

A normal uterus ovary shows a slightly lower density (CT value = 20 ~ 80 Hu) than the body of the uterus on the plain CT scan (Fig. 2.37).

2.2.1.4 Uterine Ligaments

Due to the significant contrast provided by the fat in the pelvic cavity, the normal uterine ligaments appear to be con-

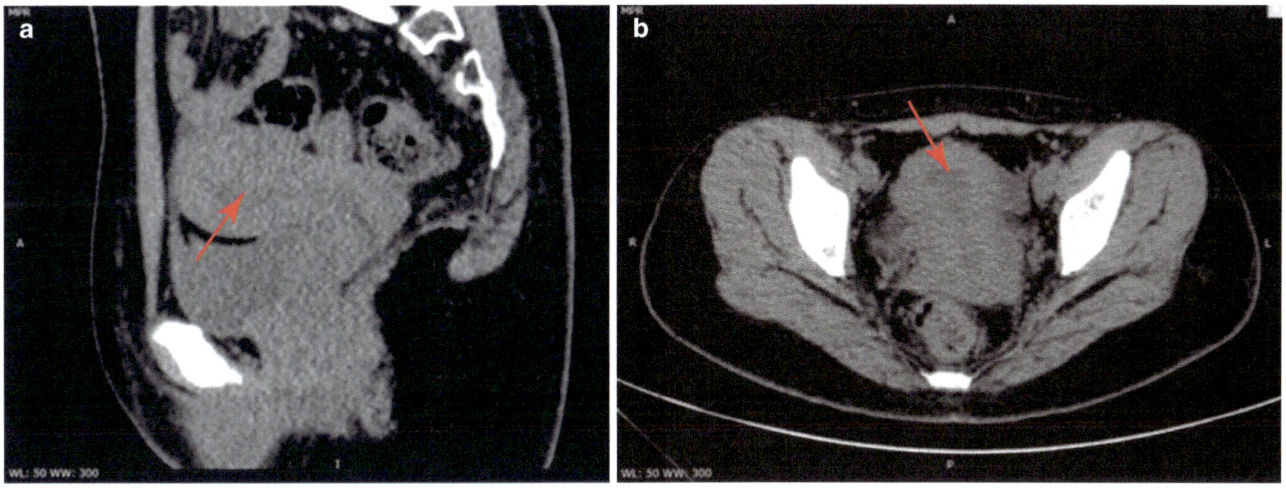

Fig. 2.35 Plain CT scan of a normal uterine body. (**a**) sagittal; (**b**) axial

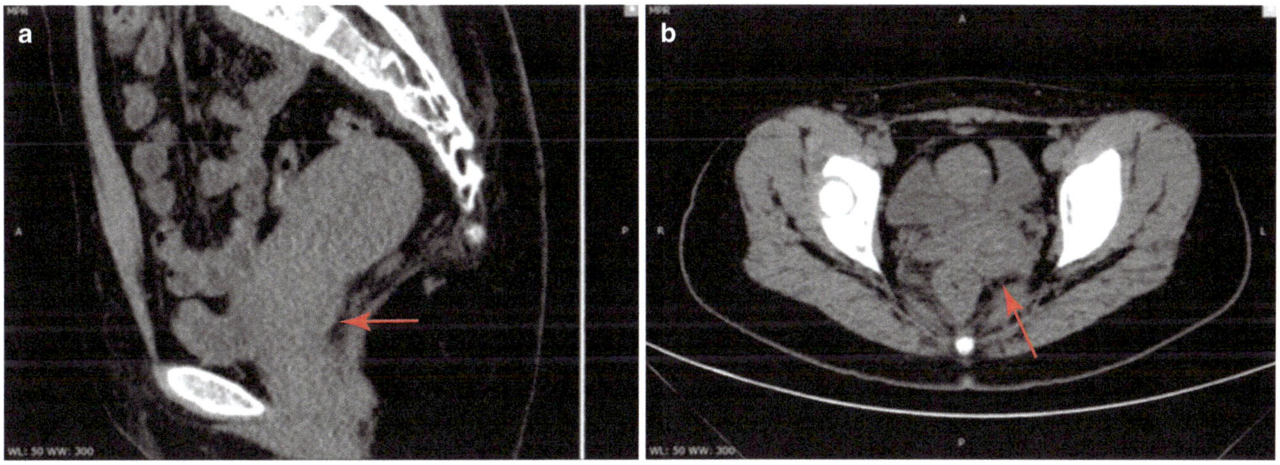

Fig. 2.36 Plain CT scan of a normal uterine cervix. (**a**). sagittal; (**b**) Axial

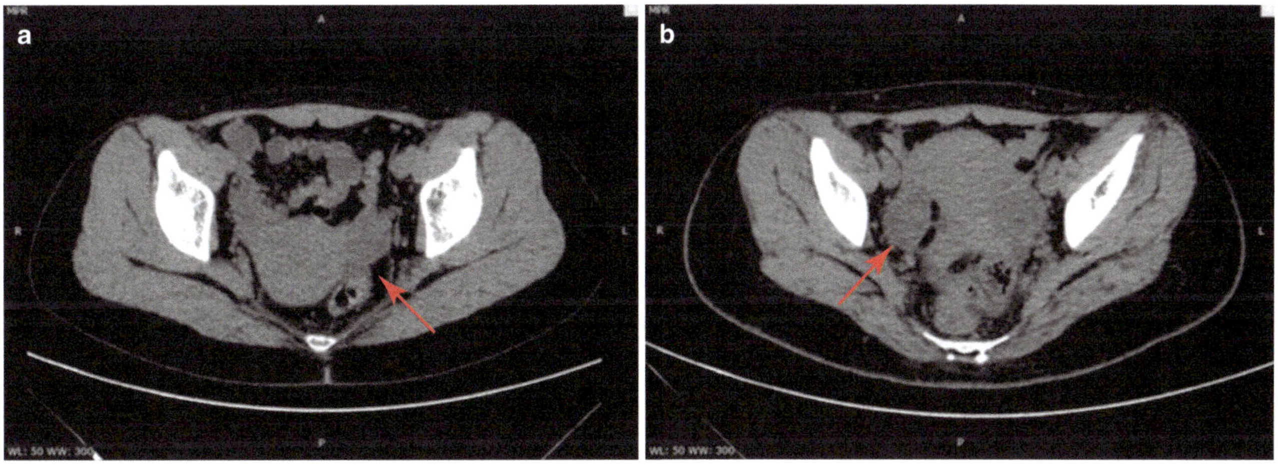

Fig. 2.37 Plain CT scan of a normal ovary. (**a**, **b**) axial

nected to the body of the uterus in a fibrous strip on the plain CT scan, and the specific types of ligaments are indistinguishable (Fig. 2.38).

2.2.1.5 Contrast-Enhanced CT Scan of the Uterus

Due to the low fat density in the pelvic cavity and the significant contrast provided by the contrast agent, the comparison between the contrast enhanced CT scan and the plain CT scan of a normal uterus can significantly improve the contrast between various tissue structures. The body of the uterus, cervix, ovary, and ligaments can be clearly displayed. However, compared with MRI, the contrast enhanced CT scan is still difficult to distinguish the various layers of the body of the uterus (Fig. 2.39).

2.2.2 Uterine Fibroids

CT examination is of certain significance for the diagnosis of uterine fibroids, but it is difficult to distinguish their types and subtypes. It requires the diagnostician to have rich clinical and imaging experiences.

2.2.2.1 Submucosal Uterine Fibroids

CT Findings

1. **Plain CT scan:** Submucosal fibroids show an enlarged uterus with an enlarged and deformed uterine cavity, and the enlarged uterine cavity shows a roundish mass with a density roughly equivalent to that of the uterus (Fig. 2.40a).
2. **Contrast Enhanced CT scan:** Submucosal fibroids are significantly and homogeneously enhanced, with "pseudocapsules" visible on the edges (Fig. 2.40b).

Differential Diagnosis

Endometrial Polyps Contrast enhanced CT scan shows endometrial defects with inhomogeneous density, but it is difficult to distinguish from submucosal uterine fibroids and often requires clinical diagnosis and biopsy confirmation.

2.2.2.2 Intramural Uterine Fibroids

CT Findings

1. **Plain CT scan:** Small intramural uterine fibroids are usually difficult to find on plain CT scans. Fibroids hardly change the morphology of the corresponding muscle layer. The density of fibroids is the same as or slightly lower than that of the normal uterine wall. Various low-density shadows can be seen in them (Fig. 2.41a). Large-volume intramural uterine fibroids are characterized by the inhomogeneous enlargement or contour deformation of the uterus. In addition, the surrounding normal tissues and organs can be moved. The fibroids on the plain CT scan are usually of similar density to the myometrium, with ill-defined boundaries. The density of tumors is relatively homogeneous, and the cystic degeneration or necrosis among them can be patchy and show low density (Fig. 2.41c, e).
2. **Contrast Enhanced CT scan:** The contrast enhanced CT scan of smaller fibroids shows low-density non-enhanced roundish shadows (Fig. 2.41b). For the ones with larger volumes, the contrast enhanced CT scan usually shows the same density as the myometrium, with ill-defined boundaries and sometimes visible vascular shadows. Due to the difference in the size of the fibroids and the blood supply, all fibroids may have a slightly lower density relative to the muscle layer, and a lower density of degenerated tissue components can be seen in them (Fig. 2.41d, f).

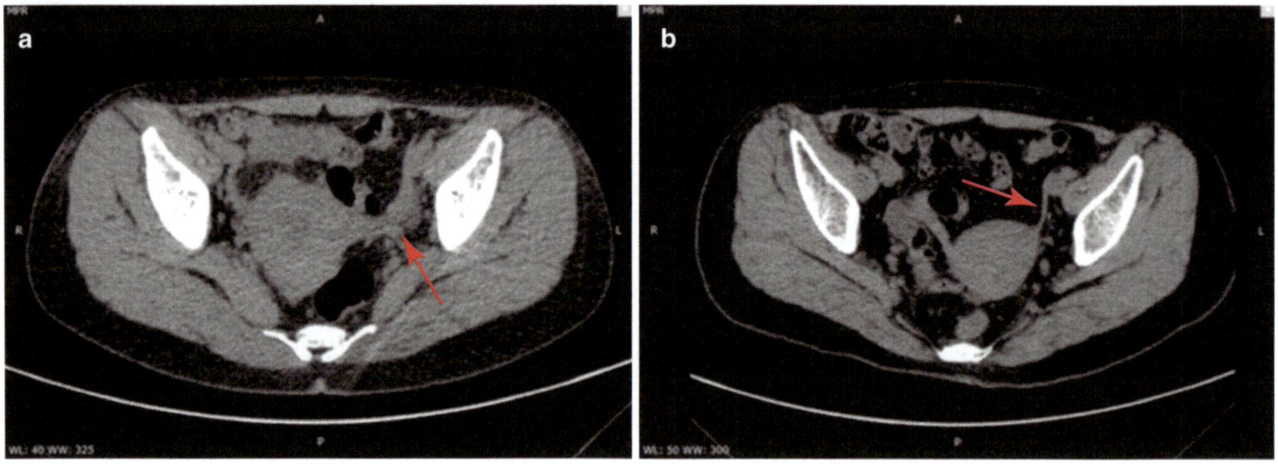

Fig. 2.38 Plain CT scan of normal uterine ligaments. (**a**, **b**). axial

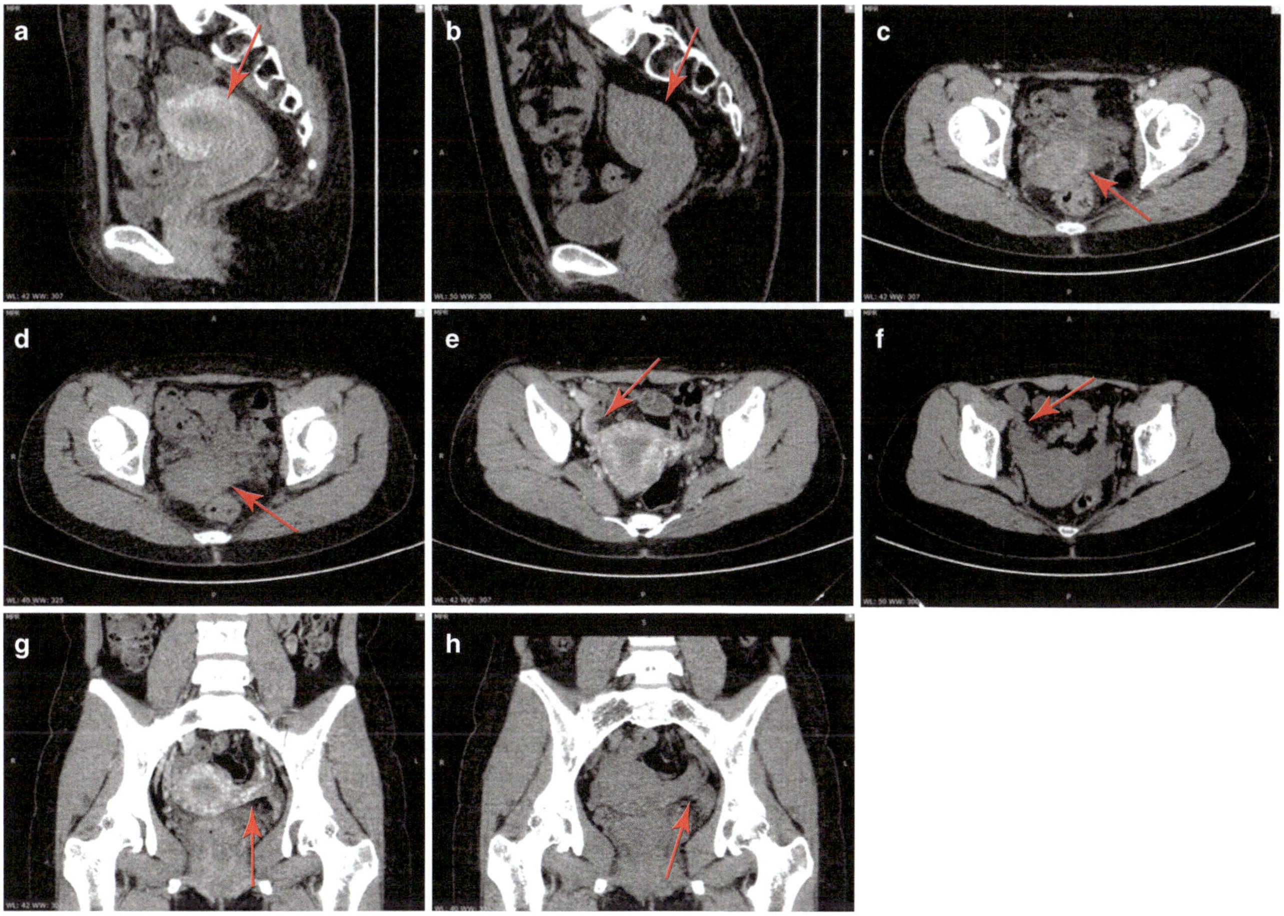

Fig. 2.39 CT images of a normal uterus. (**a**) Contrast enhanced CT scan, sagittal; (**b**) Plain CT scan, sagittal; (**c/e**) Contrast enhanced CT scan, axial; (**d/f**). Plain CT scan, axial; (**g**) Contrast enhanced CT scan, coronal; (**h**) Plain CT scan, coronal

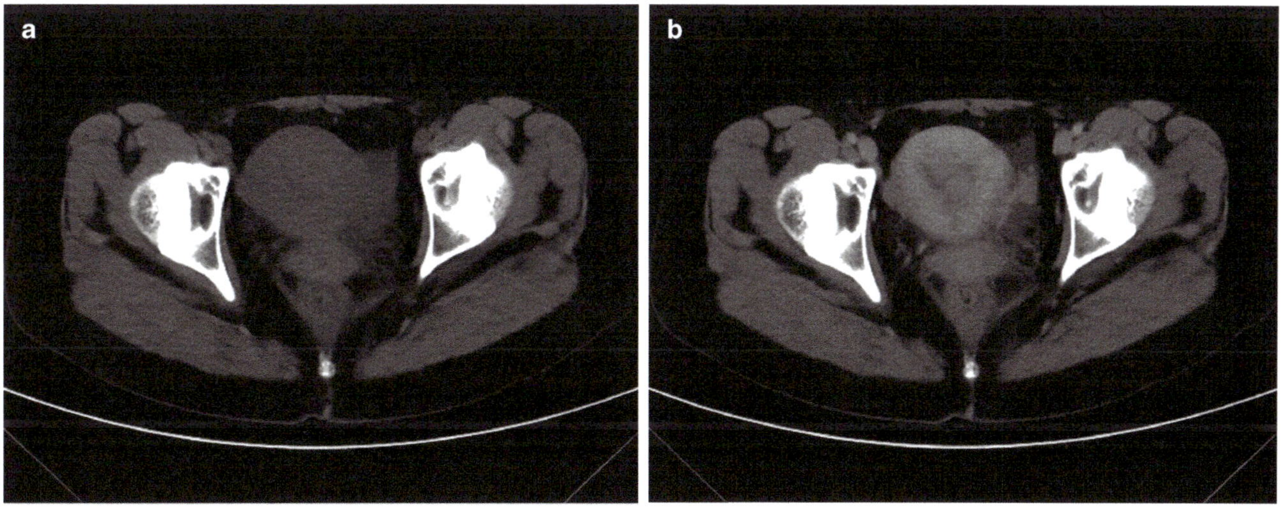

Fig. 2.40 Submucosal uterine fibroids. (**a**) plain CT scan, axial; (**b**) Contrast enhanced CT scan, axial

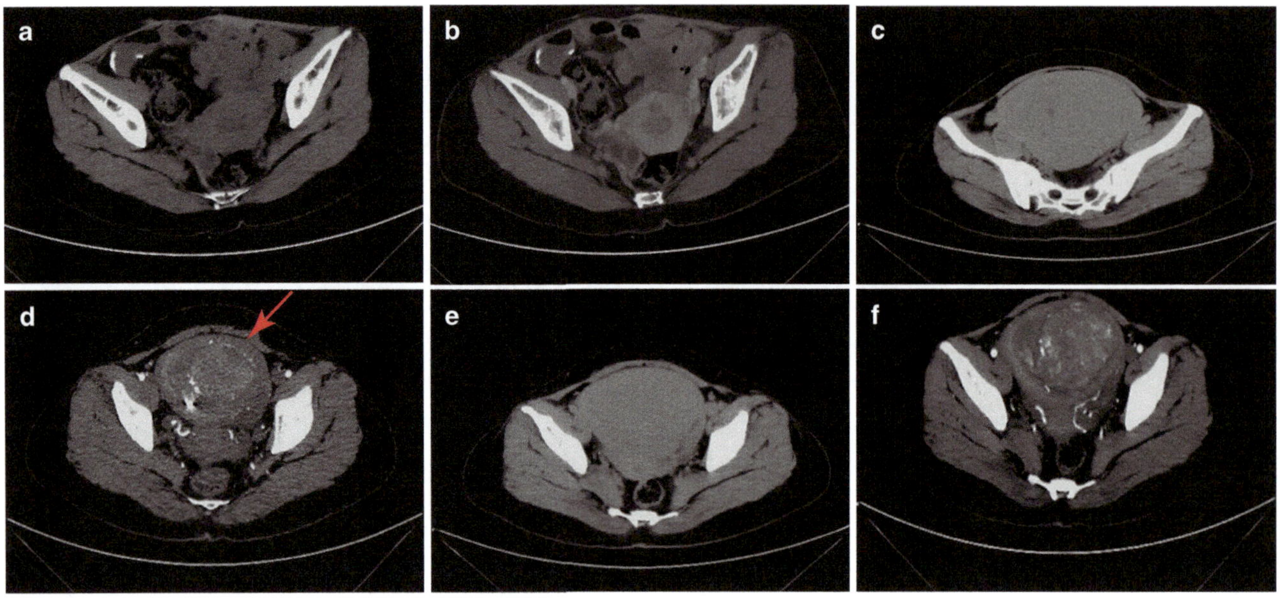

Fig. 2.41 Intramural uterine fibroids. **(a/c/e)** Plain CT scan, axial; **(b/d/f)** Contrast-enhanced CT scan, axial

Differential Diagnosis

- **Adenomyosis:** Plain CT scan shows the diffuse homogeneous enlargement of the body of the uterus and thickened uterine wall. The CT value is 50–70 Hu. The contrast enhanced CT scan shows inhomogeneous enhancement, and spot-like non-enhanced foci are seen inside. Focal adenomyosis is similar to intramural uterine fibroids. However, adenomyosis has secondary dysmenorrhea, and the uterus is mostly homogeneously enlarged. It seldom exceeds the size of a 3-months gravid uterus.
- **Uterine sarcoma:** Plain CT scan shows an irregularly enlarged uterus with a lobulated shape. The tumor density is inhomogeneous, related to tumor degeneration and necrosis. Contrast enhanced CT scan shows inhomogeneous tumor enhancement. Neighboring organs in the pelvic cavity are sometimes invaded, and swollen lymph nodes can be seen. It shows rapid growth, often accompanied by abdominal pain, abdominal masses, and irregular vaginal bleeding.

2.2.2.3 Subserosal Uterine Fibroids

CT Findings

1. **Plain CT scan**: Subserosal uterine fibroids usually appear as roundish or lobulated masses protruding from the surface of the uterus on plain CT scans, with well-defined and smooth boundaries. They are connected to the broad base of the uterus or connected by pedicles. The morphology of a normal body of uterus is less affected, with occasional signs of body compression on one side. The density of fibroids is usually similar to the normal muscle layer or slightly lower than that of the myometrium of the uterus. The density of fibroids is relatively inhomogeneous, sometimes with patchy low-density shadows [7] (Fig. 2.42a, c).
2. **Contrast Enhanced CT scan:** After an enhanced CT scan of subserosal uterine fibroids, the density is usually close to or slightly higher than that of normal myometrium. The early appearance of enhancement is significant, showing obvious homogeneous or inhomogeneous enhancement (including low-density necrotic area). These low-density areas are not enhanced or slightly enhanced. Due to the difference in the origin and blood supply of the subserosal uterine fibroids and the normal muscle layer, sometimes it can be seen that the subserosal uterine fibroids appear as low-density masses in the muscle layer, and the density of fibroids is relatively homogeneous (Fig. 2.42b, d).

[Differential Diagnosis]

- **Ovarian thecoma-fibroma group:** They are benign ovarian tumors. A plain CT scan shows a homogeneous solid mass in the appendage area on one side, with well-defined boundaries and possible shallow lobes. Most tumors are large, and the uterus is displaced. As the contact area between the tumor and the uterus increases, the contact angle with the uterus is mostly obtuse or surrounds the uterus. On the contrast enhanced CT scan, it can be seen that the fine arteries inside the mass are developed, and the solid mass is not significantly enhanced (fibrovascular sign), which is a characteristic manifesta-

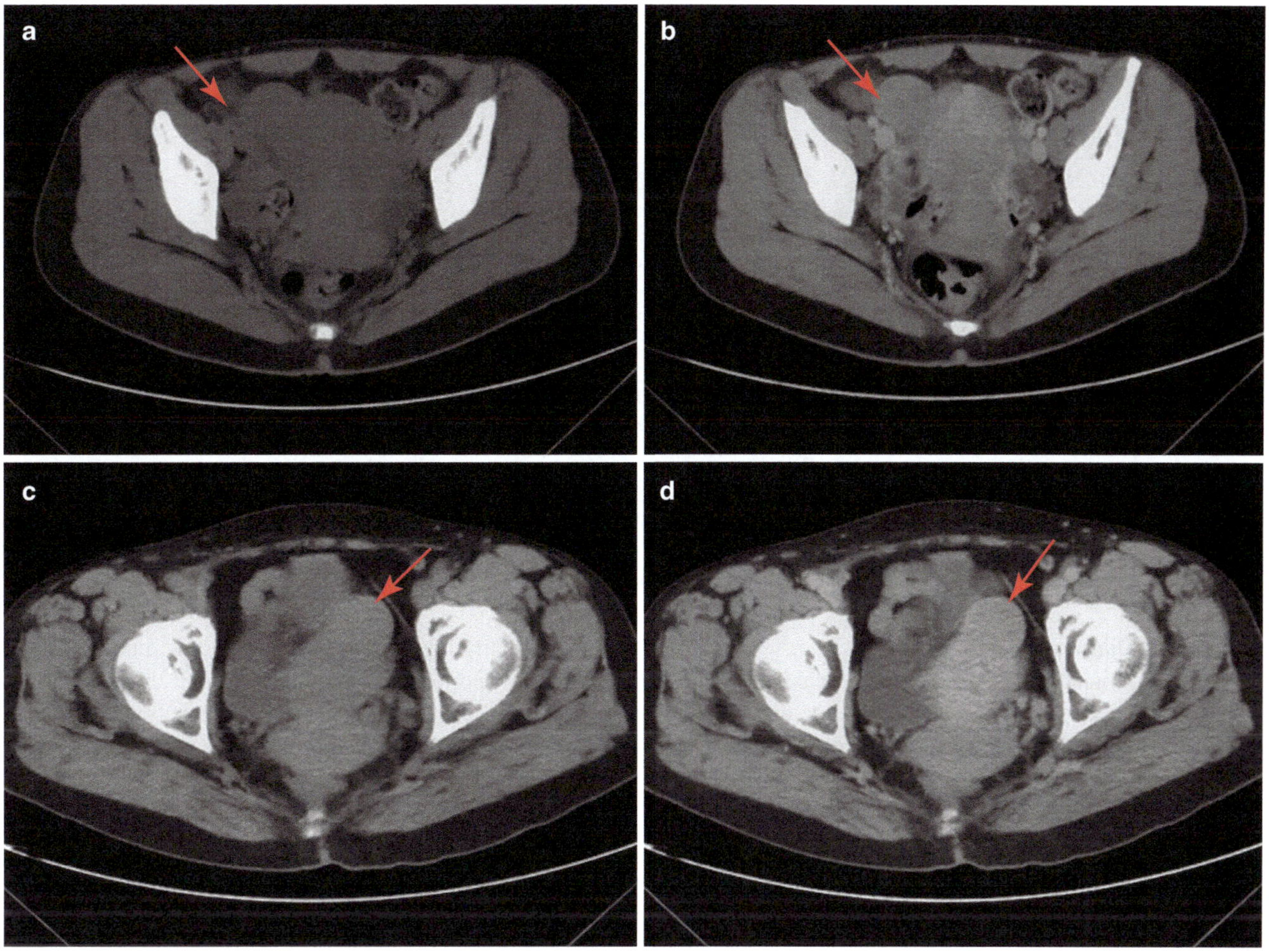

Fig. 2.42 Subserosal uterine fibroids. (**a/c**) Plain CT scan, axial; (**b/d**) Contrast enhanced CT scan, axial

tion [8]. This type of tumor is difficult to distinguish from larger subserosal uterine fibroids. Still, the characteristic manifestations on the contrast-enhanced CT is helpful for the diagnosis and differential diagnosis of the two.

- **Malignant tumors of the ovary:** CT shows that the lesions are more common on both sides, the contours are irregular, with lobulated edges, and often invade the surrounding organs. The scope of the lesions is wide and spreads over the abdominal cavity [9]. Infiltration characteristics and enlarged pelvic lymph nodes help the differential diagnosis of the two.

2.2.3 Special Types of Uterine Fibroids

2.2.3.1 Uterine Cervical Fibroids

CT diagnosis also has certain difficulties in the differential diagnosis of special types of uterine fibroids. For example, the diagnosis of fibroids at the cervix, broad ligament, and other areas is still not as obvious and intuitive as MRI. Multiple uterine fibroids are sometimes seen with multiple roundish masses, and uterine fibroids are difficult to distinguish.

CT Findings

1. **Plain CT scan**: Uterine cervical fibroids can grow in the interstitium of the anterior, posterior, and lateral walls of the cervix, with a complete capsule with a swelling. They can also grow submucosa, protruding into the vagina or occupying the pelvis or upper middle parts of the vagina. Uterine cervical fibroids show homogeneous density on the plain CT scan and are usually difficult to identify. Due to the low-density contrast sometimes provided by endometrial fluid, the boundaries of fibroids are occasionally visible but ill-defined (Fig. 2.43a).
2. **Contrast Enhanced CT scan:** Compared with a plain CT scan, contrast enhanced CT has a certain value in the diagnosis at the cervix. Due to the non-perfusion and low-density signal of endometrial fluid, it can highlight the contrast and boundaries of the cervical fibroids (Fig. 2.43b).

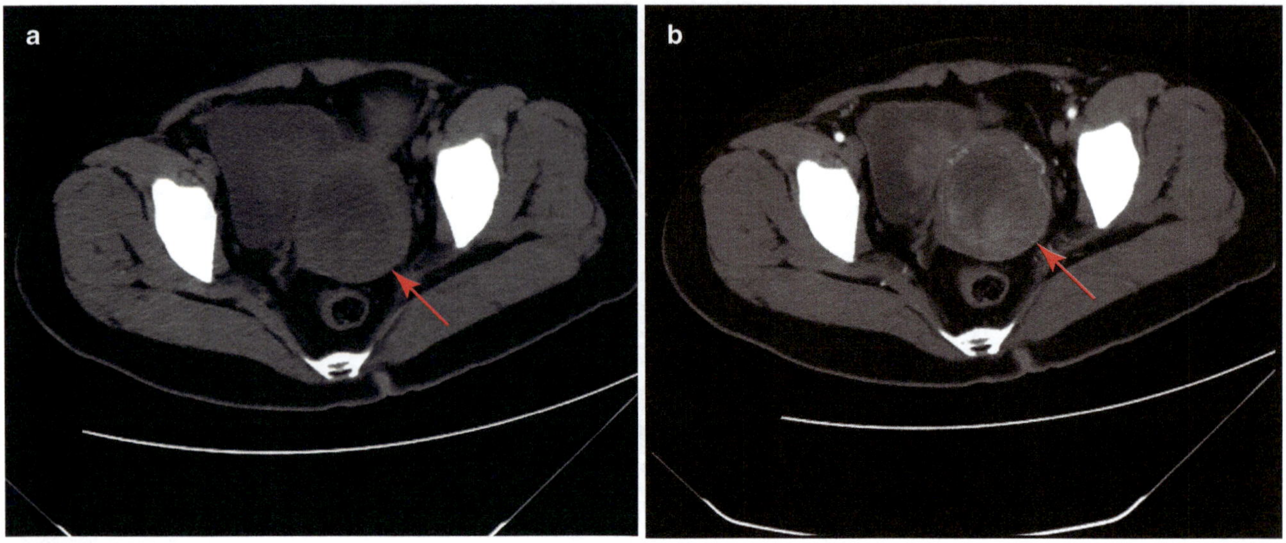

Fig. 2.43 Uterine cervical fibroids. (**a**) Plain CT scan, axial; (**b**) Contrast-enhanced CT scan, axial

Differential Diagnosis

- **Cervical cancer:** The CT scan of cervical cancer shows an enlarged cervix with irregular edges, and medium-density masses can be seen. If necrosis occurs, low-density foci can be seen. Irregular or homogeneous enhancement can be seen after contrast enhancement [10].

2.2.3.2 Multiple Uterine Fibroids

CT Findings

1. **Plain CT scan**: Multiple uterine fibroids usually appear as an asymmetric enlargement of the body of uterus. There are multiple round-like protrusions on the surface of the body of the uterus. The surrounding tissues and organs are subject to a certain degree of displacement. Fibroids usually exhibit the same density as the muscle layer. The boundary is ill-defined, and sometimes patchy low-density shadows can be seen (Fig. 2.44a, c, e).
2. **Contrast Enhanced CT scan:** The image of multiple uterine fibroids has certain signal characteristics. Due to the difference in the blood supply of different types and parts of fibroids, it can be expressed as multiple round masses with different densities, and the boundaries between different fibroids can be relatively well-defined, sometimes visible high-density vascular shadows (Fig. 2.44b, d, f).

Differential Diagnosis

- **Uterine leiomyosarcoma:** Patients are usually elderly, showing similar CT imaging findings as uterine fibroids, but the tumor is larger in size, irregular in shape, lobulated, necrosis in the tumor is more obvious, blood vessels are abundant, and enhancement is significant.
- **Metastasis:** Irregular lobed masses with mainly solid properties, mostly affected on both sides, ill-defined boundary, extremely inhomogeneous density, and often involve the uterine rectal fossa and subserous membrane, which may be accompanied by "omental cake sign." The contrast enhanced CT scan shows obvious inhomogeneous enhancement and is commonly associated with ascites. Because of the above characteristic findings, it is easy to differentiate from multiple uterine fibroids [11].

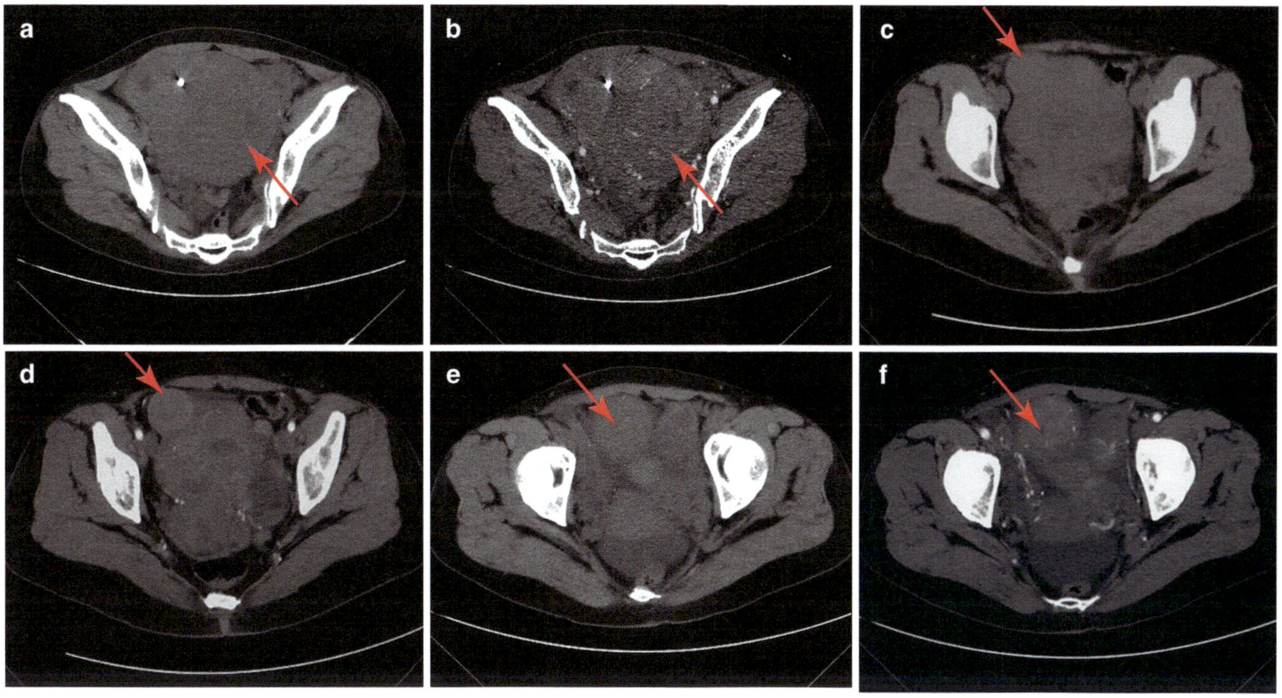

Fig. 2.44 Multiple uterine fibroids. (**a/c/e**) Plain CT scan, axial; (**b/d/f**) Contrast-enhanced CT scan, axial

2.3 Ultrasound Diagnosis of Uterine Fibroids

Ultrasonography is a non-invasive diagnostic technique [12], which stays in the first line to evaluate the endometrium and myometrium, and has commonly been used to diagnose the presence and monitor the growth of uterine fibroids by providing the number, size, position, and blood supply of fibroids.

2.3.1 Submucosal Uterine Fibroids

2.3.1.1 US Manifestation

Color Doppler shows a characteristic circumferential pattern of vascularity around the fibroid, which helps to differentiate it from endometrial polyps; they usually have a vascular pedicle with a central feeding vessel [13, 14], also show circumferential vascularity, blood flow, and arterial supply of the fibroid; necrotic fibroids or those that undergo torsion do not present any blood flow. Characteristics of submucosal fibroids include finding hypoechoic masses by ultrasound (US), immediately subjacent to the endometrium, that project into the endometrial cavity. These masses are classified as to whether or not they are 100% (Fig. 2.45a), greater than 50% (Fig. 2.45b), or less than 50% intracavitary (Fig. 2.45c) and have the typical sonographic appearance of fibroids that appear in other locations. An echogenic "cap" of the endometrium may be observed outlining the endometrial surface of a submucosal fibroid, especially during the periovulatory stage of the menstrual cycle or if there is fluid within the endometrial cavity. However, a 100% intracavitary submucosal fibroid may be indistinguishable from other endometrial masses.

2.3.1.2 Differential Diagnosis

- **Endometrial polyps:** Endometrial polyps are typically smaller and echogenic, often indistinguishable from the surrounding endometrium. These will not extend into the myometrium or disrupt the subendometrial halo (Fig. 2.46a). A vascular pedicle with a single feeding vessel is often identified on color Doppler imaging. However, if there is necrotic tissue present, there will be no increase in color flow. The presence of a single feeding vessel

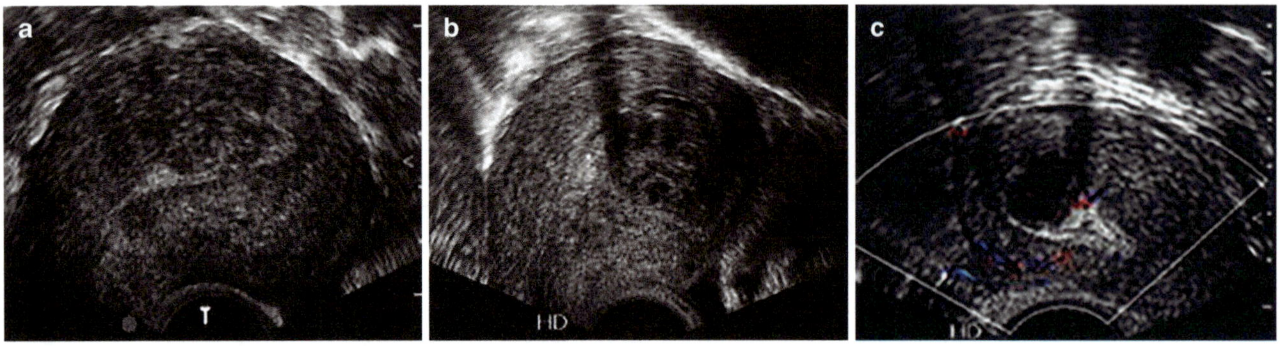

Fig. 2.45 Submucosal fibroids. (**a**) submucosal fibroid; (**b**) submucosal fibroid; (**c**) submucosal fibroids

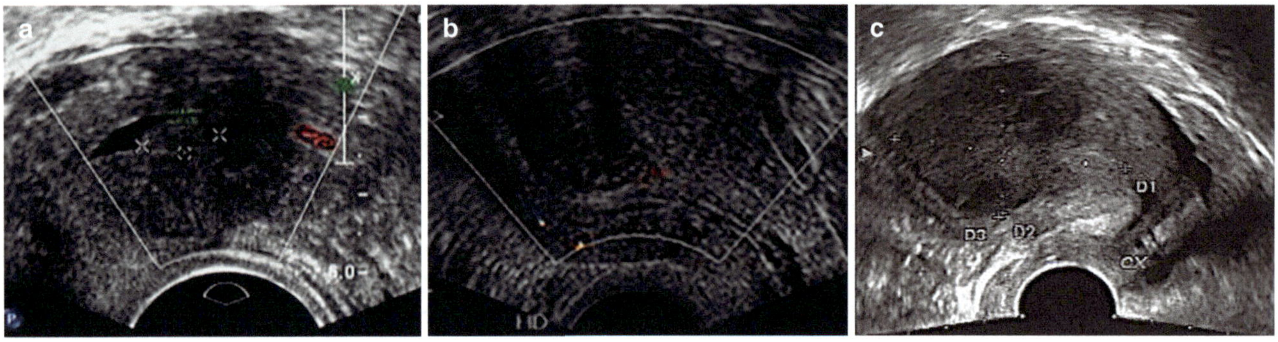

Fig. 2.46 Differential diagnosis of intramural fibroids. (**a**) endometrial polyps; (**b**) submucosal uterine fibroids; (**c**) uterine carcinosarcoma

favors the diagnosis of a benign entity, such as an endometrial polyp. Sonohysterography may be useful to outline endometrial polyps and differentiate them from submucosal fibroids.

- **Submucosal uterine fibroids:** The myometrial echogenicity of uterine fibroids may vary and be hypoechogenic, isoechogenic, hyperechogenic, or mixed, depending on the size and nature of the fibroid. In contradistinction, submucosal fibroids are more likely to be round, sharply marginated, and hypoechoic (Fig. 2.46b). Although a submucosal fibroid can be partially located in the myometrium, and the infiltrative border would not be observed, nor would the mass be irregular or multifocal, and would less likely be echogenic and vascular.
- **Endometrial cancer:** The most specific ultrasound finding for endometrial cancer is an invasion of the mass into the adjacent myometrium and/or disruption of the subendometrial halo by the mass (Fig. 2.46c), visualization of an irregular, lobular, or poorly defined endometrial mass with an increased number of irregularly oriented and disorganized blood vessels.

2.3.2 Submucosal Uterine Fibroids

2.3.2.1 US Manifestation

Uterine fibroids have a variety of appearances on ultrasound examination, ranging from sharply marginated, hypoechoic round masses to echogenic and heterogenous masses, with or without calcifications or cystic areas and with posterior acoustic shadowing. Uterine fibroids most commonly exist in the intramural location. Histologic variants may affect both echotexture and posterior acoustic properties; for example, a cellular fibroid is often more homogeneous and echogenic with less posterior acoustic shadowing, and larger fibroids (>3–5 cm in diameter) are often heterogenous in echotexture, due to the propensity for developing areas of degeneration, particularly if growth has been rapid (Fig. 2.47a). Areas of cystic degeneration will appear relatively anechoic, whereas areas of hemorrhagic degeneration may range from anechoic to echogenic, depending on the time course since the hemorrhage occurred (Fig. 2.47b). On the contrary, a lipofibroid variant will be extremely echogenic with posterior attenuation due to the fat content (Fig. 2.47c). Conversely, fibroids typically shrink in size and develop calcifications after menopause, as estrogen levels subside (Fig. 2.47d). The blood supply is abundant during uterine fibroids with red degeneration (Fig. 2.47e), and it grows rapidly in a short time. A cellular fibroid is often more homogeneous and echogenic with less posterior acoustic shadowing (Fig. 2.47f).

2.3.2.2 Differential Diagnosis

- **Uterine adenomyoma:** The uterus is enlarged to varying degrees. The shape is most irregular. The tumor has no obvious boundary with the myometrium, the uterine cavity line is arcuate, and there is no obvious vortex-like structure in the internal echo (Fig. 2.48a). Significant sound attenuation, with scattered punctate blood flow signals, was seen.
- **Uterine sarcoma:** The uterus is enlarged and irregular in shape. The lesions are located in different locations. When the size is large, the uterine cavity and the myometrium can be involved (Fig. 2.48b). The internal echo is uniform, or the internal echo is mixed due to hemorrhage, necrosis, or cystic degeneration. The demarcation between the mass and the myometrium is unclear (Fig. 2.48c), the internal echo is uniform, or the internal echo is mixed due to hemorrhage, necrosis, or cystic degeneration. Color Doppler shows abundant strip and dendritic blood flow in the mass.

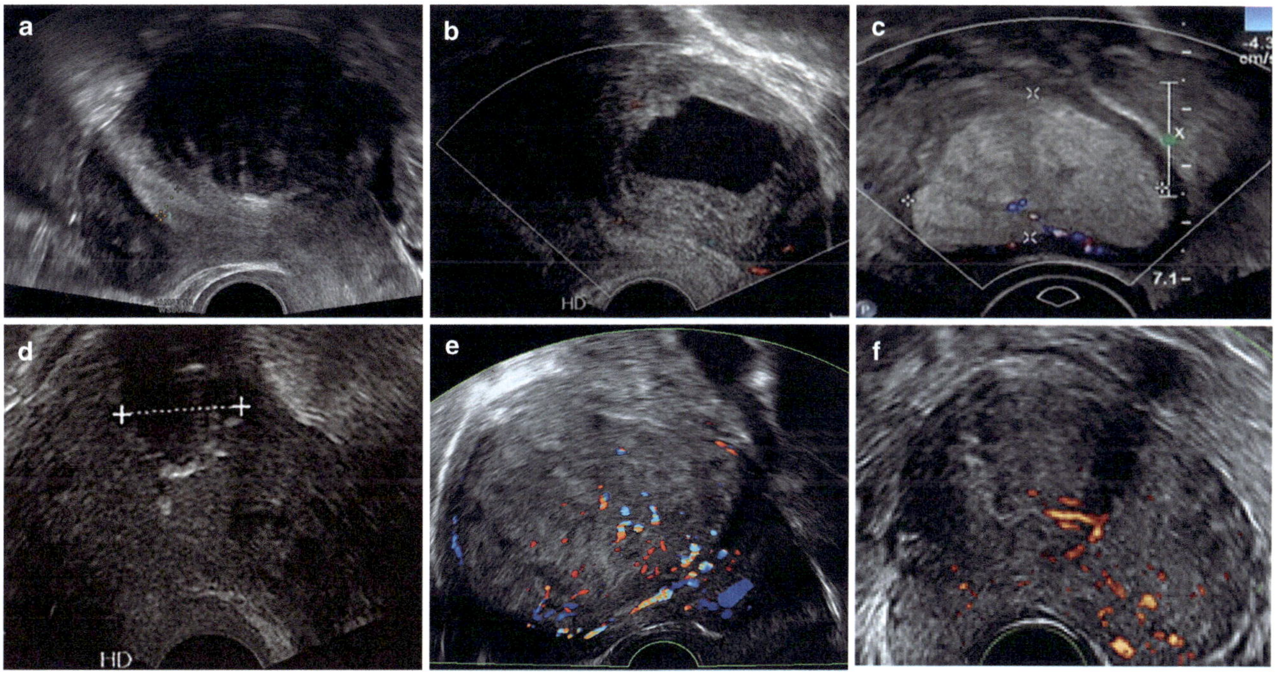

Fig. 2.47 Submucosal uterine fibroids. (**a**) submucosal fibroid; (**b**) submucosal fibroid with cystic degeneration; (**c**) submucosal fibroid with fat degeneration; (**d**) submucosal fibroid with calcification; (**e**) submucosal fibroid with red degeneration; (**f**) cellular submucosal fibroid

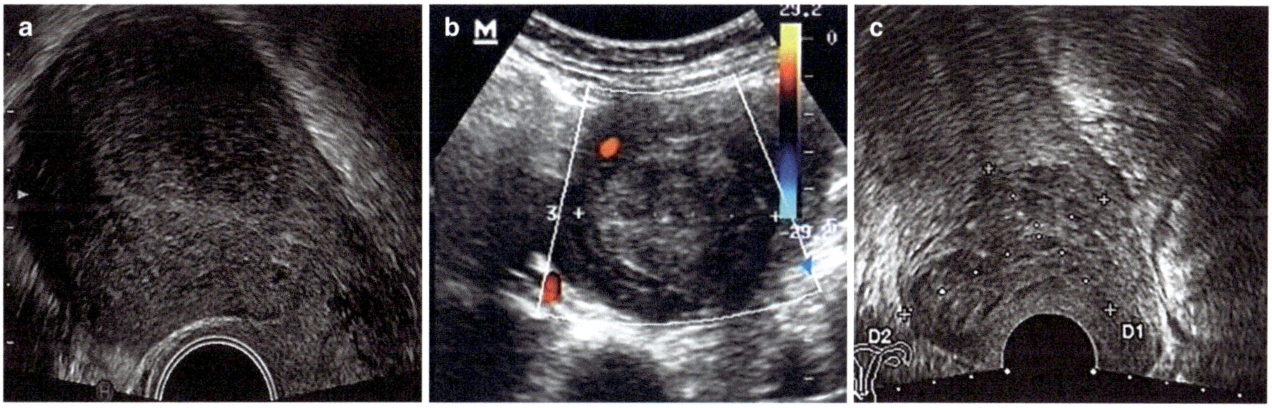

Fig. 2.48 Differential diagnosis of submucosal uterine fibroids. (**a**) uterine adenomyoma; (**b**) endometrial stromal sarcoma; (**c**) uterine leiomyosarcoma

2.3.3 Pedunculated Subserosal Fibroid

2.3.3.1 US Manifestation

These stromal tumors are distinguished from a pedunculated fibroid by several features, including the absence of a connecting pedicle from the solid adnexal mass to the uterine surface and the visualization of ovarian parenchyma surrounding them that clearly indicates its origin was not from the ovary, and extremely dense posterior shadowing from the tumor. The demonstration of the ovary separate from the tumor cements the diagnosis of a pedunculated fibroid. On transvaginal scanning, gentle pressure on the mass, either with the probe or manual compression of the anterior abdominal wall (Fig. 2.49a) and the posterior abdominal wall (Fig. 2.49b), may also help determine if the mass can be separated from the uterus or ovary; the blood supply could be easily shown by color Doppler (Fig. 2.49c). If the ultrasound is nondiagnostic, pelvic MRI will more clearly define these features, allowing a more confident diagnosis.

2.3.3.2 Differential Diagnosis

- **Adnexal ovarian mass:** Pedunculated subserosal fibroid can be confused with solid ovarian mass, lymphadenopathy, gastrointestinal stromal tumor, intestinal masses, and schwannoma. If the solid mass is not related and the activity is inconsistent with the uterus, it may originate from the ovary (Fig. 2.50a). For a pedunculated subserous fibroid, there will be an ovary with normal shape and size on the ipsilateral side. An ovarian thecal cell tumor has a dense posterior shadowing, often much denser than that of a fibroid, due to the presence of extensive fibrous tissue.
- **Broad ligament fibroid:** If the mass after probe compression is consistent with the uterine activity, it may be broad ligament fibroids with the normal ovary also found on the same side. The tumor is accompanied by cystic degeneration (Fig. 2.50b), and multiple anechoic areas appear inside.
- **Remnant horn uterine malformation:** Remnant horn uterine malformation without uterine cavity needs to be differentiated from subserosal fibroids. A solid mass can appear on one side of the uterus (Fig. 2.50c), but the uterus is observed without pedicle connection and pedicle blood supply.

2.3.4 Cervical Fibroids

2.3.4.1 US Manifestation

Fibroids may occasionally be found in the cervix, appearing on ultrasound as cervical masses. Typically, their epicenter

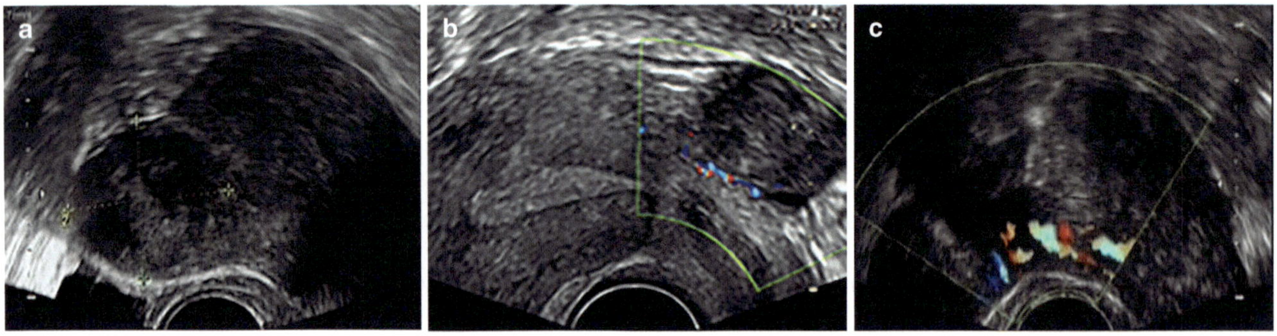

Fig. 2.49 Pedunculated subserosal fibroid. (**a**) anterior protrusion of subserosal fibroids; (**b**) the protrusion of the posterior wall of the subserosal fibroids; (**c**) the blood supply of the pedicle of the subserosal fibroids

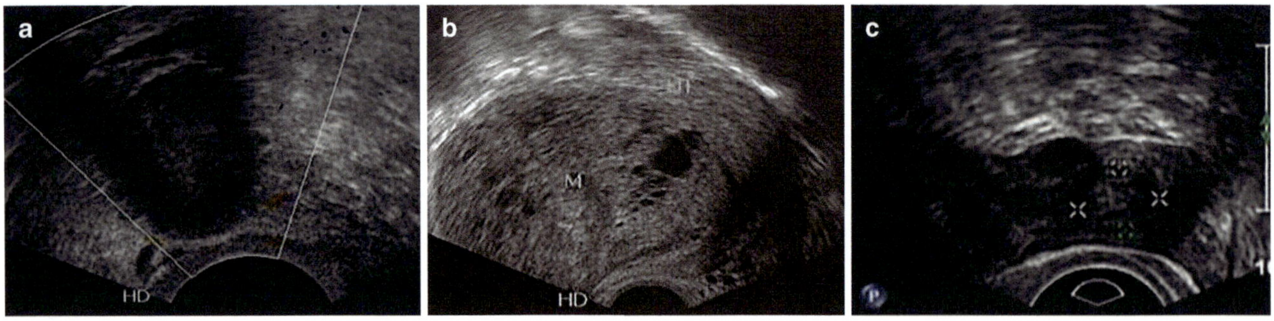

Fig. 2.50 Differential diagnosis of pedunculated subserosal fibroid (**a**) ovarian theca cell tumor; (**b**) cystic degeneration; (**c**) left residual horn uterus with fibroids

will originate in the cervical wall or within the muscular tissue, but some may be exophytic (similar to subserosal fibroids), and others have been known to protrude into the endocervical canal (submucosal). The US most commonly depicts cervical fibroids as round, well-marginated hypoechoic masses. However, cervical cancer may also have a nearly identical appearance, though rarely seen. On the sonographic image, the cervical fibroid appears as an oval or round-like hypoechoic mass (Fig. 2.51a), clearly demarcated with surrounding tissues. Its colored peripheral blood flow or internal strip suggested blood flow from the pedicle (Fig. 2.51b). Hyperechoic plaques may be seen around or inside caused by combined steatosis (Fig. 2.51c).

2.3.4.2 Differential Diagnosis

- **Cervical cancer:** In contrast, cervical cancers are more likely to have their epicenter at the junction of the endocervical lining, with hypoechoic cervical stroma, and are more likely to be polypoid with an irregular margin. Masses that appear to prolapse through the cervical os invade surrounding parametrical tissues, obstruct the endometrial canal, distend the endometrial cavity with fluid, or invade the lower uterine segment more likely represent cervical cancers. Cervical cancer is hypoechoic (Fig. 2.52a), with unclear boundaries, irregular shape, and blurred with the surrounding tissues (Fig. 2.52b). It may infiltrate to surrounding lymph nodes, bladder, or bowel.
- **Cervical polyps:** Cervical polyps are medium-high echoes (Fig. 2.52c), with uniform internal echoes and clear boundaries. In some polyps, a strip-shaped blood flow signal connected to the basal layer of the endocervix was seen. In a few cases, a short rod-shaped and strip-shaped blood flow signal was seen at the root of the polyp. The RI was greater than 0.6, or the low-velocity venous blood flow spectrum.

2.3.5 Broad Ligament Fibroids

2.3.5.1 US Manifestation

Broad ligament fibroids are often located on the side of the uterus, with a larger volume and a spheroid or irregular shape, mainly solid hypoechoic or medium-low echoes (Fig. 2.53a), with homogeneous or inhomogeneous echoes, showing a swirling structure, and the "fence sign" can be seen, which is prone to degeneration and complicated the echo performance inside the tumor, which may have irregular anechoic (Fig. 2.53b), strong echo, and hyperechoic areas (Fig. 2.53c); there are often different degrees of echo attenuation in the rear, clear or indistinct borders, and pseudocapsules. The size

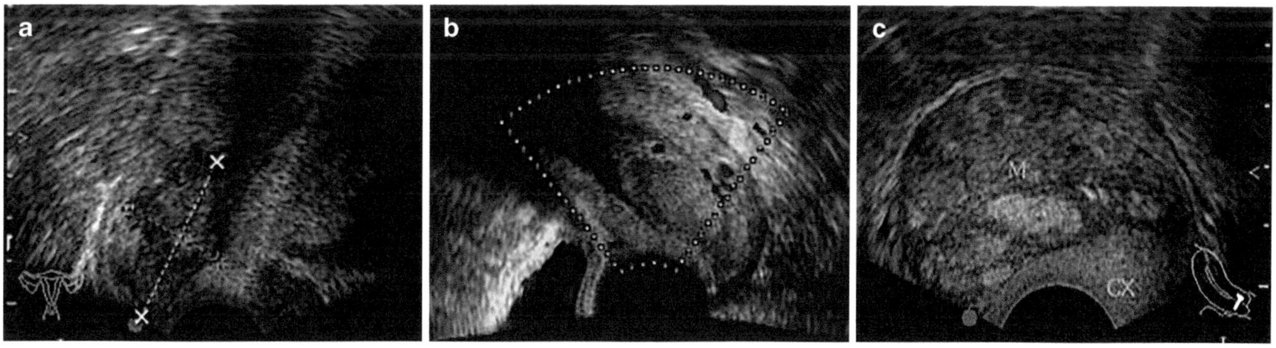

Fig. 2.51 Cervical Fibroids. (**a**) Subserous cervical fibroids; (**b**) cervical fibroids by color Doppler; (**c**) cervical fibroids with steatosis

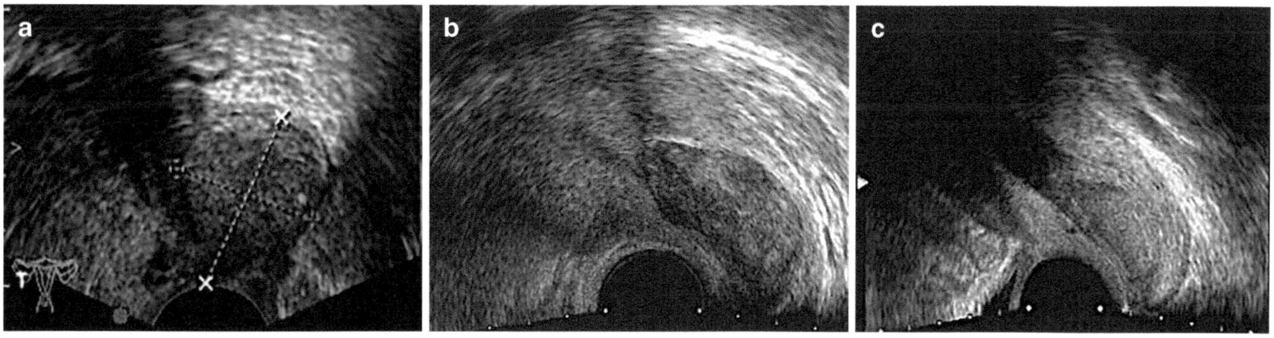

Fig. 2.52 Differential diagnosis of cervix fibroids. (**a**) cervical carcinoma; (**b**) cervical carcinoma; (**c**) cervical polyp

of the uterus is normal, and the uterus and cervix are easily pushed to the healthy side by the tumor and become long and narrow. Color Doppler could show the blood flow not communicated with the uterus, and spectral Doppler can detect the low resistance arterial spectrum.

2.3.5.2 Differential Diagnosis

- **Ovarian tumor:** If the solid mass is not related to the uterus with inconsistent activity, it may originate from the ovary. It may be a broad ligament fibroid if the mass moves consistent with the uterine movement revealed by probe pressure. A broad ligament fibroid can often show an ipsilateral normal ovary, while a larger ovarian tumor may present with irregular shapes without a pseudocapsule.
- **Pedunculated subserosal uterine fibroids:** A pedunculated subserosal fibroid protrudes from the uterus (Fig. 2.54a). The movement is large, and the blood flow can be shown by the color Doppler communicating with the uterus (Fig. 2.54b).
- **Broad ligament adenomyoma:** Endometriosis to the broad ligament can form broad ligament adenomyoma, manifested as a hypoechoic mass on one side of the uterine body, and multiple anechoic areas are seen inside, which is an endometriotic lesion (Fig. 2.54c).
- **Retroperitoneal and small intestinal stromal tumors:** Retroperitoneal tumors have poor activity and are not closely related to the uterus. Small intestinal stromal tumors have an abundant blood supply, and color blood flow signals are mainly peripheral.

2.3.6 Rare Uterine Fibroid

2.3.6.1 Diffuse Uterine Leiomyomatosis (DUL)

US Manifestation

Diffuse uterine leiomyomatosis (DUL) is a specific growth pattern of uterine fibroids, first described as "complete uterine fibromyomatosis" in 1924 [15] and was named diffuse uterine leiomyomatosis in 1979 [16]. The main feature of DUL is the diffuse enlargement of the uterus, and the myometrium is filled with numerous ill-defined hypoechoic masses, most of which are less than 3 cm in diameter (Fig. 2.55a).

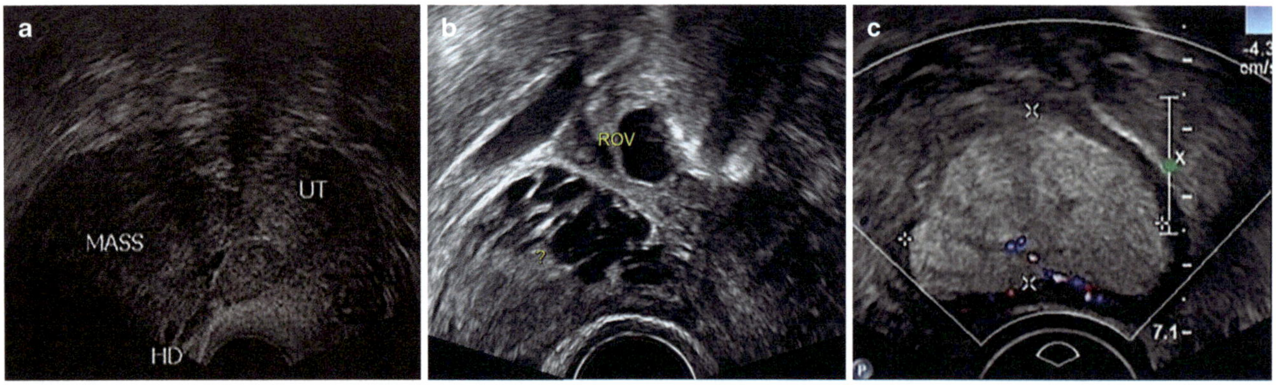

Fig. 2.53 Ultrasound Diagnosis of Broad ligament fibroids. (**a**) broad ligament fibroids; (**b**) broad ligament fibroids with cystic degeneration; (**c**) broad ligament fibroids with steatosis

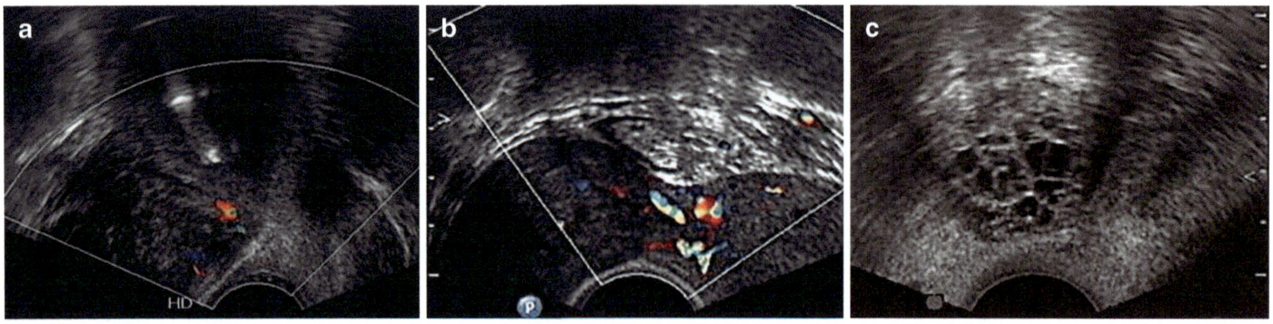

Fig. 2.54 Ultrasound Differential diagnosis of broad ligament fibroids. (**a**) Pedunculated subserosal fibroids; (**b**) Pedunculated subserosal fibroids (color Doppler); (**c**) Broad ligament adenomyoma

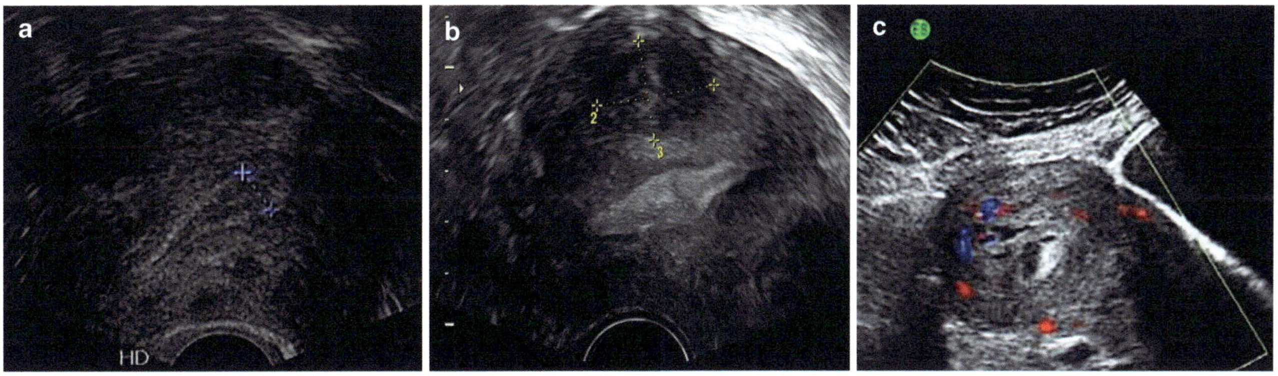

Fig. 2.55 Ultrasound Diagnosis and identification of diffuse uterine leiomyomatosis. (**a**) multiple uterine fibroids; (**b**) multiple intramural fibroids; (**c**) endometrial stromal sarcoma

Differential Diagnosis

- **Multiple uterine fibroids:** The uterus is enlarged, the echo is uneven, the fibroids have complete capsules, with typical spiral or palisade-like structures, and their boundaries with the myometrium are clear (Fig. 2.55b).
- **Intravenous leiomyomatosis (IVL):** IVL patients are mostly between 40 and 50 years old. More than half of these fibroids have extrauterine growth, mostly involving the broad ligament vein. A few extend to the inferior vena cava and the heart and tend to recur after surgery.
- **Endometrial stromal sarcoma:** It is an enlarged uterus with an irregular shape and at different locations of the uterus. When it is larger, both the uterine cavity and the myometrium can be involved. The location of the lesion can change with the progression of the disease, and the boundary with the myometrial layer is unclear. The US scan shows uniform (Fig. 2.55c) or mixed echoes.
- **Myometrial hypertrophy:** The uterus is enlarged, and the myometrium is diffusely thickened, but no nodular manifestations are present.
- **Adenomyosis:** It shows diffuse thickening of the myometrium. The adenomyoma is visible as a hypoechoic structure with minimal mass effect and has no obvious boundary with the myometrium [17].

2.3.7 Uterine Angioleiomyomatosis

2.3.7.1 US Manifestation

Fibroids are commonly seen as benign smooth muscle tumors of the uterus. Smooth muscle tumors with unusual growth patterns are rare and include three primary neoplasms: intravenous leiomyomatosis (IVL), benign metastasizing leiomyoma (BML), and disseminated peritoneal leiomyomatosis (DPL). DPL is a rare benign disease, often presenting metastatic ovarian or peritoneal carcinoma. Its risk of malignant transformation is 2–5%. According to the WHO (2014) histological classification of female reproductive organ tumors, uterine venous angioleiomyomatosis has adverse biological behaviors such as invasive growth and easy recurrence along the uterine vein and the iliac vein, sometimes involving the inferior vena cava. A few tumors can spread to the right atrium and pulmonary artery. The disease usually occurs in 40–50 years old. It is divided into three types according to the shape and distribution of the tumor: (1) Solid type, solid hypoechoic mass in the uterine body, or paracervical location, in which many thick-walled blood vessels of different sizes are found (Figure 2.56a); (2) Venous type, beaded multiple nodules running along the uterine vein; (3) Active thrombotic type, the mass runs along the uterine vein in a cord shape. Figure 2.56b shows the recurrence of uterine venous angioleiomyomatosis after hysterectomy, and multiple hypoechoic masses are seen in the pelvis (Fig. 2.56c).

2.3.7.2 Differential Diagnosis

- **Uterine fibroid:** Solid-type uterine venous angioleiomyomatosis occurs in the cervix and parametrial region and must be differentiated from cervical fibroids, uterine subserosal fibroids, and broad ligament fibroids. Cleft-like anechoic patterns are often seen in the former mass, CDFI: venous blood flow can be measured. The venous type and active thrombosis type often show echoes of the tumor in the venous lumen, while uterine fibroids do not have this feature.
- **Ovarian tumor:** Solid uterine venous angioleiomyomatosis can be manifested as a solid mass in the adnexal area, which needs to be differentiated from ovarian tumors. Multiple internal cleft anechoic tumors must be differentiated from ovarian tumors derived from sex cords (Fig. 2.56c). At the same time, the former can detect normal-shaped ovarian tissue on both sides through careful observation, and the use of transvaginal ultrasonography is helpful for the differential diagnosis between the two.

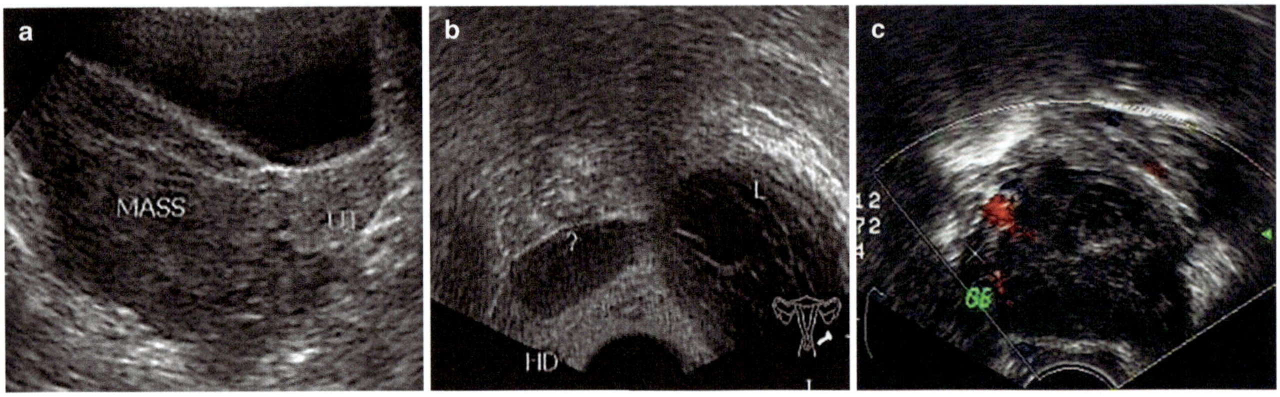

Fig. 2.56 Ultrasound Diagnosis and identification of uterine angioleiomyomatosis. (**a**) uterine Intravenous leiomyomatosis; (**b**) uterine intravenous angioleiomyomatosis; (**c**) peritoneal disseminated Peritoneal leiomyomatosis

- **Venous thrombosis:** The clinical manifestations of venous thrombosis, combined with the detection of D-dimer, are helpful for differential diagnosis.

References

1. Munro MG, Critchley HO, Broder MS, et al. FIGO classification system (PALM-COEIN) for causes of abnormal uterine bleeding in nongravid women of reproductive age. Int J Gynaecol Obstet. 2011;113(1):3–13.
2. The diagnosis and treatment of uterine fibroids by Chinese experts consensus expert group. Chin J Obstet Gynecol. 2017;12(52):793–800.
3. Zhao WP, Chen JY, Zhang L, et al. Feasibility of ultrasound-guided high intensity focused ultrasound ablating uterine fibroids with hyperintense on T2-weighted MR imaging. Eur J Radiol. 2013;82(1):e43–9.
4. Yamashita Y, Torashima M, Takahashi M, et al. Hyperintense uterine leiomyoma at T2-weighted MR imaging: differentiation with dynamic enhanced MR imaging and clinical implications [J]. Radiology. 1993;189(3):721–5.
5. Oguchi O, Mori A, Kobayashi Y, et al. Prediction of histopathologic features and proliferative activity of uterine leiomyoma by magnetic resonance imaging prior to GnRH analogue therapy: correlation between T2 weighted images and effect of GnRH analogue. J Obstet Gynaecol. 1995;21(2):107–17.
6. Shuo X, Lin Z. Clinical analysis of 42 cases of uterine fibroid red degeneration associated abdominal pain during pregnancy. J Clin Military Med. 2017;45(8):845–7.
7. Huan J, Zhang B, Zhang W, et al. CT diagnosis and differential diagnosis of huge subserous hysteromyoma. J Practical Radiol. 2010;26(9):1308–11.
8. Yen P, Khong K, Lamba R, et al. Ovarian fibromas and fibrothecomas: sonographic correlation with CT and MRI. J Ultrasound Med. 2013;32:13–8.
9. Ding CQ, Shi ZW, Dai XY. CT diagnosis of primary malignant ovarian tumors. J Chin Pract Diagnosis Ther. 2006;20(4):263–4.
10. Pannu HK, Corl FM, Fishman EK. CT evaluation of cervical cancer: spectrum of disease. Radiographics. 2001;21(5):1155–68.
11. Husband JE. CT/MRI of nodal metastases in pelvic cancer. Cancer Imaging. 2002;2:123–9.
12. Robbins JBB, et al. ACR appropriateness criteria® abnormal uterine bleeding. J Am Coll Radiol. 2020;17(11s):S336–45.
13. Woźniak A, Woźniak S. Ultrasonography of uterine fibroids. Prz Menopauzalny. 2017;16(4):113–7.
14. Timmerman D, et al. The pedicle artery sign based on sonography with color doppler imaging can replace second-stage tests in women with abnormal vaginal bleeding. Ultrasound Obstet Gynecol. 2003;22(2):166–71.
15. Murray HL, Glynn E. A case of complete fibromyomatosis of the corpus uteri. J Obstet Gynecol Br Emp. 1924;31:398–401.
16. Lapan B, Solomon L. Diffuse fibroidtosis of the uterus precluding myomectomy. Obstet Gynecol. 1979;53:82–4.
17. Sakhel K, Abuhamad A. Sonography of adenomyosis. J Ultrasound Med. 2012;31:805–8.

Imaging Diagnosis of Adenomyosis (Adenomyoma)

3

Lixia Yang, Felix Wong, Yonghua Xu, Zhongxiang Fu, and Liqun Sun

Abstract

The presence of ectopic endometrial glands within the myometrium and the clinical features of adenomyosis are described. The MRI, CT, and transvaginal US (TVUS) findings of adenomyoma and diffuse adenomyosis are illustrated. MRI presents an accurate diagnosis, especially T2-weighted sequences that highlight the uterine zonal anatomy. The ultrasonic tips for diagnosing adenomyosis and distinguishing it from various mimics are described by TVUS.

Keywords

MRI · CT · Transvaginal US · Adenomyoma Adenomyosis · Uterus · Diagnosis

The clinical signs and symptoms of adenomyosis (adenomyoma) are similar to those of uterine fibroids. Its comorbidity is the same as uterine fibroids in some cases, so it is difficult to diagnose solely based on clinical signs and symptoms. Pathological diagnosis has always been the gold standard in diagnosing adenomyosis. With the rapid development of high-resolution imaging technologies, the diagnostic accuracy of suspected adenomyosis can be improved with the help of clinical symptoms, imaging, and other non-surgical examinations. The diagnosis and differential diagnosis can be achieved with imaging examinations, which will be instrumental in formulating therapeutic regimens, determining the range and extent of lesions, and investigating the relationship between lesions and symptoms. The therapeutic effects of conservative treatment can be monitored dynamically. At present, MRI and ultrasound, especially transvaginal ultrasound, are the ideal non-invasive methods for the diagnosis of adenomyosis. This chapter mainly introduces the application of MRI, CT, and ultrasound in adenomyosis.

L. Yang (✉) · Y. Xu · Z. Fu
Zhongshan-Xuhui Hospital, Fudan University, Shanghai, China

F. Wong
The University of New South Wales, Sydney, NSW, Australia

L. Sun
Department of Ultrasound, International Peace Maternity & Child Health Hospital, School of Medicine, Shanghai Jiao Tong University, Shanghai, China

3.1 MRI Diagnosis of Adenomyosis (Adenomyoma)

Adenomyosis, also known as endometriosis interna, is a benign disease in which ectopic endometrial tissue invades and grows in the uterine myometrium due to some factors, usually accompanied by the proliferation and hypertrophy of adjacent smooth muscle cells. According to the different growth patterns of adenomyosis, it can be classified as diffuse and focal types. The latter is often nodular, also known as adenomyoma, usually solitary with ill-defined boundary and without a pseudocapsule. The smaller adenomyoma does not change the normal uterine shape generally. Larger adenomyoma can cause a localized bulge of the body of uterus on one side. The clinical manifestations of patients with adenomyosis are similar to those with uterine leiomyoma, such as menorrhagia and prolonged menstruation. It also presented as dysmenorrhea with progressive severity, mainly due to the invasion of the endometrium into uterine myometrium and repeated bleeding of endometrium growing in myometrium during menstruation. The gynecological examination can find a homogeneous enlarged uterus or localized nodule, hard, tenderness, especially during the menstrual period. The significantly elevated serum CA125 also suggests the possibility of this disease. However, it is difficult to diagnose it clinically due to the lack of specificity and the simultaneous occurrence of many other gynecological diseases. MRI findings include: (1) The lesion is diffuse

Y. Xu et al. (eds.), *Surgical Techniques of Focused Ultrasound Ablation in Benign Uterine Diseases*,
https://doi.org/10.1007/978-981-19-7180-8_3

with an ill-defined boundary, (2) the thickness of the junction region is more than 12 mm, (3) the endometrial-myometrial interface is fussy, (4) multiple hyperintense signal spots are in the lesions on T1WI and T2WI, and (5) the morphology of uterus is smooth. These signs suggest the diagnosis of adenomyosis. Therefore, MRI examination is currently recognized as a reliable non-invasive modality for diagnosing adenomyosis.

3.1.1 Adenomyosis

3.1.1.1 MRI Findings

Routine T1WI imaging has great significance for the diagnosis of adenomyosis. Adenomyosis usually presents a slightly homogeneous low signal, with characteristic millet, scattered spotty (Fig. 3.1a), or patchy (Fig. 3.1g) hyperintensity, suggesting spotty bleeding within the ectopic endometrial tissue.

The sagittal view of adenomyosis is best on T2WI imaging. Usually, the pathway showing ectopic endometrium from the uterine cavity to the uterine wall is morphologically changed. The adjacent junction region is blurred, with the endometrial-myometrial thickness ≥ 12 mm. Adenomyosis shows diffuse growth without pseudocapsule, and the boundary is not well-defined. It can accumulate on one side of the body of uterus, accompanied by hyperplasia and hypertrophy of adjacent muscular tissue (Fig. 3.1h, i). It can involve both sides of the body of the uterus or even the entire myometrium (Fig. 3.1b, c). When the size of adenomyosis is small, the normal uterine morphology is generally not changed (Fig. 3.1m, n). When the adenomyosis is large, there will be a localized bulge over the uterine body or present with a homogeneous or spherical enlargement of the uterus (Fig. 3.1h, i). Adenomyosis usually shows relatively regular high and low mixed signals on T2WI imaging, of which the high signal is the bleeding spots (Fig. 3.1i, o).

DWI functional imaging has a certain specificity in diagnosing adenomyosis compared with uterine fibroids. Its signal characteristics are usually isointense or slightly hypointense relative to the myometrium, and slightly hyperintense punctate hemorrhages can be seen (Fig. 3.1d, j, p).

Due to adenomyosis's relatively small bleeding spots and the influence of MRI volume effect, T1WI contrast enhancement of adenomyosis usually shows relatively uniform iso-intensity (Fig. 3.1e), with some non-perfusion hypointense hemorrhage (Fig. 3.1k, l). At the same time, because adenomyosis originates from the invasion of the intima into the muscle layer, as well as the differences in the growth size and location of adenomyosis, the relatively insignificant differences in high and low signal between the normal muscle layer and the adenomyosis area can be seen in the early enhancement stage, and some of them show slightly lower signal (Fig. 3.1f) and part of it are shown as a slightly higher signal relative to the muscle layer (Fig. 3.1q, r).

3.1.2 Adenomyoma

3.1.2.1 MRI Findings

The imaging features of adenomyoma on routine T1WI are similar to those of adenomyosis. Adenomyoma showed a slightly uniform iso-low signal overall, and characteristic miliary or patchy hyperintense hemorrhages were seen in it (Fig. 3.2a, d).

T2WI imaging shows some differences between adenomyoma and adenomyosis. Adenomyoma usually has relatively limited growth and seems to have some fussy boundaries but no obvious pseudocapsule (Fig. 3.2b, e). Adenomyoma is usually solitary, quasi-round, or oval in appearance. Usually, it involves only one side of the body of the uterus, without replacing the entire myometrium, and without significant hyperplasia or hypertrophy in the adjacent tissues (Fig. 3.2j). The signal characteristics of adenomyoma on T2WI imaging are similar to those of adenomyosis, which is usually homogeneously low signal, with relatively regular scattered high-signal bleeding spots (Fig. 3.2e, f).

The signals on functional DWI imaging (Fig. 3.2c, g) and contrast enhanced T1WI imaging (Fig. 3.2h, m, n, o) are similar to adenomyosis.

3.1.2.2 Differential Diagnosis

- **Uterine fibroids:** Uterine adenomyoma is not difficult to distinguish from common uterine fibroids, and T1WI imaging features can easily distinguish the two. Uterine fibroids appear as characteristic punctate or small patchy hyperintense hemorrhagic foci on T1WI, whereas uterine fibroids usually appear homogeneous isointense on T1WI. On T2WI imaging, the characteristics of adenomyoma are mostly distributed in high-signal bleeding areas. At the same time, the uterine fibroids are relatively uniform isointensity, with some areas of flake or patchy high-intensity cystic degeneration and necrosis. Moreover, the two also show similar differences in DWI functional imaging.

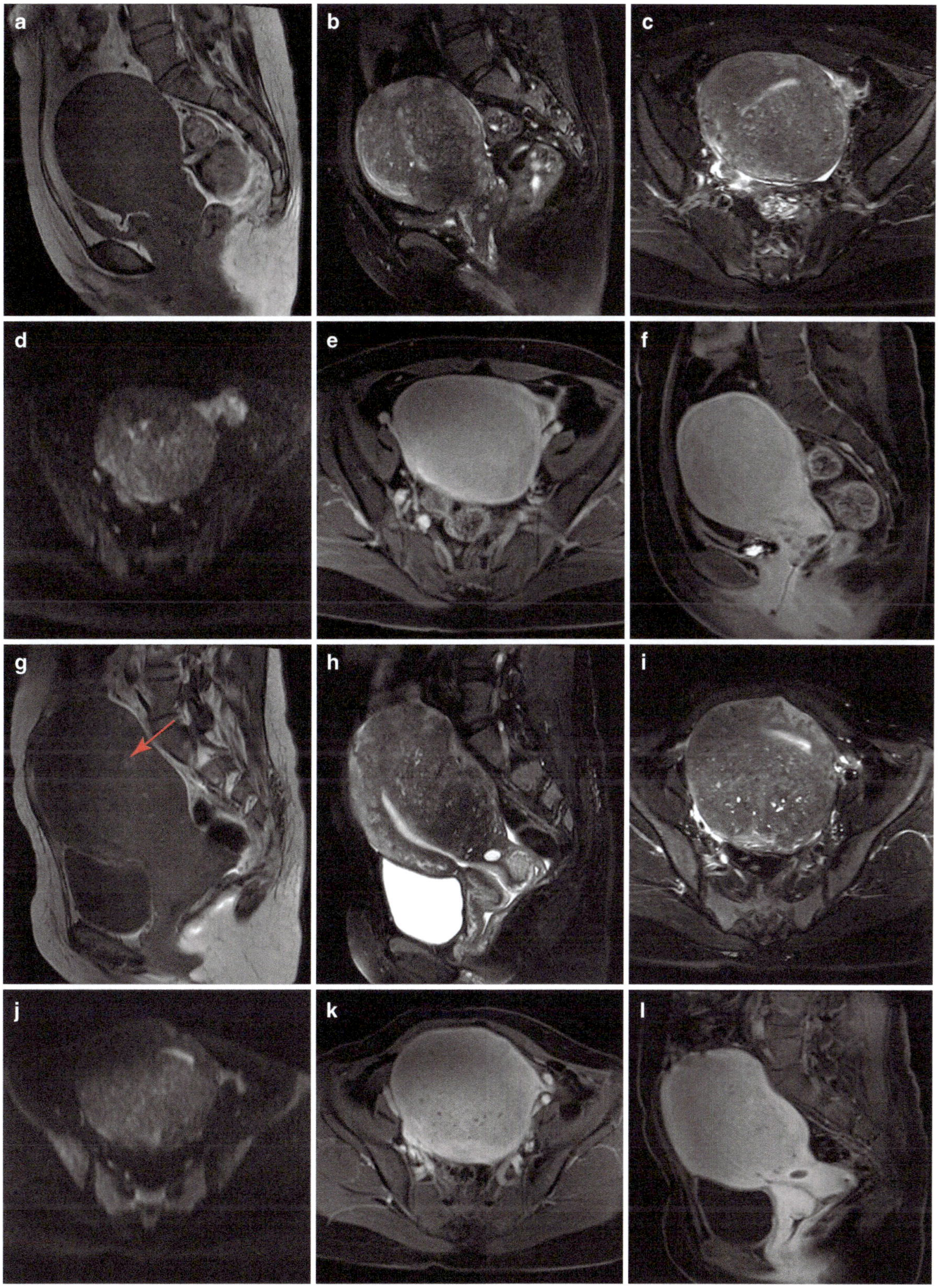

Fig. 3.1 MRI findings of adenomyosis. (**a**) T1WI sagittal; (**b**) T2WI_FS sagittal; (**c**) T2WI_FS axial; (**d**) DWI axial (b = 800 s/mm^2); (**e**) T1WI_FS + C axial; (**f**) T1WI_FS + C sagittal; (**g**) T1WI sagittal; (**h**) T2WI_FS sagittal; (**i**) T2WI_FS axial; (**j**) DWI axial (b = 800 s/mm^2); (**k**) T1WI_FS + C axial; (**l**) T1WI_FS + C sagittal; (**m**). T2WI_FS sagittal; (**n**) T1WI axial; (**o**) T2WI_FS axial; (**p**). DWI axial (b = 800 s/mm^2); (**q**) T1WI_FS + C axial; (**r**) T1WI_FS + C sagittal

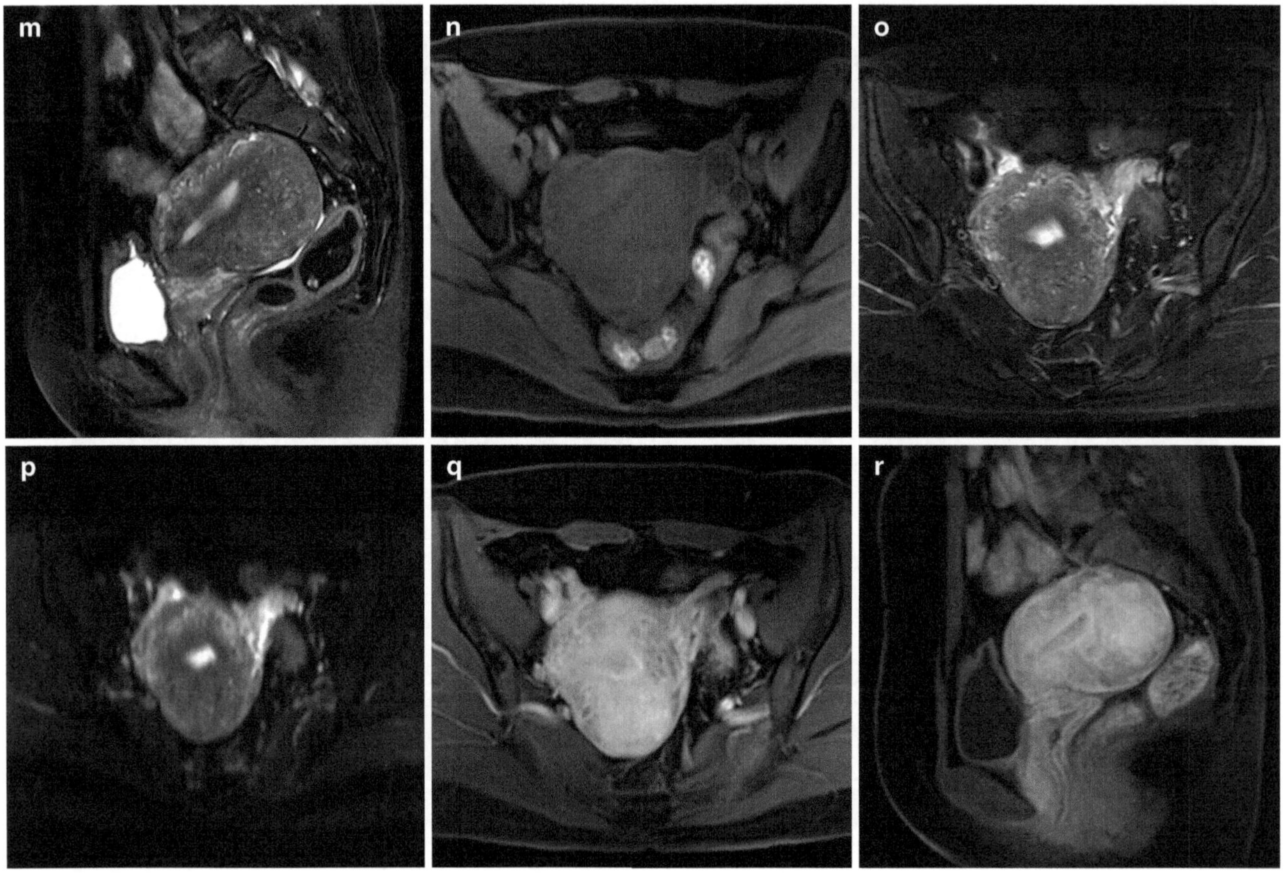

Fig. 3.1 (continued)

3.1.3 Adenomyosis (Adenomyoma) Combined with Uterine Fibroids

Studies have shown that about 30% of patients with adenomyosis (adenomyoma) also have uterine fibroids, and there is no significant correlation between adenomyosis (adenomyoma) and fibroids. It is not difficult to distinguish them by MRI diagnosis [1, 2].

3.1.3.1 MRI Findings

Routine T1WI imaging can clearly show the typical signal characteristics of adenomyosis (adenomyoma) but is insensitive to comorbid uterine fibroids that usually shows relatively homogeneous uniform iso-signal (Fig. 3.3a).

T2WI imaging can clearly show the signal characteristics of adenomyosis (adenomyoma) and concomitant fibroids. The concomitant uterine fibroids are of different types, including submucosal, intermuscular, or subserosal fibroids or multiple fibroids (Fig. 3.3).

The signal characteristics of T2WI imaging, functional DWI imaging, and contrast enhanced T1WI imaging between adenomyosis (adenomyoma) and comorbid uterine fibroids are similar to those between fibroids and adenomyosis (adenomyoma), and there is no significant correlation between the two (Fig. 3.4).

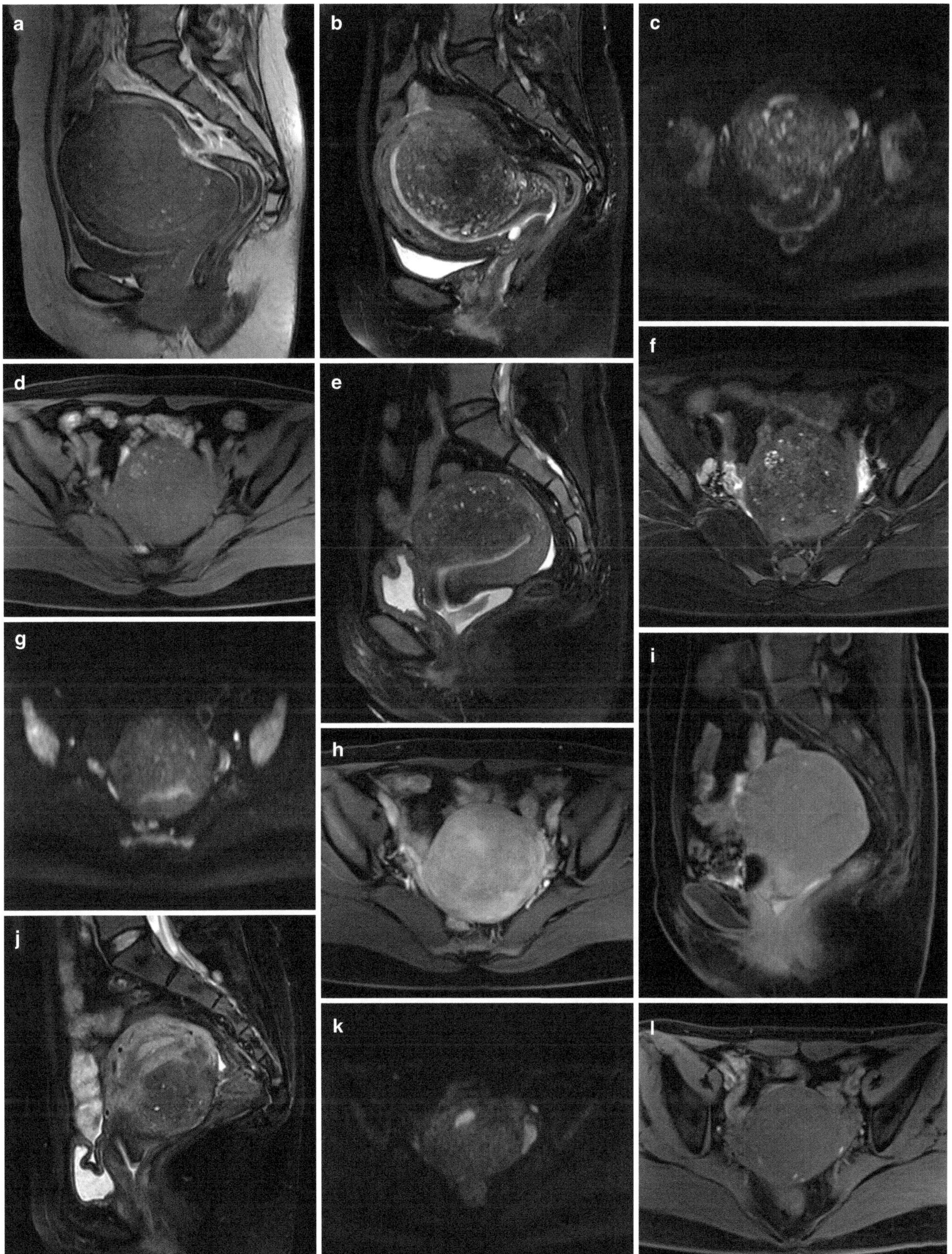

Fig. 3.2 MRI findings of adenomyoma. (**a**) T1WI sagittal; (**b**) T2WI_FS sagittal; (**c**) DWI axial (b = 800 s/mm^2); (**d**) T1WI_FS axial; (**e**) T2WI_FS sagittal; (**f**) T2WI_FS axial; (**g**) DWI axial (b = 800 s/mm^2); (**h**) T1WI_FS + C axial; (**i**) T1WI_FS + C sagittal; (**j**) T2WI_FS sagittal; (**k**) DWI axial (b = 800 s/mm^2); (**l**) T1WI_FS axial; (**m**) T1WI_FS + C sagittal; (**n**) T1WI_FS + C axial; (**o**) T1WI_FS + C coronal

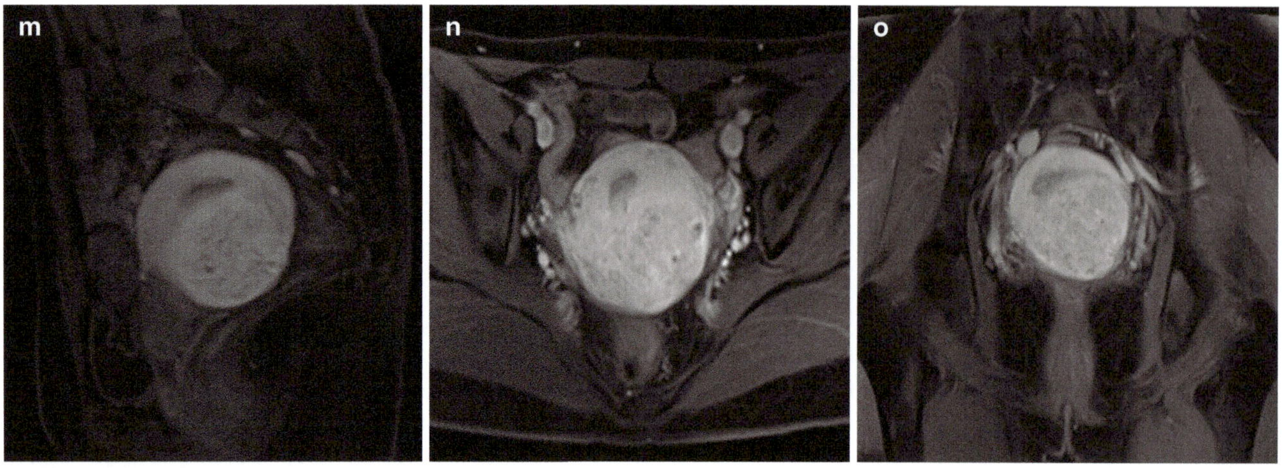

Fig. 3.2 (continued)

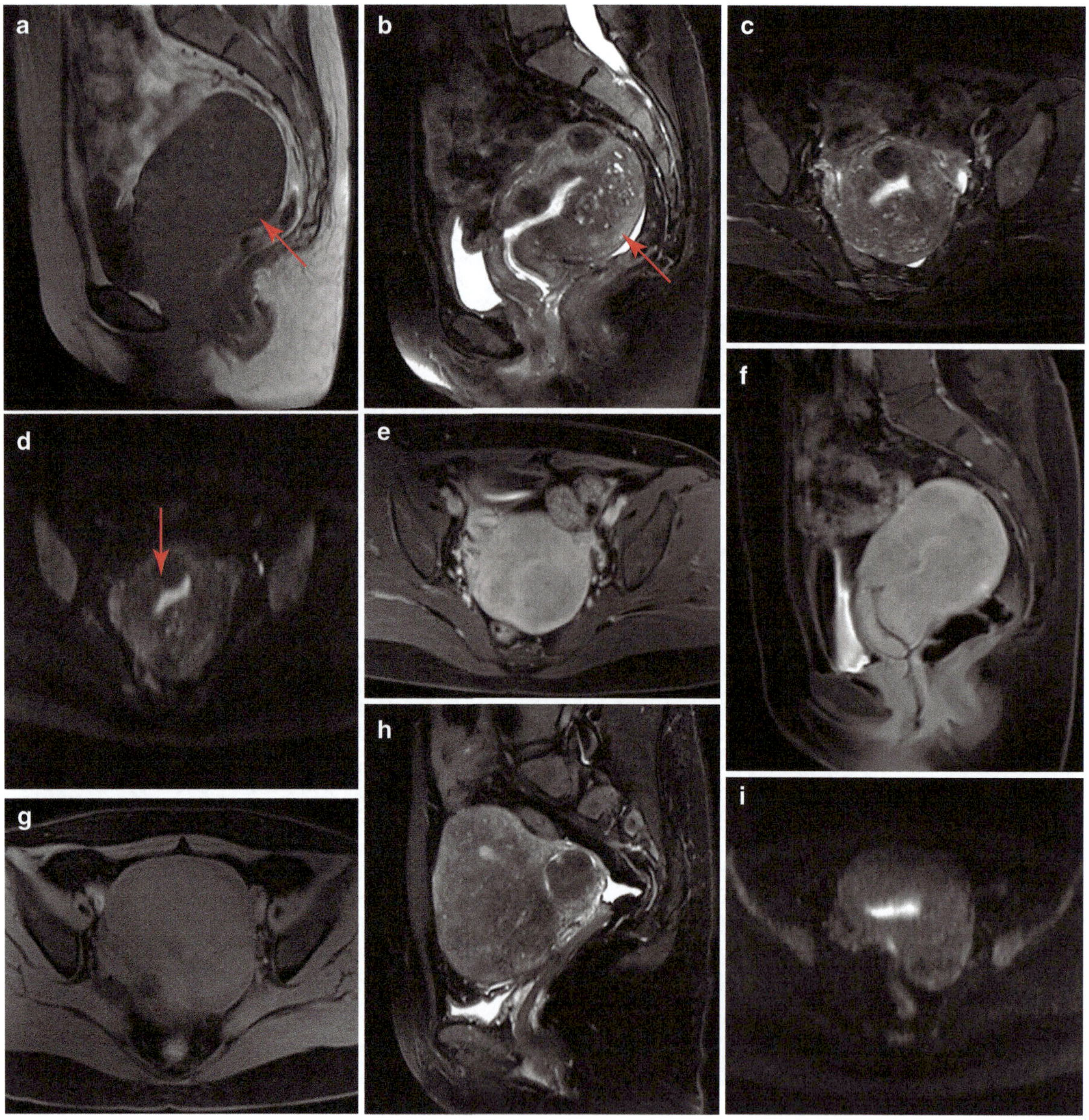

Fig. 3.3 MRI findings of adenomyosis combined with uterine fibroids. (**a**) T1WI sagittal; (**b**) T2WI_FS sagittal; (**c**) T2WI_FS axial; (**d**) DWI axial ($b = 800$ s/mm^2); (**e**) T1WI_FS + C axial; (**f**) T1WI_FS + C sagittal; (**g**) T1WI axial; (**h**) T2WI_FS axial; (**i**) DWI axial (b = 800 s/mm^2); (**j**) T2WI_FS axial; (**k**) T1WI_FS + C sagittal; (**l**) T1WI_FS + C axial; (**m**) T1WI_FS axial; (**n, o**) T2WI_FS sagittal

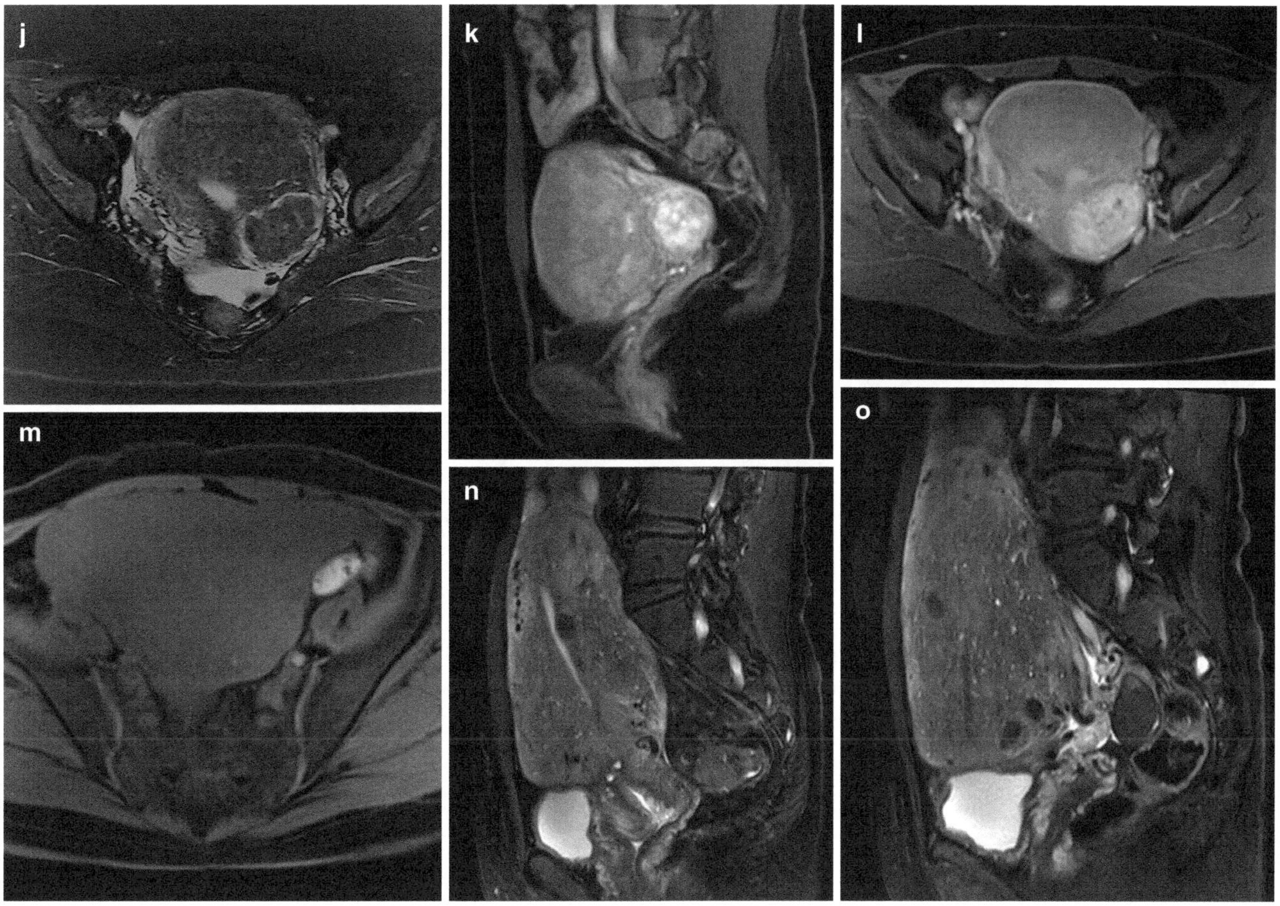

Fig. 3.3 (continued)

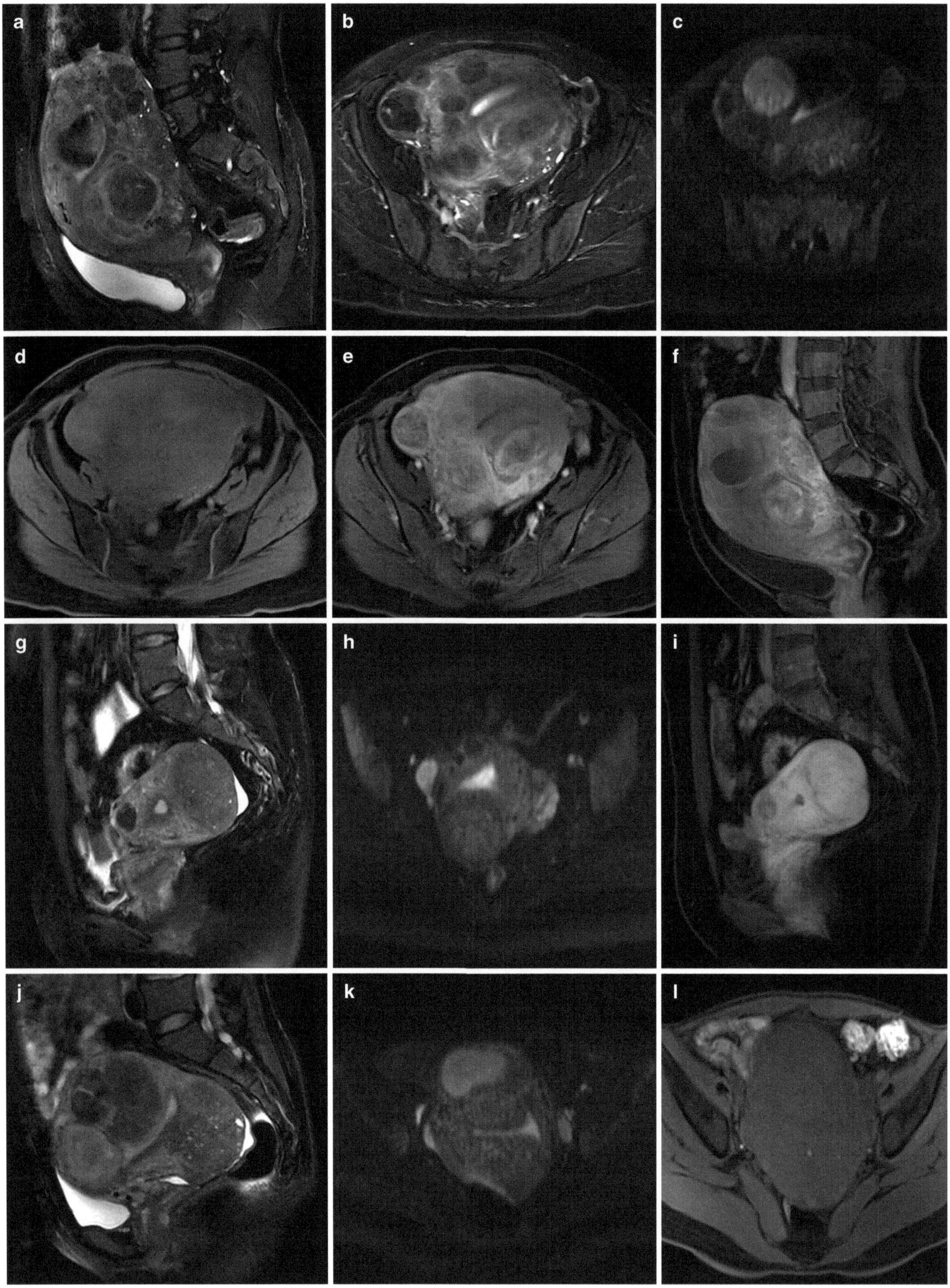

Fig. 3.4 MRI findings of adenomyoma combined with uterine fibroids. (**a**) T2WI_FS sagittal; (**b**) T2WI_FS axial; (**c**) DWI axial (b = 800 s/mm^2); (**d**) T1WI_FS axial; (**e**) T1WI_FS + C axial; (**f**) T1WI_FS + C sagittal; (**g**) T2WI_FS sagittal; (**h**) DWI axial (b = 800 s/mm^2); (**i**) T1WI_FS + C sagittal; (**j**) T2WI_FS sagittal; (**k**) DWI axial (b = 800 s/mm^2); (**l**) T1WI_FS axial

3.2 CT Diagnosis of Adenomyosis (Adenomyoma)

It is difficult to identify and diagnose adenomyosis and adenomyoma by CT. Although the advanced CT imaging has higher tissue resolution, the typical punctate or patchy high-signal hemorrhagic foci on T1WI imaging cannot be observed in CT imaging.

3.2.1 CT Findings

1. **Plain CT scan:** Adenomyosis (adenomyoma) usually manifests as irregular or diffuse homogeneous enlargement of the body of the uterus, thickened uterine wall, and homogeneous signal density in the uterus, without well-defined boundaries or pseudocapsule (Fig. 3.5a, c, e).
2. **Contrast Enhanced CT scan:** Adenomyosis (adenomyoma) shows inhomogeneous density and inhomogeneous enhancement in the myometrium on the contrast enhanced CT scan, with scattered speckled low-density foci and localized nodules with inhomogeneous enhancement density and speckled low-density areas (Fig. 3.5b, d, f).

3.2.2 Differential Diagnosis

- **Endometrial cancer:** Irregular thickening lesion in the uterine cavity has abnormal enhancement on the contrast enhanced CT. It is commonly seen in older women with a history of vaginal bleeding.
- **Liquefaction and necrosis of uterine fibroids:** Most of the necrotic areas show water-like density, and the remaining parenchymal part is enhanced synchronously with the normal myometrium on the contrast enhanced CT.

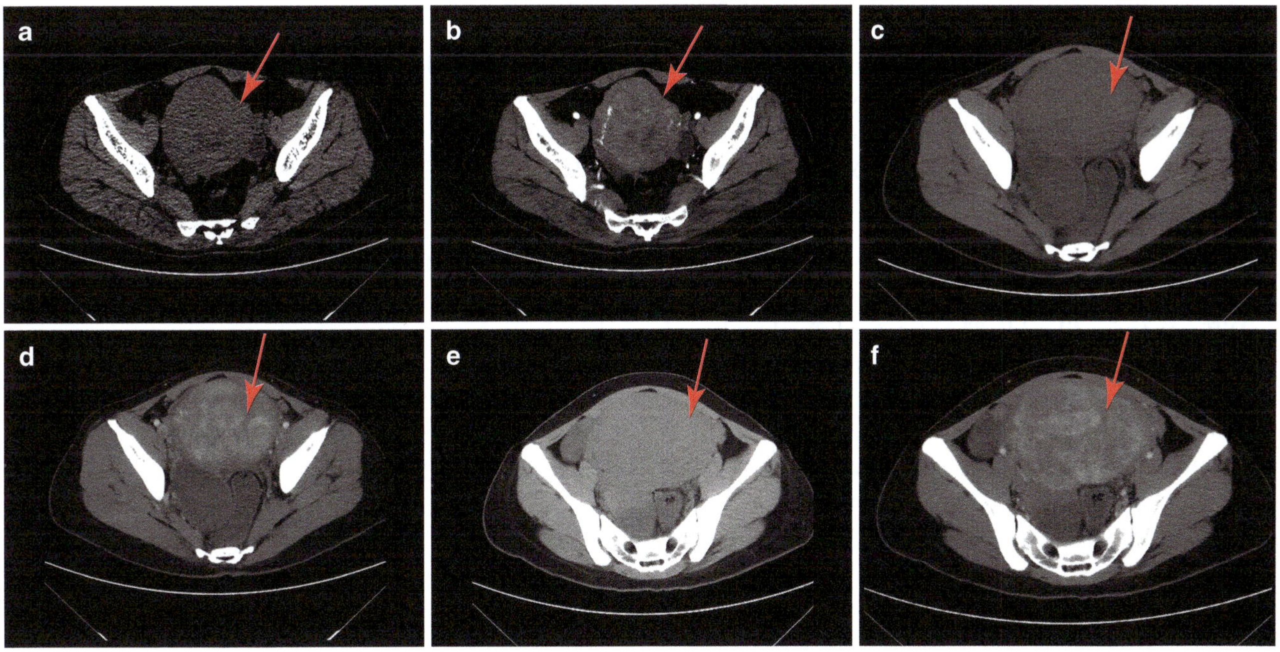

Fig. 3.5 CT findings of adenomyosis (adenomyoma). **(a/c/e)** Plain CT scan, axial; **(b/d/f)** Contrast enhanced CT scan, axial

3.3 Ultrasound Diagnosis of Adenomyosis

Adenomyosis is a benign uterine disease caused by Endometriosis, which could cause menorrhagia and dysmenorrhea. Adenomyosis usually affects most of the myometrium, common in the posterior wall, and the cervix is not easily immersed. Although the uterus is significantly enlarged, its overall outline is usually maintained, and in some cases, adenomyosis can form a localized mass called adenomyoma. Cystic adenomyosis is rare and is thought to result from repeated focal bleeding that fills the cyst with blood.

3.3.1 Diffuse Adenomyosis

3.3.1.1 US Manifestation

The uterus is enlarged and full of shape, with obvious thickening of the posterior wall of the uterus, and sometimes around the endometrium can be observed Hypoechoic halo ≥12 mm (Fig. 3.6a). Diffuse echogenicity in the inner myometrium could be symmetry and asymmetry. Endometrial echo was linear or nodular (Fig. 3.6b), myometrial hypertrophy and thickening, and the island-shaped endometrial echo were also seen. The "louvered" sign may be a linear streak formed by the proliferative reaction of the intimal tissue (Fig. 3.6c).

3.3.1.2 Differential Diagnosis

- **Diffuse uterine fibroids:** The uterus is diffusely enlarged, and the myometrium is covered with numerous small fibroids with unclear boundaries, most of which are less than 3 cm in diameter.
- **Myometrial hypertrophy:** The uterus is enlarged, and the myometrium is diffusely thickened, which is symmetrical, and there is no obvious uneven echo.

3.3.2 Adenomyoma of Uterus

3.3.2.1 US Manifestation

The uterus was enlarged to varying degrees, and it could be spherical, and a few were heterogeneously enlarged with morphological changes. The lesions are mostly located in the posterior wall. The myometrium is obviously thickened. The uterine cavity line is often arcuate due to the thickening of the posterior wall, without obvious vortex-like structure and no obvious sound attenuation. Uterine adenomyoma is mostly irregular in shape, with unclear boundary, no obvious demarcation with myometrium, and uneven internal echo (Fig. 3.7a). Color Doppler only shows scattered punctate blood flow.

3.3.2.2 Differential Diagnosis

- **Uterine intramural fibroid:** Adenomyoma has no pseudocapsule, no vortex-like structure inside, blood flow comes from normal uterine blood vessels, and there is no annular or semi-circular blood flow around the mass (Fig. 3.7b); it is necessary to observe the internal echo and the relationship with the surrounding tissues and the characteristics of blood flow signals and distinguish them based on the medical history.

The demarcation between malignant uterine tumor and the myometrium is unclear, the internal echo is uniform, or there are mixed echoes due to hemorrhage, necrosis, or cystic change, and CDFI shows that the mass is rich in strips and dendritic blood flow (Fig. 3.7c).

3.3.3 Adenomyosis Cyst

3.3.3.1 US Manifestation

Intramyometrial cyst or endometrial cyst has an uneven echo in the myometrium with a small anechoic area that can be

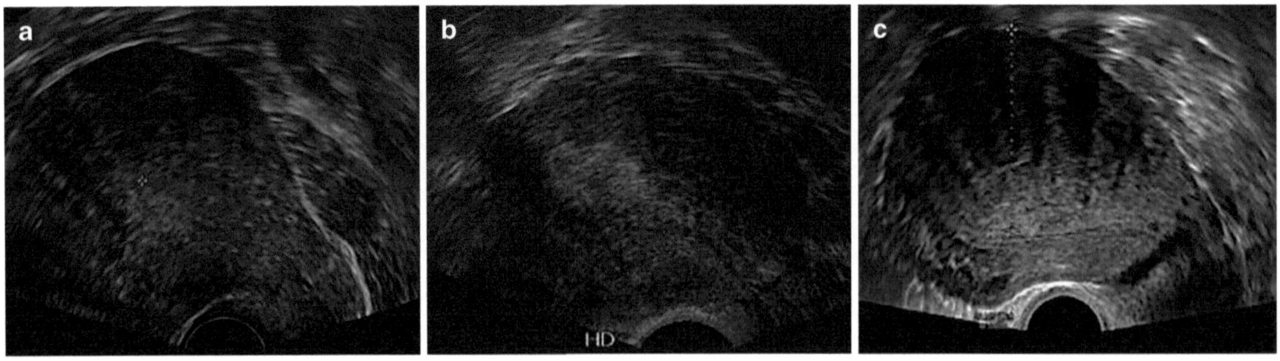

Fig. 3.6 Ultrasound Diagnosis of Adenomyosis. (**a**) Diffuse adenomyosis; (**b**) Diffuse adenomyosis (anterior); (**c**) Diffuse adenomyosis (posterior)

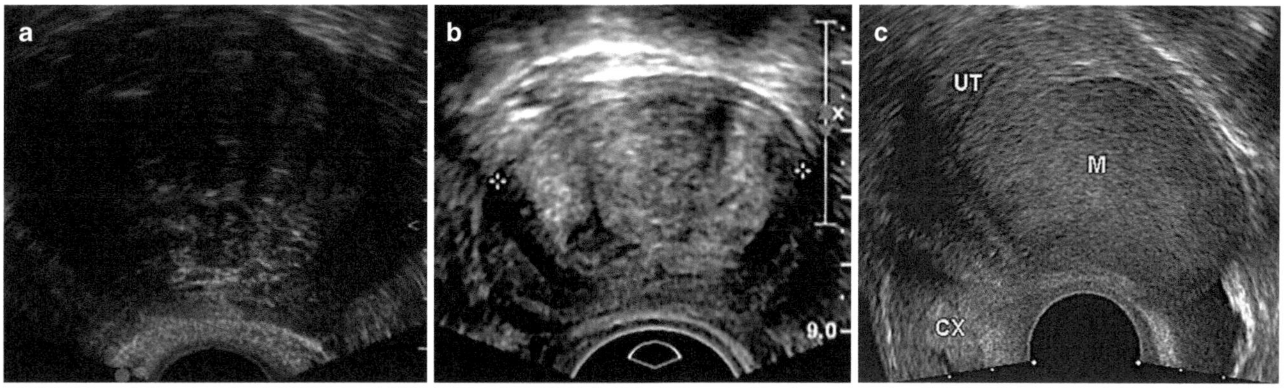

Fig. 3.7 Ultrasound Diagnosis and identification of adenomyoma of the uterus. (**a**) adenomyoma; (**b**) intramural fibroids; (**c**) endometrial stromal sarcoma

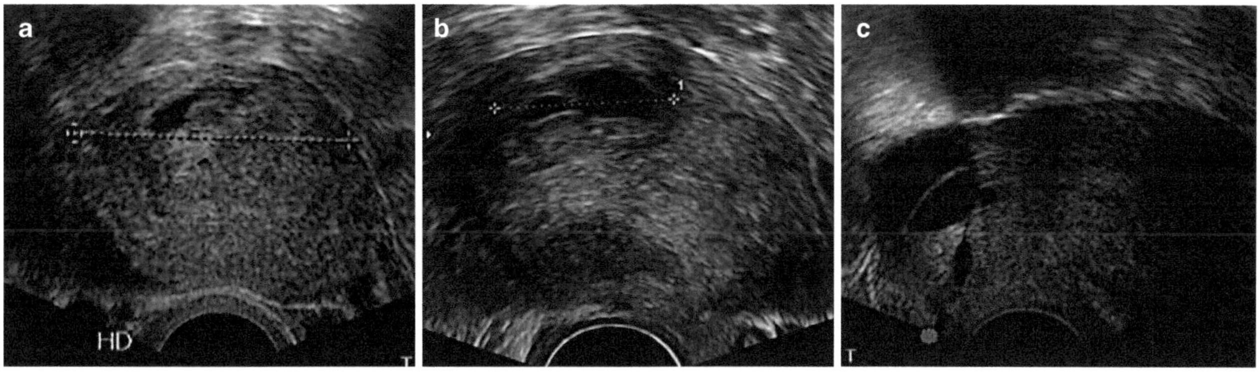

Fig. 3.8 Ultrasound Diagnosis and identification of adenomyosis cyst. (**a**) adenomyosis cyst; (**b**) cystic degeneration of intramural fibroids; (**c**) cesarean section scar diverticulum

seen like a honeycomb (Fig. 3.8a). The cyst wall is slightly thicker and is smooth. There is no separation, and it is filled with dense point-like echoes, and the peripheral blood flow signals are seen.

3.3.3.2 Differential Diagnosis

- **Uterine fibroids with cystic degeneration:** Cystic degeneration of uterine fibroids has an uneven inner wall, with many divisions in the cyst (Fig. 3.8b), and the blood flow signal is rich and semi-circular.
- **Cesarean section scar:** The lesions of the diverticulum are located in the muscle layer of the anterior uterine wall isthmus. The patient has a history of cesarean section. One or more anechoic areas, connected or non-connected to the uterine cesarean scars, can be seen, which may or may not communicate with the uterine cavity (Fig. 3.8c). The diagnosis is easier to make with the medical history and clinical symptoms.

References

1. Scarperi S, Pontrelli G, Campana C, et al. Laparoscopic radiofrequency thermal ablation for uterine adenomyosis. JSLS. 2015;19(4):00071.
2. Yavuzcan A, Caglar M, Ustün Y, et al. Evaluation of the outcomes of laparoscopic hysterectomy for normal and enlarged uterus (>280 g). Arch Gynecol Obstet. 2014;289(4):831–7.

Focused Ultrasound Ablation for Uterine Fibroids

4

Yonghua Xu, Lixia Yang, Yu Cheng, and Felix Wong

Abstract

The focused ultrasound ablation yields an encouraging therapeutic outcome for type 0-II submucosal fibroids, for which the laparatomy or/and laparoscopic surgeries have potential operative risks or tumor recurrence resulting from incomplete excision. Including the submucosal fibroids, all types of intramural uterine fibroids (type III-V), subserosal uterine fibroids with a base (≥2 cm) connecting the uterus, and special types of uterine fibroids (such as cervical uterine fibroid, broad ligament uterine fibroids, multiple uterine fibroids, diffuse uterine leiomyomatosis (DUL), and giant uterine fibroids) treated using focused ultrasound surgery are demonstrated. The therapeutic strategies, treatment techniques, focused ultrasound parameters, and MRI per-procedure assessment and posttreatment evaluation are described with a case-based approach in detail. The ablation efficacy, the corresponding outcome, and the possibility of re-treatment are discussed.

Keywords

High-intensity focused ultrasound · Ablation · Submucosal · Intramural · Subserosal · Uterine fibroids

Focused ultrasound ablation is one of the emerging treatment techniques under the minimal and non-invasiveness concept. In 2004, the FDA approved MRI-guided focused ultrasound in clinically ablation treatment of uterine fibroids. This technique has become the treatment option for uterine fibroids worldwide. Based on the non-invasiveness characteristic of focused ultrasound ablation, as well as its ability to accurately focus on the target with imaging guidance and conformal and controllable ablation, it has been originally recognized to be unsuitable or difficult to ablate various types of uterine fibroids, such as cervical myoma (special locations), uterine leiomyomatosis, giant fibroids, subserosal fibroids, broad ligament fibroids, and type 0 submucosal fibroids, but now satisfactory treatment results can be achieved. The focused ultrasound ablation of various types of uterine fibroids is described as follows.

4.1 Focused Ultrasound Ablation for Submucosal Uterine Fibroids

4.1.1 Case 1 Type 0 Submucosal Fibroid (1)

4.1.1.1 Case Description

The female patient was 41 years old without anticipating pregnancy. Two years ago, she developed prolonged menstrual periods, accompanied by increased blood volume and small amount of blood clots. She showed easy fatigue, limb weakness, and severe anemia. She had a history of several hysteroscopic operations, and recurrent submucosal fibroids were diagnosed. Focused ultrasound ablation was performed and after treatment, her symptoms of bleeding and anemia improved significantly to normal.

4.1.1.2 Pre-Treatment Assessment

MRI showed that multiple pedunculated submucosal fibroids with isointensity on T2WI were located in the uterine cavity, and the largest fibroids were about 10 mm in diameter (Fig. 4.1a). The contrast-enhanced T1WI showed that the submucosal fibroids were gradually enhanced, and the blood supply was abundant (Fig. 4.1b, c). It was difficult to predict the focused ultrasound ablation results of the pedicled submucosal myoma before treatment.

Y. Xu (✉) · L. Yang · Y. Cheng
Zhongshan-Xuhui Hospital, Fudan University, Shanghai, China

F. Wong
The University of New South Wales, Sydney, NSW, Australia

Y. Xu et al. (eds.), *Surgical Techniques of Focused Ultrasound Ablation in Benign Uterine Diseases*,
https://doi.org/10.1007/978-981-19-7180-8_4

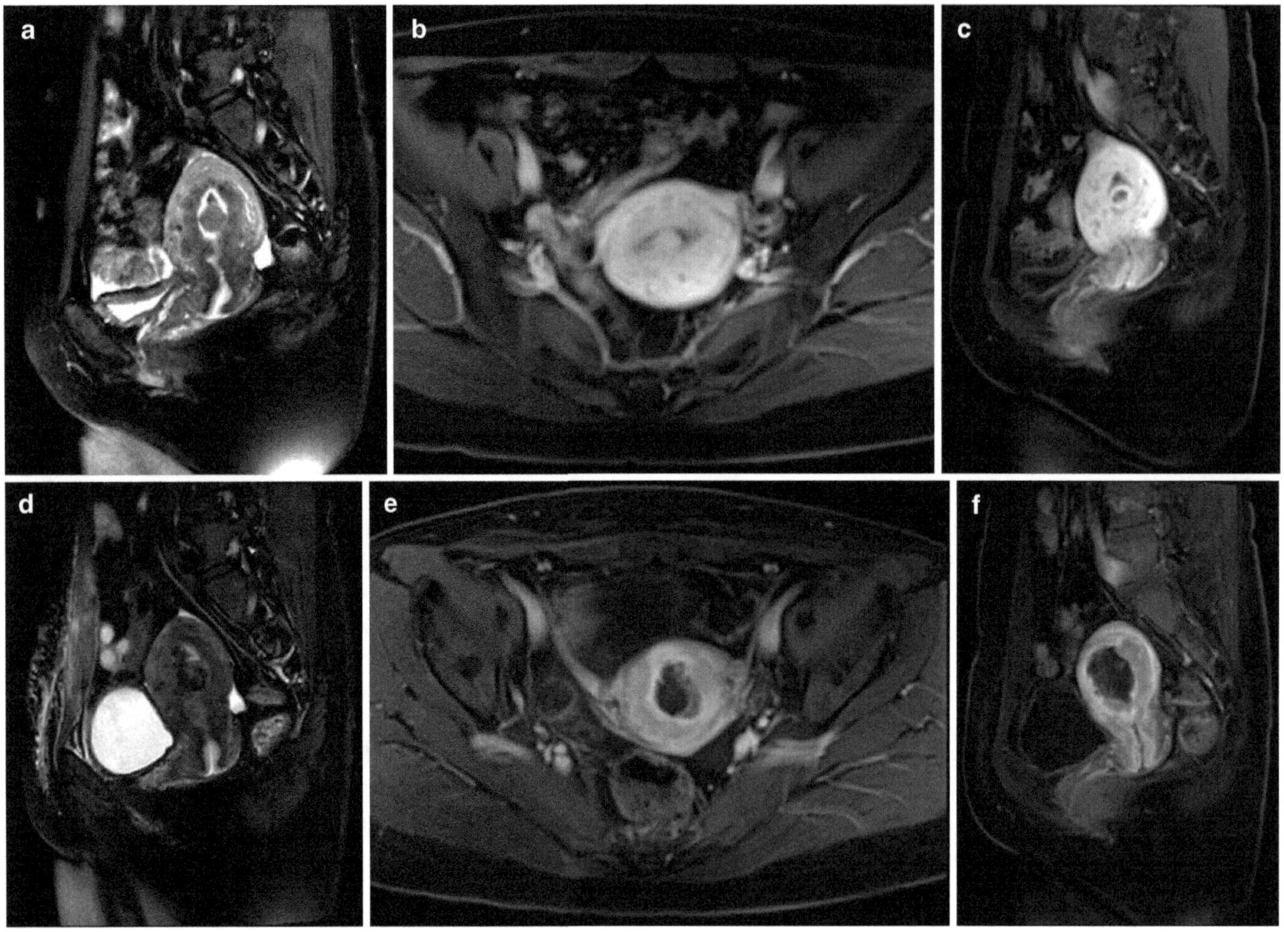

Fig. 4.1 Type 0 submucosal fibroids before treatment (**a–c**) and evaluation after treatment (**d–f**). (**a**) T2WI_FS sagittal, (**b**) T1WI_FS + C axial, (**c**) T1WI_FS + C sagittal, (**c**) T2WI_FS sagittal (**d**) T1WI_FS + C axial, (**e**) T1WI_FS + C sagittal

4.1.1.3 Treatment Techniques

1. **Focused ultrasound parameters.** Average acoustic power: 219 W, sonication time: 2703 s, duration of treatment: 153 min, total energy: 592,670 J.
2. **Focused ultrasound ablation techniques.** Generally, the energy required for ablation of submucosal fibroids is at least two times higher than that for intramural fibroids. The key to preventing the recurrence of such fibroids is to start ablation treatment from the base of the fibroids to achieve the goal of complete ablation and inactivation.

4.1.1.4 Post-Treatment Assessment

MRI Evaluation after Treatment The soft tissues of the anterior abdominal wall showed the apparent edema on T2WI with fat saturation (FS) (Fig. 4.1d). The submucosal fibroids were completely ablated, and the intima side portion of the anterior uterine wall adjacent to the fibroids was not enhanced on contrast-enhanced T1WI (Fig. 4.1e, f).

4.1.1.5 Discussion

- Uterine fibroids were located in the uterine cavity with a connecting pedicle (type 0 submucosal uterine fibroid). The most suitable treatment option should be hysteroscopic myomectomy. Since the ultrasonic mechanical shock wave during focused sonication would affect the location stability of the fibroids and might cause the focal region to move relatively, the treatment was of certain difficulty. Generally, focused ultrasound ablation is not recommended for this type of fibroid.
- This patient had a history of multiple hysteroscopic operations and was diagnosed with recurrent submucosal fibroids and severe anemia. Therefore, the aggressive strategy of focused ultrasound ablation was selected to avoid the relapses resulting in repeated operations. Based on the outcome of this case, the therapeutic effects were satisfactory.

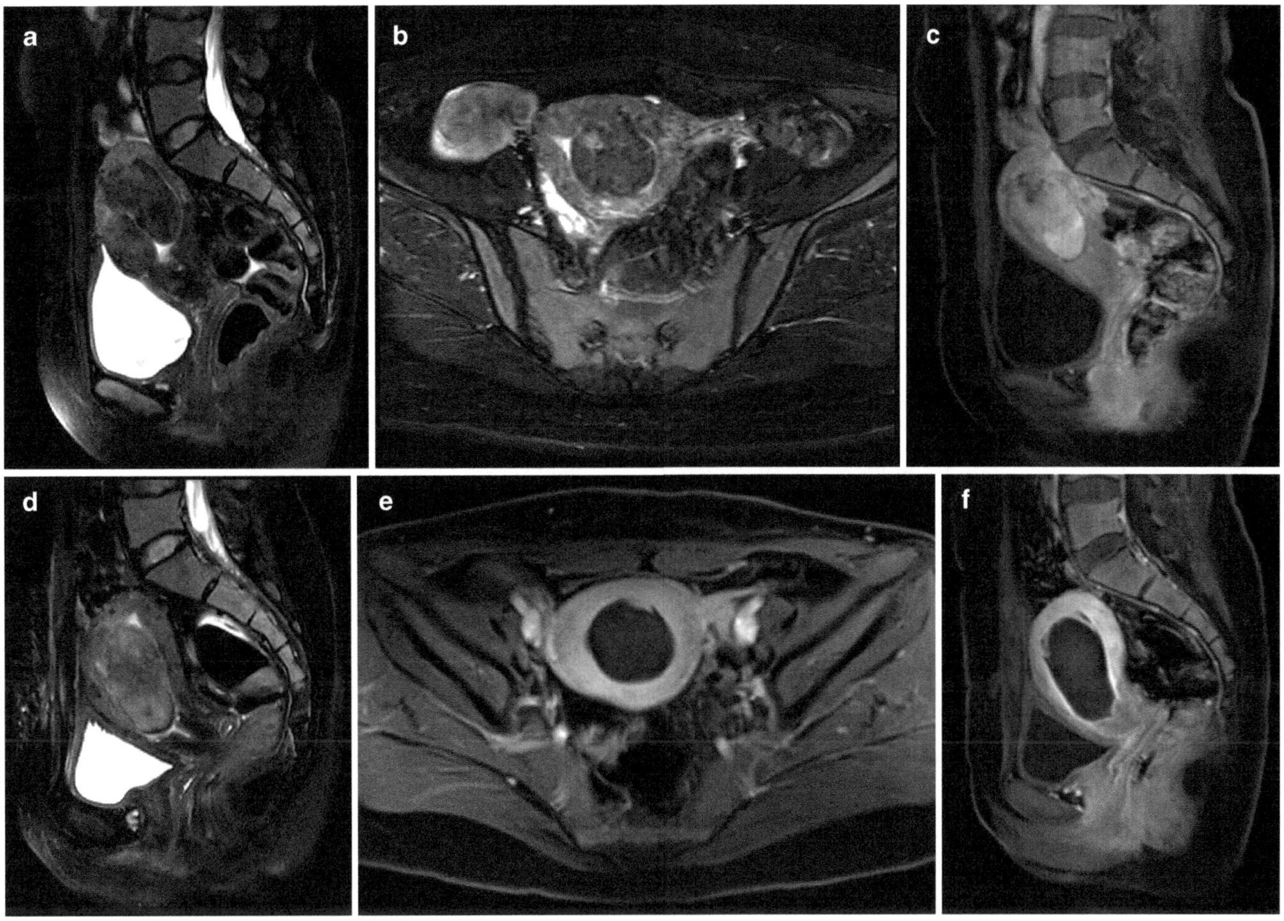

Fig. 4.2 Type 0 submucosal fibroids before treatment (**a**–**c**) and evaluation after treatment (**d**–**f**). (**a**) T2WI_FS sagittal, (**b**) T2WI_FS axial, (**c**) T1WI_FS + C axial, (**d**) T2WI_FS sagittal, (**e**) T1WI_FS + C axial, (**f**) T1WI_FS + C sagittal

4.1.2 Case 2 Type 0 Submucosal Fibroid (2)

4.1.2.1 Case Description

The female patient was 44 years old with twice the previous menstrual volumes for more than 1 year, accompanied by more blood clots. Her hemoglobin was 83 g/L, and the menstrual period was extended from 4–5 days to about 10 days. One uterine fibroid with a maximum diameter of 55 mm was found with ultrasound examination. She had anesthetic allergy and requested a nonsurgical treatment with a strong desire.

4.1.2.2 Pre-Treatment Assessment

MRI showed a pedunculated submucosal fibroid with a diameter of 54 mm and T2 hypointensity from the anterior wall into the uterine cavity (Fig. 4.2a, b). The contrast enhanced T1WI demonstrated that the type 0 submucosal fibroid with a wide pedicle had partially abundant blood supply; and it almost filled the uterine cavity, thus, its position was relatively fixed (Fig. 4.2c).

4.1.2.3 Treatment Techniques

1. **Focused ultrasound parameters.** Average acoustic power: 206 W, sonication time: 1828 seconds, duration of treatment: 78 min, total energy: 376,494 J.
2. **Focused ultrasound ablation techniques.** Because the fibroid occupying the uterine cavity was surrounded by the endometrium, the focal energy with a reduced power targeted initially the connecting base of the tumor, once the changes of ultrasonic grayscale occurred in that area, the focal regions gradually moved to the central portion of the myoma and then covered the whole volume by heating diffusion. A fully distended bladder was needed to fix the uterus in order to ensure the ablation accuracy.

4.1.2.4 Post-Treatment Assessment

MRI Evaluation after Treatment The submucosal fibroid, which had the increased signal on T2WI (Fig. 4.2d), was completely ablated with a total area of nonperfusion, and the uterine wall was intact with a little pseudoenhancement on the contrast-enhanced T1WI (Fig. 4.2e, f).

4.1.2.5 Discussion

- Most of the patients with uterine submucosal fibroids experienced severe menorrhagia followed by anemia. Although the resection of type 0 submucous fibroids under hysteroscopy remains a good choice for treatment, the indications for this patient were limited because she complained of an allergy to narcotic drugs, therefore, the focused ultrasound ablation, as a noninvasive procedure without requiring anesthesia, can be an alternative therapy.
- The treatment outcome indicated the submucosal fibroid in the uterine cavity had been complete necrosis, resulting in relief of menorrhagia. Furthermore, the necrotic tissues might be spontaneously expulsed through the vagina without complications.

4.1.3 Case 3 Type I Submucosal Fibroid (1)

4.1.3.1 Case Description

The female patient was 36 years old. She developed menorrhagia and moderate anemia for more than one year. After the ultrasound ablation, menstruation tended to be normal, and a small piece of reddish brown necrotic tissue was excluded each period.

4.1.3.2 Pre-Treatment Assessment

MRI showed that uterine fibroids expanded from the muscular layer to the uterine cavity, and the majority (>50%) were located in the uterine cavity. The largest diameter of the fibroids was about 67 mm, and the fibroids showed hypointensity on T2WI (Fig. 4.3a). The contrast-enhanced T1WI showed a rich blood supply for submucosal fibroids (Fig. 4.3b). Although the fibroids were located under the mucosa with a rich blood supply, T2WI showed that the fibroids were low-intensity and located on the uterus's anterior wall. Therefore, positive results of focused ultrasound ablation would be anticipated. However, there are many bowels between the anterior abdominal wall and the uterus, which affect the acoustic pathway of focused ultrasound (Fig. 4.3b).

4.1.3.3 Treatment Techniques

1. **Focused ultrasound parameters.** Average acoustic power: 350 W, sonication time: 1163 s, duration of treatment: 58 min, total energy: 406,870 J.
2. **Focused ultrasound ablation techniques.** The treatment target was mainly concentrated at the base of the submucosal fibroid. The purpose was to cut off the blood supply to achieve the desired ablation effect. Meanwhile, to create a clear acoustic pathway, the distended bladder and extracorporal degassed water balloon were needed to push the bowels, which lie anterior to the uterus, away from the acoustic pathway.

4.1.3.4 Post-Treatment Assessment

MRI Follow-Up at 6 Months After Treatment Most of the submucosal fibroid was discharged, and the uterus morphology returned to normal. The uterine muscle wall was intact, the endometrial lining was clear, and only a few residual fibroid tissues were visible from the lesion (Fig. 4.3c).

4.1.3.5 Discussion

- Hysteroscopic surgery or focused ultrasound ablation may be considered for type I submucosal uterine fibroids. In this case, the fibroid was large with a rich blood supply. Hysteroscopic surgery was prone to massive bleeding, and it was difficult to remove the intramural part of the fibroid.
- MRI follow-up after treatment showed that the submucosal uterine fibroid was almost completely discharged, leaving only a few residual tissues at the lesion. Focused

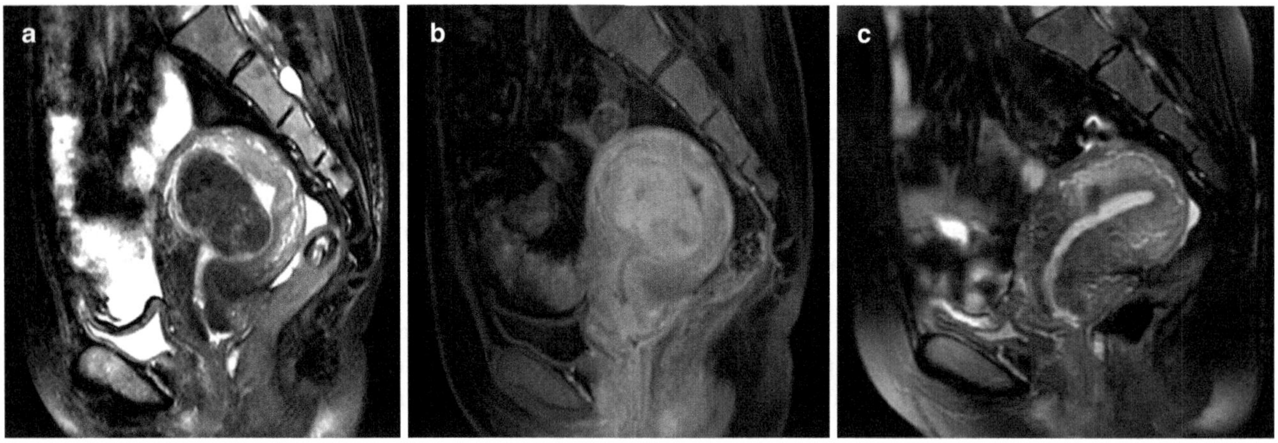

Fig. 4.3 Type I submucosal fibroid before treatment (**a**, **b**) and at 6 months after treatment (**c**). (**a**) T2WI_FS sagittal, (**b**) T1WI FS + C axial, (**c**) T2WI_FS sagittal

ultrasound ablation could ablate the entire fibroid, and the necrotic fibroid parts could be discharged through the cervix.

4.1.4 Case 4 Type I Submucosal Fibroid (2)

4.1.4.1 Case Description

The female patient was 44 years old. She developed menorrhagia with blood clots.

4.1.4.2 Pre-Treatment Assessment

MRI showed that the uterine submucosal fibroid was inhomogeneous and slightly hypointense on T2WI, about 50 mm in size (Fig. 4.4a). Contrast-enhanced T1WI showed that the fibroids had pseudocapsules and a rich blood supply (Fig. 4.4b, c). The fibroid was located on the right anterior wall, and the acoustic pathway was good, so it is relatively easy to predict focused ultrasound ablation results of the fibroids before treatment.

4.1.4.3 Treatment Techniques

1. **Focused ultrasound parameters.** Average acoustic power: 352 W, sonication time: 2400 s, duration of treatment: 128 min, total energy: 844,750 J.
2. **Focused ultrasound ablation techniques.** Sonication started with targeting the small focal region where the blood supply of the fibroid was absent (Fig. 4.4c). In this way, the released energy should be enough to achieve a better ablation effect. Still, care should be taken to protect the adjacent intima.

4.1.4.4 Post-Treatment Assessment

MRI Evaluation after Treatment Abdominal wall edema was diffuse on T2WI (Fig. 4.5a). The contrast-enhanced MR imaging showed that the non-perfused volume (NPV) ratio of the fibroids was up to 99% (Fig. 4.5b, c).

4.1.4.5 Discussion

- In this case, the broad base of the submucosal fibroids was located in the muscular layer. Hysteroscopy was prone to major bleeding, and the risk was high.
- During hysteroscopic surgery, in order to avoid perforation of the uterus, the part within the muscular walls is often not completely excised. Focused ultrasound ablation therapy can completely ablate a type I submucosal fibroid under the premise of safety.

4.1.5 Case 5 Type I Submucosal Fibroid (3)

4.1.5.1 Case Description

The female patient was 34 years old. Her disease recurred after removing uterine fibroids previously, and she developed menorrhagia with dysmenorrhea and occasional nausea and vomiting. At the 6-month follow-up after focused ultrasound ablation treatment, her dysmenorrhea disappeared, and the menstruation was normal. Three years after treatment, the menstrual volume began to increase.

4.1.5.2 Pre-Treatment Assessment

MRI demonstrated that the fibroid, measuring about 78 mm, showed a low signal on T2WI (Fig. 4.6a). Although the fibroids were located below the mucosa with abundant blood supply (Fig. 4.6b, c), it could be predicted that they were easy to be ablated before treatment.

4.1.5.3 Treatment Techniques

1. **Focused ultrasound parameters.** Average acoustic power: 253 W, sonication time: 3000 s, duration of treatment: 147 min, total energy: 757,980 J.
2. **Focused ultrasound ablation techniques.** The layout of targeted focuses was mainly concentrated at the base of the fibroids, and the blood supply was cut off. Less energy was used to achieve the ablation effect.

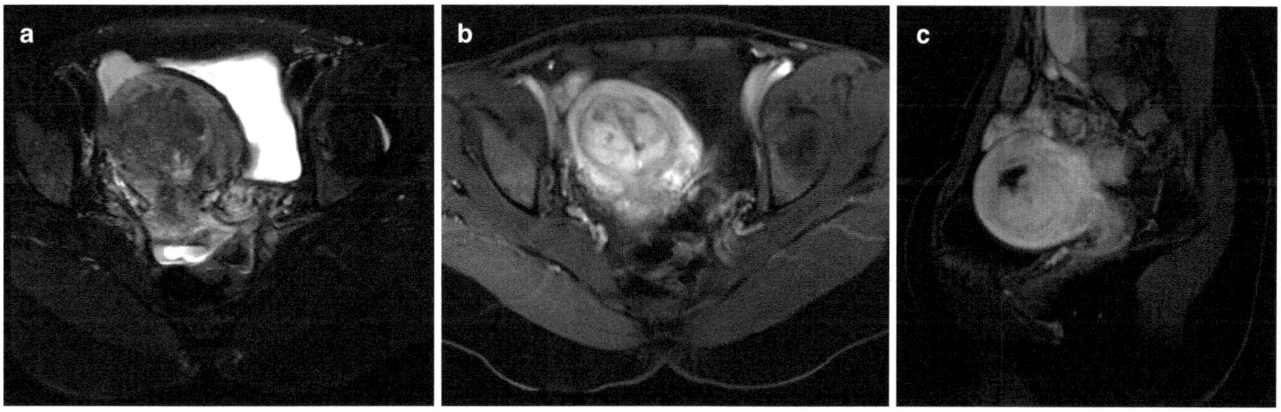

Fig. 4.4 Type I submucosal fibroids before treatment. (**a**) T2WI_FS axial (**b**) T1WI_FS + C axial, (**c**) T1WI_FS + C sagittal

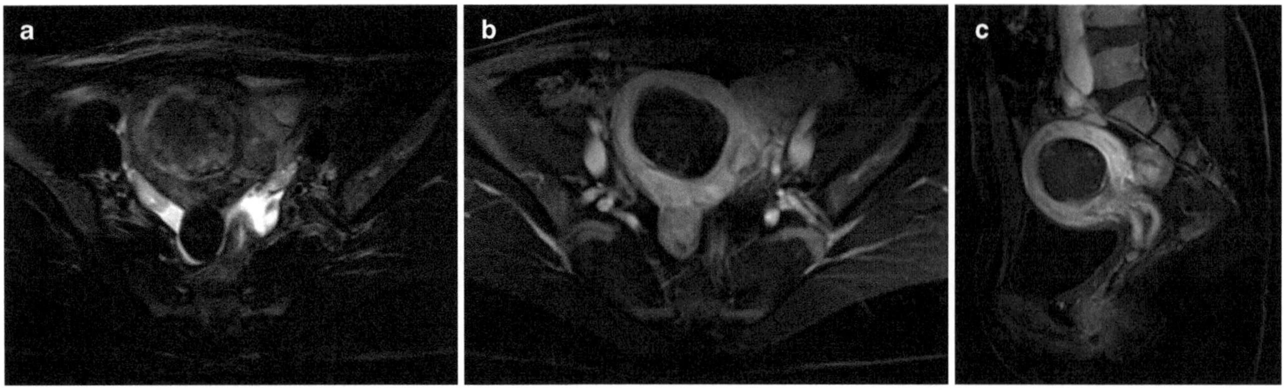

Fig. 4.5 MRI follow-up of type I submucosal fibroids immediately after treatment. (**a**) T2WI_FS axial (**b**) T1WI_FS + C axial, (**c**) T1WI_FS + C sagittal

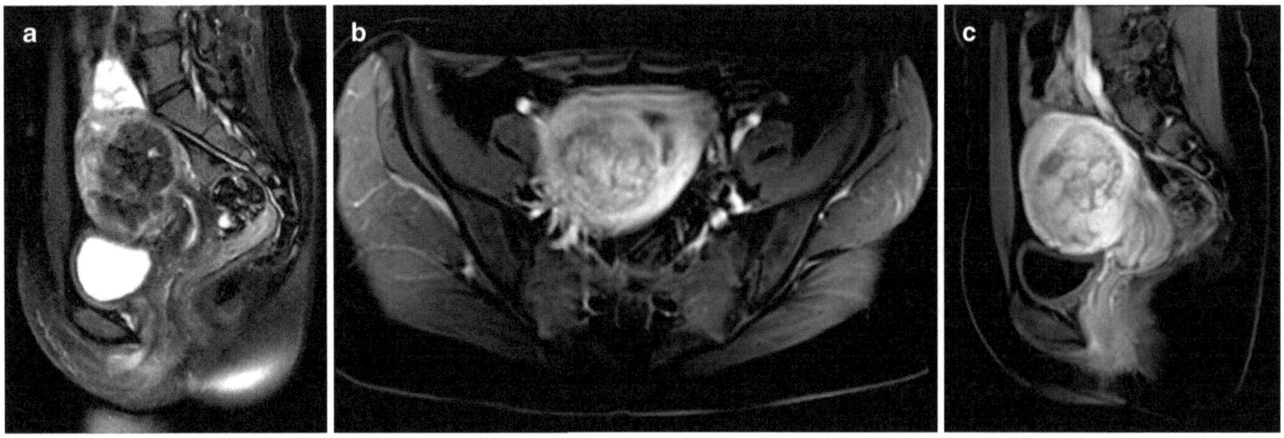

Fig. 4.6 Type I submucosal fibroids before treatment. (**a**) T2WI_FS sagittal (**b**) T1WI_FS + C axial, (**c**) T1WI_FS + C sagittal

4.1.5.4 Post-Treatment Assessment

1. **MRI evaluation after treatment.** There was no edema in the abdominal wall on T2WI (Fig. 4.7a), and the contrast-enhanced T1WI showed that the NPV ratio of the submucosal uterine fibroid was up to 99% (Fig. 4.7b, c).
2. **MRI follow-up at 6 months after treatment.** The fibroid shrank by about 70%, and it still showed no perfusion changes after enhancement (Fig. 4.7d–f).
3. **MRI follow-up at 3 years after treatment** The fibroid shrank by more than 90%, and most of them showed a high signal on T1WI. The remaining small parts showed liquid signals on T2WI (indicating no survival and recurrence of the fibroid), but new smaller fibroids were seen on the uterus's right front wall and fundus (Fig. 4.7g–i).

4.1.5.5 Discussion

- The submucosal fibroid was relatively large and compressed the uterine cavity. Focused ultrasound ablation had better cover the whole fibroid. However, the suitable treatment option for a larger submucosal fibroid was to reduce the size of the fibroid first to relieve the clinical symptoms, rather than completely ablate the entire fibroid since incarceration might occur in the cervix during discharge through the physiological cavity and require further hysteroscopy intervention for the latter.
- The fibroid was reexamined at 6 months and 3 years after treatment, and the fibroid volume was significantly reduced without symptoms. Three years after ablation treatment, new fibroids were found in the uterus of this patient. If fibroid-related symptoms appeared, a repeat non-invasive focused ultrasound ablation treatment might be more appropriate because of her history of recurrent fibroids and successful past focused ultrasound ablation treatment.

4.1.6 Case 6 Type I Submucosal Fibroid (4)

4.1.6.1 Case Description

The female patient was 30 years old. She developed menorrhagia with moderate anemia. The patient clearly indicated her fertility requirements. After ablation treatment, her menstruation was normal, and her anemia was improved.

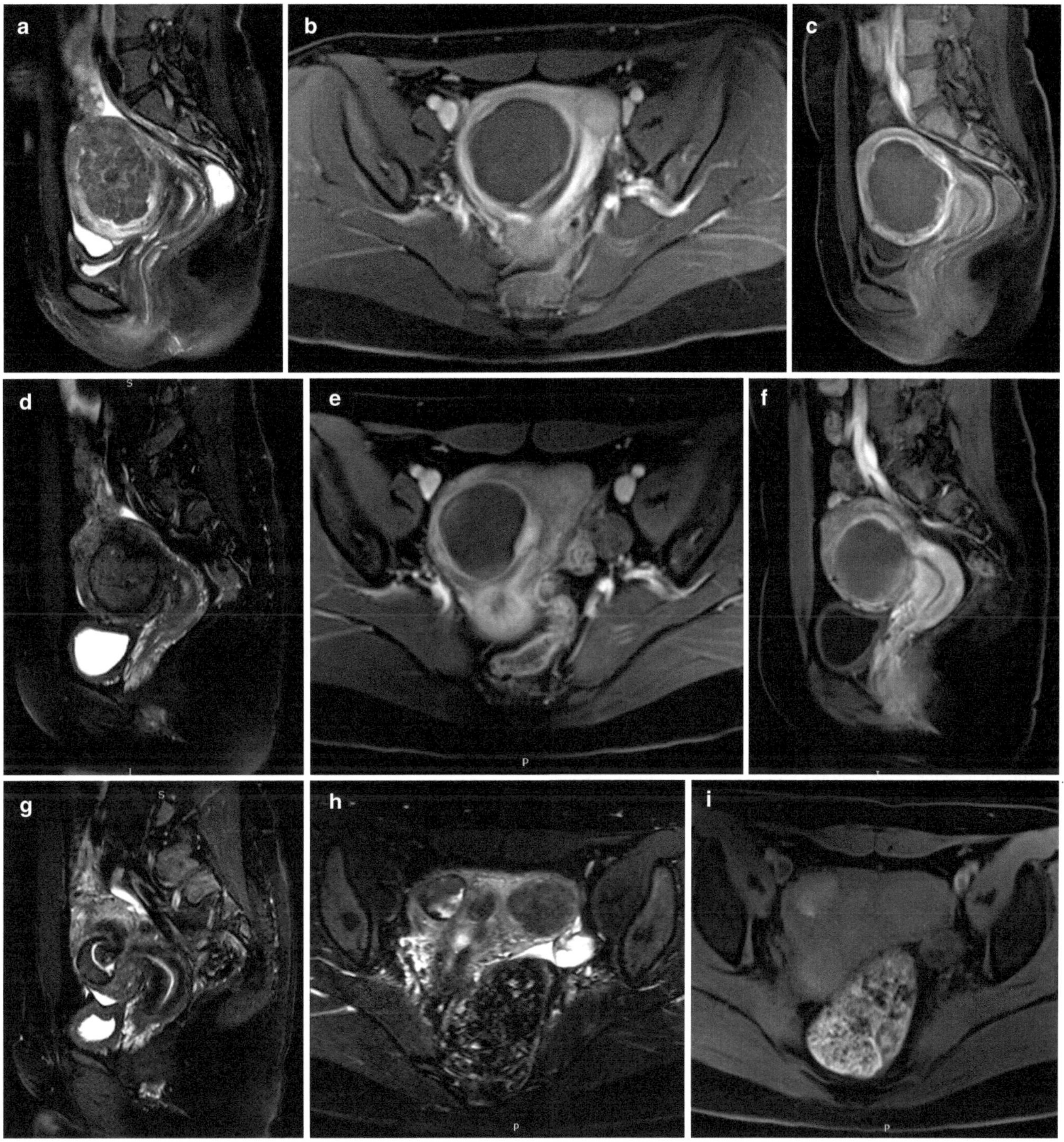

Fig. 4.7 MRI follow-up of type I submucosal fibroids immediately (**a**–**c**), at 6 months (**d**–**f**) and 3 years (**g**–**i**) after treatment. (**a**) T2WI_FS sagittal (**b**) T1WI_FS + C axial, (**c**) T1WI_FS + C sagittal, (**d**) T2WI_FS sagittal, (**e**) T1WI_FS + C axial, (**f**) T1WI_FS + C sagittal, (**g**) T2WI_FS sagittal, (**h**) T2WI_FS axial, (**i**) T1WI–FS axial

4.1.6.2 Pre-Treatment Assessment

MRI showed a submucosal fibroid and an intramural myoma with hypointensity on T2WI (Fig. 4.8a), and the submucosal fibroid was larger with an abundant blood supply (Fig. 4.8b, c). Both were located on the anterior wall of the anteverted uterus, which provided a good acoustic pathway.

4.1.6.3 Treatment Techniques

1. **Focused ultrasound parameters.** Average acoustic power: 366 W, sonication time: 2663 s, duration of treatment: 135 min, total energy: 973,370 J.
2. **Focused ultrasound ablation techniques.** The targeted region was mainly located at the base of the submucosal fibroids, and higher acoustic power might be given.

4.1.6.4 Post-Treatment Assessment

1. **MRI evaluation after treatment.** The anterior wall of the uterus showed apparent edema (Fig. 4.9a). The contrast-enhanced T1WI showed that the NPV ratio of the submucosal uterine fibroids was up to 97% (Fig. 4.9b, c).
2. **MRI follow-up at 6 months after treatment.** The submucosal uterine fibroid had been discharged, leaving only scanty tissues at the lesion site. The other intramural fibroid behind the base of the submucosal fibroids was significantly reduced. The uterine morphology returned to normal, the muscular wall was intact, and the endometrium line was well-defined (Fig. 4.10).

4.1.6.5 Discussion

- There was an intramural fibroid in the muscular wall adjacent to the type I submucosal fibroids. Surgical removal of fibroids might damage the entire anterior wall of the uterus, increasing the risk of uterine rupture. Therefore, for this type of fibroid, focused ultrasound ablation is a better option to cause less damage to the uterine wall and help women of childbearing age who have fertility requirements.

4.1.7 Case 7 Type I Submucosal Fibroid (5)

4.1.7.1 Case Description

The female patient was 39 years old. She developed increased menstrual volume and had a previous cesarean section. Follow-up at 6 months after focused ultrasound ablation for a submucous fibroid, the necrotic fibroid was discharged, and the menstrual blood flow returned to normal.

4.1.7.2 Pre-Treatment Assessment

MRI showed that a submucosal fibroid was located at the posterior wall of the uterus with a well-defined boundary, and another larger subserosal fibroid could be seen at the right posterior wall of the uterus (Fig. 4.11a–c). Both had a homogeneous low-intense signal on T2WI, suitable for ultrasound ablation.

4.1.7.3 Treatment Techniques

1. **Focused ultrasound parameters.** Average acoustic power: 260 W, sonication time: 2700 s, duration of treatment: 160 min, total energy: 702, 000 J.
2. **Focused ultrasound ablation techniques.** Firstly, the option for treating the subserosal fibroid near the right posterior pelvic wall could be chosen, and its deeper layer was initially ablated with lower acoustic power. The focal region was mainly targeted at its deeper base for the submucosal fibroid treatment. The entire tumor could be ablated through heat diffusion from the deeper to the shallow.

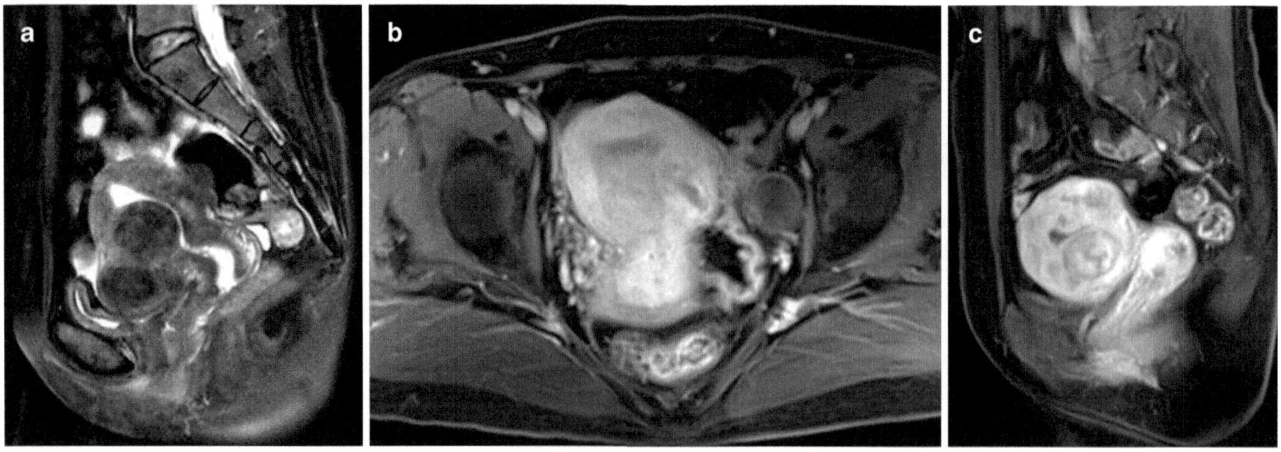

Fig. 4.8 Type I submucosal fibroid before treatment. (**a**) T2WI_FS sagittal (**b**) T1WI_FS + C axial, (**c**) T1WI_FS + C sagittal

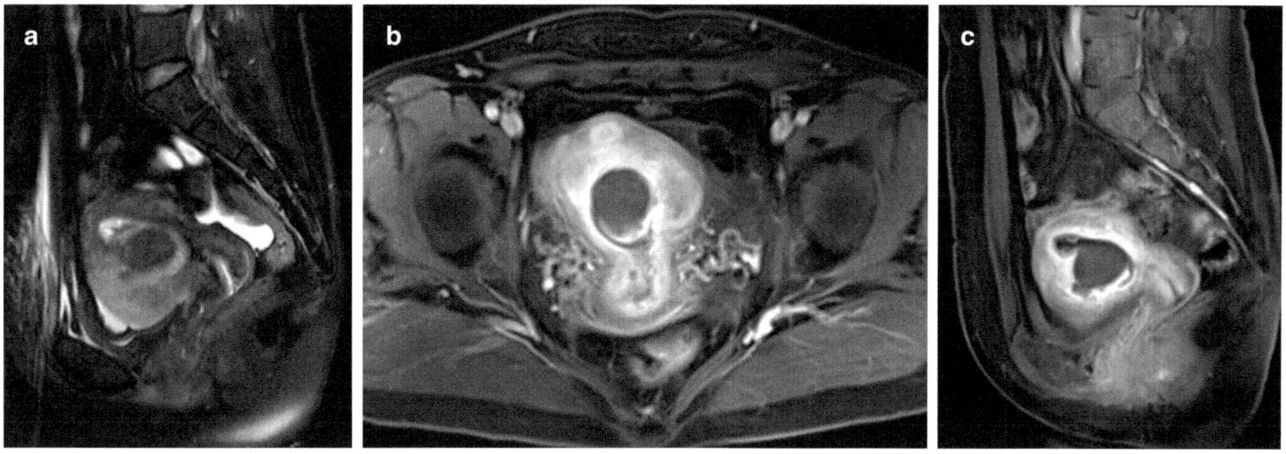

Fig. 4.9 MRI follow-up of Type I submucosal fibroid immediately after treatment. (**a**) T2WI_FS sagittal (**b**) T1WI_FS + C axial, (**c**) T1WI_FS + C sagittal

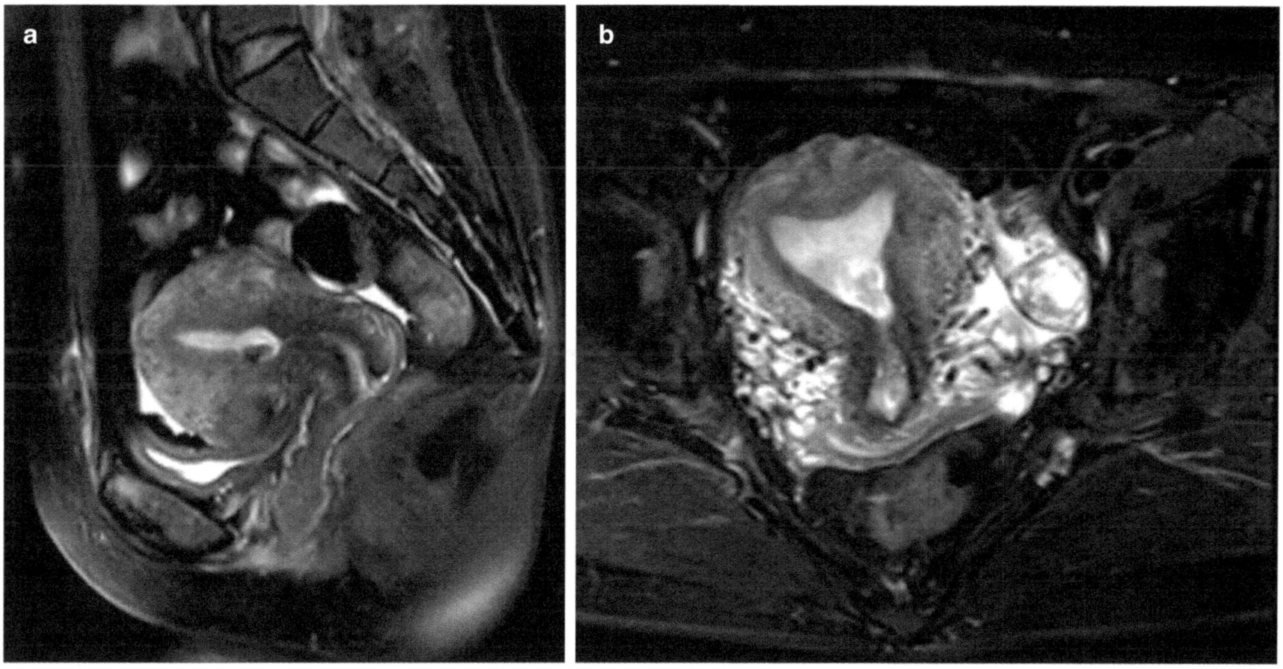

Fig. 4.10 MRI follow-up of the submucosal fibroid 6 months after treatment. (**a**) T2WI_FS sagittal (**b**) T2WI_FS axial

4.1.7.4 Post-Treatment Assessment

1. **MRI evaluation after treatment** The muscular layer of the anterior abdominal wall showed edema (Fig. 4.12a). The contrast-enhanced T1WI showed that the NPV ratios of the submucosal fibroid and the right posterior subserosal fibroid were about 98% and more than 90%, respectively (Fig. 4.12b, c).
2. **MRI follow-up at 6 months after treatment.** MRI showed that the submucosal uterine fibroid was basically discharged, only a few residual tissues left. The uterine cavity returned to normal with a well-defined endometrial line. The subserosal fibroid at the right posterior wall of the uterus shrank in size (Fig. 4.13).

4.1.7.5 Discussion

- Hysteroscopic surgery is the preferred option for type I submucosal uterine fibroid. This case also had a large subserosal fibroid, so the non-invasive focused ultrasound ablation could be useful to treat both fibroids simultaneously.
- For focused ultrasound ablation in treating submucosal fibroids, necrotic fibroids can be completely discharged and disappear. For patients who have a history of cesarean section and fertility requirements, one should avoid a surgical myomectomy so as not to cause damage to the uterine wall and affect future fertility.

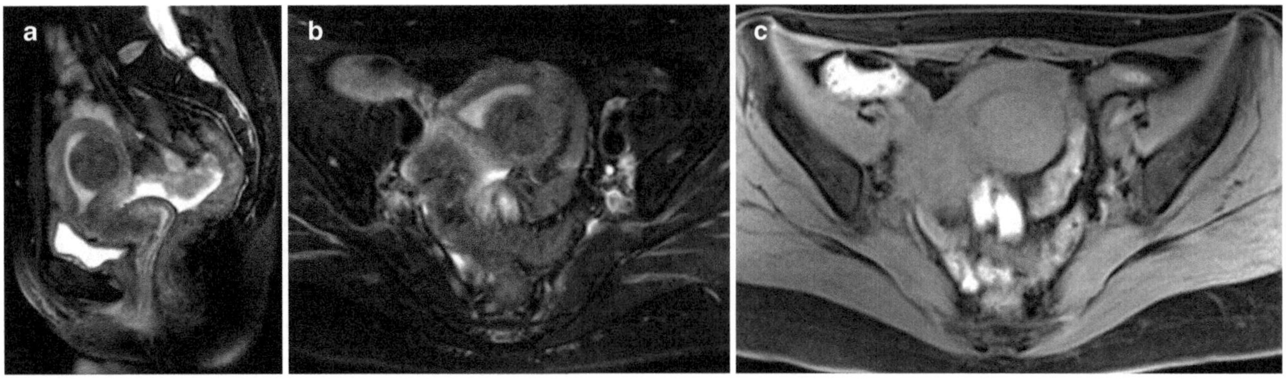

Fig. 4.11 Type I submucosal fibroid before treatment. (**a**) T2WI_FS sagittal (**b**) T2WI_FS axial, (**c**) T1WI axial

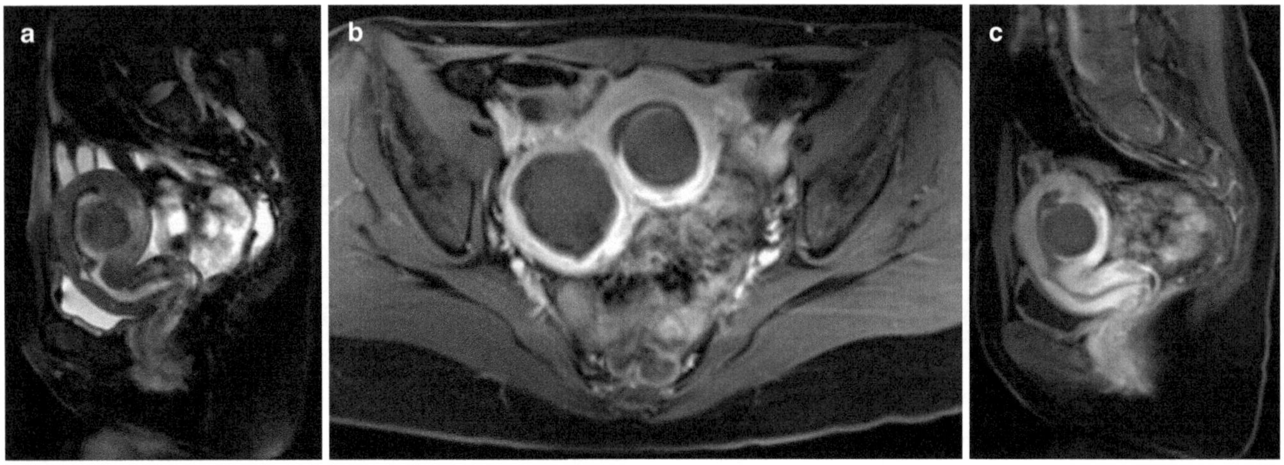

Fig. 4.12 MRI follow-up of type I submucosal fibroid immediately after treatment. (**a**) T2WI_FS sagittal (**b**) T1WI_FS + C axial, (**c**) T1WI_FS + C sagittal

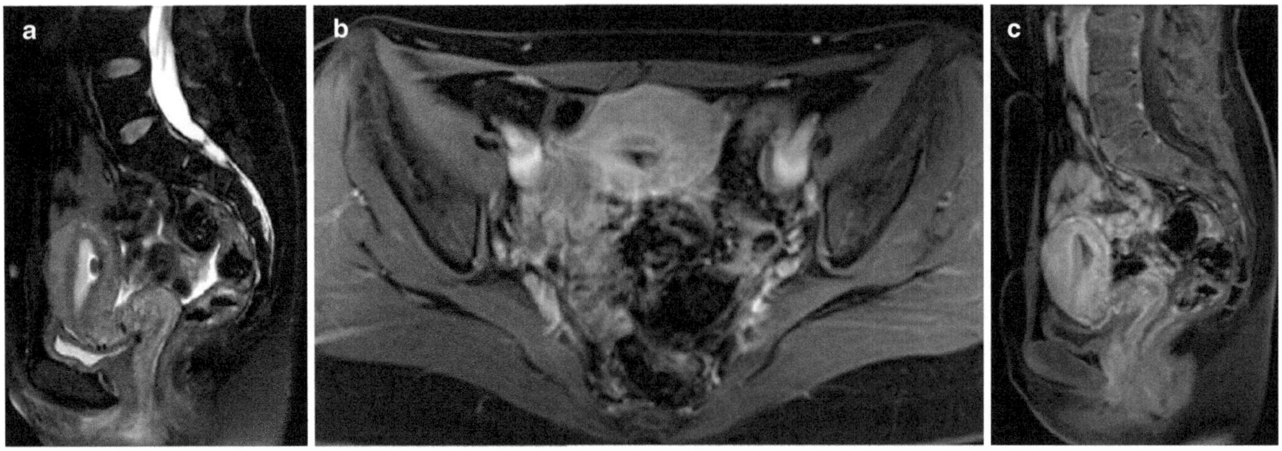

Fig. 4.13 MRI follow-up of type I submucosal fibroids at 6 months after treatment. (**a**) T2WI_FS sagittal (**b**) T1WI_FS + C axial, (**c**) T1WI_FS + C sagittal

4.1.8 Case 8 Type II Submucosal Fibroid (1)

4.1.8.1 Case Description

The female patient was 42 years old. She developed decreased menstrual volume but a prolonged menstrual cycle. She also felt lower abdominal distension. An ultrasound was performed to confirm a diagnosis of submucosal fibroid.

4.1.8.2 Pre-Treatment Assessment

MRI demonstrated that a submucosal fibroid with hypointensity was located at the anterior wall of the uterus on T2WI, and the contrast-enhanced T1WI showed the fibroid with poor blood supply (Fig. 4.14a–c). There was a clear acoustic pathway. It was preferred focused ultrasound ablation to hysteroscopic or laparoscopic myomectomy for this case.

4.1.8.3 Treatment Techniques

1. **Focused ultrasound parameters.** Average acoustic power: 240 W, sonication time: 1454 s, duration of treatment: 99 min, total energy: 210,100 J.
2. **Focused ultrasound ablation treatment technique.** The fibroid with hypointensity and poor blood supply was located at the anterior wall of the anteverted uterus and was small in size. The ultrasonic power might be reduced.

4.1.8.4 Post-Treatment Assessment

1. **MRI evaluation after treatment.** The edema of the anterior abdominal wall was not apparent on T2WI (Fig. 4.15a). The contrast-enhanced MRI showed that the NPV ratio of submucosal uterine fibroids was up to 99% (Fig. 4.15b, c).
2. **MRI follow-up 5 months after treatment.** The fibroid volume was significantly reduced, and the contrast-enhanced T1WI still showed non-perfusion in the whole tumor without any signs of residual recurrence (Fig. 4.16).

4.1.8.5 Discussion

- Type II submucosal uterine fibroids have more than 50% of their bodies in the uterine muscular wall, so hysteroscopic surgery has limitations for their complete removal.
- Focused ultrasound ablation treatment can lead to the necrosis of the entire fibroid while protecting and causing minimal damage to the intact intima. Therefore, focused ultrasound ablation is suitable for treating type II submucosal fibroids and may have curative efficacy.

4.1.9 Case 9 Type II Submucosal Fibroid (2)

4.1.9.1 Case Description

The female patient was 45 years old. She developed increased menstrual blood flow and had a history of dysmenorrhea, which had aggravated recently, for more than 3 years.

4.1.9.2 Pre-Treatment Assessment

MRI showed that a submucosal fibroid at the fundus of the uterus protruded into the uterine cavity, with a slightly hyperintense signal on T2WI (Fig. 4.17a). The contrast-enhanced MRI showed that the fibroids had an intact pseudocapsule with moderate blood perfusion (Fig. 4.17b, c). The fibroid was located at the fundus of the anteverted uterus adjacent to the anterior abdominal wall, in which there was a good acoustic pathway. However, as the posterior boundary of the fibroid was close to the sacrum, care must be taken during ablation. Endometriosis and multiple chocolate cysts could be seen in the pelvic cavity.

4.1.9.3 Treatment Techniques

1. **Focused ultrasound parameters.** Average acoustic power: 300 W, sonication time: 499 s, duration of treatment: 37 min, total energy: 149,700 J.

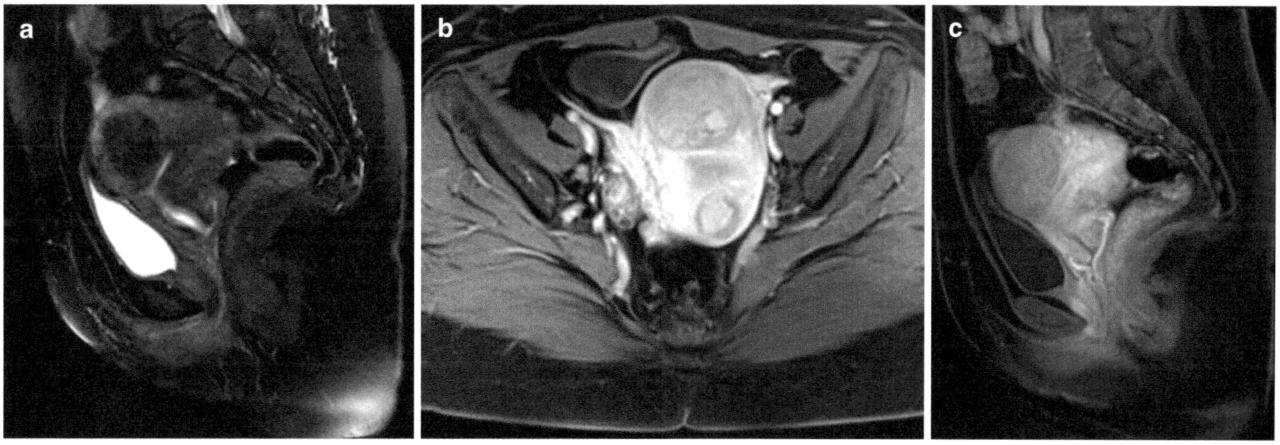

Fig. 4.14 Type II submucosal fibroid before treatment. (**a**) T2WI_FS sagittal (**b**) T1WI_FS + C axial, (**c**) T1WI_FS + C sagittal

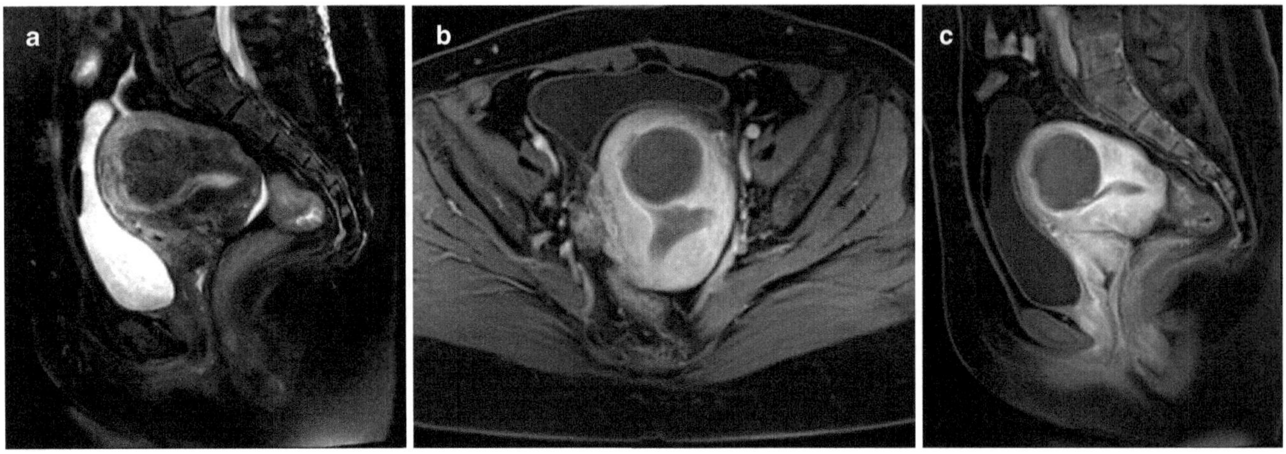

Fig. 4.15 MRI follow-up of type II submucosal fibroid immediately after treatment. (**a**) T2WI_FS sagittal (**b**) T1WI_FS + C axial, (**c**) T1WI_FS + C sagittal

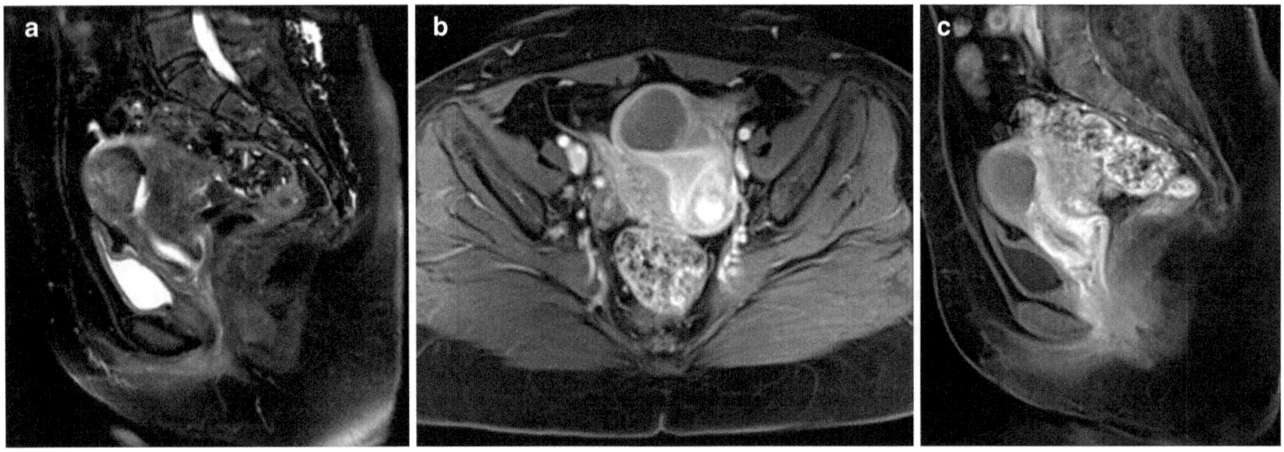

Fig. 4.16 MRI follow-up of type II submucosal fibroid at 5 months after treatment. (**a**) T2WI_FS sagittal (**b**) T1WI_FS + C axial, (**c**) T1WI_FS + C sagittal

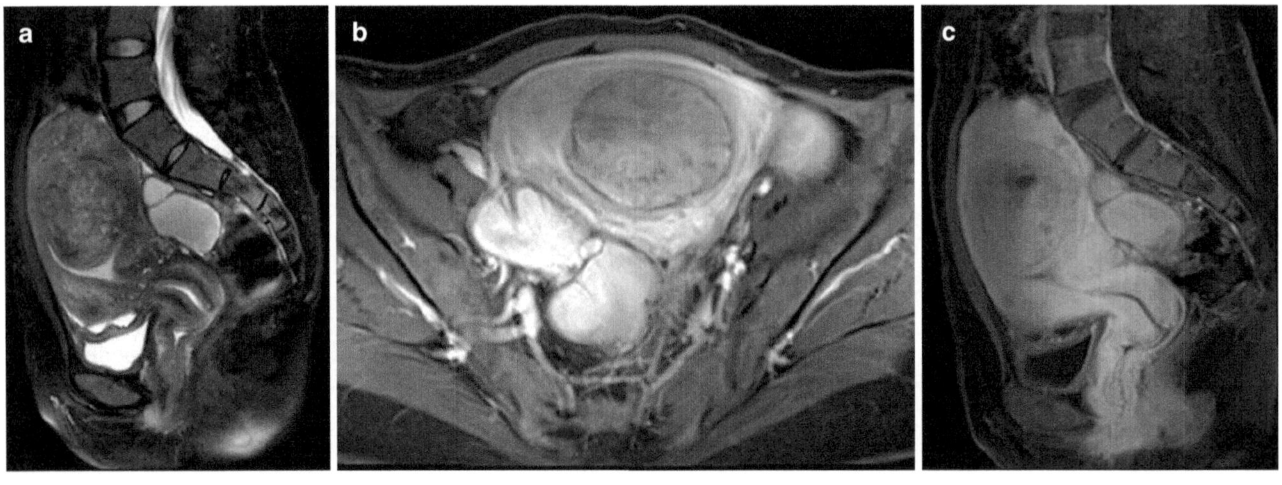

Fig. 4.17 Type II submucosal fibroid before treatment. (**a**) T2WI_FS sagittal (**b**) T1WI_FS + C axial, (**c**) T1WI_FS + C sagittal

2. **Focused ultrasound ablation techniques.** The fibroid was initially treated on a deep layer with lower acoustic power since its posterior edge was close to the lumbar sacrum. After an "acoustic barrier" was formed at the deep layer, the acoustic power irradiation was increased on its shallow layer.

4.1.9.4 Post-Treatment Assessment

MRI Evaluation after Treatment The ablated fibroid showed an increased signal on T2WI (Fig. 4.18a). The contrast-enhanced T1WI showed that the fibroid was completely ablated without perfusion, and the intimal layer was intact (Fig. 4.18b, c).

4.1.9.5 Discussion

- When focused ultrasound ablation is used to treat submucosal fibroids, any damage to the endometrium should be avoided and minimized as much as possible. In this case, after focused ultrasound ablation treatment, the fibroids were completely ablated with the corresponding endometrium well protected. If focused ultrasound ablation is used properly, it can completely ablate a submucosal fibroid safely and effectively.

4.1.10 Case 10 Type II Submucosal Fibroid (3)

4.1.10.1 Case Description

The female patient was 49 years old. She developed increased menstrual flow and anemia.

4.1.10.2 Pre-Treatment Assessment

MRI indicated a submucosal fibroid at the fundus and posterior wall of the uterus with heterogenous hyper- and hypointensity on T2WI (Fig. 4.19a). The contrast-enhanced MRI showed that the fibroid's blood supply was partially abundant, but one-third of myoma was non perfused (Fig. 4.19b, c). Since the fibroid showed mixed signals on T2WI and the acoustic pathway was clear, a better ablation outcome would be anticipated before treatment.

4.1.10.3 Treatment Techniques

1. **Focused ultrasound parameters.** Average acoustic power: 385 W, sonication time: 2000 s, duration of treatment: 105 min, total energy: 770,620 J.
2. **Focused ultrasound ablation techniques.** The targeted focal region for treatment was initially concentrated at the low-T2WI signal area of the fibroid to reduce the irradiation energy to ablate the fibroid completely.

4.1.10.4 Post-Treatment Assessment

MRI Evaluation after Treatment A slight edema was seen at the muscular layer of the anterior abdominal wall (Fig. 4.20a). The contrast-enhanced T1WI showed that the NPV ratio of the submucosal fibroid was up to 98%, and the endometrium and serous membrane were intact (Fig. 4.20b, c).

4.1.10.5 Discussion

- For uterine fibroids with mixed hyper- and hypointensity on T2WI, a favorable ablation can be achieved by ultrasound ablation.
- Before treatment, the area of uterine fibroids with hyperintensity on T2WI but no enhancement on the enhanced MRI may indicate fibroid degeneration. Follow-up observation is required after focused ultrasound ablation in such cases.

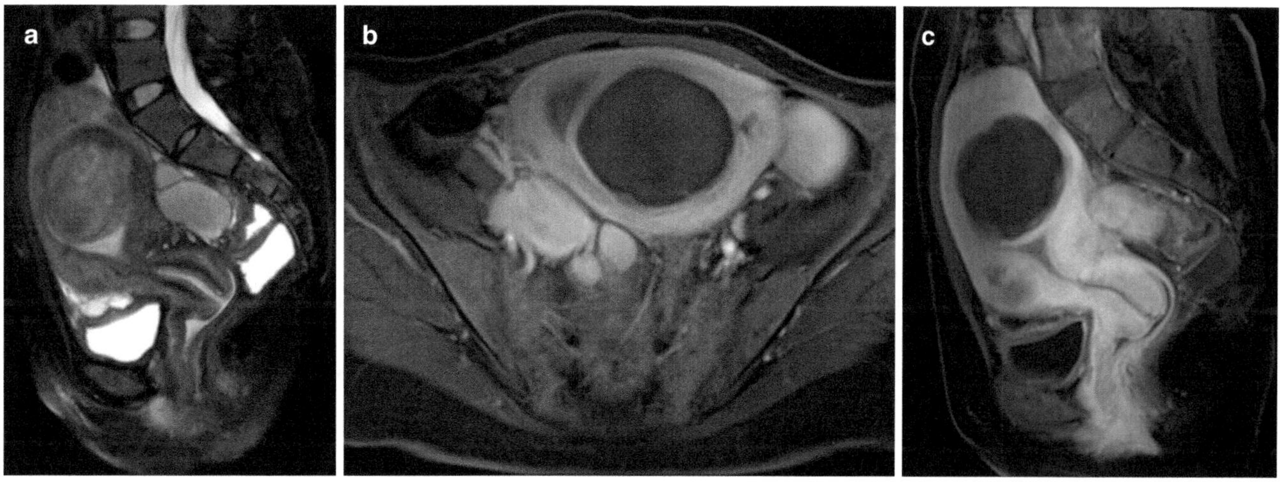

Fig. 4.18 MRI follow-up of type II submucosal fibroid immediately after treatment. (**a**) T2WI_FS sagittal (**b**) T1WI_FS + C axial, (**c**) T1WI_FS + C sagittal

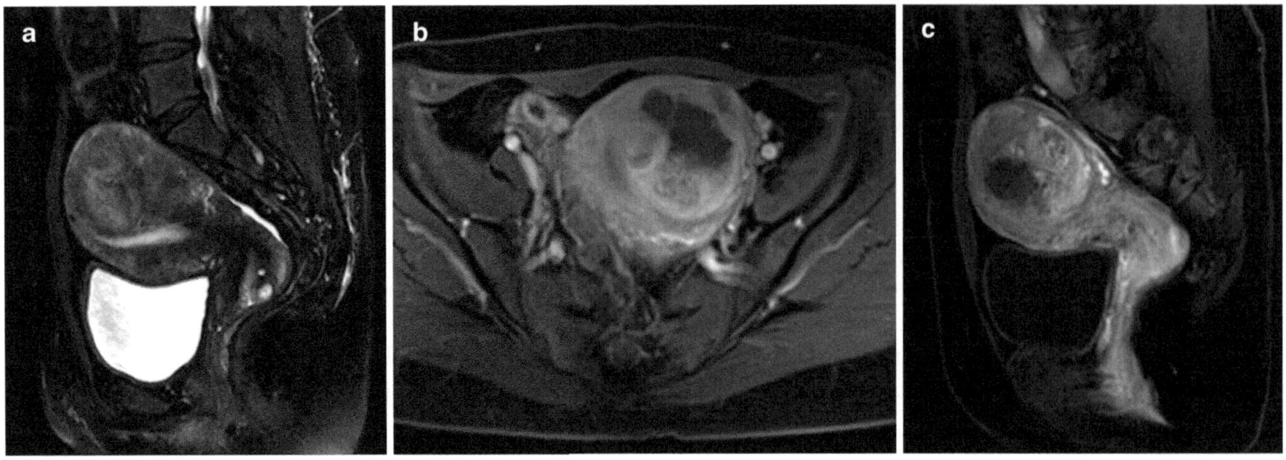

Fig. 4.19 Type II submucosal fibroid before treatment. (**a**) T2WI_FS sagittal. (**b**) T1WI_FS + C axial, (**c**) T1WI_FS + C sagittal

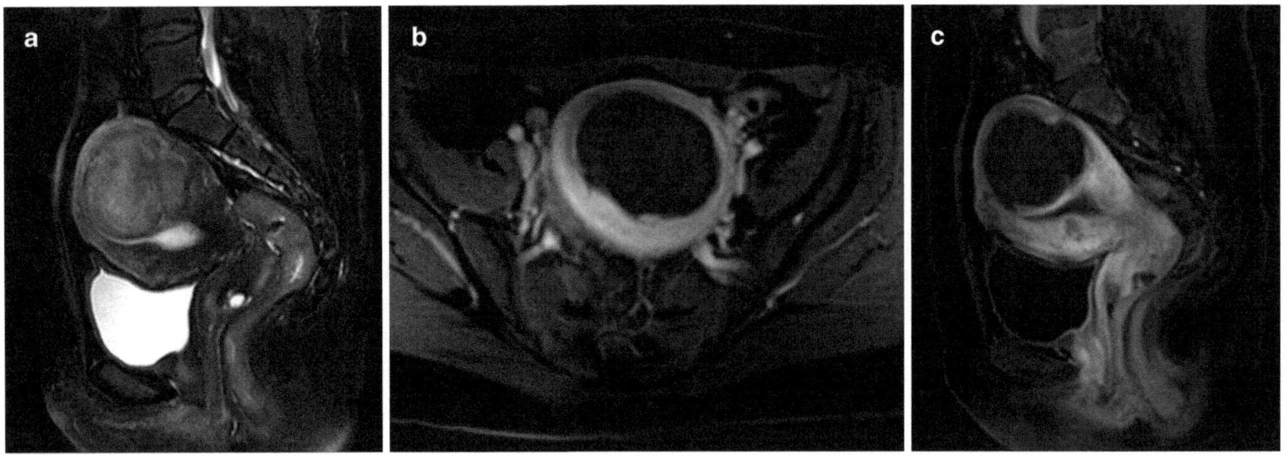

Fig. 4.20 MRI follow-up of type II submucosal fibroid immediately after treatment. (**a**) T2WI_FS sagittal, (**b**) T1WI_FS + C axial, (**c**) T1WI_FS + C sagittal

4.1.11 Case 11 Type II Submucosal Fibroid (4)

4.1.11.1 Case Description

The female patient was 42 years old. Physical examination revealed uterine fibroids for more than 5 years and increased menstrual blood flow for nearly 1 year. At follow-up after the focused ultrasound ablation treatment, the menstrual volume significantly reduced.

4.1.11.2 Pre-Treatment Assessment

MRI showed that the submucosal fibroids in the anterior wall of the uterus were mixed signal on T2WI, most of which were low signal in the middle and high signal in the periphery (Fig. 4.21a). The contrast-enhanced MRI showed fibroids had poor blood supply with some non-perfused areas (Fig. 4.21b, c). Although the fibroid was located at the anterior wall of the anteverted uterus, the space between the abdominal wall and the uterus was filled with bowels. The full distended bladder and an extracorporal degassing water balloon were needed to push the bowels away to achieve a clear acoustic pathway.

4.1.11.3 Treatment Techniques

1. **Focused ultrasound parameters.** Average acoustic power: 209 W, sonication time: 1763 s, duration of treatment: 79 min, total energy: 368,700 J.
2. **Focused ultrasound ablation techniques.** For focused ultrasound ablation of the submucosal fibroid at the anterior wall of the uterus, the targeted focus should be deployed 10 mm away from the endometrium. And the acoustic power for treatment should be reduced (the acoustic power at the deeper face of the fibroids was not more than 200 W) to protect the endometrium while achieving ablation of the fibroid.

4.1.11.4 Post-Treatment Assessment

MRI Evaluation after Treatment There was no edema in the anterior abdominal wall (Fig. 4.22a). The contrast-

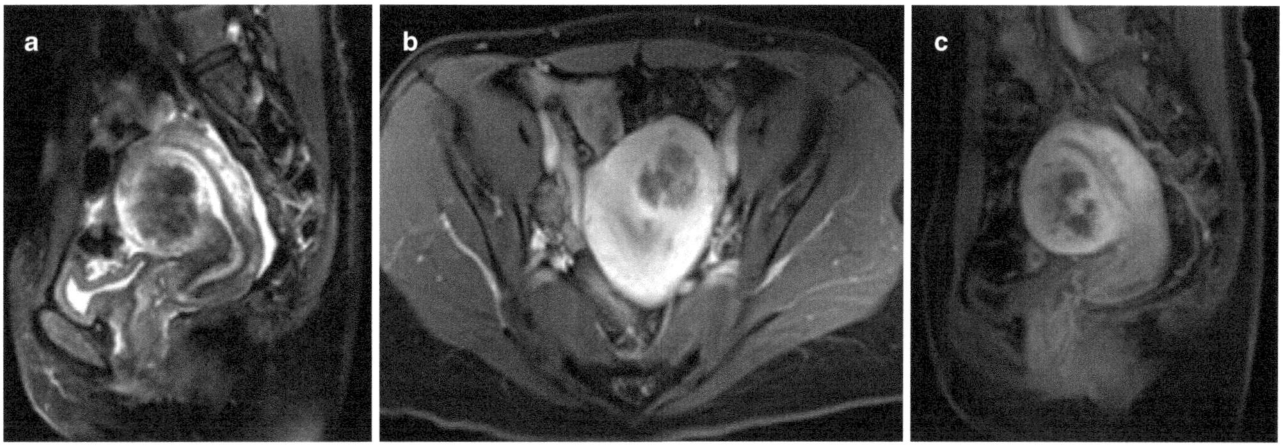

Fig. 4.21 Type II submucosal fibroid before treatment. (**a**) T2WI_FS sagittal (**b**) T1WI_FS + C axial, (**c**) T1WI_FS + C sagittal

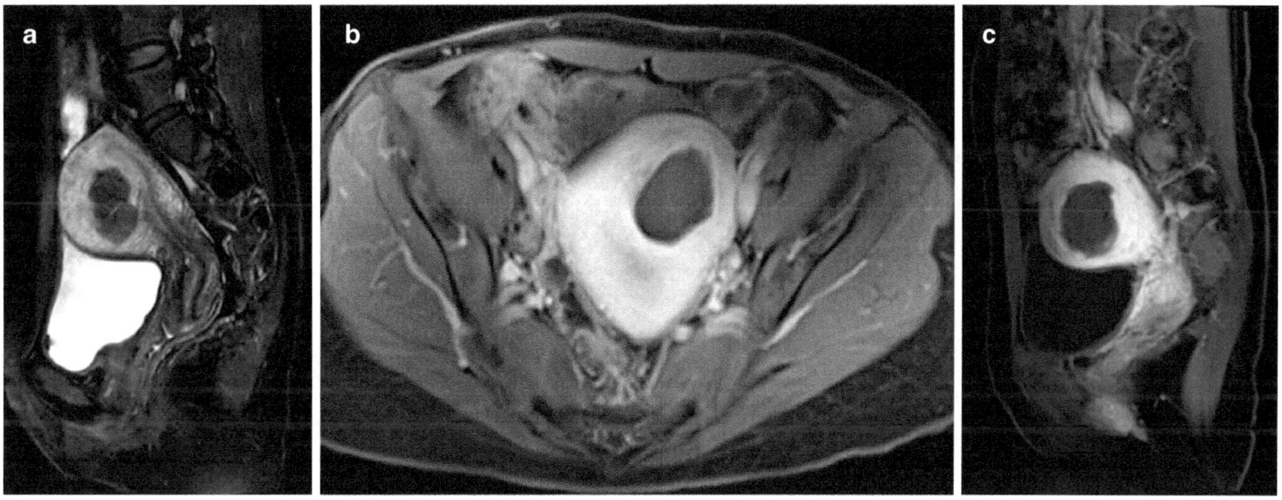

Fig. 4.22 MRI follow-up of type II submucosal fibroid immediately after treatment. (**a**) T2WI_FS sagittal (**b**) T1WI_FS + C axial, (**c**) T1WI_FS + C sagittal

enhanced MRI showed that the NPV ratio of the submucosal fibroid was more than 90%, and the endometrium was intact (Fig. 4.22b, c).

4.1.11.5 Discussion

- Type II submucosal fibroid grows and protrudes into the uterine cavity, which could cause dysmenorrhea and/or increased menstrual blood flow. Focused ultrasound ablation therapy can improve the clinical symptoms by ablating the fibroid.

4.1.12 Case 12 Type II Submucosal Fibroid (5)

4.1.12.1 Case Description

The female patient was 41 years old and expecting fertility. She developed significantly increased menstrual blood flow with blood clots. She had prolonged menstrual periods with severe anemia and abdominal pain before menstruation in the past 6 months.

4.1.12.2 Pre-Treatment Assessment

MRI showed that the submucosal fibroids in the anterior wall of the retroverted uterus showed low signal on T2WI (Fig. 4.23a). The contrast-enhanced T1WI showed that the central part of the fibroid lacked blood supply, and its periphery with abundant blood supply (Fig. 4.23b, c). It is predicted that the central part of the fibroid was easy to be ablated.

4.1.12.3 Treatment Techniques

1. **Focused ultrasound parameters.** Average acoustic power: 315 W, sonication time: 2001 s, duration of treatment: 111 min, total energy: 629, 660 J.
2. **Focused ultrasound ablation techniques.** Focused ultrasound targeted the deep layer of the fibroid about

10 mm away from the endometrial margin to protect the endometrium from damage. There were more bowels between the uterus and the anterior abdominal wall. A full bladder and extracorporeal water balloon were needed to push these bowels away to create a safe acoustic pathway during treatment.

4.1.12.4 Post-Treatment Assessment

1. **MRI evaluation after treatment** The anterior abdominal wall showed slight edema, and the intense signal of the fibroid had no change on T2WI (Fig. 4.24a). The contrast-enhanced T1WI showed that the NPV ratio of uterine submucosal fibroids was about 85%, and the fibroid showed residual fibroid under the endometrium that remained intact (Fig. 4.24b, c).
2. **MRI follow-up at 6 months after treatment.** The fibroid volume was significantly reduced, and there was blood supply to the residual fibroid that was not ablated next to the endometrium. No significant increase in size was observed in this residual fibroid (Fig. 4.25).

4.1.12.5 Discussion

- For submucosal fibroids located at the anterior wall of the uterus, in order to protect the endometrium from damage, the target focal region of the focused ultrasound is placed 10 mm beneath the endometrium, which might leave subendometrial residual fibroid unablated.
- The MRI follow-up of this case for half a year showed that the fibroid volume was significantly reduced, and there was no obvious growth of residual fibroid under the endometrium. It should be noted that focused ultrasound ablation therapy does not necessarily pursue a perfect ablation, which is especially important for the patient with reproductive needs. Damage to the endometrium should be reduced and avoided as much as possible, in line with the rules of minimally noninvasive treatment.

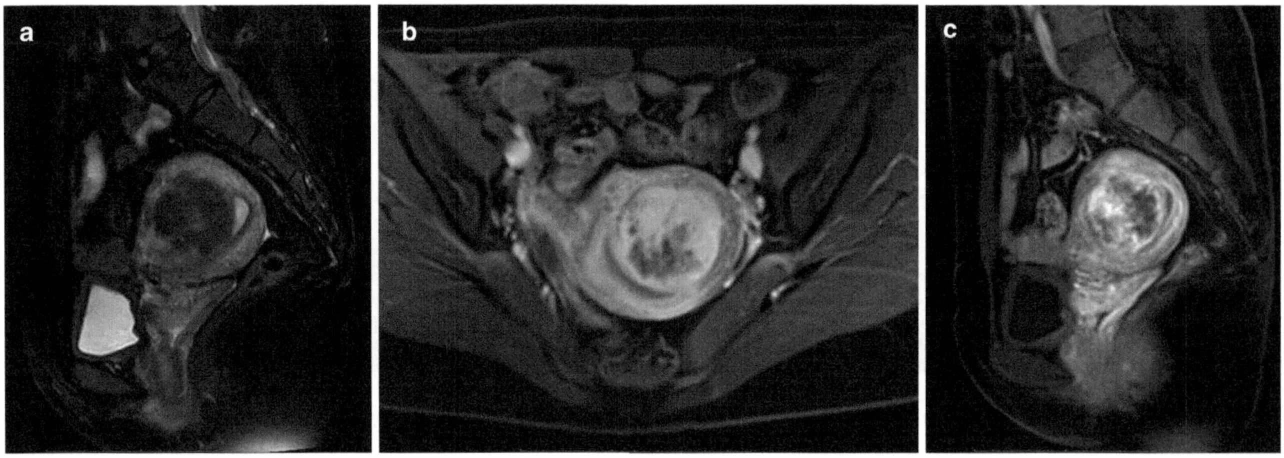

Fig. 4.23 Type II submucosal fibroid before treatment. (**a**) T2WI_FS sagittal (**b**) T2WI + C axial, (**c**) T1WI_FS + C sagittal

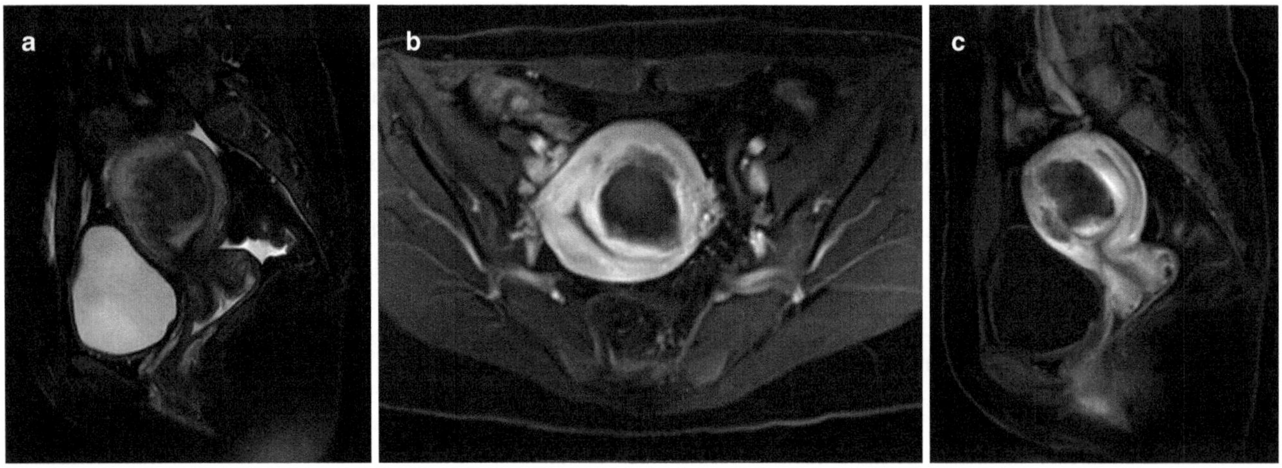

Fig. 4.24 MRI follow-up of type II submucosal fibroid immediately after treatment. (**a**) T2WI_FS sagittal (**b**) T1WI_FS + C axial, (**c**) T1WI_FS + C sagittal

4.1.13 Case 13 Type II Submucosal Fibroid (6)

4.1.13.1 Case Description

The female patient was 25 year old and unmarried. She had progressively increased menstrual blood flow, prolonged menstrual period, and mild anemia.

4.1.13.2 Pre-Treatment Assessment

MRI showed a type II submucosal fibroids in the right anterior wall of the uterus with hypointensity on T2WI, measuring the largest diameter of 96 mm (Fig. 4.26a). The contrast-enhanced MRI showed a larger fibroid with poor blood supply (Fig. 4.26b, c), and the acoustic pathway was clear. Given the above, a good result of focused ultrasound ablation would be anticipated.

4.1.13.3 Treatment Techniques

1. **Focused ultrasound parameters.** Average acoustic power: 347 W, sonication time: 2271 s, duration of treatment: 115 min, total energy: 788,600 J.
2. **Focused ultrasound ablation techniques.** For submucosal fibroids with a good acoustic pathway and low intense signal on T2WI, the focal point must be ≥10 mm away from the endometrium during treatment. While protecting the endometrium, give enough acoustic energy to ablate the tumor fully.

4.1.13.4 Post-Treatment Assessment

1. **MRI evaluation after treatment.** There was no apparent edema in the anterior abdominal wall (Fig. 4.27a). The contrast-enhanced MRI showed that the NPV ratio of the

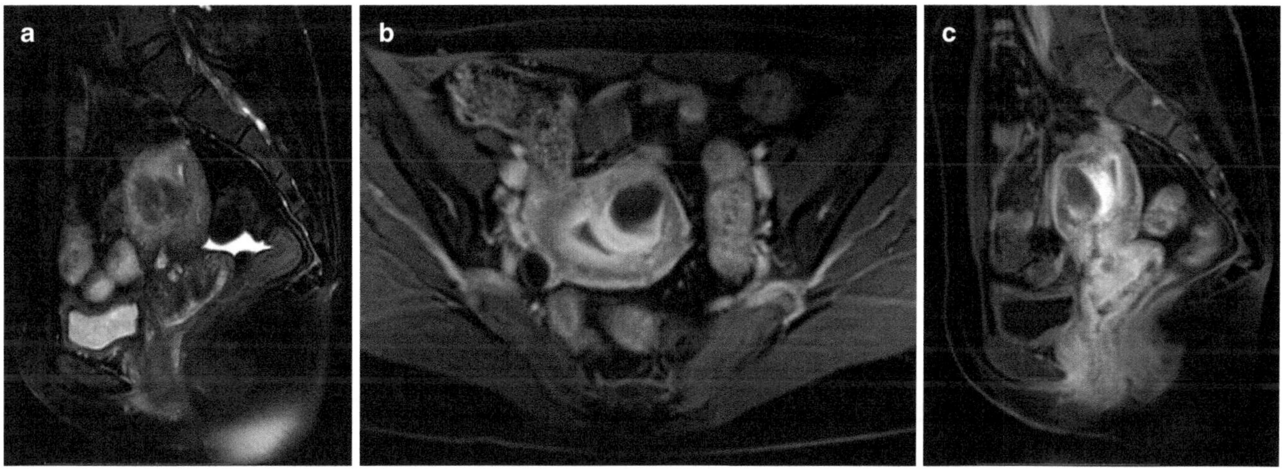

Fig. 4.25 MRI follow-up of type II submucosal fibroid at 6 months after treatment. (**a**) T2WI_FS sagittal, (**b**) T1WI_FS + C axial, (**c**) T1WI_FS + C sagittal

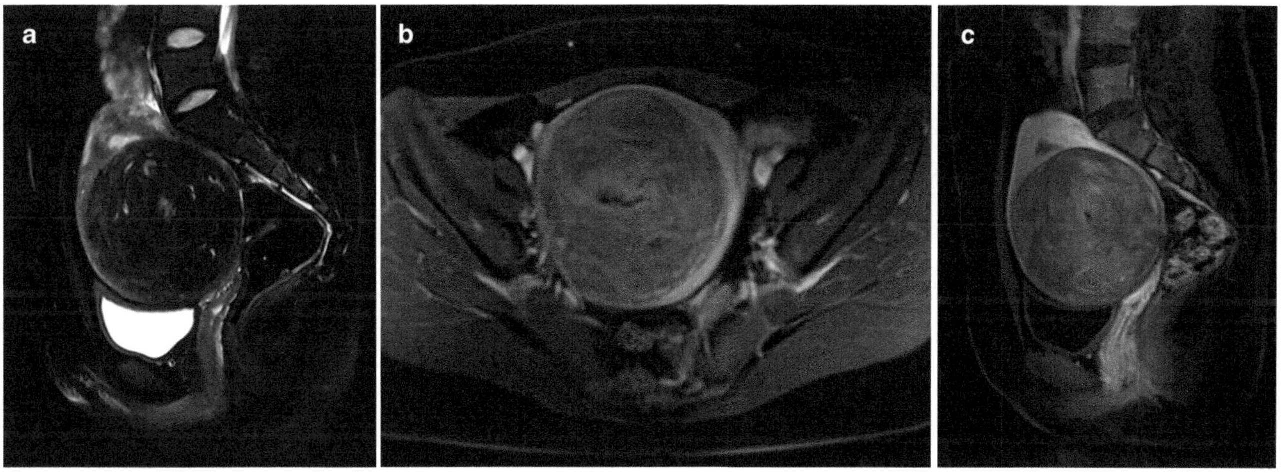

Fig. 4.26 Type II submucosal fibroid before treatment. (**a**) T2WI_FS sagittal, (**b**) T2WI + C axial, (**c**) T1WI_FS + C sagittal

submucosal fibroids was about 98%, and only an arc thin layer of enhancement remained at the posterior margin of the fibroid. The endometrium was intact (Fig. 4.27b, c).

2. **MRI follow-up at 6 months after treatment.** It showed that the volume of uterine fibroids was reduced by about 57%. Contrast-enhanced MR imaging showed the residual enhancement at the posterior margin of the fibroid disappeared, and the NPV ratio of the tumor was 100% (Fig. 4.28).

4.1.13.5 Discussion

- Focused ultrasound ablation treatment of submucosal uterine fibroid requires attention to protect the endometrium, especially for unmarried and nonparous patients. Since the targeted focal region needs to be ≥10 mm from the endometrium, complete ablation and necrosis of the fibroid might not be obtained after treatment.
- In this case, the few residual enhancement portions disappeared after half a year, representing a pseudoenhance-

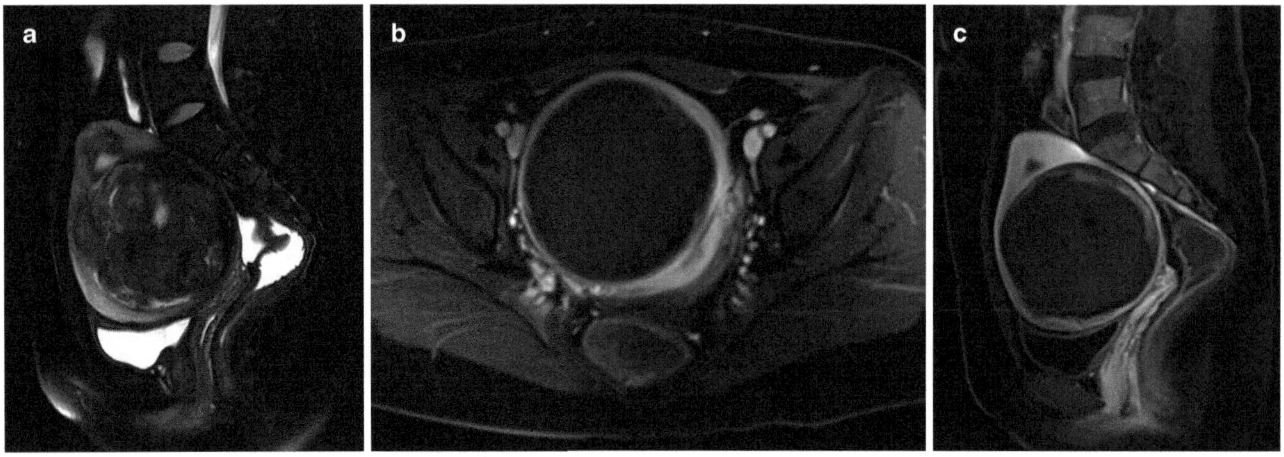

Fig. 4.27 MRI follow-up of type II submucosal fibroid immediately after treatment. (**a**) T2WI_FS sagittal, (**b**) T1WI_FS + C axial, (**c**) T1WI_FS + C sagittal

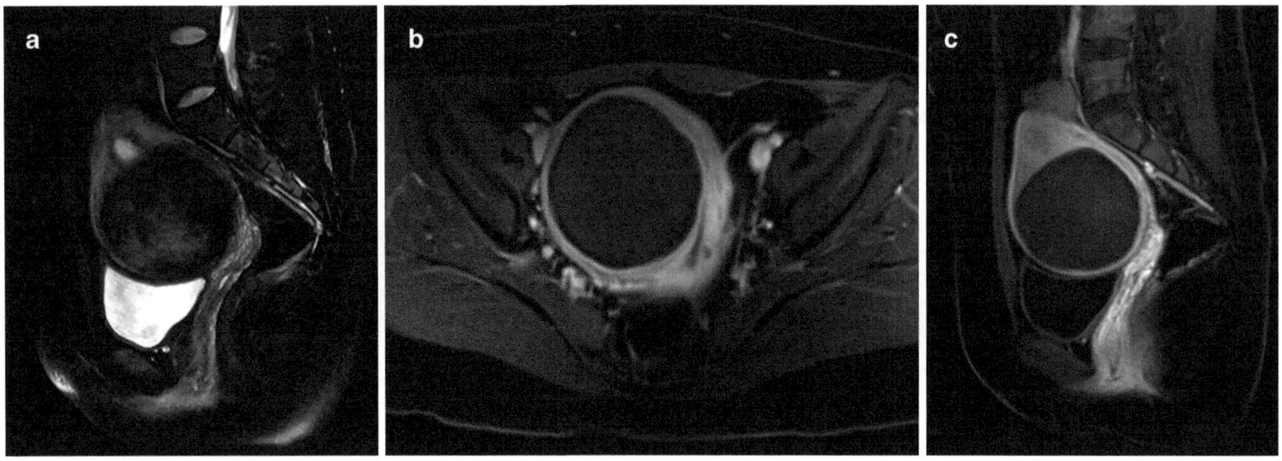

Fig. 4.28 MRI follow-up of type II submucosal fibroid at 6 months after treatment. (**a**) T2WI_FS sagittal, (**b**) T1WI_FS + C axial, (**c**) T1WI_FS + C sagittal

ment appearance from leaky capillaries at the treatment margin that can be seen immediately after thermal ablation.

4.2 Focused Ultrasound Ablation for Intramural Uterine Fibroids

4.2.1 Case 1 Type III Intramural Fibroid (1)

4.2.1.1 Case Description

The female patient was 38 years old. She had a recurrent fibroid after a hysteroscopic myomectomy.

4.2.1.2 Pre-Treatment Assessment

T2WI showed a posterior wall uterine fibroid with inhomogeneous hyper- and hypointensity, compressing the uterine cavity (Fig. 4.29a). It was accompanied by uterine posterior wall adenomyosis. The contrast-enhanced T1WI showed that the fibroid had an abundant blood supply with a pseudocapsule (Fig. 4.29b, c). The focused ultrasound near-field was good for ablation treatment.

4.2.1.3 Treatment Techniques

1. **Focused ultrasound parameters.** Average acoustic power: 383 W, sonication time: 2599 s, treatment time: 134 min, total energy: 994, 800 J.
2. **Focused ultrasound ablation techniques.** The posterior uterine fibroid was adjacent to the bowels behind the uterus; therefore, treatment of the deeper part of the fibroid requires a distance of 15 mm or more from the posterior uterine serosa.

4.2.1.4 Post-Treatment Assessment

1. **MRI evaluation after treatment.** There is no sign of edema in the anterior abdominal wall, and the T2WI signal intensity increased in the posterior portion of fibroid (Fig. 4.30a). The contrast-enhanced MRI showed that the NPV ratio of the fibroid was about 95%, and only a small amount of residual fibroid in the left and posterior margin of the fibroid (Fig. 4.30b, c).
2. **MRI follow-up at 9 months after treatment.** The fibroid volume was significantly reduced, with the necrotic tissues being absorbed. The uterus had reduced size (Fig. 4.31).

4.2.1.5 Discussion

- For the focused ultrasound ablation treatment of uterine posterior wall fibroids, even if the focal region is away from the endometrium, it might have the risk of endometrial injury. The ultrasound energy accumulation at the focal region would be dispersed within the acoustic near-field, which may damage the endometrium leading to the shedding and discharge of some necrotic fibroid tissues through the damaged endometrial defect. Therefore, the targeted focal region should be put at the deeper layer of fibroid during treatment. Whereas, for the posterior wall uterine fibroid adjacent to the intestine behind the uterus, the focus distribution must be at a certain distance ≥15 mm from the posterior serosa of the uterus to avoid bowel injury, which may lead to the residual un-ablated portion at the tumor edge.

4.2.2 Case 2 Type III Intramural Fibroid (2)

4.2.2.1 Case Description

The female patient was 36 years old. Physical examination revealed a large uterine fibroid. She recently felt that her abdomen was gradually enlarged, accompanied by increased menstrual blood flow, frequent urination, urgency, and severe anemia.

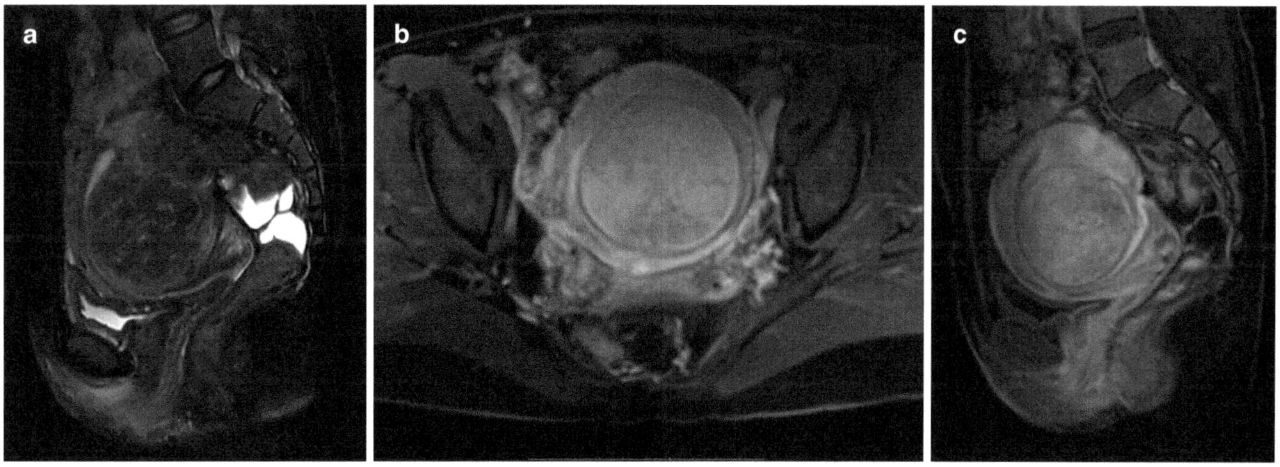

Fig. 4.29 Type III intramural fibroid before treatment. (**a**) T2WI_FS sagittal, (**b**) T1WI_FS + C axial, (**c**) T1WI_FS + C sagittal

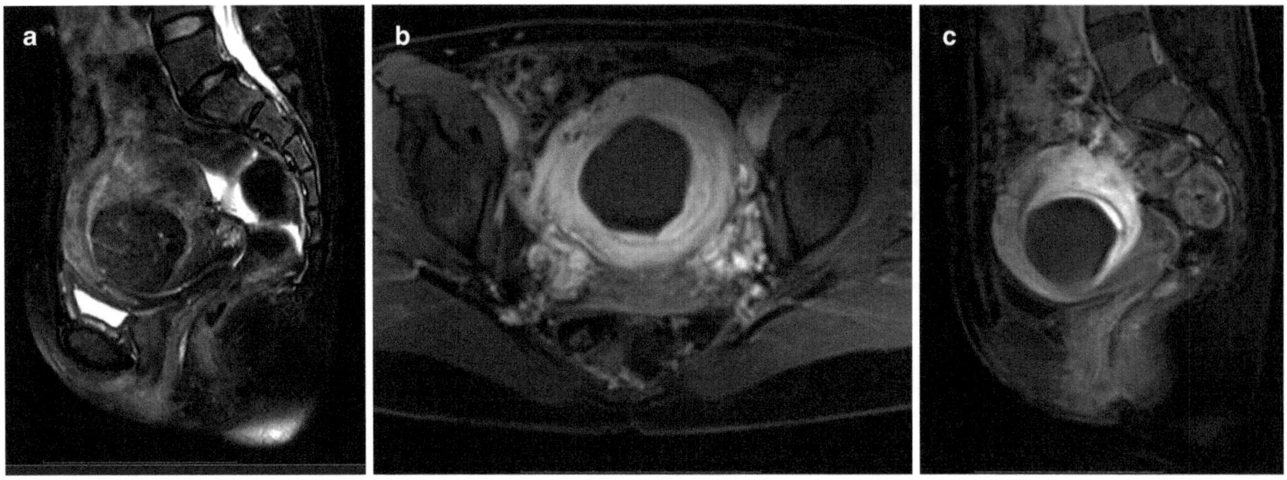

Fig. 4.30 MRI follow-up of type III intramural fibroid immediately after treatment. (**a**) T2WI_FS sagittal, (**b**) T1WI_FS + C axial, (**c**) T1WI_FS + C sagittal

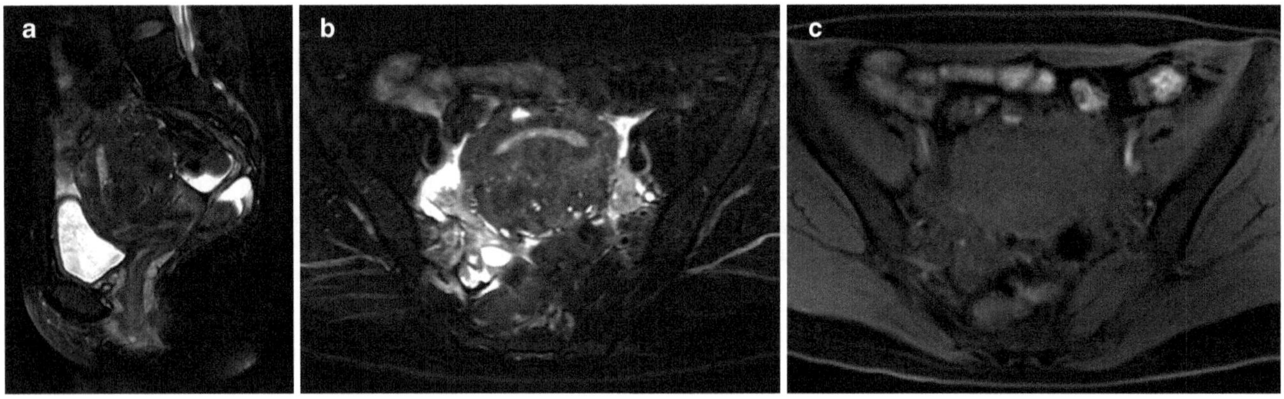

Fig. 4.31 MRI follow-up of type III intramural fibroid at 9 months after treatment. (**a**) T2WI_FS sagittal, (**b**) T2WI_FS axial, (**c**) T1WI axial

4.2.2.2 Pre-Treatment Assessment

T2WI imaging showed a large intramural fibroid with inhomogeneous hyperintensity and a size of about 80 mm × 131 mm × 122 mm (Fig. 4.32a). T1WI imaging without contrast and with contrast indicated the fibroid had a poor blood supply and a clear acoustic near-field (Fig. 4.32b–d). Considering the above characteristics, a better outcome could be anticipated for focused ultrasound ablation of the fibroid.

4.2.2.3 Treatment Techniques

1. **Focused ultrasound parameters.** Average acoustic power: 351 W, sonication time: 3270 s, duration of treatment: 188 min, total energy: 1,147,620 J.
2. **Focused ultrasound ablation techniques.** The fibroid is relatively large, and the acoustic pathway is good. There is no need to compress the abdominal wall during treatment; simply immerse the anterior abdominal wall in low-temperature degassed water. The higher sonication energy and ultrasonic contrast agent, the microbubble to enhance ultrasound ablation, can be used. However, attention should be paid to avoiding abdominal wall skin burn or scald.

4.2.2.4 Post-Treatment Assessment

1. **MRI evaluation after treatment.** The subcutaneous soft tissue and muscles of the abdominal wall showed significant edematous changes (Fig. 4.33a). The contrast-enhanced T1WI showed that the NPV ratio of the uterine fibroids reached 95% (Fig. 4.33b, c). The T1WI showed high intense signals inside the necrotic fibroid, considered to be hemorrhagic necrosis (Fig. 4.33d).
2. **MRI follow-up at 8 months after treatment.** MRI follow-up showed that the fibroid volume was significantly reduced, and the uterus gradually returned to a smaller size (Fig. 4.34).

4.2.2.5 Discussion

- When the acoustic pathway is good for treating large uterine fibroids, higher acoustic power can be used, assisted

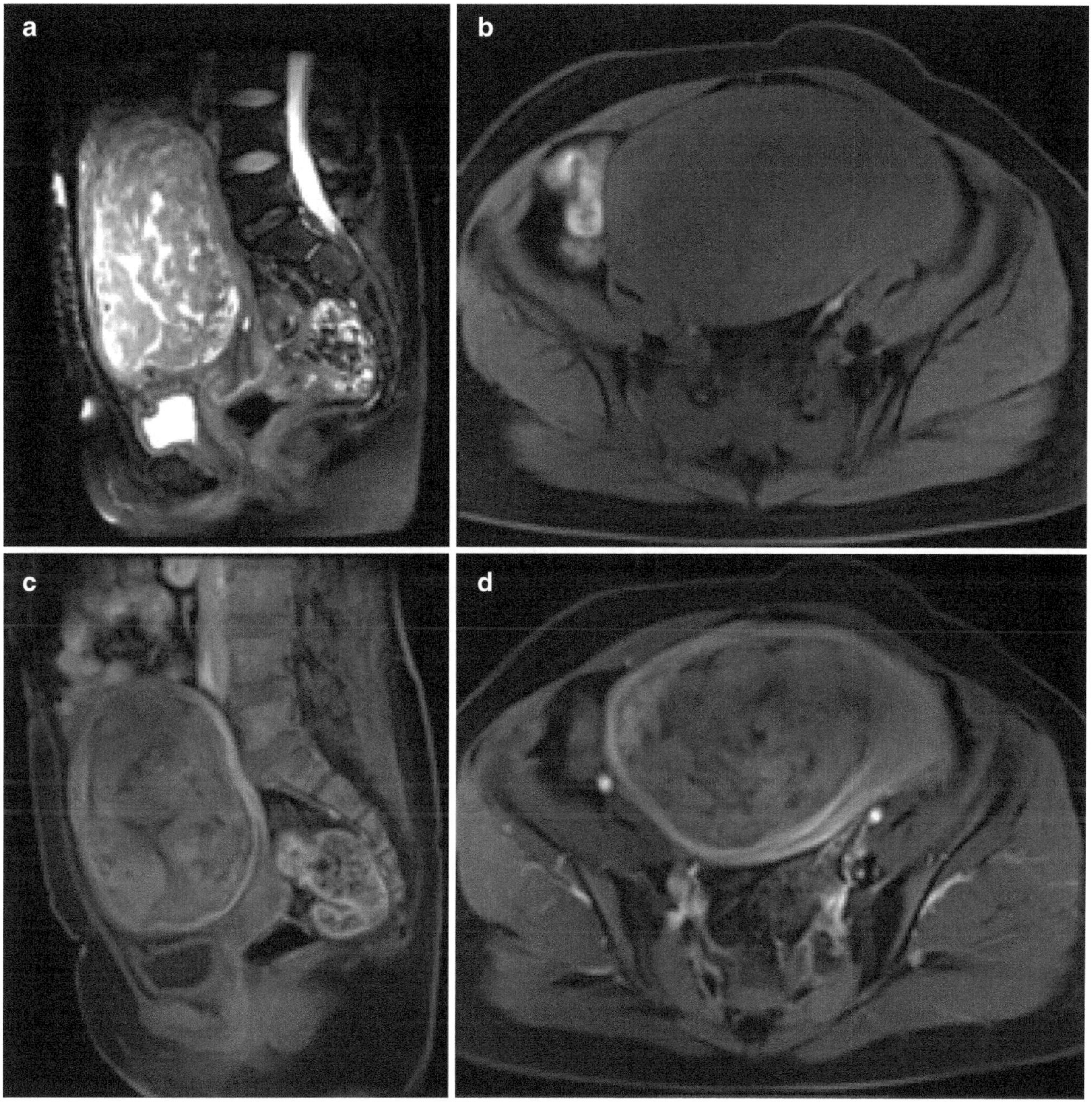

Fig. 4.32 Type III intramural fibroid before treatment. (**a**) T2WI_FS sagittal, (**b**) T1WI_FS axial, (**c**) T1WI_FS + C sagittal, (**d**) T1WI_FS + C axial

with the ultrasound contrast agent—microbubble to enhance the ablation effect, improve treatment efficiency, and avoid excessive treatment time.

- For a large fibroid treatment, pay attention to the follow-up results after treatment. Surgical removal is recommended once the uterine fibroid continues to grow despite treatment.

4.2.3 Case 3 Type III Intramural Fibroid (3)

4.2.3.1 Case Description

The female patient was 47 years old. She presented with increased menstrual blood flow and bladder pressure symptoms such as urinary frequency. After treatment, menstruation returned to normal, and urinary frequency improved gradually.

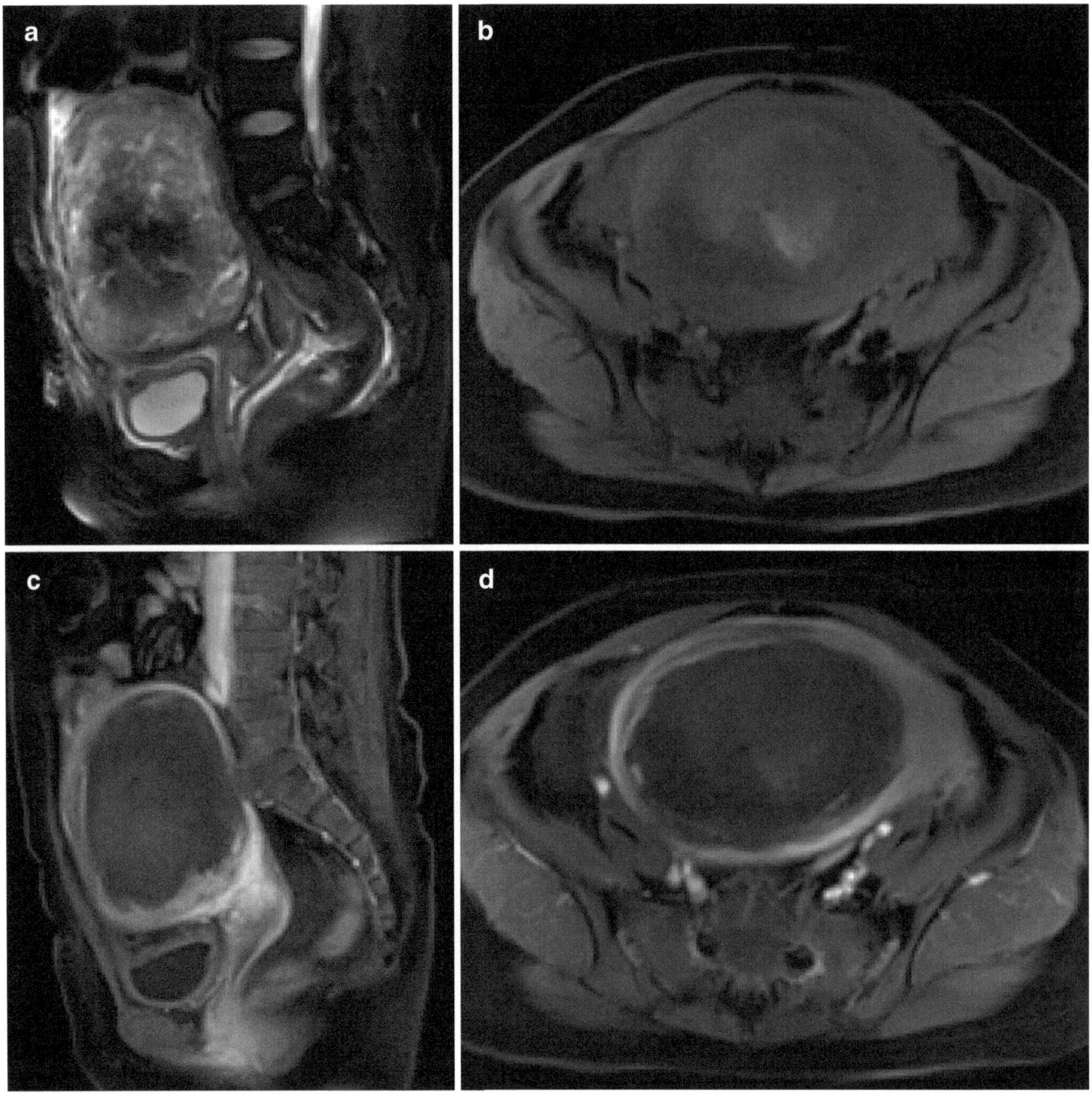

Fig. 4.33 MRI follow-up of type III intramural fibroids immediately after treatment. (**a**) T2WI_FS sagittal, (**b**) T1WI _FS axial, (**c**) T1WI_FS + C sagittal, (**d**) T1WI_FS + C axial

4.2.3.2 Pre-Treatment Assessment

MRI showed an intramural fibroid of the anterior wall with inhomogeneous hyperintensity on T2W. The contrast-enhanced T1WI showed that the fibroid was inhomogeneously enhanced, the blood supply was abundant, and the vascular flowing void effect was seen (Fig. 4.35), which indicated the fibroid could be difficult to be ablated.

4.2.3.3 Treatment Techniques

1. **Focused ultrasound parameters.** Average acoustic power: 386 W, sonication time: 2700 s, duration of treatment: 145 min, total energy: 1,043,020 J.
2. **Focused ultrasound ablation techniques.** Uterine fibroids are located on the anterior uterine wall of an anteverted uterus, with a good acoustic pathway; however, the

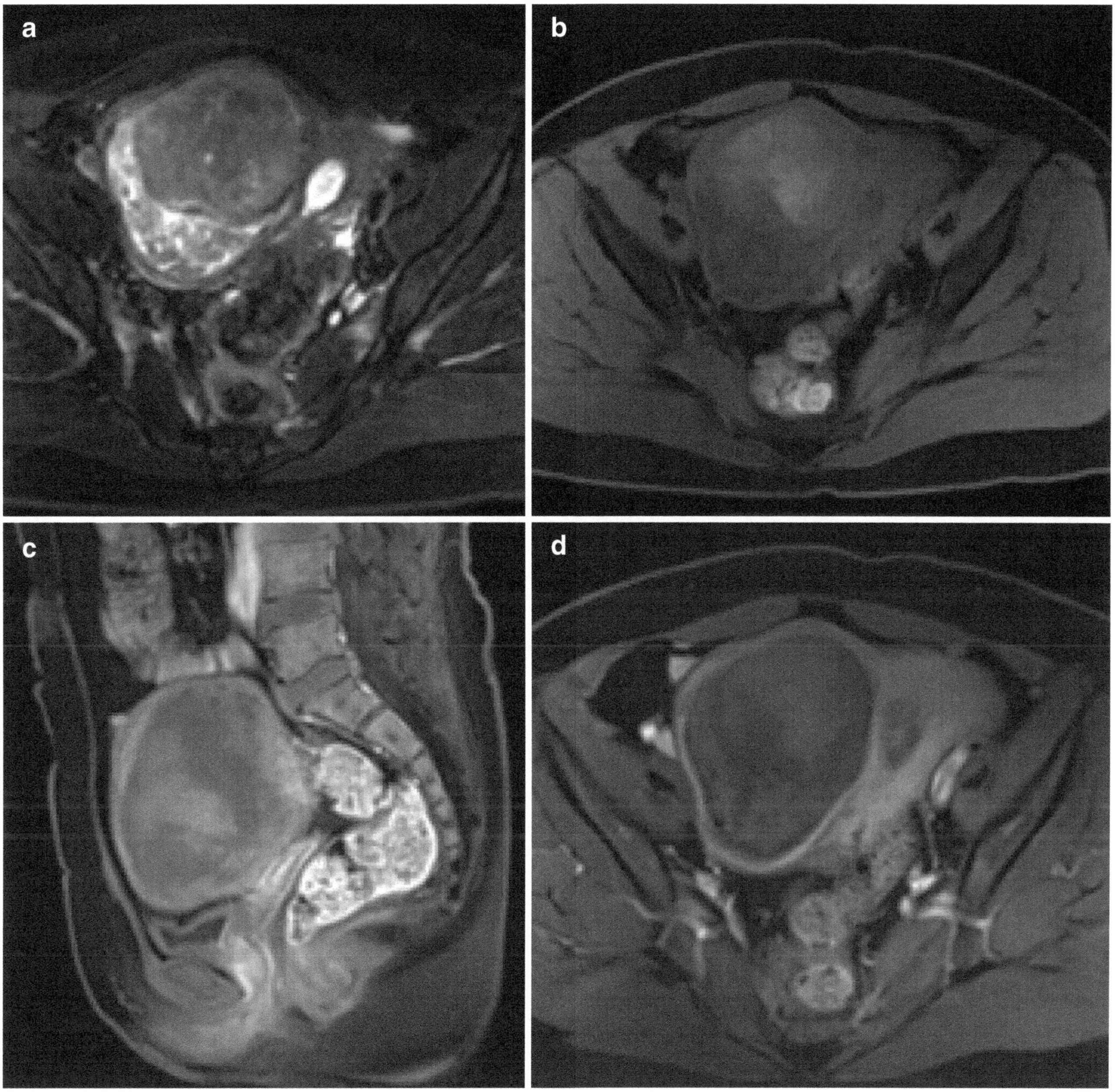

Fig. 4.34 MRI follow-up of type III intramural fibroids at 8 months after treatment. (**a**) T2WI_FS axial, (**b**) T1WI_FS axial, (**c**) T1WI_FS + C sagittal, (**d**) T1WI_FS + C axial

T2WI signal intensity is inhomogeneous and high, accompanied by the abundant blood supply. Therefore, high acoustic power and longer irradiation time were required to achieve sufficient ultrasonic energy deposited in the planned treatment area.

4.2.3.4 Post-Treatment Assessment

1. **MRI evaluation after treatment.** There was local subcutaneous soft tissue edema above the pubic symphysis (Fig. 4.36a), and the Contrast-enhanced T1WI MRI showed complete ablation of the fibroid and intact endometrium (Fig. 4.36b, c).
2. **MRI follow-up 6 months after treatment** MRI reexamination showed that fibroid volume was reduced by about 60%. Contrast-enhanced T1WI MRI showed no residual un-ablated portion in the fibroid. The subcutaneous edema of the abdominal wall had been absorbed (Fig. 4.37).

4.2.3.5 Discussion

- The intramural fibroid protrudes onto the endometrium and compresses the endometrium. It increases its surface area. Most of these patients would have symptoms of increased menstrual blood flow. This fibroid cannot be

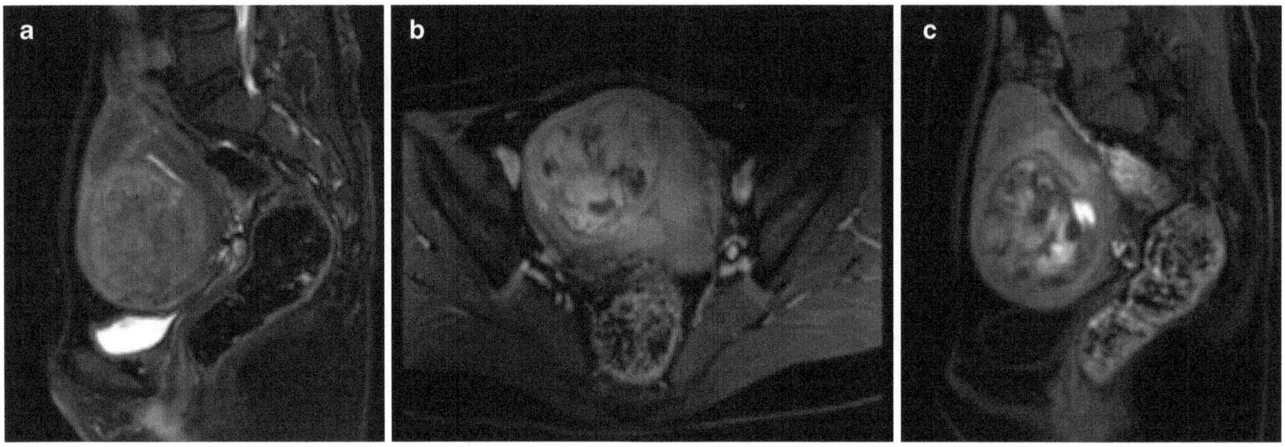

Fig. 4.35 A Type III intramural fibroid before treatment. (**a**) T2WI_FS sagittal, (**b**) T1WI_FS + C axial, (**c**) T1WI_FS + C sagittal

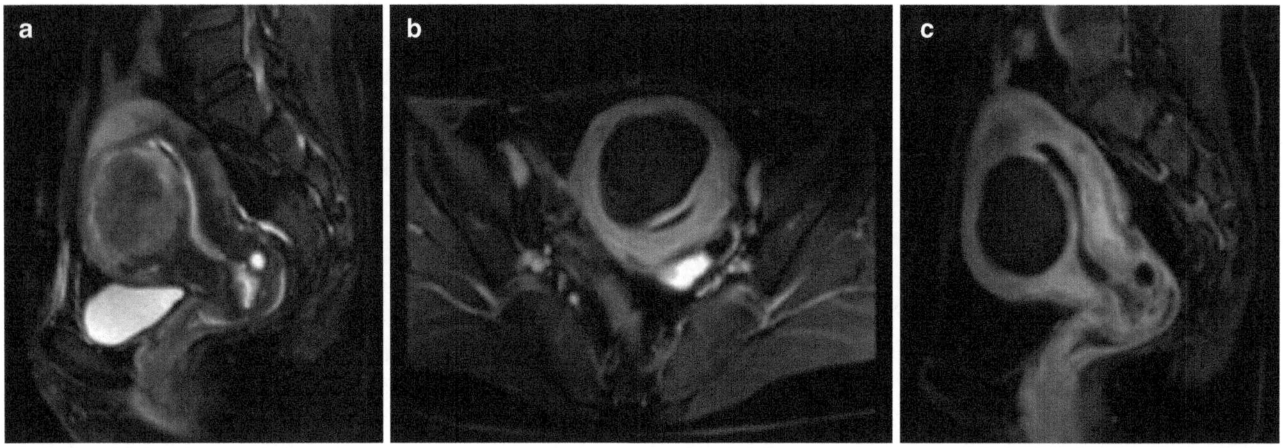

Fig. 4.36 MRI follow-up of type III intramural fibroid immediately after treatment. (**a**) T2WI_FS sagittal, (**b**) T1WI_FS + C axial, (**c**) T1WI_FS + C sagittal

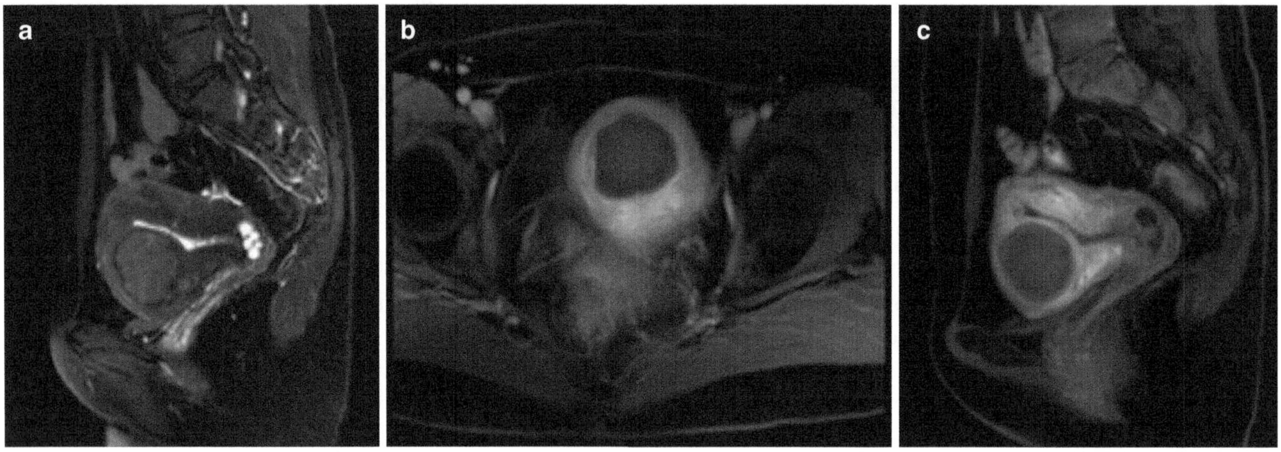

Fig. 4.37 MRI follow-up of type III intramural fibroid at 6 months after treatment. (**a**) T2WI_FS sagittal, (**b**) T1WI_FS + C axial, (**c**) T1WI_FS + C sagittal

treated with hysteroscopic surgery only. Laparoscopic surgery can also easily damage the endometrium and even causes iatrogenic adenomyosis.
- Focused ultrasound ablation is to inactivate the fibroid in situ. In this case, the fibroids were completely ablated while the endometrium was not damaged.

4.2.4 Case 4 Type III Intramural Fibroids (4)

4.2.4.1 Case Description

The female patient was 48 years old. She had symptoms of pelvic compression and frequent constipation. The clinical symptoms had improved significantly after the focused ultrasound ablation treatment.

4.2.4.2 Pre-Treatment Assessment

MRI showed that a fibroid was located on the posterior wall of the retroverted uterus, with slightly hyperintense signal on T2WI, compressing the rectum backward (Fig. 4.38a). The contrast-enhanced T1WI MRI showed that the fibroids were of a moderate blood supply with small areas of degeneration and necrosis (Fig. 4.38b, c). The fibroid was located next to the rectum and sacrococcygeal plexus, and the abdominal wall was thick. Therefore, it was predicted that it might be difficult to ablate the fibroid.

4.2.4.3 Treatment Techniques

1. **Focused ultrasound parameters.** Average acoustic power: 397 W, sonication time: 944 s, duration of treatment: 131 min, total energy: 375,100 J.
2. **Focused ultrasound ablation techniques.** The area of necrosis in the fibroid could serve as a breakthrough point for ablation treatment. The focal region was placed initially in that area as the deep layer of the uterine fibroid, which can heat the ischemic necrosis to quickly accumulate energy to disperse into the surrounding area for achieving an ideal thermal effect.

4.2.4.4 Post-Treatment Assessment

1. **MRI evaluation after treatment.** The signal intensity of the fibroid was significantly increased with a peripheral low signal ring on T2WI (Fig. 4.39a). The contrast-enhanced MRI showed that the overall ablation effect of the fibroid was good, completely ablated without perfusion, the boundary was clear and smooth, the NPV ratio was as high as 99%, and the endometrium was well protected (Fig. 4.39b, c).
2. **MRI follow-up at 7 months, 5 years and 8 months, and 7 years after treatment.** It showed that the volume of uterus and fibroid were significantly reduced, about 50%, 60%, and 80%, respectively, with no signs of recurrence (Fig. 4.39d–l).

4.2.4.5 Discussion

- The uterine fibroids with T2WI homogeneous slight hyperintensity are generally considered difficult to be ablated by HIFU. The patient should be fully communicated before treatment. Because the patient had only symptoms of constipation and was close to her perimenopausal period, she had refused surgical removal of the fibroid but required non-invasive focused ultrasound ablation treatment.
- In this case, the effect of focused ultrasound ablation of the fibroid was satisfactory. There was no recurrence in long-term follow-up, indicating that focused ultrasound ablation can also treat the homogeneously and slightly

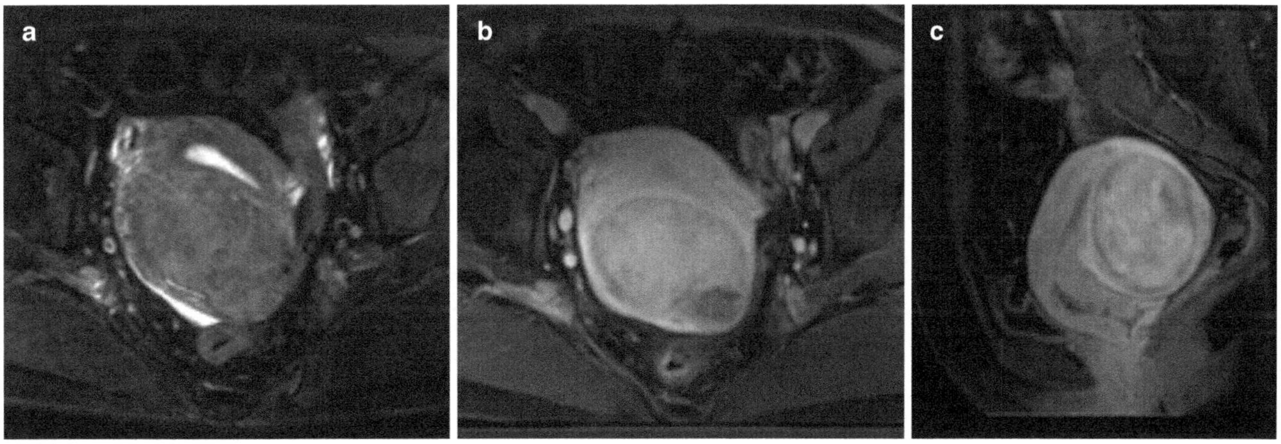

Fig. 4.38 A Type III intramural fibroid before treatment. (**a**) T2WI_FS sagittal, (**b**) T1WI_FS + C axial, (**c**) T1WI_FS + C sagittal

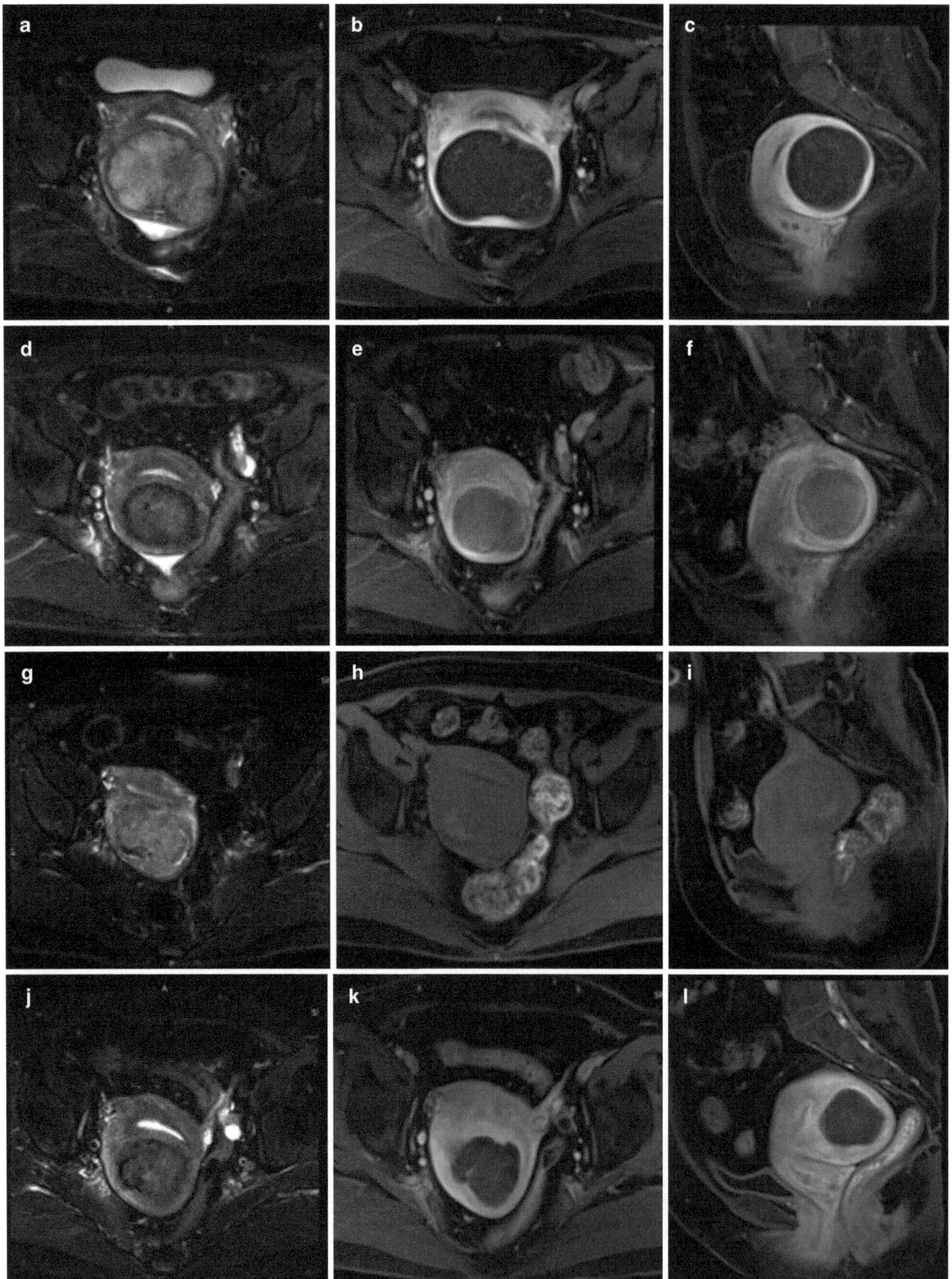

Fig. 4.39 MRI follow-up of type III intramural fibroids immediately (**a**–**c**), at 7 months (**d**–**f**), 5 years, and 8 months (**g**–**i**), and 7 years (**j**–**l**) after treatment. (**a**) T2WI_FS axial, (**b**) T1WI_FS + C axial, (**c**) T1WI_FS + C sagittal, (**d**) T2WI_FS axial, (**e**) T1WI_FS + C axial, (**f**) T1WI_FS + C sagittal, (**g**) T2WI_FS axial, (**h**) T1WI axial, (**i**) T1WI sagittal, (**j**) T2WI_FS axial, (**k**) T1WI_FS + C axial, (**l**) T1WI_FS + C sagittal

hyperintense fibroids on T2WI. Thus, magnetic resonance examination before treatment to predict the treatment effect still needs further research and exploration.

4.2.5 Case 5 Type III Intramural Fibroid (5)

4.2.5.1 Case Description

The female patient was 39 years old. Physical examination revealed uterine fibroids for more than 4 years. She had increased menstrual blood flow with blood clots for more than 2 years, associated with prolonged menstrual periods. She also had anemia for more than 1 year.

4.2.5.2 Pre-Treatment Assessment

MRI showed that the fibroid with inhomogeneous and slight hyperintensity was located in the anterior wall of the anteverted uterus on T2WI. The uterine cavity and endometrium were compressed (Fig. 4.40a). The contrast-enhanced T1WI showed that the fibroids had abundant blood supply and a small area of degeneration and necrosis in the center (Fig. 4.40b, c). Although the acoustic pathway was clear, it was predicted that it could be difficult for the fibroid to be ablated.

4.2.5.3 Treatment Techniques

1. **Focused ultrasound parameters.** Average acoustic power: 387 W, sonication time: 4400 s, duration of treatment: 215 min, total energy: 1,704,450 J.
2. **Focused ultrasound ablation techniques.** Since the fibroid was located on the anterior wall, in order to protect the endometrium, the focal region of ablation was more than 10 mm away from the endometrium. As it is predicted that the fibroid is difficult to ablate, increasing the initial ultrasound irradiation intensity (400 W, 2:1). While using the high-power ultrasound ablation, the pelvic nerve damage is at high risk. Therefore during the treatment process, keep observing the treatment while mastering the treatment timing to prevent any damage.

4.2.5.4 Post-Treatment Assessment

1. **MRI evaluation after treatment.** Localized soft tissue edema occurred under the umbilicus of the anterior abdominal wall, and the fibroid showed mixed signals with low central signals but high intense signals at the periphery on T2WI (Fig. 4.41a). The contrast-enhanced T1WI showed that the NPV ratio of the fibroid was about 75%, and there were more non-ablated residual tissues adjacent to the endometrium (Fig. 4.41b, c).
2. **MRI follow-up at 4 months after treatment.** The soft tissue edema of the anterior abdominal wall had disappeared, and the size of the fibroid was slightly reduced. The contrast-enhanced T1WI showed that the necrotic area of the fibroids was significantly reduced, but the residual area increased and recurred with the clearer tumor pseudocapsule(Fig. 4.42).

4.2.5.5 Discussion

- High T2WI signals in the uterine fibroid often suggest the possibility of richer water content and fewer collagen fibers. Focused ultrasound ablation is not conducive to energy deposition, so this type of fibroid may be difficult to ablate.
- Although this case was irradiated with high acoustic power of focused ultrasound for more than 4000 seconds, the NPV ratio was still only 75%. The residual un-ablated fibroid is prone to recur and re-grow. The outcome needs further research and exploration. It is recommended that minimally invasive surgery should be performed in 3–6 months after ablation treatment, when the fibroid shrinks in size, together with reduced vascularity and distinct fibroid edge after the disappearance of abdominal wall edema.

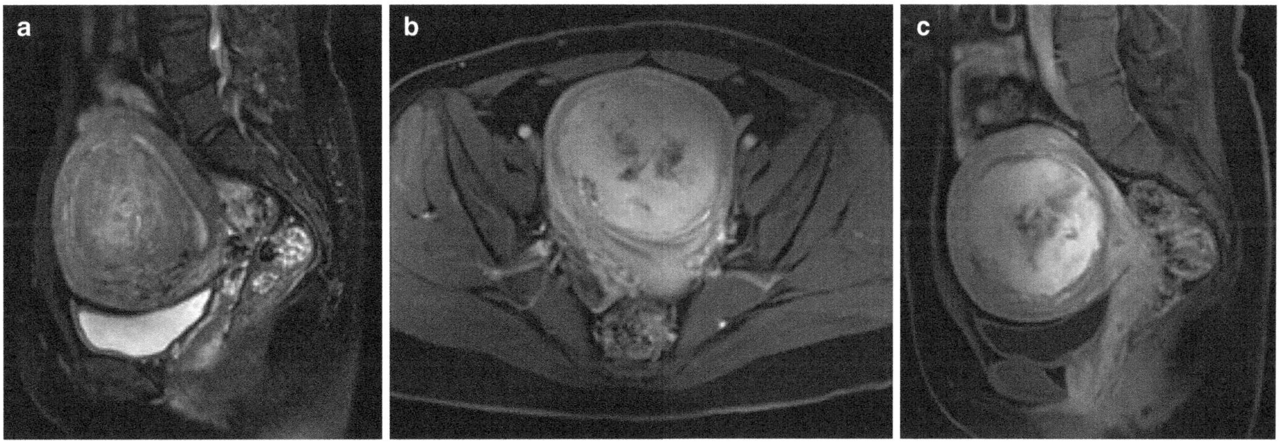

Fig. 4.40 A Type III intramural fibroid before treatment. (**a**) T2WI_FS sagittal, (**b**) T1WI_FS + C axial, (**c**) T1WI_FS + C sagittal

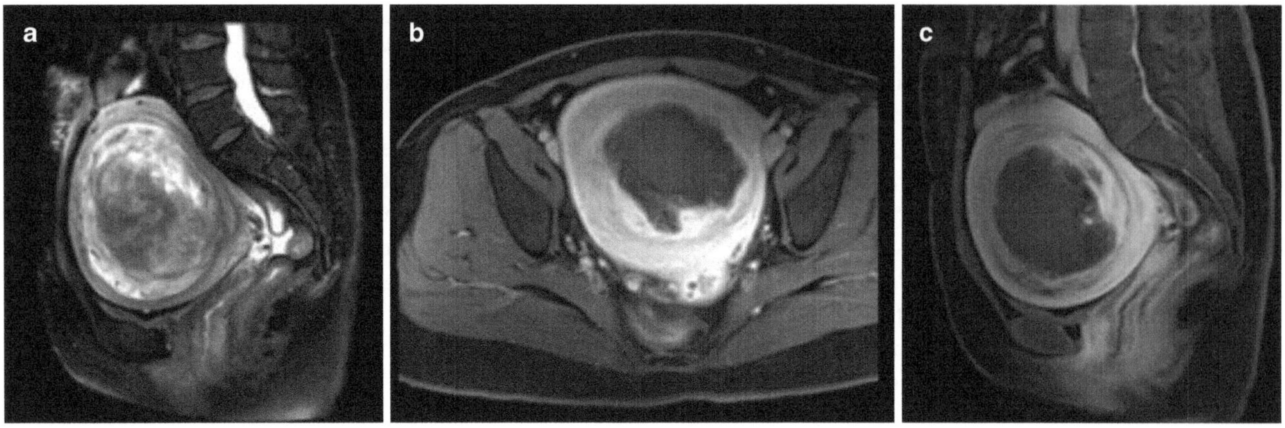

Fig. 4.41 MRI follow-up of type III intramural fibroid immediately after treatment. (**a**) T2WI_FS sagittal, (**b**) T1WI_FS + C axial, (**c**) T1WI_FS + C sagittal

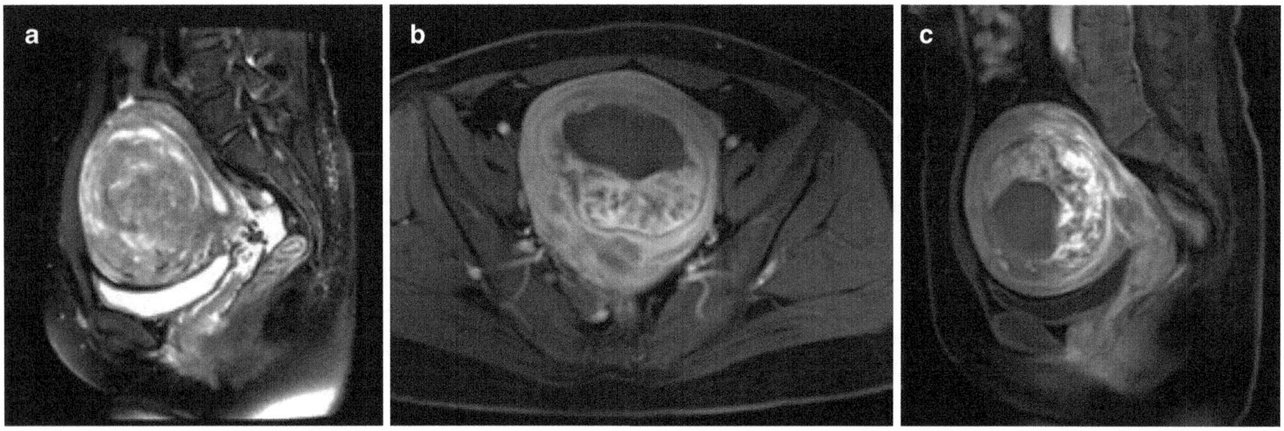

Fig. 4.42 MRI follow-up of type III intramural fibroid at 4 months after treatment. (**a**) T2WI_FS sagittal, (**b**) T1WI_FS + C axial, (**c**) T1WI_FS + C sagittal

4.2.6 Case 6 Type III Intramural Fibroid (6)

4.2.6.1 Case Description

The female patient was 47 years old. She presented with increased menstrual blood flow and infertility. She received two focused ultrasound ablation (HIFU) treatments 6 months apart. Her menstrual volume decreased after treatments.

4.2.6.2 Pre-Treatment Assessment

MRI showed an anterior wall fibroid with mixed high and isointense signals on T2WI, and the uterine cavity was significantly compressed and flattened. The contrast-enhanced T1WI showed that the fibroid had an abundant blood supply with a pseudocapsule that could be seen on the edges (Fig. 4.43a, b). The part of the fibroid adjacent to the endometrium had abundant blood supply, which was likely to recur after ablation treatment.

4.2.6.3 Treatment Techniques

1. **Focused ultrasound parameters**. The first average acoustic power: 400 W, sonication time: 709 s, duration of treatment: 102 min, total energy: 283,600 J. The second average acoustic power: 366 W, sonication time: 1398 s, duration of treatment: 124 min, and total energy: 273,370 J.
2. **Focused ultrasound ablation techniques**. The fibroid was located on the anterior uterine wall, but the small bowels lay between the abdominal wall and uterus. After filling the bladder, a good acoustic pathway was established. The ultrasound-focused region could be placed ≥10 mm from the endometrium. Thus, high-power sonication was used.

4.2.6.4 Post-treatment Assessment

1. **MRI evaluation after treatment**. The contrast-enhanced T1WI showed that the NPV ratio of the fibroids was about 95%, and the endometrium was intact. Some parts of the un-ablated fibroid were left next to the endometrium (Fig. 4.43c).
2. **MRI follow-up at 3 and 6 months after treatment**. The contrast-enhanced T1WI showed that the area of necrosis was gradually reduced, but the residual tumor tissue adjacent to the endometrium gradually thickened and recurred (Fig. 4.44a, b, red arrows).
3. **MRI evaluation after the second ablation treatment at 6 months intervals**. The contrast-enhanced T1WI showed that the residual and recurring portion of the fibroid showed complete ablation without perfusion, no obvious marginal residual, and the endometrium was well protected (Fig. 4.44c).

4.2.6.5 Discussion

- To preserve the patient's fertility or avoid continuous vaginal fluid discharge, the endometrium is always protected as much as possible during focused ultrasound ablation of the fibroid that is adjacent to the endometrium. Suppose there is a large part of the fibroid next to the endometrium or the fibroid has an abundant blood supply; in that case, any residual un-ablated fibroid can continue to grow and recur after focused ultrasound ablation surgery.
- If the residual fibroid regrows after surgery, focused ultrasound ablation can be performed again. Because there were some necrotic areas after past ablation, the ultrasound energy can be deposited well, and the recurrent fibroid can be relatively easy to ablate.

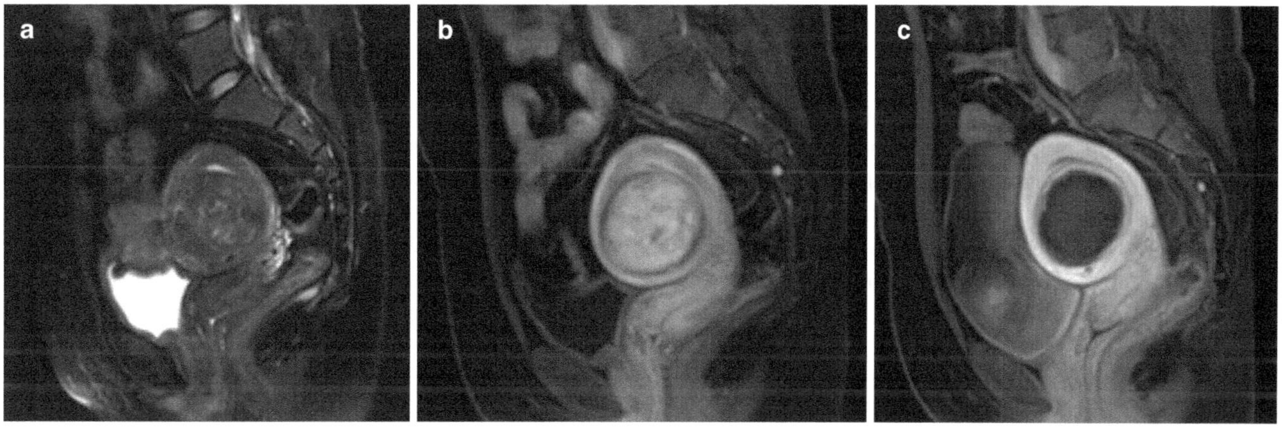

Fig. 4.43 Type III intramural fibroid before treatment (**a**, **b**) and immediately after treatment (**c**). (**a**) T2WI_FS sagittal, (**b**) T1WI_FS + C sagittal, (**c**) T1WI_FS + C sagittal

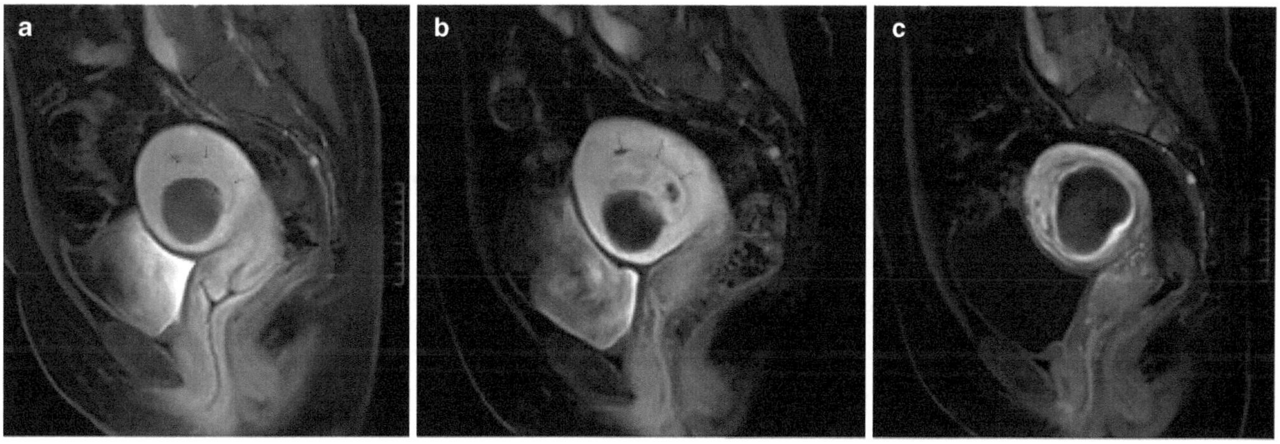

Fig. 4.44 Type III intramural fibroid at 3 months (**a**), 6 months (**b**), and immediately after the second treatment (**c**). (**a**) T1WI_FS + C sagittal, (**b**) T1WI_FS + C sagittal, (**c**) T1WI_FS + C sagittal

4.2.7 Case 7 Type III Intramural Fibroid (7)

4.2.7.1 Case Description

The female patient was 37 years old with uterine fibroids 3 years ago. She presented with heavy menstrual blood flow, and without dysmenorrhea and low back pain.

4.2.7.2 Pre-Treatment Assessment

MRI showed a uterine fibroid of the left lateral wall with hypo-intense signals on T2WI, and the uterine cavity was significantly compressed (Fig. 4.45a, b). The contrast-enhanced T1WI revealed that the fibroid had a moderate blood supply with a pseudocapsule that could be seen on the edges (Fig. 4.45c). The part of the fibroid adjacent to the endometrium had blood supply, which was easy to recur after ablation treatment.

4.2.7.3 Treatment Techniques

1. **Focused ultrasound parameters.** Average acoustic power: 249 W, sonication time: 3216 s, duration of treatment: 146 min., total energy: 800,460 J.
2. **Focused ultrasound ablation techniques.** The fibroid with T2WI hypointense signals and moderate blood supply was suitable for focused ultrasound ablation treatment; however, it was close to the endometrium. The key issue was how to avoid the intima injury and obtain the curative effect of complete ablation without need for re-intervention.

4.2.7.4 Post-Treatment Assessment

1. **MRI evaluation after treatment.** The contrast-enhanced T1WI showed that non-perfusion area covered all of fibroid without any residual (Fig. 4.46a–c).
2. **MRI follow-up at 6 months and 9 months after treatment.** The volume of the abated fibroid decreased significantly without any perfusion on the contrast-enhanced T1WI (Fig. 4.46d–f).

4.2.7.5 Discussion

- The fibroid was close to the endometrium, so the acoustic power should be reduced so as to avoid the intima broken; meanwhile, it is necessary to release enough energy for complete ablation of the fibroid. Thus, the accumulated sonication time would be relatively longer.
- After ablation treatment, the residual tissue of the ablated fibroid is easy to recur, resulting in relapse, which influences its long-term efficacy. Therefore, the complete ablation or almost complete ablation is preferred if the fibroid is suitable for the focused ultrasound ablation.

4.2.8 Case 8 Type III Intramural Fibroid (8)

4.2.8.1 Case Description

The female patient was 47 years old without a fertility requirement. She presented with heavy menstrual blood flow, and menstrual cramps started at the age of 14 and gradually worsened.

4.2.8.2 Pre-Treatment Assessment

MRI showed two fibroids with hypointensity in the anterior wall of the uterus on T2WI (Fig. 4.47a). The contrast-enhanced T1WI showed that they were of poor blood supply (Fig. 4.47b, c). Due to the anteversion of the uterus, the fibroids were close to the anterior abdominal wall. Thus, the acoustic pathway was good. It was predicted to be relatively easy to ablate.

4.2.8.3 Treatment Techniques

1. **Focused ultrasound parameters.** Average acoustic power: 295 W, sonication time: 1401 s, duration of treatment: 100 min, total energy: 413, 400 J.
2. **Focused ultrasound ablation techniques.** According to the patient's response to the focused ultrasound ablation and the grayscale changes of ultrasound echo in the tar-

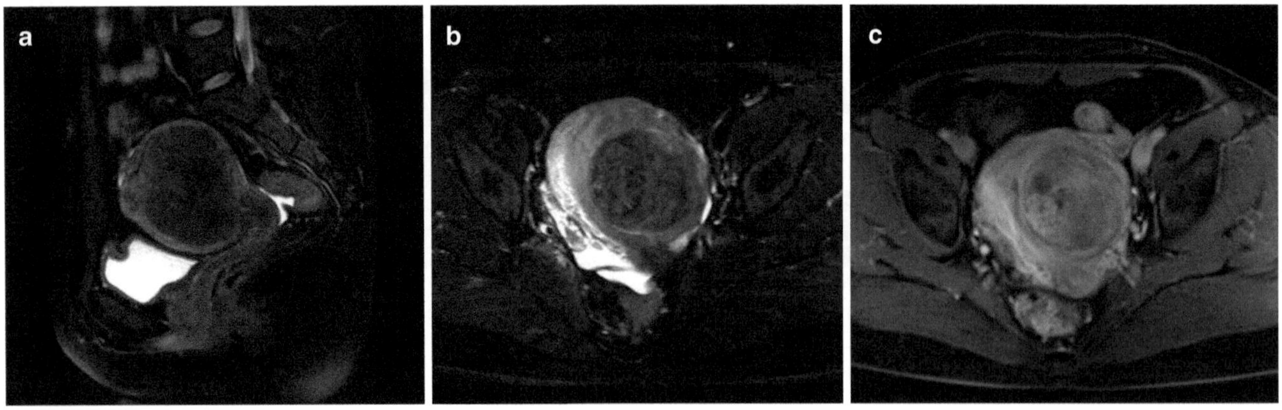

Fig. 4.45 Type III intramural fibroid before treatment. (**a**) T2WI_FS sagittal, (**b**) T2WI_FS axial, (**c**) T1WI_FS + C sagittal

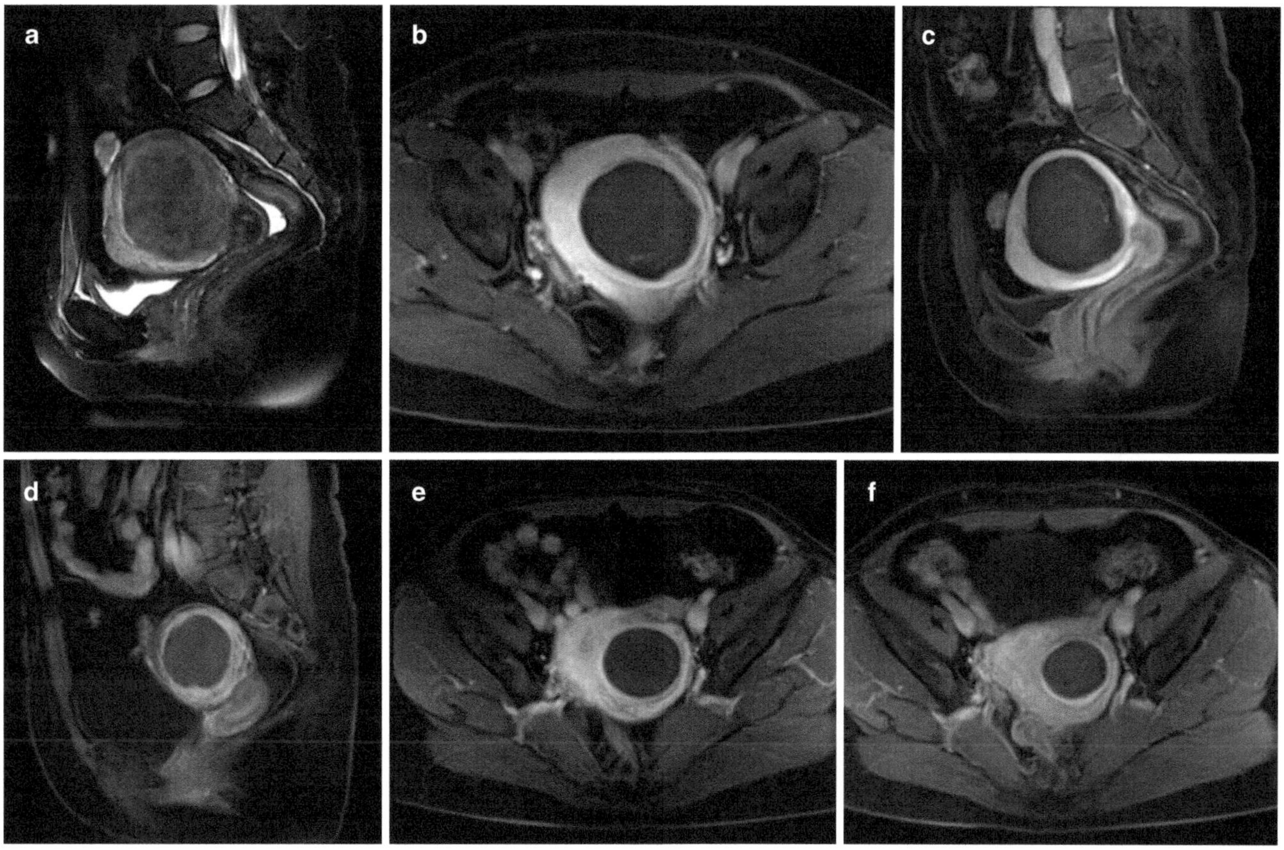

Fig. 4.46 MRI follow-up of type III intramural fibroids immeidately (**a**–**c**), 6 months (**d**, **e**) and 9 months (**f**) after treatment. T2WI_FS sagittal, (**b**) T1WI_FS + C axial, (**c**) T1WI_FS + C sagittal, (**d**) T1WI_FS + C sagittal, (**e**, **f**) T1WI_FS + C axial

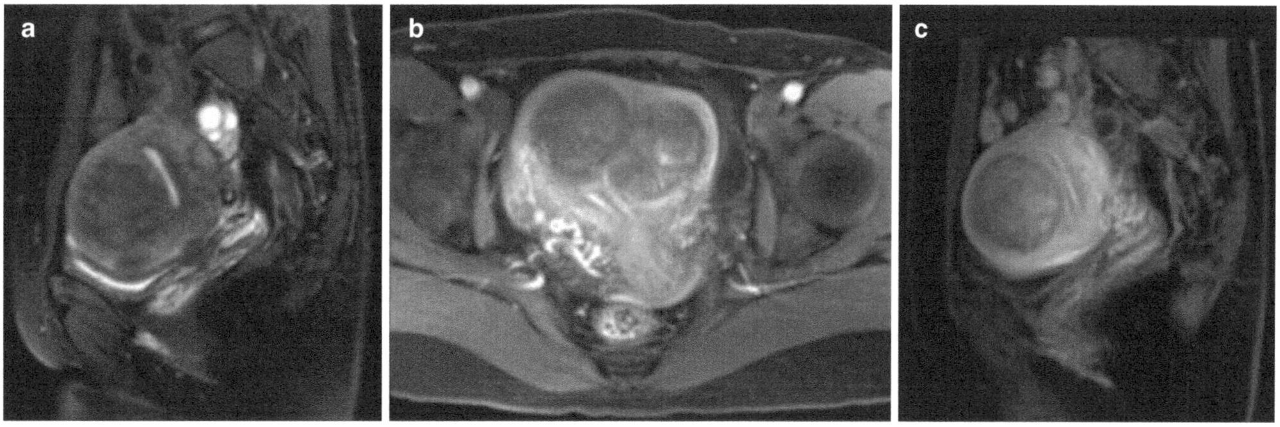

Fig. 4.47 A Type III intramural fibroid before treatment. (**a**) T2WI_FS sagittal, (**b**) T1WI_FS + C axial, (**c**) T1WI_FS + C sagittal

geted area, the treatment needed to adjust the acoustic power and time of radiation for the two fibroids.

4.2.8.4 Post-Treatment Assessment

1. **MRI evaluation after treatment.** There was no edema in the anterior abdominal wall, and there was mild sacrococcygeal fascial edema on T2WI (Fig. 4.48a). The contrast-enhanced T1WI showed the NPV ratio of the two fibroids exceeded 95%, and there were two small damages on the endometrial surface of the anterior wall of the uterus (Fig. 4.48b, c).
2. **MRI follow-up at 3 years after treatment.** The two fibroids were significantly reduced to about 10 mm (Fig. 4.49b), but new small fibroids of about 10 mm

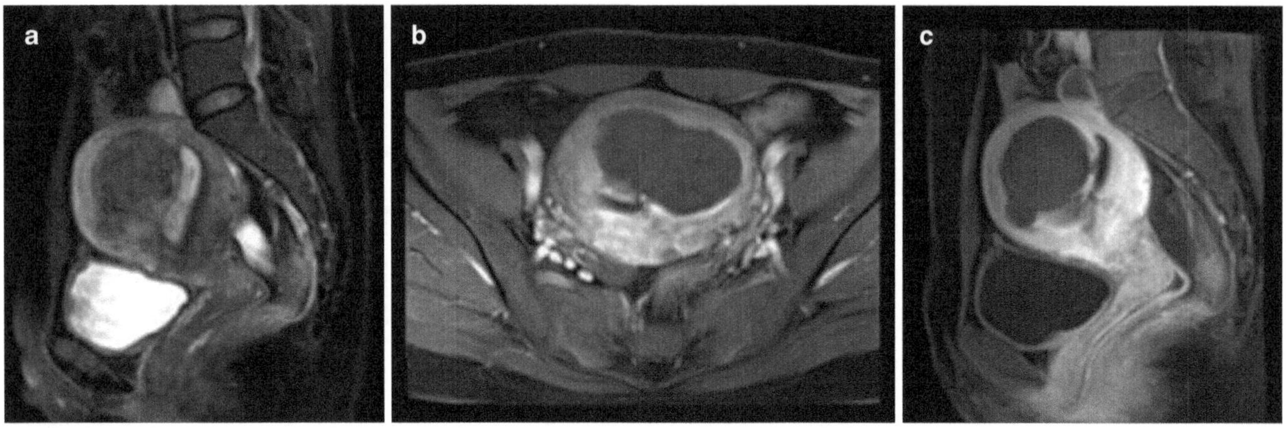

Fig. 4.48 MRI evaluation of type III intramural fibroids after treatment. (**a**) T2WI_FS sagittal, (**b**) T1WI_FS + C axial, (**c**) T1WI_FS + C sagittal

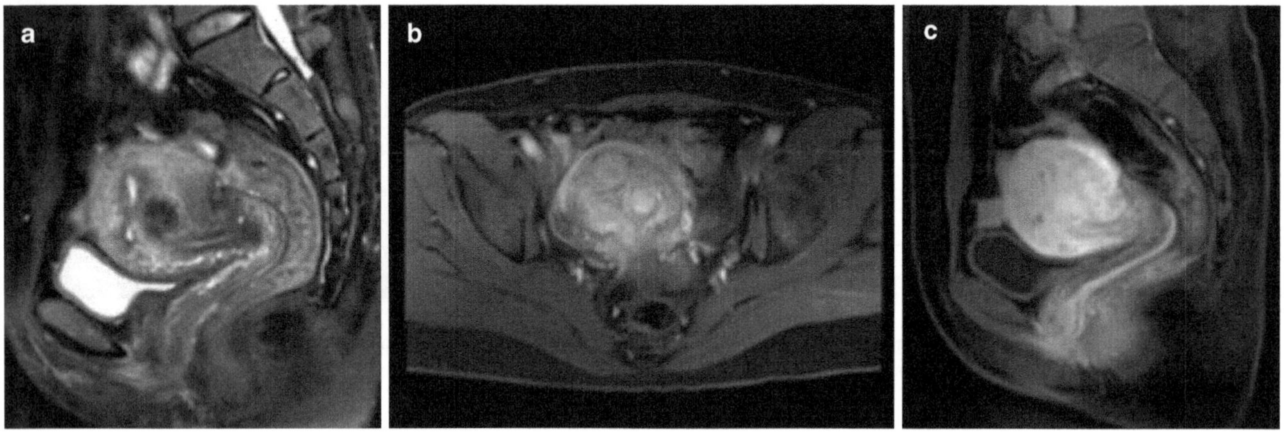

Fig. 4.49 MRI follow-up of type III intramural fibroid at 3 years after treatment. (**a**) T2WI_FS sagittal, (**b**) T1WI_FS + C axial, (**c**) T1WI_FS + C sagittal

appeared in the posterior wall of the uterus, the endometrial damages were completely repaired to normal shape, and the sacrococcygeal fascial edema disappeared (Fig. 4.49a, c).

4.2.8.5 Discussion

- After focused ultrasound ablation of fibroids, the size of fibroids gradually decreases over time. However, new fibroids will appear even after surgeical removal of multiple uterine fibroids. Focused ultrasound ablation can be repeated as a non-invasive treatment method. Thus, it is more suitable for multiple uterine fibroids.
- The pelvic fascia edema was related to the injury caused by ultrasound ablation, which may irritate or compress the adjacent nerves causing pain or paresthesia in the corresponding area.

4.2.9 Case 9 Type III Intramural Fibroid (9)

4.2.9.1 Case Description

The female patient was 39 years old. Her menstruation was prolonged, irregular, and with mild anemia. More than 1 month after focused ultrasound ablation treatment, she experienced persistent abdominal pain with paroxysmal aggravation after strenuous activity, accompanied by a low fever. Her blood test showed increased white blood cells. MRI follow-up showed the necrotic fibroid was partially discharged through the cervix. Colposcopy showed a large piece of necrotic fibroid at the cervix. The protruding fibroid was removed. Then the abdominal pain was relieved, and other related symptoms disappeared altogether.

4.2.9.2 Pre-Treatment Assessment

T2WI showed a large anterior wall uterine fibroid with inhomogeneous, mixed high and low intense signals, compressing the uterine cavity (Fig. 4.50a). The contrast-enhanced MR imaging showed that the fibroid had moderate blood supply (its peripheral area had abundant blood supply), with obvious pseudocapsule on the edges (Fig. 4.50b, c). It is predicted that it would be relatively not easy to ablate, although there was a clear acoustic pathway for ultrasound ablation.

4.2.9.3 Treatment Techniques

1. **Focused ultrasound parameters.** Average acoustic power: 241 W, sonication time: 4650 s, duration of treatment: 167 min, total energy: 1,120,320 J.
2. **Focused ultrasound ablation techniques.** High ultrasonic energy was needed for ablating this type of fibroid. If the patient has poor pain tolerance, the acoustic power and irradiation intensity can be appropriately reduced with a longer sonication time for accumulating more ultrasonic doses in the treated area.

4.2.9.4 Post-Treatment Assessment

1. **MRI evaluation after treatment.** The anterior abdominal wall was edematous (Fig. 4.51a). The contrast-enhanced MRI showed that the fibroid was completely ablated and showed no perfusion area, with the edges clear and smooth. The endometrium was preserved intact (Fig. 4.51b, c).
2. **MRI follow-up at 1.5 months, 2 months, and 3 months after treatment.** The endometrial lining was incomplete, part of the fibroids protruded into the uterine cavity, and the necrotic fibroids were gradually discharged (Fig. 4.52a). The endometrium presented a "V"-shaped gap, and the necrotic fibroids were completely discharged and disappeared (Fig. 4.52b). After another month, the endometrium was reexamined, showing complete healing

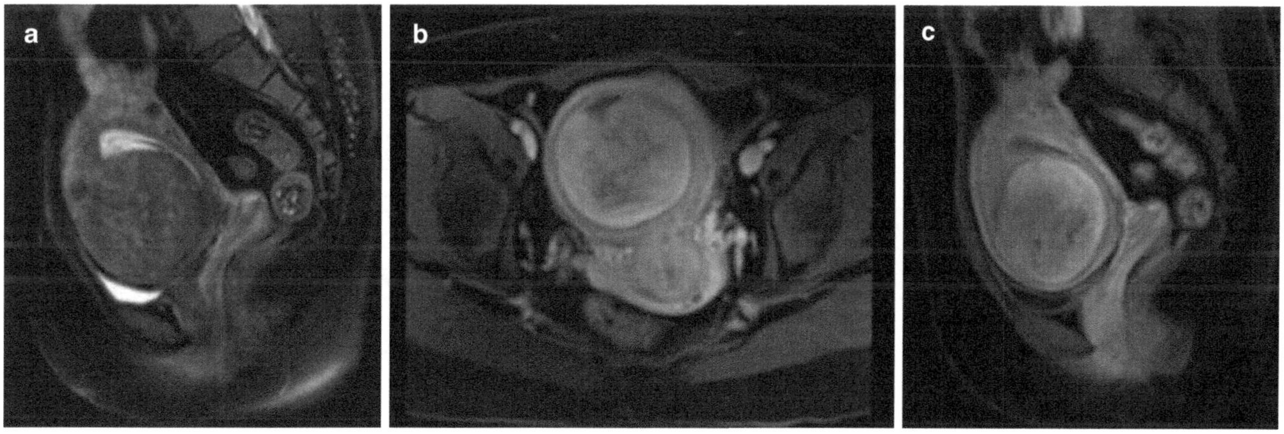

Fig. 4.50 A Type III intramural fibroid before treatment. (**a**) T2WI_FS sagittal, (**b**) T1WI_FS + C axial, (**c**) T1WI_FS + C sagittal

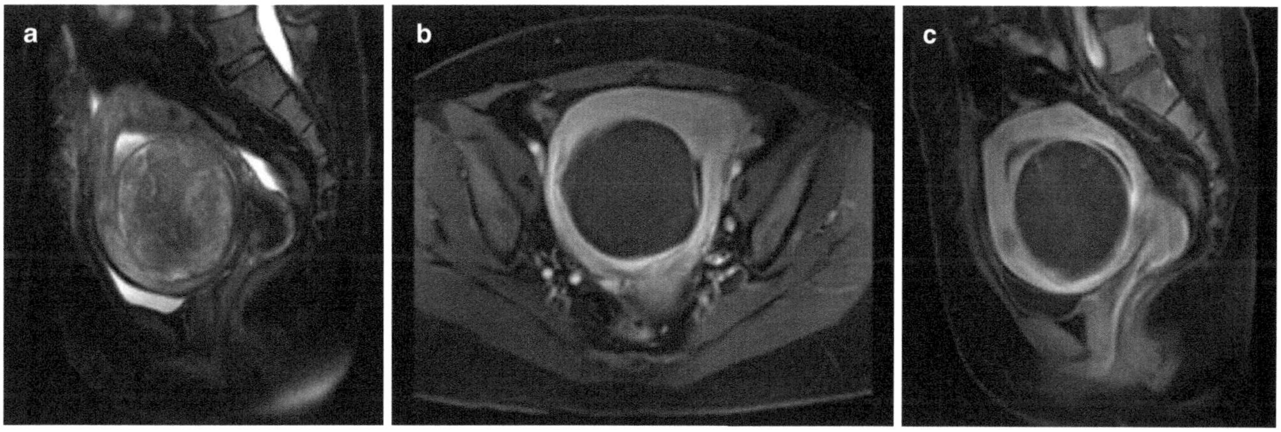

Fig. 4.51 MRI evaluation of type III intramural fibroid after treatment. (**a**) T2WI_FS sagittal, (**b**) T1WI_FS + C axial, (**c**) T1WI_FS + C sagittal

of the endometrium (Fig. 4.52c). There was no change in the size of some small intramural fibroids.

4.2.9.5 Discussion

- In addition to submucosal fibroids, the necrotic intramural fibroids will also be discharged through the physiological cavity after focused ultrasound ablation treatment. When the necrotic tissue of a larger fibroid is discharged, it may be blocked at the cervix and it requires the help of hysteroscopy.

4.2.10 Case 10 Type IV Intramural Fibroids (1)

4.2.10.1 Case Description

A 39-year-old female patient was found to have uterine fibroids for 3 years. She was asymptomatic and required treatment because of her anxiety.

4.2.10.2 Pre-Treatment Assessment

MRI showed two fibroids with homogeneous hypointensity at the posterior wall of the uterus on T2WI (Fig. 4.53a, b). The contrast-enhanced T1WI showed that one fibroid had a poor blood supply, and the other had a moderate blood supply (Fig. 4.53c). It was predicted before treatment that focused ultrasound ablation would achieve good results. But these fibroids were located in the posterior wall of the uterus, and there were many bowels in the space between the anterior abdominal wall and the uterus; thus, the focused ultrasound ablation could be technically difficult.

4.2.10.3 Treatment Techniques

1. **Focused ultrasound parameters.** Average acoustic power: 396 W, sonication time: 1025 s, duration of treatment: 80 min, total energy: 405,830 J.
2. **Focused ultrasound ablation techniques.** The technique was to push the bowel in front of the uterus out of

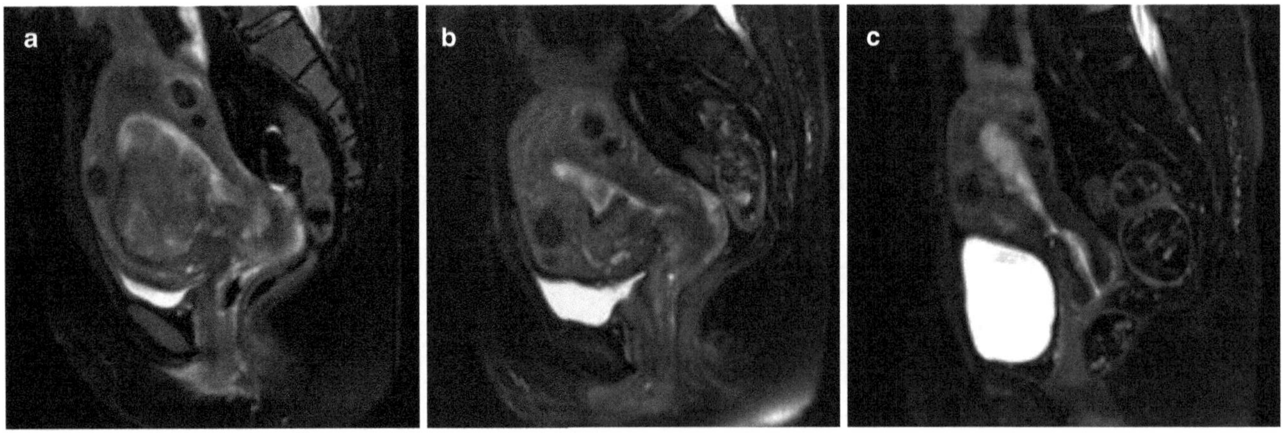

Fig. 4.52 MRI follow-up of type III intramural fibroid at 1.5 months (**a**), 2 months (**b**), and 3 months (**c**) after treatment. (**a**) T2WI_FS sagittal, (**b**) T2WI_FS sagittal, (**c**) T2WI_FS sagittal

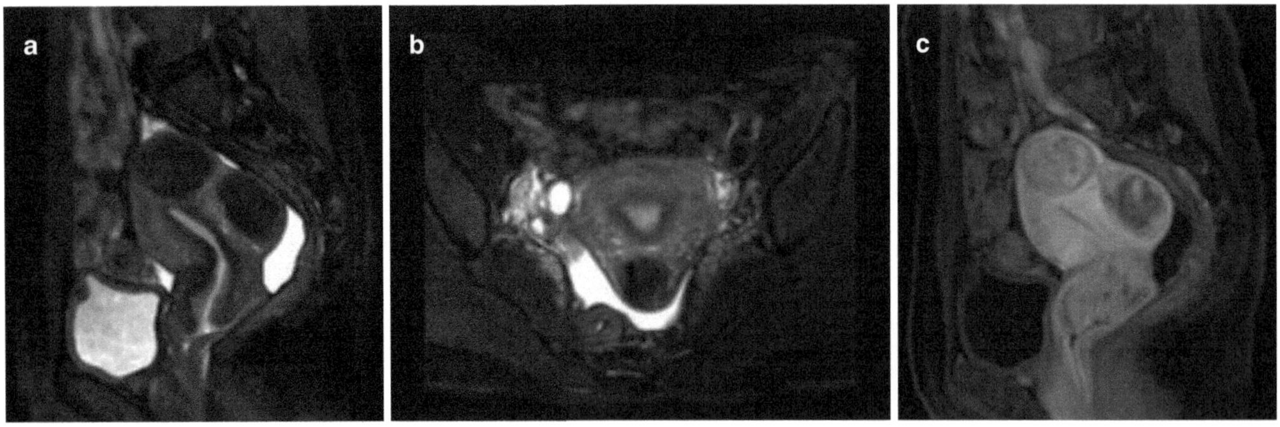

Fig. 4.53 Two type IV intramural fibroids before treatment. (**a**) T2WI_FS sagittal, (**b**) T2WI_FS axial, (**c**) T1WI_FS + C sagittal

the acoustic pathway by distending the urinary bladder. Since the intramural fibroids of the posterior wall were located in the deep part of the pelvic cavity, the ultrasound focal point may not reach the deep layer of the fibroid. A higher acoustic power was used.

4.2.10.4 Post-Treatment Assessment

MRI Evaluation after Treatment The T2WI signal of two treated fibroids increased, and the sacrococcygeal fascia was edematous (Fig. 4.54a, b). The contrast-enhanced T1WI showed that the cephalic fibroid was completely ablated, and the uterine serosa and endometrium were well protected and intact. The NPV ratio of the caudal fibroid near the cervix was about 94%, with a residual un-ablated fibroid seen at its lower edge (Fig. 4.54c).

4.2.10.5 Discussion

- There are many bowels in front of the uterus in this case; besides, they are posterior uterine fibroids for focused ultrasound ablation treatment. The bladder needs to be distended to push the intestine out of the acoustic pathway, which is the key to a successful treatment.
- In this case, the bladder is distended with 700 mL of normal saline, which pushes the bowels to form a good acoustic pathway (Fig. 4.54c). At the same time, attention must be paid to the significant edema of the sacrococcygeal fascia after treatment. Although a good technique can avoid damage to the sacrococcyx and nerves, it is recommended that the acoustic power be reduced to treat fibroids close to the posterior uterine serosa.

4.2.11 Case 11 Type IV Intramural Fibroids (2)

4.2.11.1 Case Description

The female patient was 35 years old. She had uterine fibroids with a fertility desire. After focused ultrasound ablation of her fibroids, she became pregnant after more than 1 month and eventually gave birth to a healthy girl.

4.2.11.2 Pre-Treatment Assessment

MRI showed multiple intramural fibroids with a larger fibroid on the right side wall of the uterus and small subserosal fibroids at the fundus of the uterus. All had low intense signals on T2WI (Fig. 4.55a). The contrast-enhanced T1WI showed that these fibroids had abundant blood supply (Fig. 4.55b, c). The acoustic pathway was clear. Thus, focused ultrasound ablation would be performed.

4.2.11.3 Treatment Techniques

1. **Focused ultrasound parameters.** Average acoustic power: 179 W, sonication time: 2015 seconds, duration of treatment: 146 minutes, total energy: 361,350 J.
2. **Focused ultrasound ablation techniques.** Fibroids with low signal on T2WI and the large fibroid were adjacent to the right posterior wall fascia, which could require lower acoustic power and reduce sonication time for ablation treatment.

4.2.11.4 Post-Treatment Assessment

1. **MRI evaluation after treatment.** The fibroids had inhomogeneously increased signals on T2WI. There was no edema in the abdominal wall and posterior wall fascia, and the bladder was distended to push the bowels away (Fig. 4.56a). The contrast-enhanced T1WI showed that the fibroids were almost completely ablated with intact capsules (Fig. 4.56b, c).
2. **MRI follow-up at 3 years and 5 months after treatment.** The size of fibroids was significantly reduced, shrinking by about 85%. The contrast-enhanced T1WI showed that most of the larger fibroid was in a non-perfusion state. However, there were new small intramural fibroids on the left anterior wall of the uterus (Fig. 4.57).

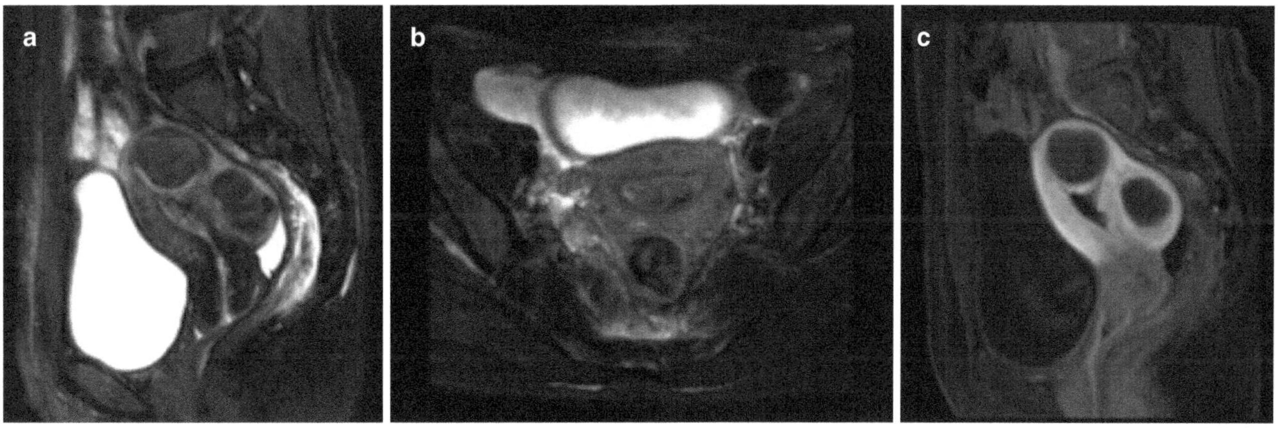

Fig. 4.54 MRI evaluation of type IV intramural fibroids after treatment. (**a**) T2WI_FS sagittal, (**b**) T2WI_FS axial, (**c**) T1WI_FS + C sagittal

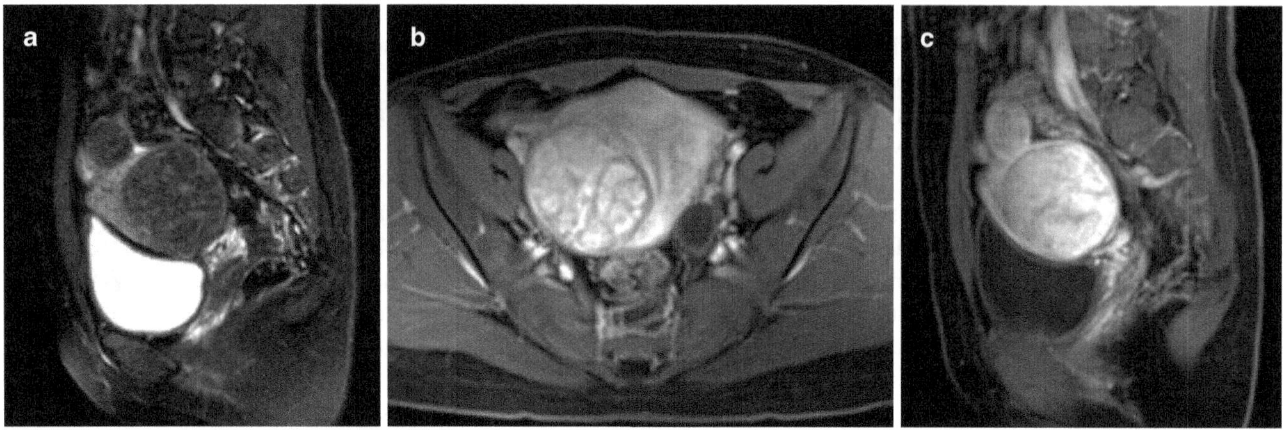

Fig. 4.55 Type IV intramural fibroids before treatment. (**a**) T2WI_FS sagittal, (**b**) T1WI_FS + C axial, (**c**) T1WI_FS + C sagittal

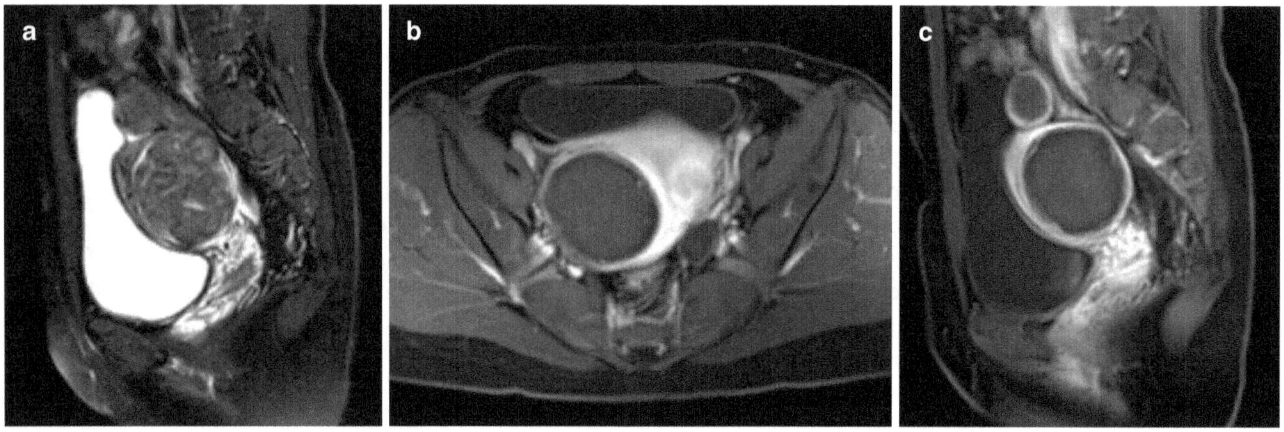

Fig. 4.56 MRI evaluation of type IV intramural fibroids after treatment. (**a**) T2WI_FS sagittal, (**b**) T1WI_FS + C axial, (**c**) T1WI_FS + C sagittal

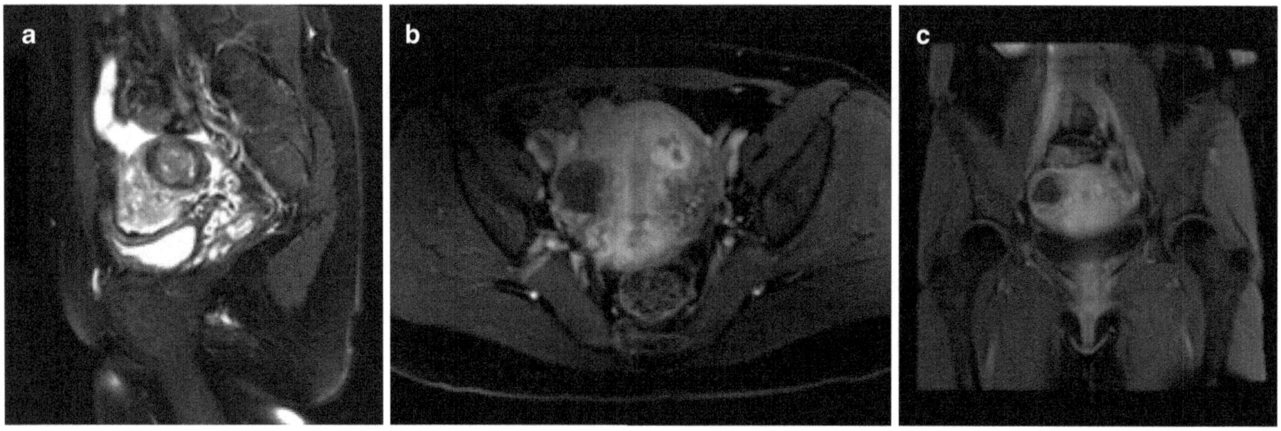

Fig. 4.57 MRI follow-up of type IV intramural fibroids at 3 years and 5 months after treatment. (**a**) T2WI_FS sagittal, (**b**) T1WI_FS + C axial, (**c**) T1WI_FS + C coronal

4.2.11.5 Discussion

- This case is a typical case of focused ultrasound ablation treatment to assist pregnancy. The patient successfully conceived more than 1 month after focused ultrasound ablation treatment and gave birth to a healthy child at full term.
- Pre-pregnancy patients with multiple uterine fibroids could expect to conceive shortly after a few months after non-invasive focused ultrasound ablation of the fibroids. Compared to surgical myomectomy, the wait for pregnancy would be for nearly 1–2 years, during which there may be new fibroids.

4.2.12 Case 12 Type IV Intramural Fibroids (3)

4.2.12.1 Case Description

The female patient was 43 years old. She presented with long-term constipation. The patient had a previous caesarean section and tended to form a keloid scar.

4.2.12.2 Pre-Treatment Assessment

MRI showed a posterior wall uterine fibroid with hypointensity on T2WI, and it was located in the deep part of the pelvic cavity (Fig. 4.58a). The contrast-enhanced T1WI showed that the fibroid had poor blood supply with degeneration in the fibroid center (Fig. 4.58b, c). There were bowels in front of the uterus, and the fibroid was deep in the pelvis. The operation would be difficult technically.

4.2.12.3 Treatment Techniques

1. **Focused ultrasound parameters.** Average acoustic power: 388 W, sonication time: 769 s, duration of treatment: 72 min, total energy: 298,200 J.
2. **Focused ultrasound ablation treatment technique.** The intestine in front of the uterus was pushed out of the acoustic pathway through the distended bladder and an extracorporeal water balloon. Careful attention should be paid to the skin burns during treatment, especially at the previous cesarean section scar. It was necessary to pause and cool the skin through the system's cold water circulation regularly from time to time.

4.2.12.4 Post-Treatment Assessment

MRI Evaluation after the Treatment The subcutaneous tissue edema at the cesarean section scar of the anterior abdominal wall was significant (Fig. 4.59a). The contrast-enhanced T1WI showed that the NPV ratio of the fibroid was as high as 95%, and the adjacent endometrium and serosa were well protected and intact (Fig. 4.59b, c).

4.2.12.5 Discussion

- The protection of the skin at the cesarean section scar is very important. The edema of the subcutaneous soft tissue can be completely absorbed within 1 to 3 months. Since the posterior edge of uterine fibroids is adjacent to the sacral plexus and sacrococcyx, the ultrasound focal point must be at a certain distance away from the serosa of the posterior edge of the uterus (≥15 mm), so there may be residual un-ablated fibroid on the posterior edge of the fibroid. Then there was a probability of fibroid recurrence, but it may vary among individuals.

4.2.13 Case 13 Type IV Intramural Fibroid (4)

4.2.13.1 Case Description

The female patient was 38 years old with a uterine fibroid >5 cm in diameter. She had a uterine fibroid with symptoms of bladder pressure for 2 years. She presented with lower abdominal pain during the menstrual period. There is no incentive to extend the menstrual period to about 12 days this month, and there is no dizziness.

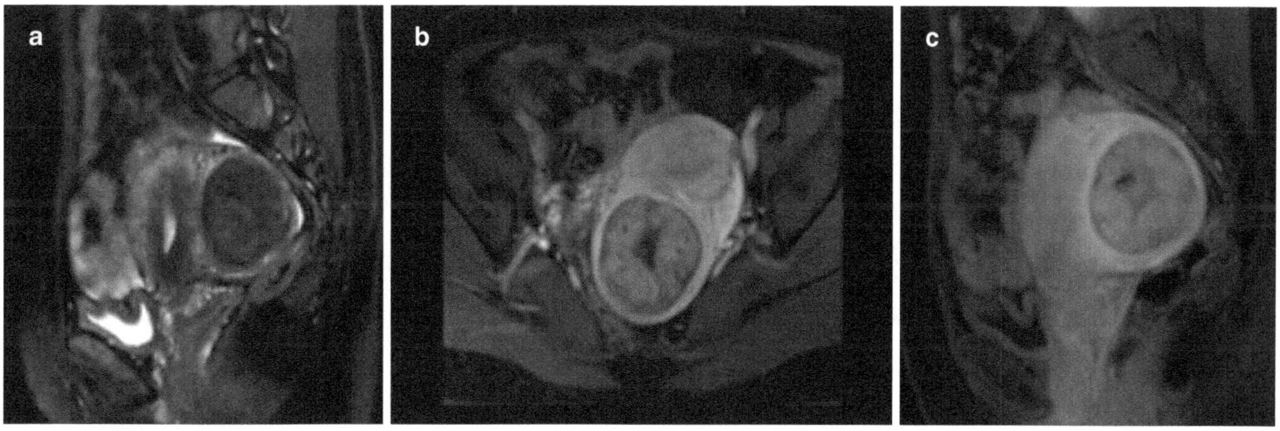

Fig. 4.58 A Type IV intramural fibroid before treatment. (**a**) T2WI_FS sagittal, (**b**) T1WI_FS + C axial, (**c**) T1WI_FS + C sagittal

4.2.13.2 Pre-Treatment Assessment

MRI showed the bicornate uterus with an intermural fibroid of its left side that was homogeneously hypointense with clear boundary on T2WI (Fig. 4.60a, b); the contrast-enhanced T1WI demonstrated that the fibroid had a moderate blood supply with a pseudocapsule (Fig. 4.60c). It is predicted that focused ultrasound ablation is relatively easy.

4.2.13.3 Treatment Techniques

1. **Focused ultrasound parameters.** Average acoustic power: 245 W, sonication time: 1504 s, duration of treatment: 85 min., total energy: 367,830 J.
2. **Focused ultrasound ablation techniques.** The acoustic pathway was clear, and the fully distended bladder was avoided to prevent the fibroid from approaching the sacrococcygeal side.

4.2.13.4 Post-Treatment Assessment

1. **MRI evaluation after treatment.** There was no edema at the anterior abdominal wall and the fibroid was completely ablated with the intact capsule on contrast-enhanced T1WI (Fig. 4.61a).
2. **MRI follow-up at 6 months after treatment.** The volume of the fibroid significantly decreased, and it revealed hypointensity mixed with high signal on T2WI (Fig. 4.61b). The contrast-enhanced T1WI demonstrated 100% of NPV ratio of the treated fibroid without any residual (Fig. 4.61b).

4.2.13.5 Discussion

- Normally the distended bladder was recommended to push the bowels out of the acoustic pathway. However, the acoustic pathway had been good with semi-filled

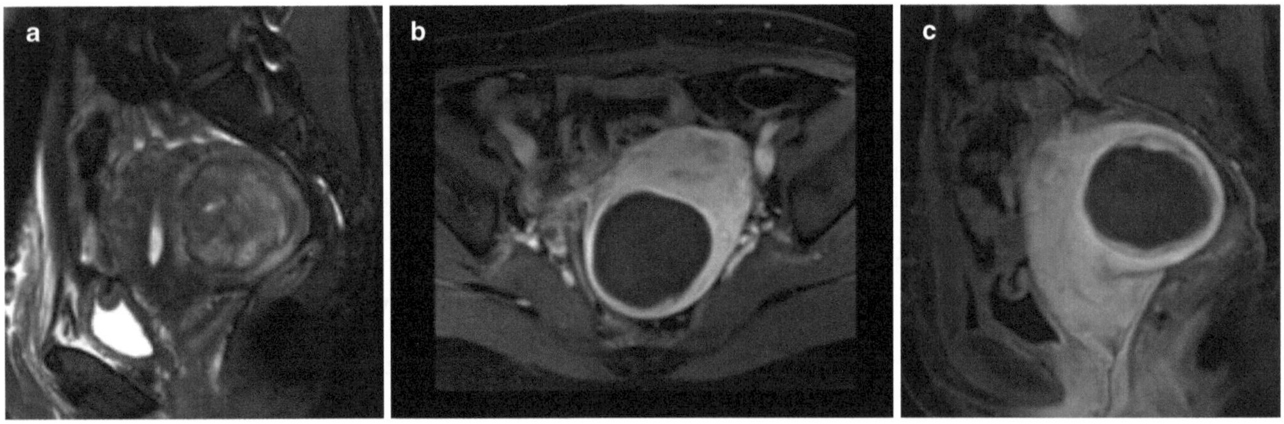

Fig. 4.59 MRI evaluation of type IV intramural fibroid after treatment. (**a**) T2WI_FS sagittal, (**b**) T1WI_FS + C axial, (**c**) T1WI_FS + C sagittal

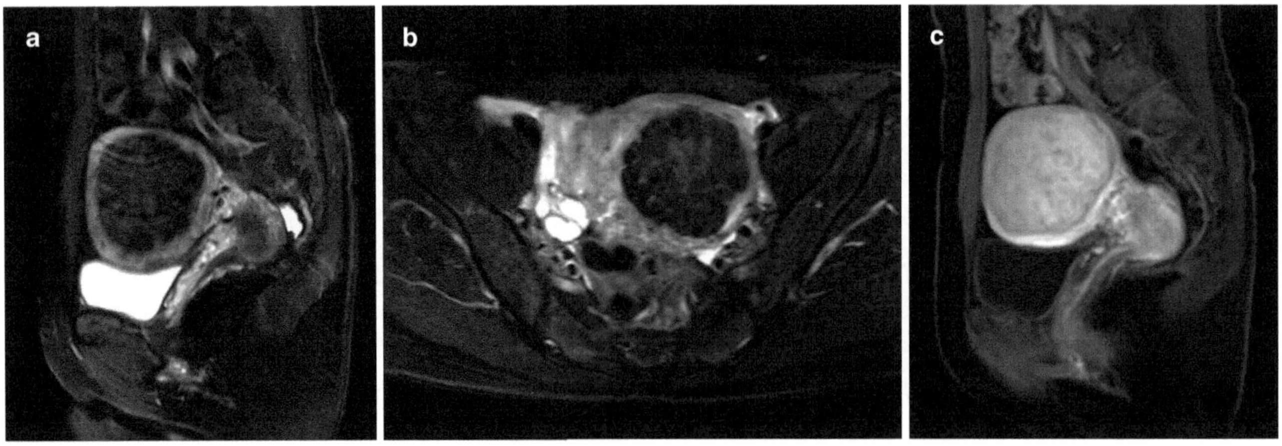

Fig. 4.60 A Type IV intramural fibroid before treatment. (**a**) T2WI_FS sagittal, (**b**) T2WI_FS axial, (**c**) T1WI_FS + C sagittal

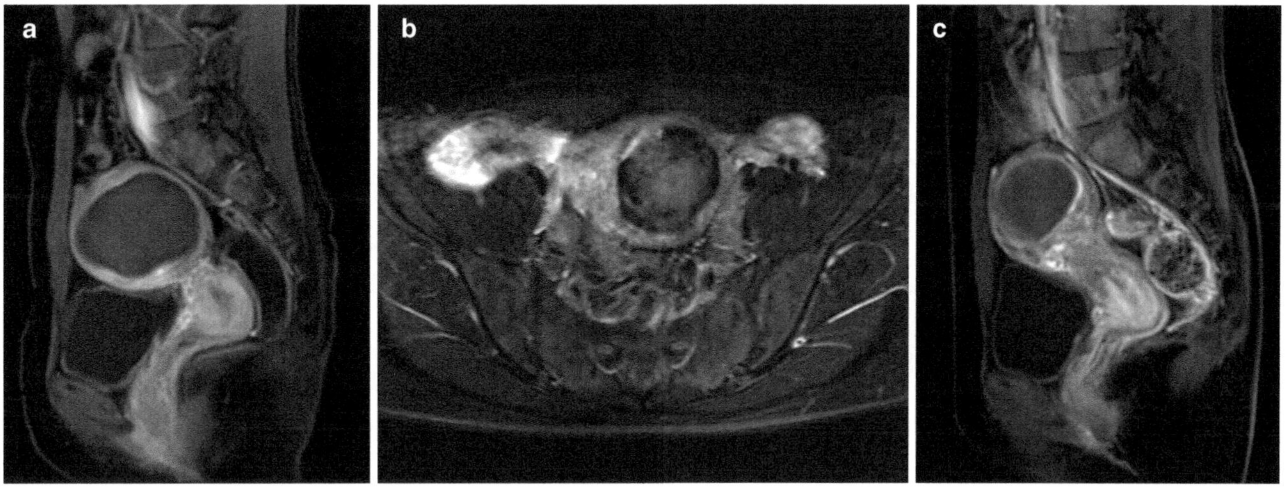

Fig. 4.61 MRI evaluation of type IV intramural fibroid (**a**) and follow-up at 6 months after treatment. (**a**) T1WI_FS + C sagittal, (**b**) T2WI_FS axial, (**c**) T1WI_FS + C sagittal

bladder for this patient. An excessive distended bladder might increase the treatment risk of nerve injury because the sacral plexus was behind the fibroid.

- The bicornate uterus with fibroid is a relatively rare disease. The therapeutic strategy should be formulated according to the patient's situation and requirements.

4.2.14 Case 14 Type IV Intramural Fibroid (5)

4.2.14.1 Case Description

The female patient was 37 years old with fibroids. Two years ago, she menstruated profusely, accompanied by lumbar acid for 7 days after the menstruate period. This patient had presented with dizziness and fatigue for 1 year, and her hemoglobin was 103 g/L. She planned for a second child, thus seeking an intervention therapy.

4.2.14.2 Pre-Treatment Assessment

MRI showed a fibroid (about 68 mm × 61 mm × 59 mm) with hypointense signal at the lateral wall of uterus on T2WI (Fig. 4.62a). The contrast-enhanced T1WI showed that the fibroid had a moderate blood supply with a pseudocapsule (Fig. 4.62b). It is predicted that the fibroid would be relatively easy to ablate.

4.2.14.3 Treatment Techniques

1. **Focused ultrasound parameters.** Average acoustic power: 247 W, sonication time: 2231 s, duration of treatment: 90 min, total energy: 550,390 J.
2. **Focused ultrasound ablation techniques.** Although the fibroid was located at the right lateral wall of the uterus, the acoustic pathway was clear. The concerning issue was the fibroid close to rectum. The bladder was distended to push the fibroid far away from the colorectum to avoid damage to the intestinal wall. Thus, the fibroid had been adjacent to the lumbosacral vertebrae, nerves and vessels behind, the acoustic power had to be reduced (Fig. 4.63).

4.2.14.4 Post-Treatment Assessment

1. **MRI evaluation after treatment.** The rectus abdominis muscle of the anterior abdominal wall was swollen. The NPV ratio of the fibroid was more than 95%, and small amounts of thin-layer enhancement remained on its anterior edge (Fig. 4.63).
2. **MRI follow-up at 6 months after treatment.** The swollen rectus abdominis of the anterior abdominal wall returned to normal. The size of the uterine fibroid was significantly smaller than that before treatment (the volume reduction rate is about 60%), and the residual enhancement layer had disappeared, with no recurrence (Fig. 4.64).

4.2.14.5 Discussion

- The contrast-enhanced T1WI follow-up can differentiate the pseudoenhancement and residual tissues after the fibroid ablation treatment. The enhancement layer at the front edge of the fibroid often did not recur or even disappeared because it received higher acoustic energy in the near-field of the focal region.
- For the uterine fibroid with T2WI hypointensity and adjacent to the nerves and vessels behind, the acoustic power must be reduced with an increase in sonication time while paying attention to the sensory activity of the patient's lower limb during treatment.

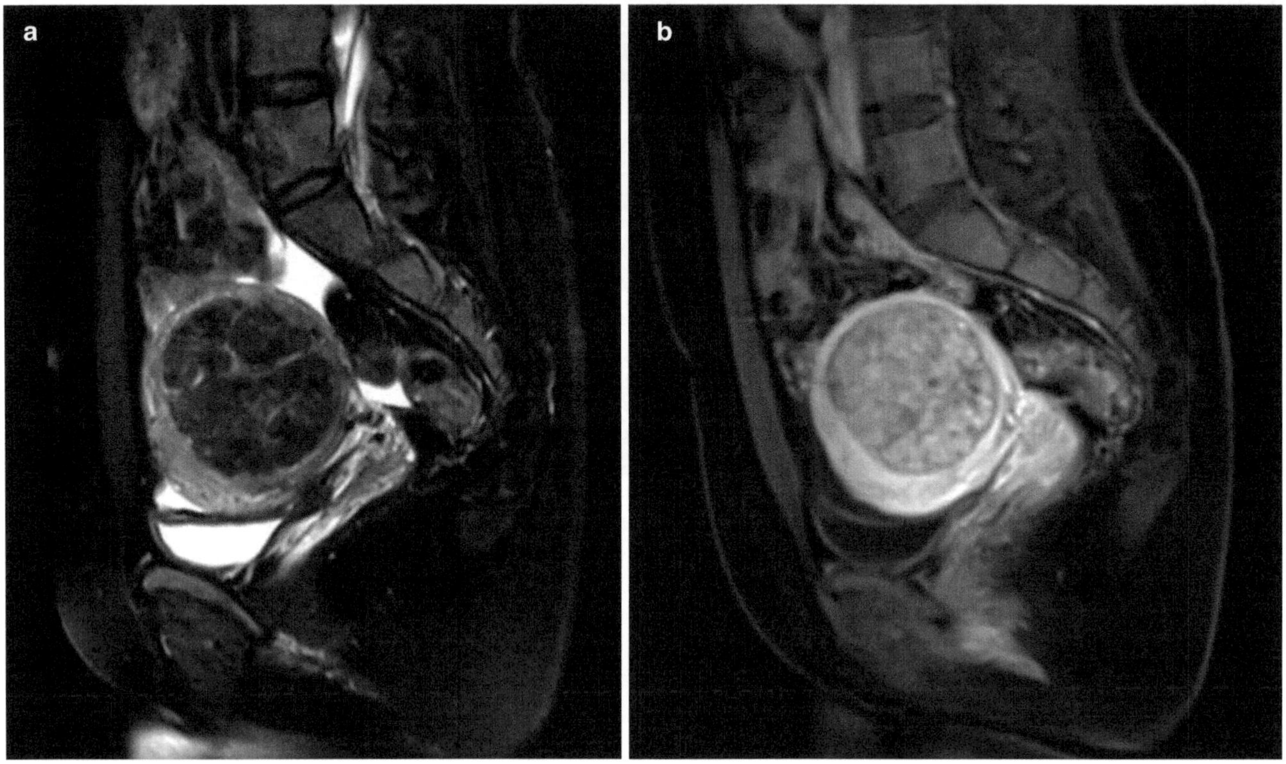

Fig. 4.62 A Type IV intramural fibroid before treatment. (**a**) T2WI_FS sagittal, (**b**) T1WI_FS + C sagittal

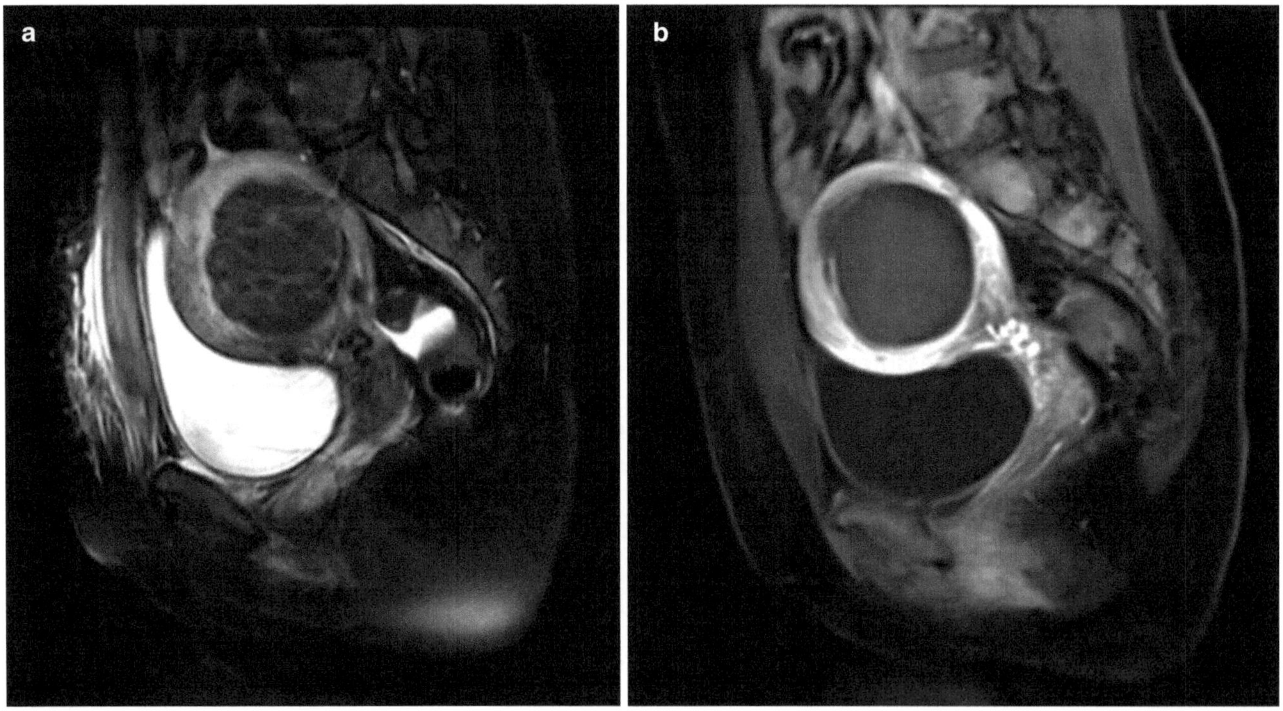

Fig. 4.63 MRI evaluation of type IV intramural fibroid after treatment. (**a**) T2WI_FS sagittal, (**b**) T1WI_FS + C sagittal

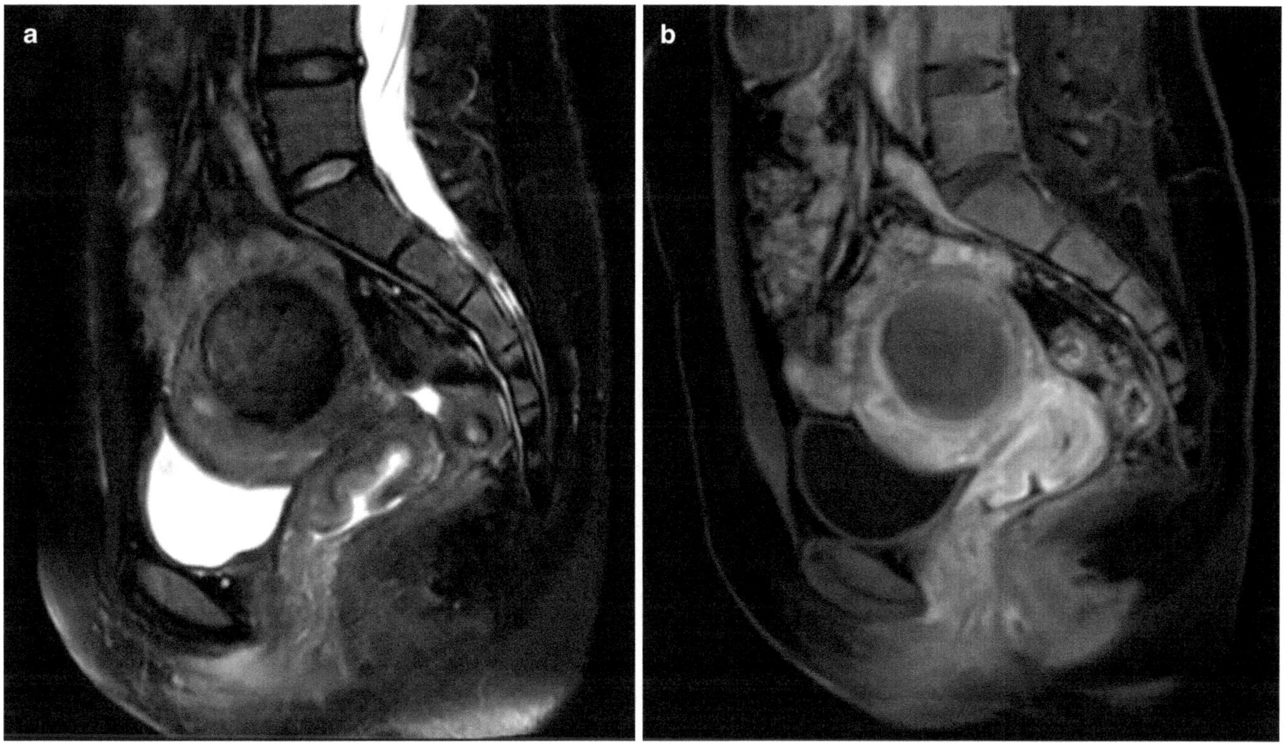

Fig. 4.64 MRI follow-up of type IV intramural fibroids at 6 months after treatment. (**a**) T2WI_FS sagittal, (**b**) T1WI_FS + C sagittal

4.2.15 Case 15 Type IV Intramural Fibroid (6)

4.2.15.1 Case Description

The female patient was 36 years old with a uterine fibroid about 8 cm in diameter, which was detected 5 years ago and grew up rapidly in the past 2 years. She came to hospital for treatment of her frequent urination and urgency.

4.2.15.2 Pre-Treatment Assessment

MRI showed a fibroid of the uterine fundus with hyper- and hypointensity on T2WI (Fig. 4.65a). The contrast-enhanced T1WI showed that the enhancement of the fibroid was significantly higher than that of the uterine muscle wall, suggesting rich blood supply (Fig. 4.65b). The fibroid was larger (8.4 cm in diameter) and close to the anterior abdominal wall with a good acoustic pathway.

4.2.15.3 Treatment Techniques

1. **Focused ultrasound parameters.** Average acoustic power: 253 W, sonication time: 1331 seconds, duration of treatment: 70 min, total energy: 336,890 J.
2. **Focused ultrasound ablation techniques.** The fibroid with hypervascularity might have the "heat sink effect" during the thermal ablation, which could influence the thermal ablation effect. The ultrasound microbubble contrast could be applied in focused ultrasound ablation. It would produce the cavitation that damages the small blood vessels to block blood flow. Thus, the treatment efficiency would be increased while the acoustic power could be reduced.

4.2.15.4 Post-Treatment Assessment

1. **MRI evaluation after treatment.** The abdominal wall had obvious edema, and most of the surrounding edges of the fibroid were edematous on T2WI (Fig. 4.66a). The contrast-enhanced T1WI showed that the fibroid was almost completely ablated with a small amount of thin-layer enhancement at the posterior edge of the fibroid (Fig. 4.66b).
2. **MRI follow-up at 6 months after treatment.** T2WI showed the subcutaneous edema at the abdominal wall decreased in extent and localized with a small amount of liquid high signal, and the signal intensity of the fibroid increased. The skin showed normal structure and signal (Fig. 4.66c). The contrast-enhanced T1WI demonstrated that the volume of the fibroid significantly decreased with 100% of NPV ratio without residual, and the local subcutaneous soft tissue and the rectus abdominis closed to the treated fibroid partially ablated (Fig. 4.66d).

4.2.15.5 Discussion

- Basically, the hypervascular tumors required more thermal energy deposit with higher acoustic power to achieve focused ultrasound ablation. The microbubbles can

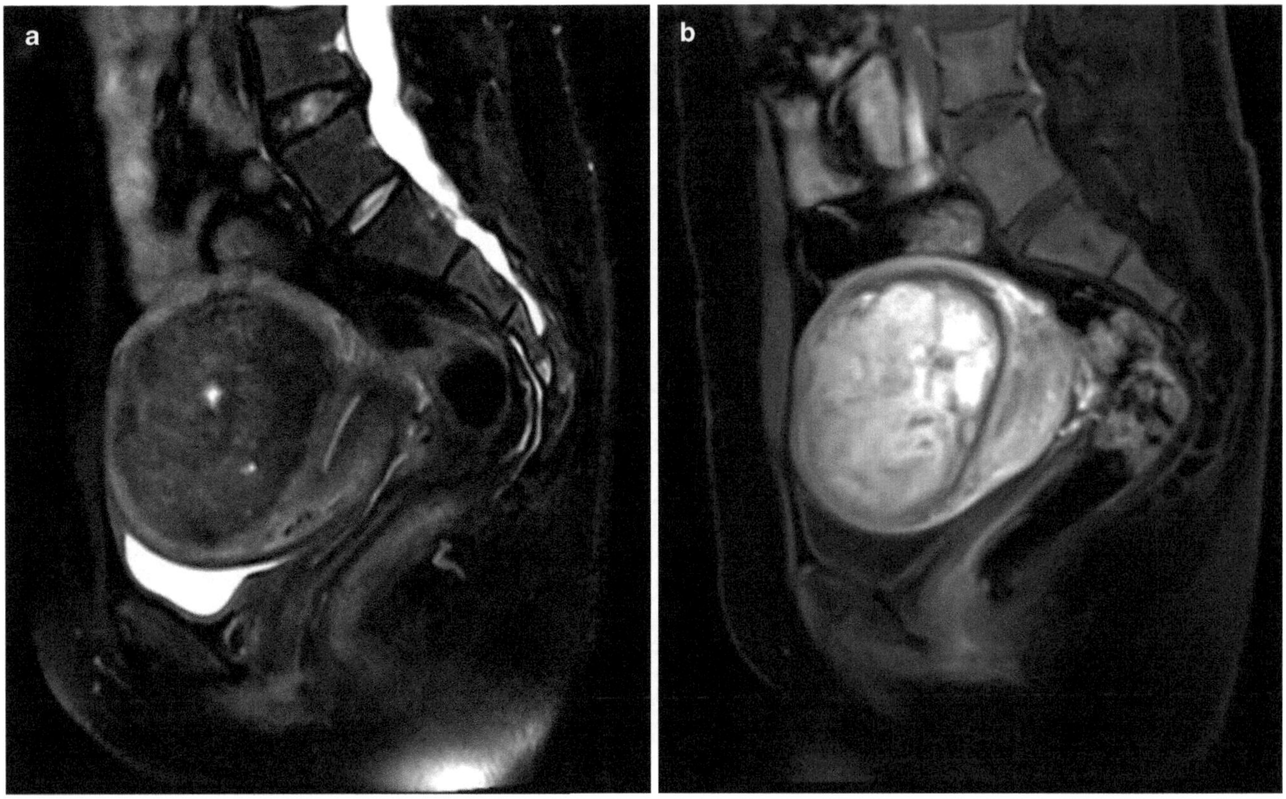

Fig. 4.65 A type IV intramural fibroid before treatment. (**a**) T2WI_FS sagittal, (**b**) T1WI_FS + C sagittal

enhance the heating effect and reduce acoustic power requirements. The SonoVue (an ultrasound contrast agent) was used to enhance the focused ultrasound ablation effects for the fibroid with an abundant blood supply in this case. The therapeutic parameters indicated treatment duration and sonication time were shortened, and the acoustic power and energy decreased.

- It is imperative that physicians know when the microbubble concentration is too high, the focused ultrasound may ablate the pre-focal region along the path of the acoustic source. The patient had injuries to the subcutaneous soft tissue and rectus abdominis of the abdominal wall, fortunately, her skin in the acoustic pathway was intact.
- The residual tissue at the rear edge of the fibroid might recur because of less energy deposition in the far-field of the focal region. This fibroid, after treatment, showed a thin-layer enhancement at its posterior edge that disappeared at the follow-up, which indicated that it was not the residual tissues. Although it was located at the far-field, the acoustic waves were reflected by the lumbosacral bone, which increased the energy deposit at the post-focal region.

4.2.16 Case 16 Type IV Intramural Fibroid (7)

4.2.16.1 Case Description

The female patient was 41 years old. She presented with a history of uterine fibroids, symptoms of pelvic pressure, and constipation.

4.2.16.2 Pre-Treatment Assessment

MRI showed a posterior wall uterine fibroid with low intense signals on T2WI mixed with hyperintensity in the center of the fibroid, and it was located close to the sacrum (Fig. 4.67a). The contrast-enhanced T1WI showed that the fibroid had a poor blood supply (Fig. 4.67b, c). There were many bowels between the uterus and the anterior abdominal wall, and the acoustic pathway was poor. Together its location was also close to the sacral plexus; it is predicted that it would be technically difficult for focused ultrasound ablation treatment.

4.2.16.3 Treatment Techniques

1. **Focused ultrasound parameters.** Average acoustic power: 289 W, sonication time: 1466 s, duration of treatment: 104 min, total energy: 424,350 J.

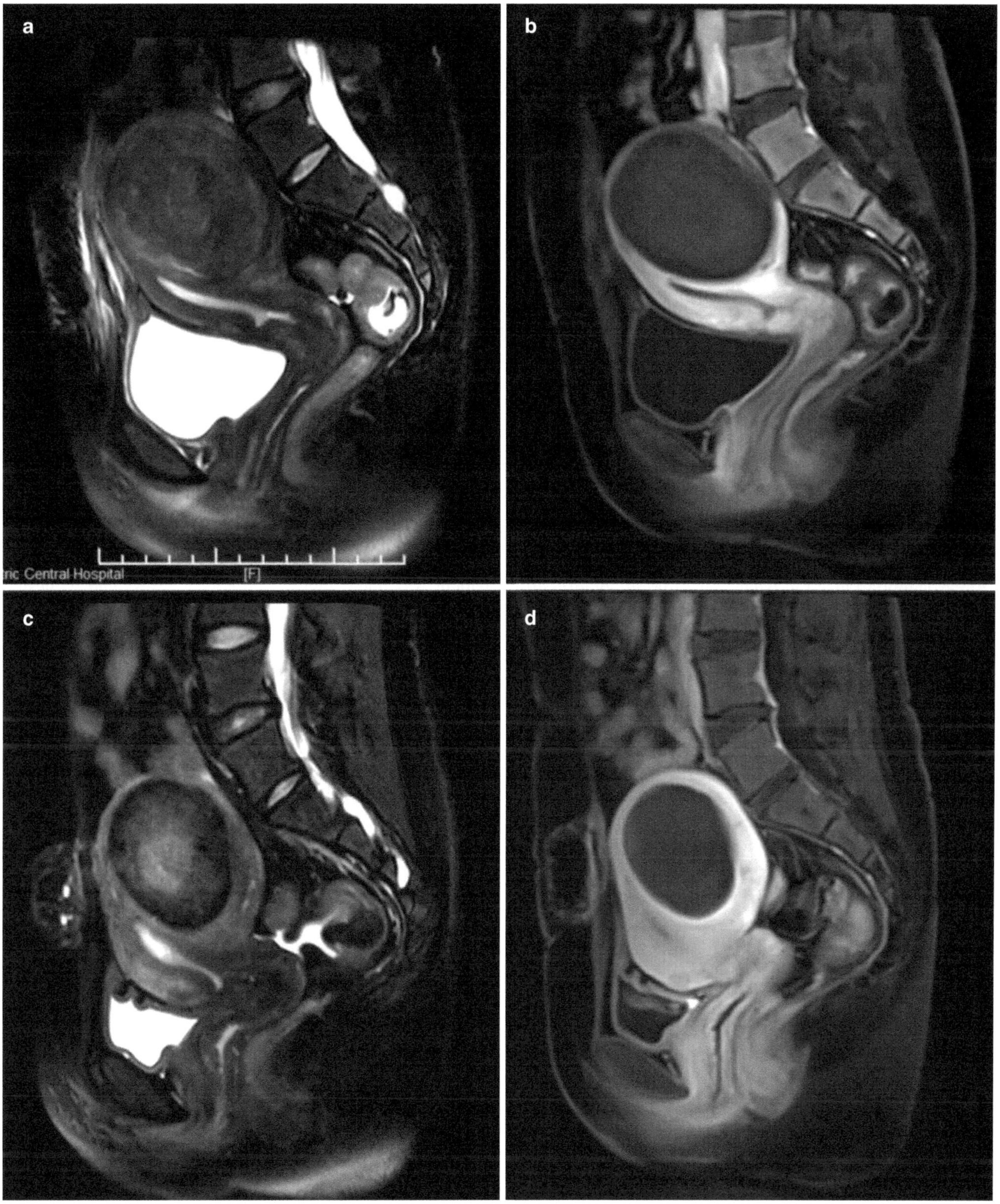

Fig. 4.66 MRI evaluation of type IV intramural fibroid (**a**, **b**) and follow-up at 6 months after treatment (**c**, **d**). (**a**) T2WI_FS sagittal, (**b**) T1WI_FS + C sagittal, (**c**) T2WI_FS sagittal, (**d**) T1WI_FS + C sagittal

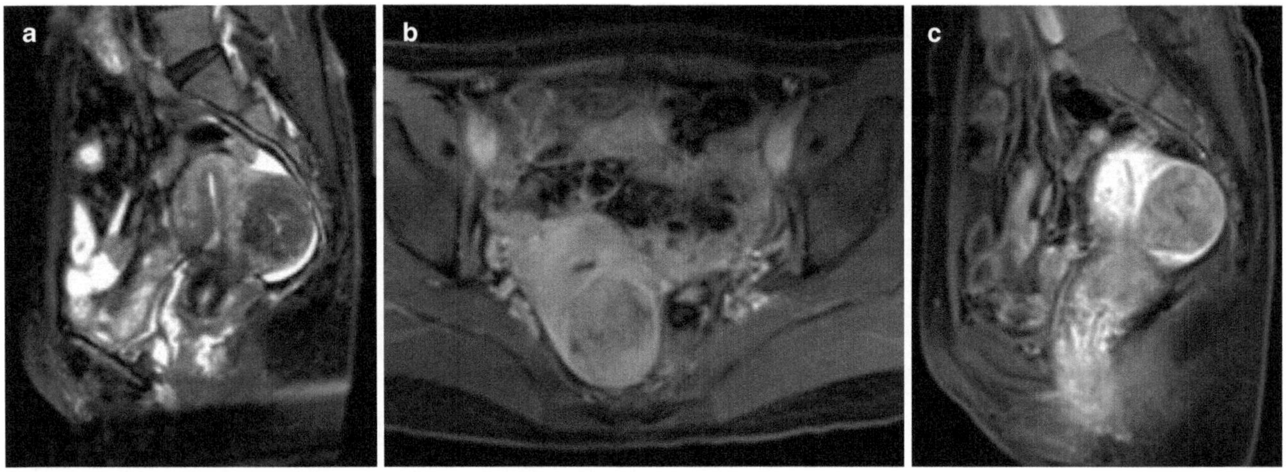

Fig. 4.67 A Type IV intramural fibroid before treatment. (**a**) T2WI_FS sagittal, (**b**) T1WI_FS + C axial, (**c**) T1WI_FS + C sagittal

2. **Focused ultrasound ablation techniques.** The distended bladder and extracorporeal water balloon were used to push the bowels out of the acoustic pathway. Because the fibroid was located in the deep part of the pelvis and adjacent to the sacrum, the ultrasound focal regions had to be reasonably arranged to balance the fibroid ablation efficacy and treatment safety. At the same time, pay close attention to the patient's response during treatment to avoid nerve damage.

4.2.16.4 Post-Treatment Assessment

1. **MRI evaluation after treatment.** The T2WI signal of the posterior edge of the fibroid increased, and the fascia of the posterior pelvic wall was edematous (Fig. 4.68a). The contrast-enhanced T1WI showed that the fibroid was completely ablated, and the uterine serosa was intact (Fig. 4.68b, c).
2. **MRI follow-up at 6 months after treatment.** The fibroid shrank by about 65% without recurrence (Fig. 4.68d–f), and the fascia edema of the posterior pelvic wall disappeared.

4.2.16.5 Discussion

- This case is a uterine posterior wall fibroid located deep in the pelvic cavity, close to the sacrum and sacral plexus. The acoustic pathway between the anterior abdominal wall and the uterus is filled with many bowels. It is technically challenging to ablate the uterine fibroid completely.
- The fascia edema of the posterior pelvic wall could be completely recovered, but the patient's response should be closely monitored during the procedure to ensure treatment safety.

4.2.17 Case 17 Type IV Intramural Fibroid (8)

4.2.17.1 Case Description

The female patient was 40 years old. Physical examination revealed uterine fibroids without clinical symptoms. The patient was under high psychological stress and requested focused ultrasound ablation treatment.

4.2.17.2 Pre-Treatment Assessment

MRI showed a right anterior wall fibroid on the retroverted uterus. It had homogeneous hypointensity on T2WI (Fig. 4.69a). The contrast-enhanced T1WI showed that the fibroid had a moderate blood supply and a pseudocapsule (Fig. 4.69b, c). There were many bowels between the uterus and the anterior abdominal wall, which would be technically difficult for focused ultrasound ablation treatment.

4.2.17.3 Treatment Techniques

1. **Focused ultrasound parameters.** Average acoustic power: 300 W, sonication time: 2499 s, duration of treatment: 144 min, total energy: 149,700 J.
2. **Focused ultrasound ablation techniques.** The uterus and fibroid are located deep in the pelvic cavity. The bowels should be pushed away using a distended bladder and an extracorporeal water balloon. Since the fibroid had a low intense signal on T2WI, lower focused ultrasound energy could be used to achieve ablation. However, we had to use increased acoustic power during treatment because the acoustic path from the ultrasound transducer to the fibroid was longer.

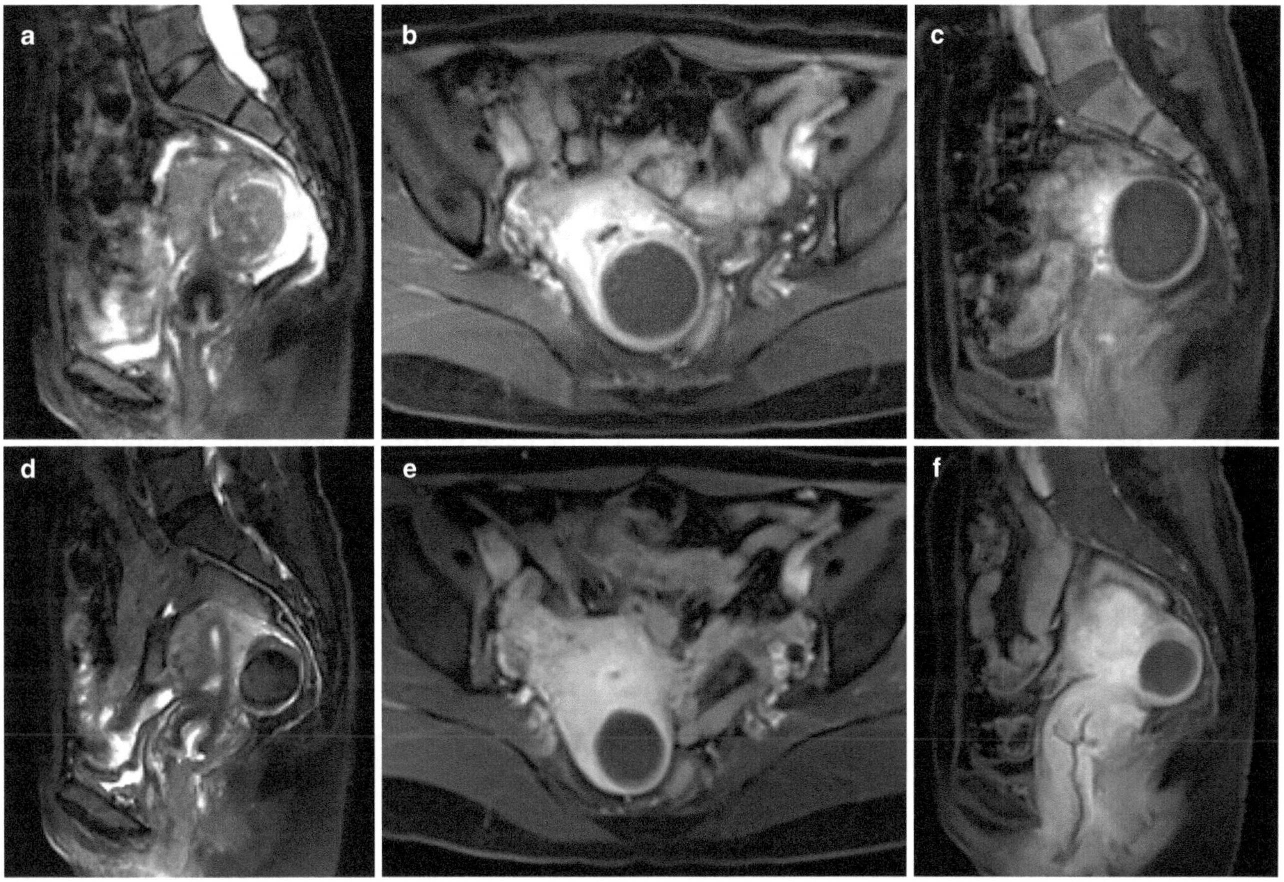

Fig. 4.68 MRI evaluation of type IV intramural fibroids immediately (**a**–**c**) and at 6 months (**d**–**f**) after treatment. (**a**) T2WI_FS sagittal, (**b**) T1WI_FS + C axial, (**c**) T1WI_FS + C sagittal, (**d**) T2WI_FS sagittal, (**e**) T1WI_FS + C axial, (**f**) T1WI_FS + C sagittal

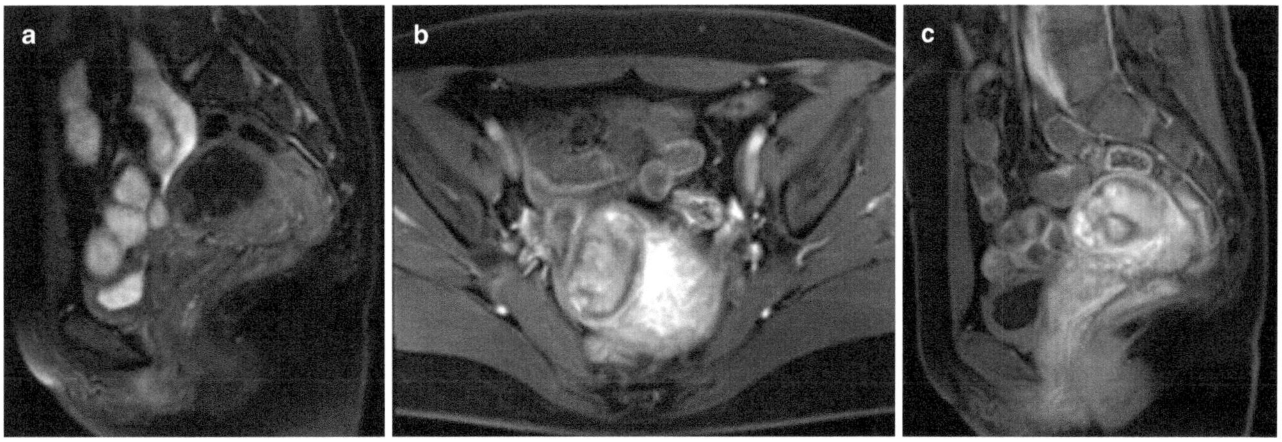

Fig. 4.69 A Type IV intramural fibroid before treatment. (**a**) T2WI_FS sagittal, (**b**) T1WI_FS + C axial, (**c**) T1WI_FS + C sagittal

4.2.17.4 Post-Treatment Assessment

1. **MRI evaluation after treatment.** The T2WI signals around the fibroid were higher than before treatment. There was no edema in the anterior abdominal wall; the bladder was distended to push the bowels away (Fig. 4.70a). The contrast-enhanced T1WI showed that the fibroid was completely ablated, and the adjacent uterine serosas were intact (Fig. 4.70b, c).
2. **MRI follow-up at 6 months after treatment.** The fibroid treated by focused ultrasound ablation showed no sign of fibroid recurrence with a reduction of fibroid volume by about 70% (Fig. 4.71).

4.2.17.5 Discussion

- It is very important for the real-time ultrasound to monitor the focused ultrasound ablation efficacy and safety. 70% to 80% of tumors can show enhanced echo in the treatment area during the procedure, but some tumors may show a reduced echo in the treatment area or no significant change in echo. It may be the result of the following situations: The treatment dose is not enough, or the treatment area is edematous, leading to reduced echo; the treatment area is moved, resulting in the false echo images; the tissue swells and thickens in the acoustic near-field causing the distance to increase from the treatment area to the skin surface, which leads to reduced echo (pseudo-echo) in the treatment area; lastly, the tissue structure on the acoustic path is damaged, which increases the ultrasound attenuation, then reducing the echo signals at the treatment area to become low intense signals.

4.2.18 Case 18 Type IV Intramural Fibroid (9)

4.2.18.1 Case Description

The female patient was 47 years old. She had undergone a myomectomy with regular follow-up, and the myoma recurred. Before focused ultrasound ablation treatment, MRI showed the fibroid had high intense signals on T2WI

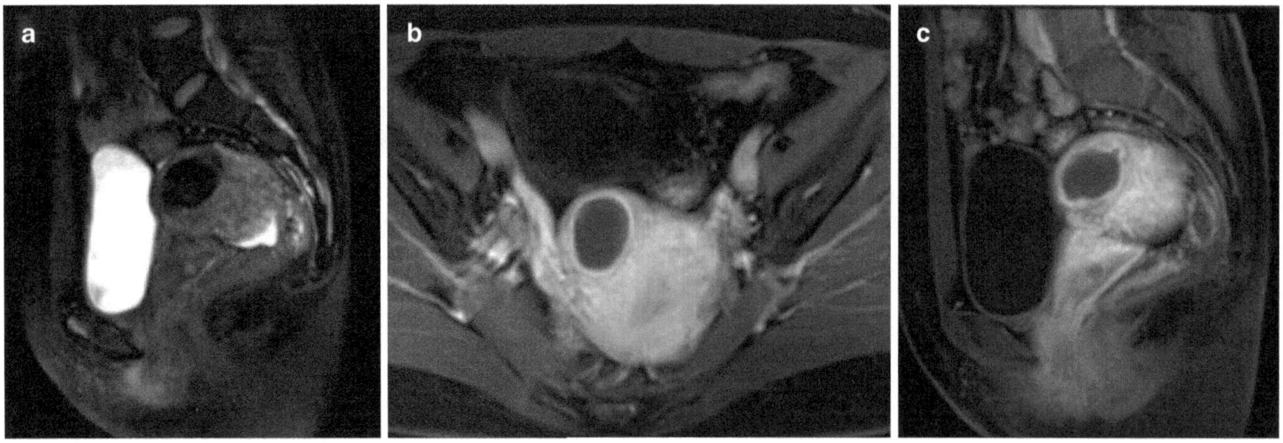

Fig. 4.70 MRI evaluation of type IV intramural fibroid after treatment. (**a**) T1WI sagittal, (**b**) T1WI_FS + C axial, (**c**) T1WI_FS + C sagittal

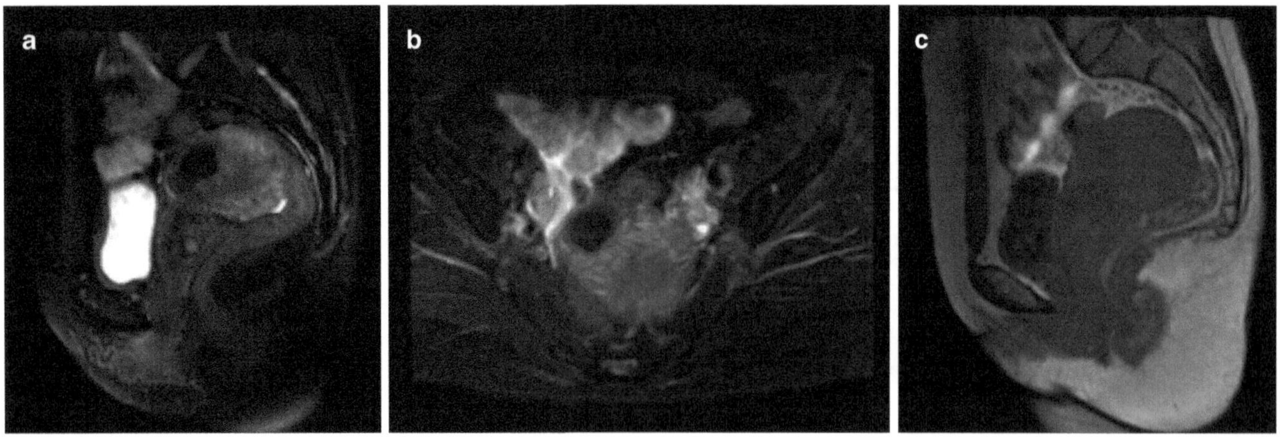

Fig. 4.71 MRI follow-up of type IV intramural fibroid at 6 months after treatment. (**a**) T2WI_FS sagittal, (**b**) T2WI_FS axial, (**c**) T1WI sagittal

(Fig. 4.72a). Low-dose mifepristone was administered orally to induce menopause (1.0–2.5 mg/d), and focused ultrasound ablation was performed half a year later.

4.2.18.2 Pre-Treatment Assessment

MRI showed a large fibroid at the left lateral wall of the uterus with homogeneous, slight hyperintensity on T2WI. The contrast-enhanced MRI showed that the fibroid had an abundant blood supply (Fig. 4.72b, c). It was predicted to be difficult to ablate. After 6 months of oral low-dose mifepristone, the fibroid was slightly reduced in size and showed inhomogeneous T2WI high signals with cystic degeneration (Fig. 4.73), which could be feasible for ultrasound ablation.

4.2.18.3 Treatment Techniques

1. **Focused ultrasound parameters.** Average acoustic power: 356 W, sonication time: 3159 s, duration of treatment: 175 min, total energy: 1,123,220 J.
2. **Focused ultrasound ablation techniques.** Because the fibroid was large and slight hyperintensity on T2WI, focused ultrasound ablation could be relatively difficult. High acoustic power was required to improve the thermal energy deposit and enhance treatment efficacy.

4.2.18.4 Post-Treatment Assessment

1. **MRI evaluation after treatment.** The T2WI signal of the fibroid increased significantly(Fig. 4.74a). The contrast-enhanced MRI showed that the NPV ratio of the fibroid was about 95%, leaving only a thin enhanced layer along the edge of the fibroid (Fig. 4.74b, c).
2. **MRI follow-up at 6 months after treatment.** The whole fibroid had high signal changes on the T1WI plain scan (Fig. 4.74d). The contrast-enhanced MRI showed that the fibroid had complete necrosis without the signs of recurrence, and the fibroid volume was reduced by about 74% (Fig. 4.74e, f).

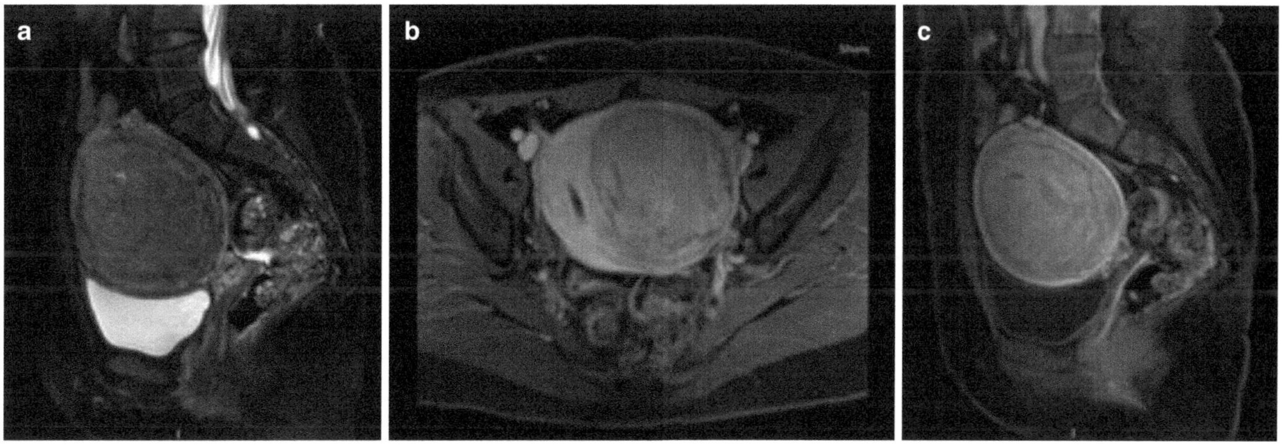

Fig. 4.72 MR imaging of the type IV intramural fibroid before oral mifepristone. (**a**) T2WI_FS sagittal, (**b**) T1WI_FS+C axial, (**c**) T1WI_FS+C sagittal

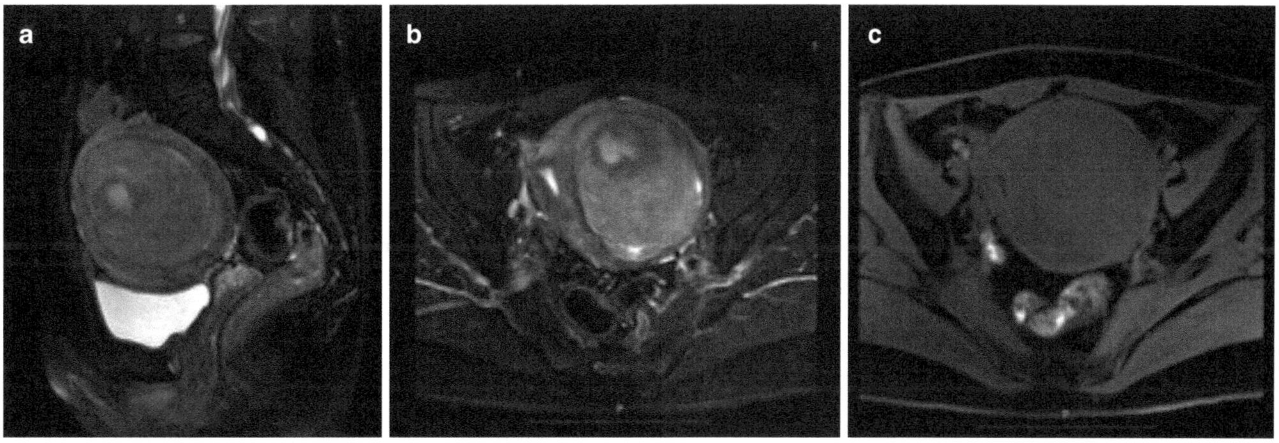

Fig. 4.73 MRI follow-up after oral mifepristone of the type IV intramural fibroid before ultrasound ablation. (**a**) T2WI_FS sagittal, (**b**) T2WI_FS axial, (**c**) T1WI axial

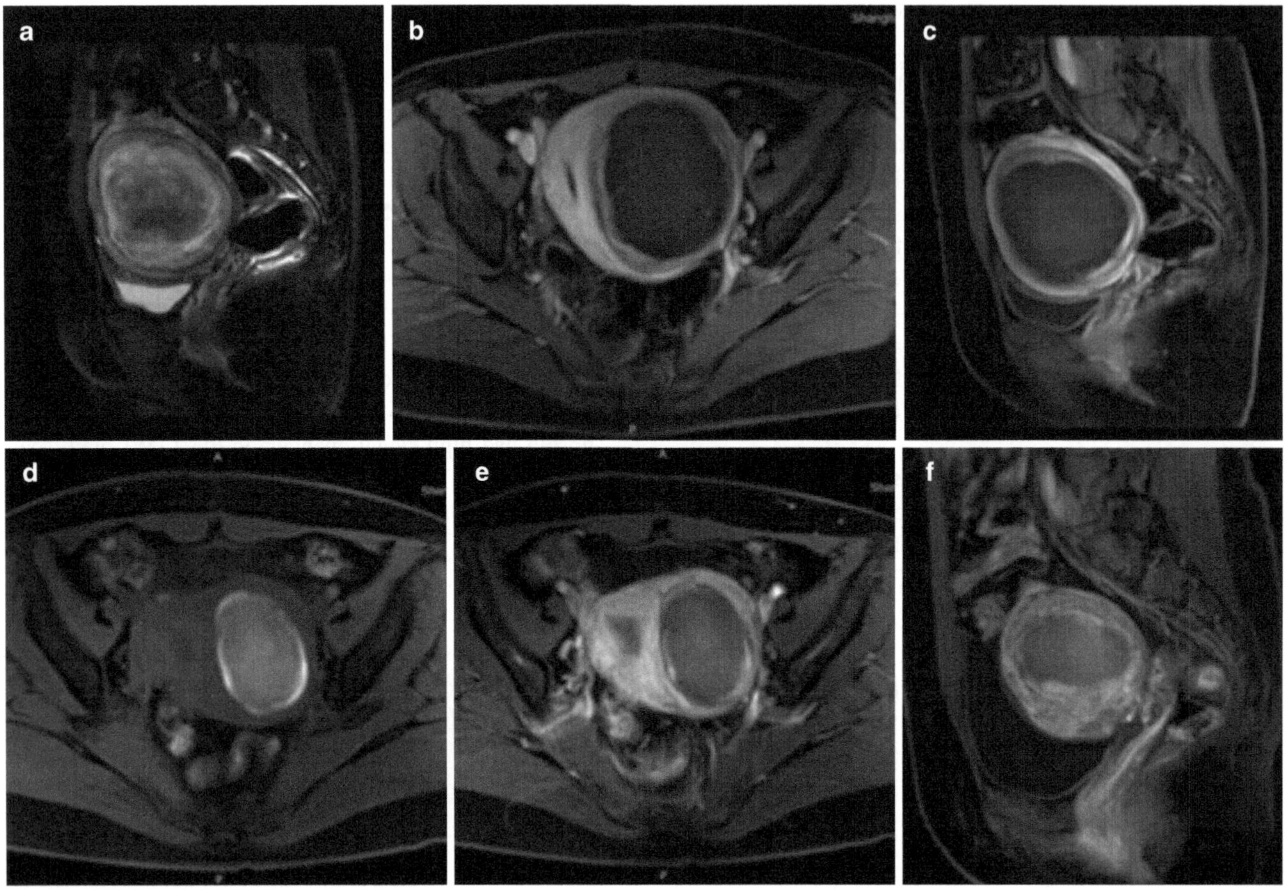

Fig. 4.74 MRI evaluation of type IV intramural fibroid immediately (**a**–**c**) and at 6 months (**d**–**f**) after treatment. (**a**) T2WI_FS sagittal, (**b**) T1WI_FS + C axial, (**c**) T1WI_FS + C sagittal, (**d**) T1WI_FS axial, (**e**) T1WI_FS + C axial, (**f**) T1WI_FS + C sagittal

4.2.18.5 Discussion

- It is reported in the literature that mifepristone can reduce the size of fibroids, shorten the operation time, reduce intraoperative blood loss, induce temporary amenorrhea, and correct anemia. It is a safe, effective, and economical preoperative adjuvant drug for uterine fibroids.
- Uterine fibroids with homogeneous T2WI high signal and abundant blood supply are difficult to be ablated by focused ultrasound. In this case, oral mifepristone before treatment can change the characteristics of the fibroid, such as necrosis with cysts formation, making them suitable for focused ultrasound ablation treatment.
- Contrast-enhanced T1WI demonstrated a thin enhancement zone along the edge of the fibroid immediately after ultrasound ablation, suggesting the leaky capillaries at the treated area margin or the physiologic response to thermal injury (initially, reactive hyperemia; subsequently, fibrosis and giant cell reaction). This transient finding can be seen immediately after ablation and can last for up to 6 months, which does not represent the remaining residual of the ablated fibroid.
- The T2WI homogeneously slight hyperintense uterine fibroid had been thought to be excluded for focused ultrasound ablation treatment. The focused ultrasound ablation efficacy should have been poor, but it was significantly improved after oral mifepristone.

4.2.19 Case 19 Type V Intramural Fibroid (1)

4.2.19.1 Case Description

The female patient was 33 years old. Physical examination revealed uterine fibroids for more than 3 years.

4.2.19.2 Pre-Treatment Assessment

MRI showed that the intramural uterine fibroid on the left anterior wall of the uterus had low signals on T2WI, protruded into the uterine cavity, and a small fibroid was adjacent to the uterine cervix (Fig. 4.75a). The contrast-enhanced T1WI showed that the two fibroids had abundant blood supply (Fig. 4.75b, c). There was a good acoustic pathway for the ultrasound ablation. However, the larger fibroid was adja-

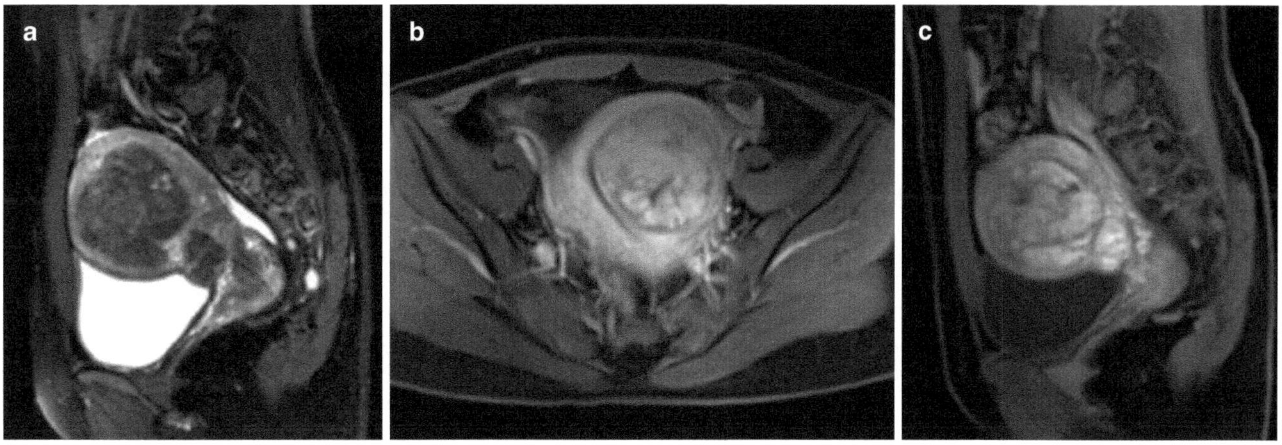

Fig. 4.75 Type V intramural fibroids before Focused ultrasound ablation treatment. (**a**) T2WI_FS sagittal, (**b**) T1WI_FS + C axial, (**c**) T1WI_FS + C sagittal

cent to the endometrium and the left sciatic nerve area; care should be taken to protect the endometrium and the posterior serosal layer during treatment. Uterine cervical fibroids could be treated simultaneously as long as a safe acoustic pathway allowed.

4.2.19.3 Treatment Techniques

1. **Focused ultrasound parameters.** Average acoustic power: 378 W, sonication time: 1601 s, duration of treatment: 80 min, total energy: 605,871 J.
2. **Focused ultrasound ablation techniques.** The sonication could begin at the sagittal middle slice of the larger fibroid. Thus, even if the initial ablation started at the deep layer of the fibroid, there was enough distance from the focal regions to the endometrium and the left sciatic nerve area. Then the heat diffusion would spread to both sides, trying to cover the whole tumor volume.

4.2.19.4 Post-Treatment Assessment

1. **MRI evaluation after treatment.** Although there was no edema on the abdominal wall, the fascia of the left pelvic wall was slightly edematous on T2WI (Fig. 4.76a). The contrast-enhanced T1WI showed that the NPV ratio of the larger fibroid was about 97%, with a thin layer remaining on its left edge. The endometrium was intact. The small cervical fibroid was completely ablated (Fig. 4.76b, c).
2. **MRI follow-up at 6 months after treatment** The uterine size was significantly reduced, the larger fibroids shrank by about 85%, and the smaller fibroid volume significantly decreased (Fig. 4.76d–f).

4.2.19.5 Discussion

- The intramural fibroid of the uterus enlarges and protrudes toward the uterine cavity. Pay attention to avoid endometrial damage during focused ultrasound ablation of such fibroids.
- Small fibroids (<3 cm) in the cervix of the uterus are not suitable for focused ultrasound ablation due to the poor acoustic pathway. In this case, the cervical fibroid has a better acoustic pathway after distending the bladder, so both intramural fibroids are treated together.

4.2.20 Case 20 Type V Intramural Fibroid (2)

4.2.20.1 Case Description

The female patient was 44 years old. Her menstrual blood flow increased for 2 years and aggravated for 2 months.

4.2.20.2 Pre-Treatment Assessment

MRI from another clinic showed a right anterior intramural fibroid (type V) with homogeneous hypointensity on the T2WI. It was predicted to be relatively easy to ablate.

4.2.20.3 Treatment Techniques

1. **Focused ultrasound parameters.** Average acoustic power: 243 W, sonication time: 1560 s, duration of treatment: 89 min, total energy: 379,820 J.
2. **Focused ultrasound ablation techniques.** The large anterior fibroid had many bowels lying within the acoustic pathway. Therefore, the bladder needed to be distended to push them away into the cephalic direction to form a good acoustic pathway for treatment.

4.2.20.4 Post-Treatment Assessment

1. **MRI evaluation after treatment.** The T2WI signal of the fibroid was homogeneously increased (Fig. 4.77a); the contrast-enhanced T1WI showed that the fibroid was completely ablated, and the anterior portion of uterine serosa was protected and intact (Fig. 4.77b, c).
2. **MRI follow-up at 1, 3, 5 years after treatment.** One year later, the size of the fibroid was significantly reduced,

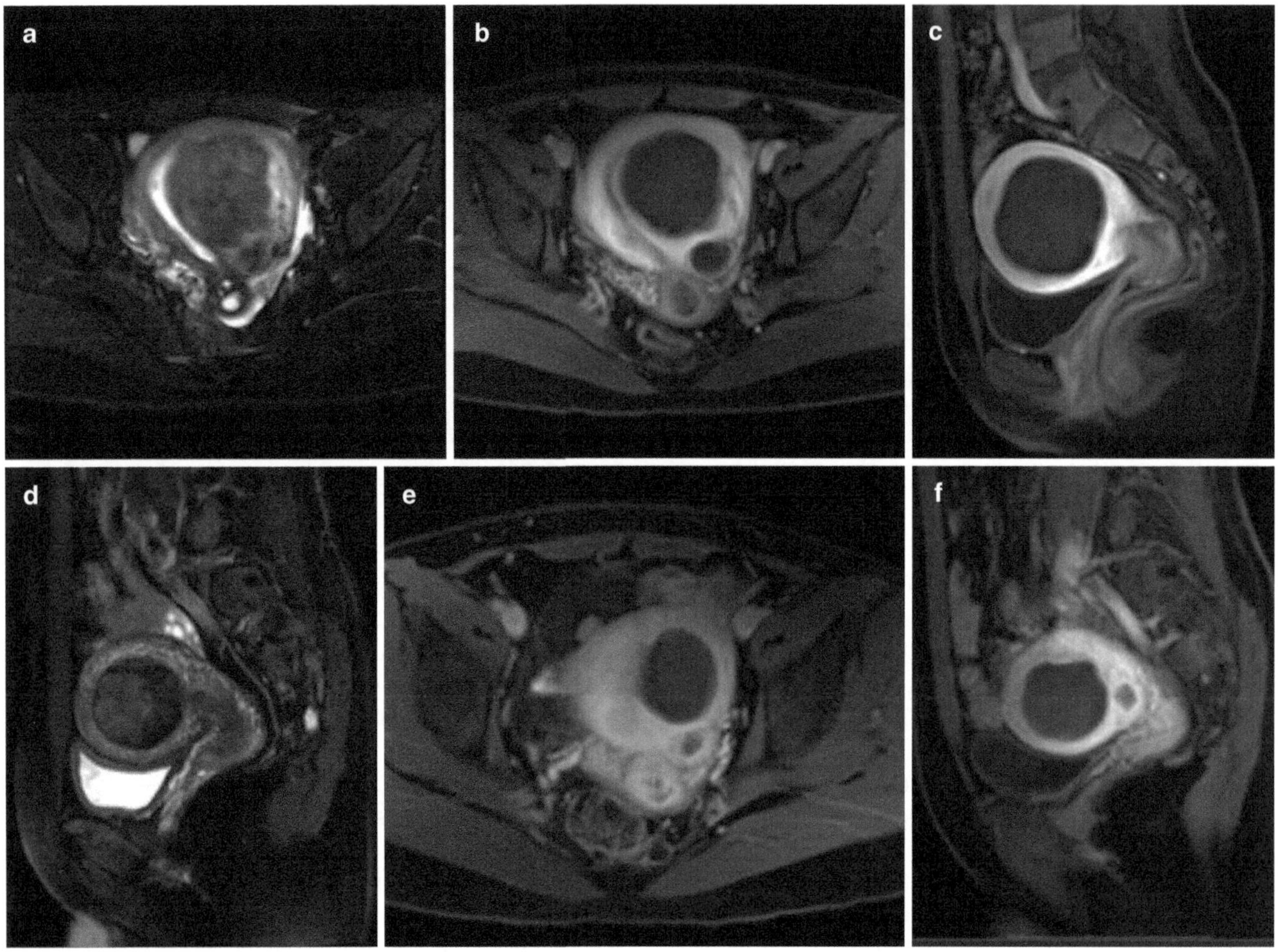

Fig. 4.76 MRI evaluation of type V intramural fibroids immediately and at 6 months after treatment. (**a**) T2WI_FS axial, (**b**) T1WI_FS + C axial, (**c**) T1WI_FS + C sagittal, (**d**) T2WI_FS sagittal, (**e**) T1WI_FS + C axial, (**f**) T1WI_FS + C sagittal

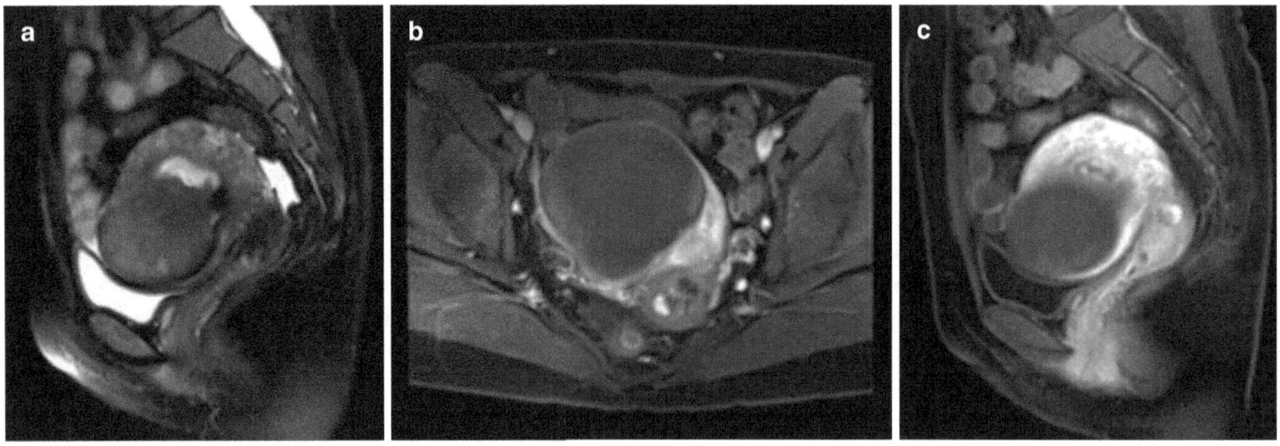

Fig. 4.77 MRI evaluation of a type V intramural fibroids after treatment. (**a**) T2WI_FS sagittal, (**b**) T1WI_FS + C axial, (**c**) T1WI_FS + C sagittal

and some tissues of the necrotic fibroid were gradually discharged through the uterine cavity (Fig. 4.78). At the 3-year follow-up, the size of the fibroid was significantly reduced, the uterine body returned to normal, and the endometrium was intact and clearly visible (Fig. 4.79). At the 5-year follow-up, the fibroid became very small and showed no recurrence (Fig. 4.80).

4.2.20.5 Discussion

- This case is a typical uterine fibroid with follow-up for 5 years after focused ultrasound ablation treatment, and the long-term results are satisfactory without recurrence.

4.2.21 Case 21 Type V Intramural Fibroid (3)

4.2.21.1 Case Description

The female patient was 49 years old. She had increased menstrual blood flow, accompanied by lower abdominal pain.

4.2.21.2 Pre-Treatment Assessment

MRI showed inhomogeneous, mixed high and low T2WI signals of a uterine fibroid, and the boundary was unclear (Fig. 4.81a). The contrast-enhanced MRI showed that the fibroid had an abundant blood supply (Fig. 4.81b, c). The fibroid was located on the right anterior wall of the uterus; thus, the acoustic pathway was clear. It was predicted that the acoustic energy needed to be increased for ablating this fibroid compared with those with low intense signals on T2WI.

4.2.21.3 Treatment Techniques

1. **Focused ultrasound parameters.** Average acoustic power: 300 W, sonication time: 2435 s, duration of treatment: 157 min, total energy: 731,340 J.
2. **Focused ultrasound ablation techniques.** It needed to increase the power and sonication time appropriately to reduce thermal damage to the skin and subcutaneous soft tissue because the fibroid was close to the anterior abdominal wall.

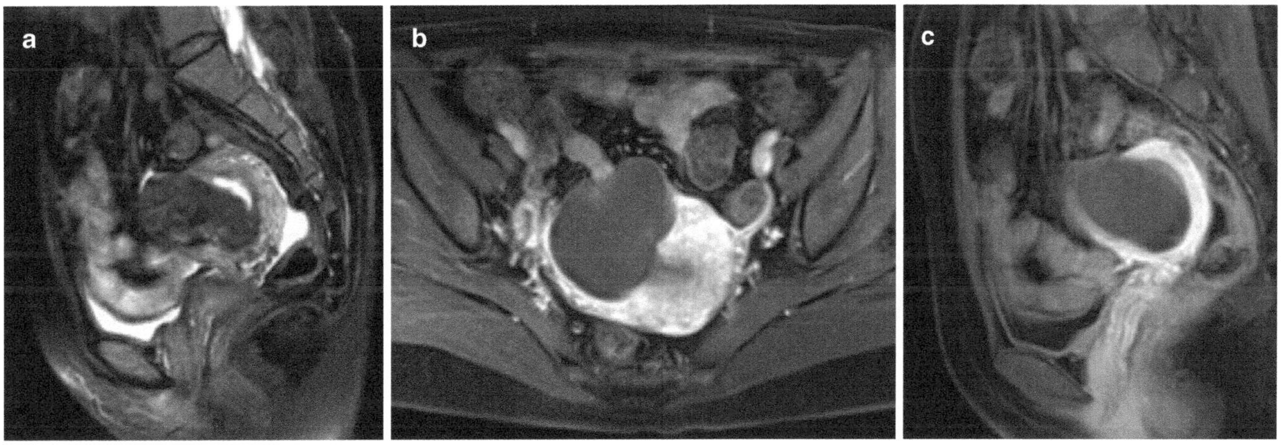

Fig. 4.78 MRI follow-up of type V intramural fibroids at 1 year after treatment. (**a**) T2WI_FS sagittal, (**b**) T1WI_FS + C axial, (**c**) T1WI_FS + C sagittal

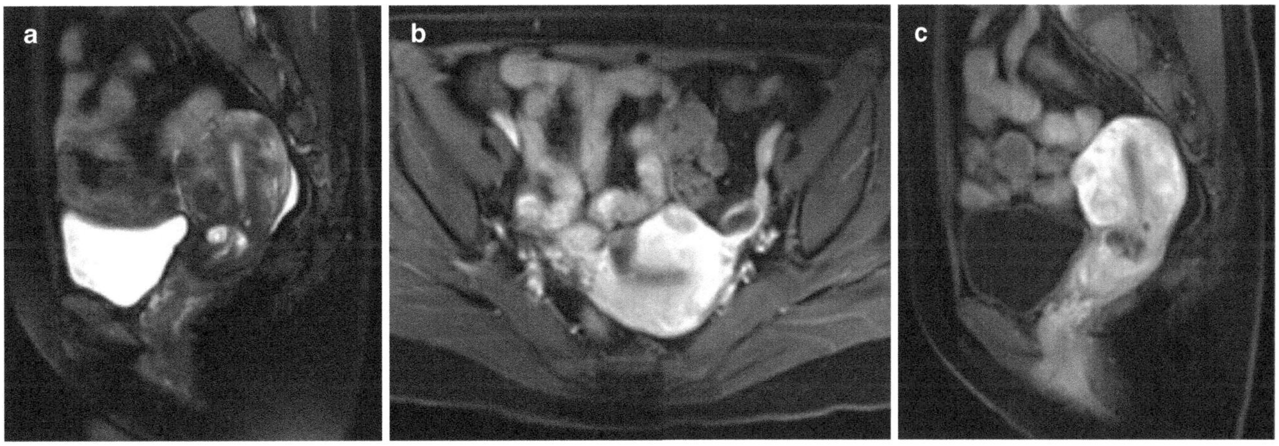

Fig. 4.79 MRI follow-up of type V intramural fibroid at 3 years after treatments. (**a**) T2WI_FS sagittal, (**b**) T1WI_FS + C axial, (**c**) T1WI_FS + C sagittal

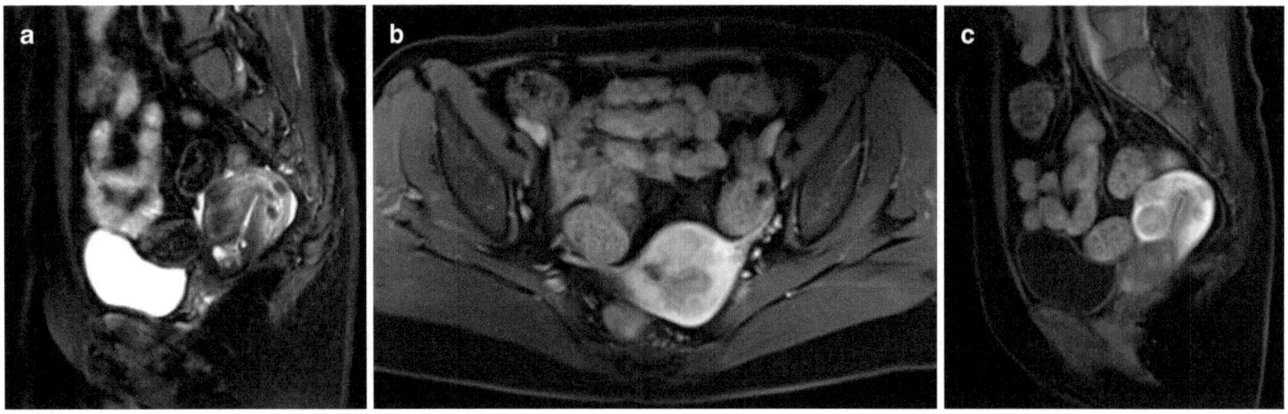

Fig. 4.80 MRI follow-up of type V intramural fibroids at 5 years after treatment. (**a**) T2WI_FS sagittal, (**b**) T1WI_FS + C axial, (**c**) T1WI_FS + C sagittal

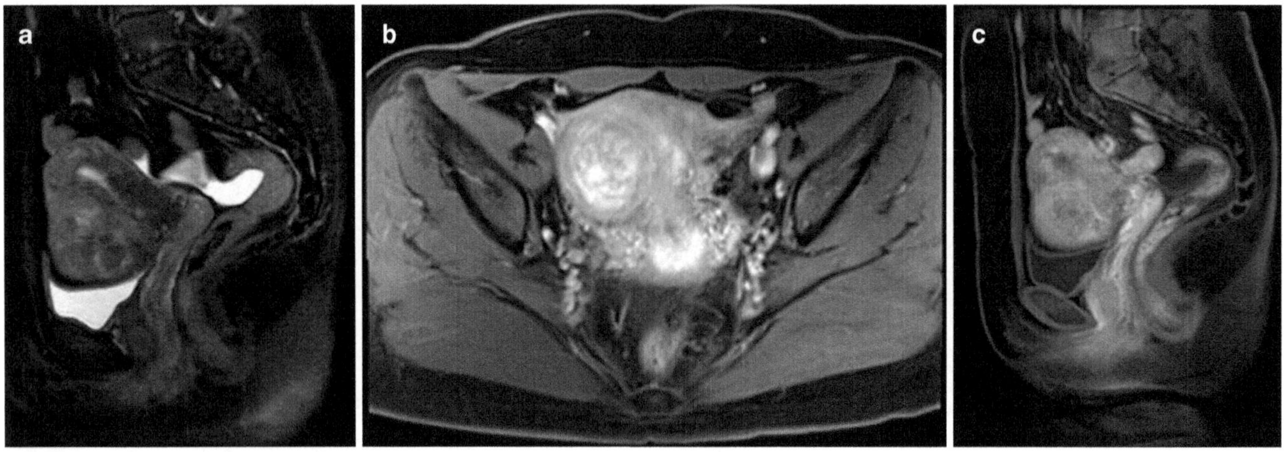

Fig. 4.81 A type V intramural fibroid before treatment. (**a**) T2WI_FS sagittal, (**b**) T1WI_FS + C axial, (**c**) T1WI_FS + C sagittal

4.2.21.4 Post-Treatment Assessment

MRI Evaluation after Treatment The T2WI signals of the fibroid increased, and the anterior abdominal wall showed localized edema (Fig. 4.82a). The contrast-enhanced T1WI showed that the fibroid was completely ablated with a distinct non-perfusion area (Fig. 4.82b, c).

4.2.21.5 Discussion

- Although the blood supply of uterine fibroid is abundant and the T2WI signal is high, as long as the T2WI signal is inhomogeneous, good ablation treatment effects may be achieved. However, attention should be paid to cooling the local accumulated heat through extracorporeal surface circulation water to avoid skin burn.

4.2.22 Case 22 Type V Intramural Fibroid (4)

4.2.22.1 Case Description

The female patient was 37 years old. She had a fibroid found more than 2 years ago. It was gradually increasing in size with symptoms of pelvic pressure.

4.2.22.2 Pre-Treatment Assessment

MRI showed a uterine fibroid with low signals on the T2WI. It had a small central area of high signals. The fibroid was adjacent to the vascular nerve plexus on the right pelvic sidewall (Fig. 4.83a). The contrast-enhanced T1WI showed that the fibroid had abundant blood supply with a pseudocapsule (Fig. 4.83b, c). The fibroid was located on the right pos-

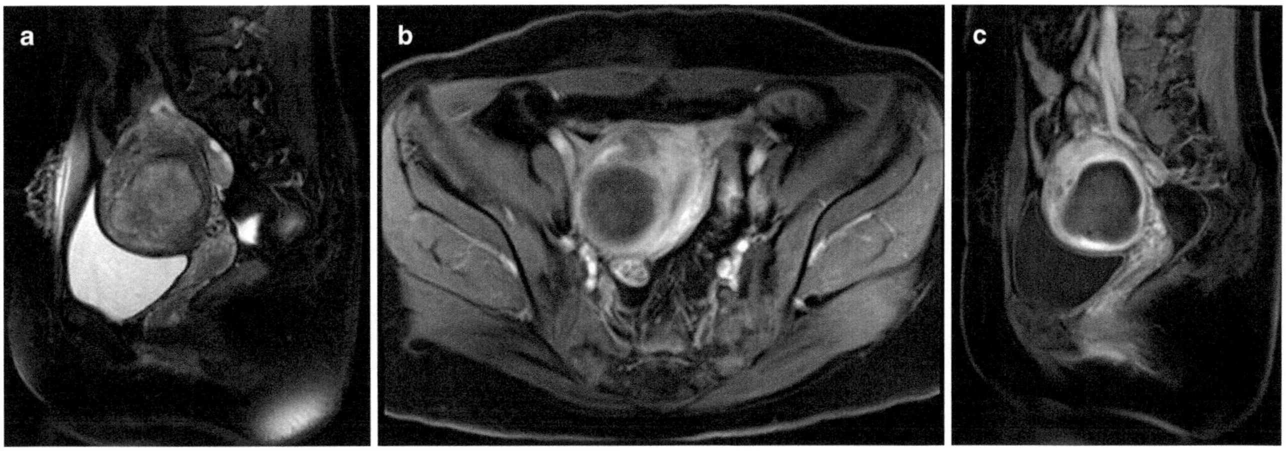

Fig. 4.82 MRI evaluation of type V intramural fibroid after treatment. (**a**) T2WI_FS sagittal, (**b**) T1WI_FS + C axial, (**c**) T1WI_FS + C sagittal

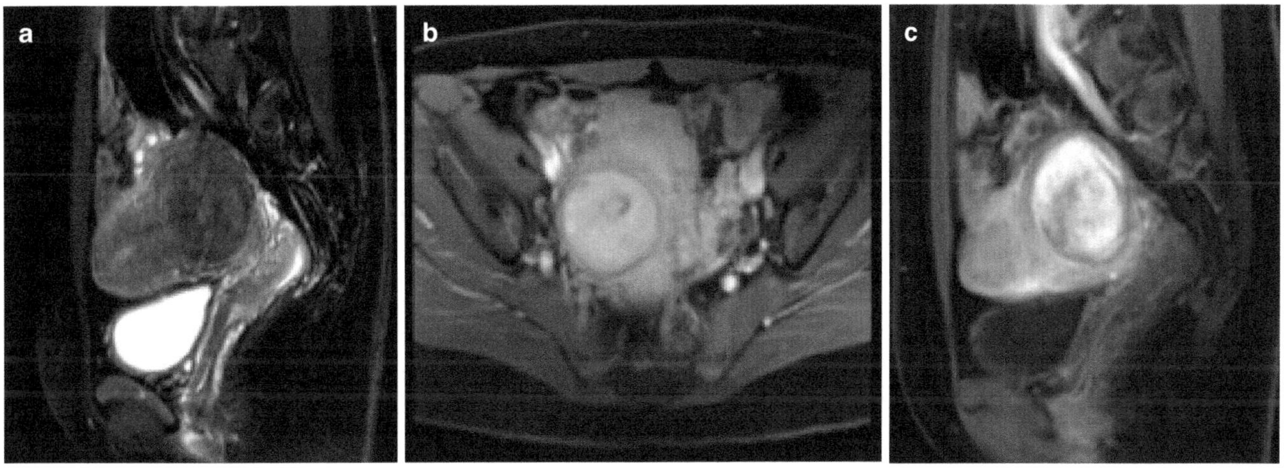

Fig. 4.83 Type V intramural fibroids before treatment. (**a**) T2WI_FS sagittal, (**b**) T1WI_FS + C axial, (**c**) T1WI_FS + C sagittal

terior wall near the cervix, with a poor acoustic pathway and close to the vascular nerve sacral plexus. Therefore, it is technically challenging for this fibroid to be ablated. However, this fibroid is mainly of low T2WI signal, which may be an indication for focused ultrasound ablation therapy.

4.2.22.3 Treatment Techniques

1. **Focused ultrasound parameters.** Average acoustic power: 252 W, sonication time: 2469 s, duration of treatment: 100 min, total energy: 621,850 J.
2. **Focused ultrasound ablation techniques.** During treatment, the acoustic power was appropriately reduced. Pay close attention to whether the patient had any symptoms such as pain and numbness in the right leg to avoid nerve damage caused by ultrasound ablation.

4.2.22.4 Post-Treatment Assessment

1. **MRI evaluation after treatment.** Only the front edge of the fibroid showed an increased T2WI signal (Fig. 4.84a). The contrast-enhanced T1WI showed that the fibroid was completely ablated. The adjacent serosa was intact. There were no obvious signs of edema in the anterior abdominal wall and the posterior pelvic wall fascia (Fig. 4.84b, c).
2. **MRI follow-up at 6 months after treatment.** The size of the necrotic fibroid was reduced by about 60% in the MRI follow-up. Only a thin enhanced layer could be seen on the upper edge of the fibroid, which could be the healing fibrous tissue after necrosis (Fig. 4.85a–c).
3. **MRI follow-up at 20 months after treatment.** The fibroid shrank to less than 2 cm. The non-perfusion area was no longer significant, and the uterus returned to its normal shape (Fig. 4.85d–f).

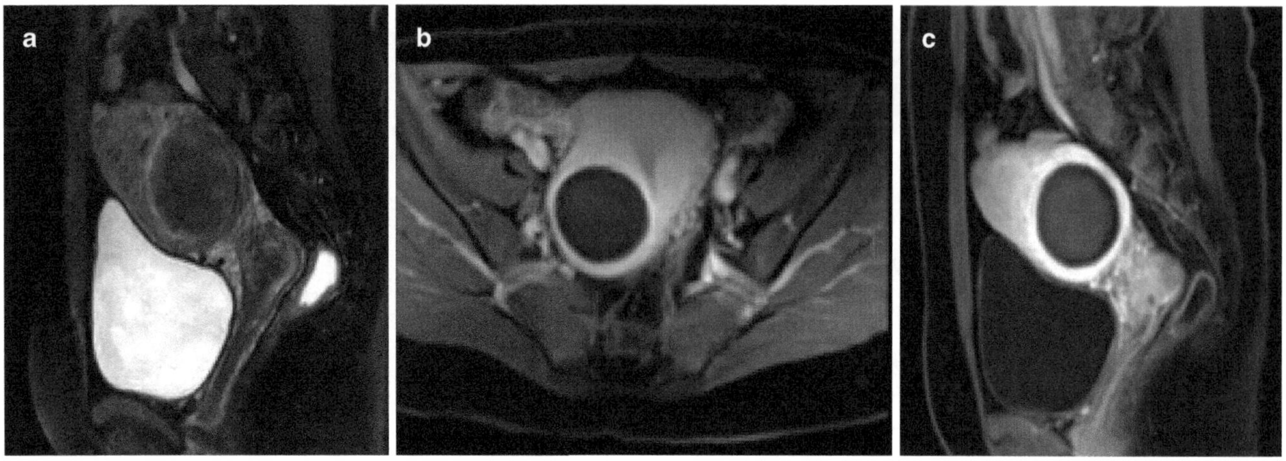

Fig. 4.84 MRI evaluation of type V intramural fibroids after treatment. (**a**) T2WI_FS sagittal, (**b**) T1WI_FS + C axial, (**c**) T1WI_FS + C sagittal

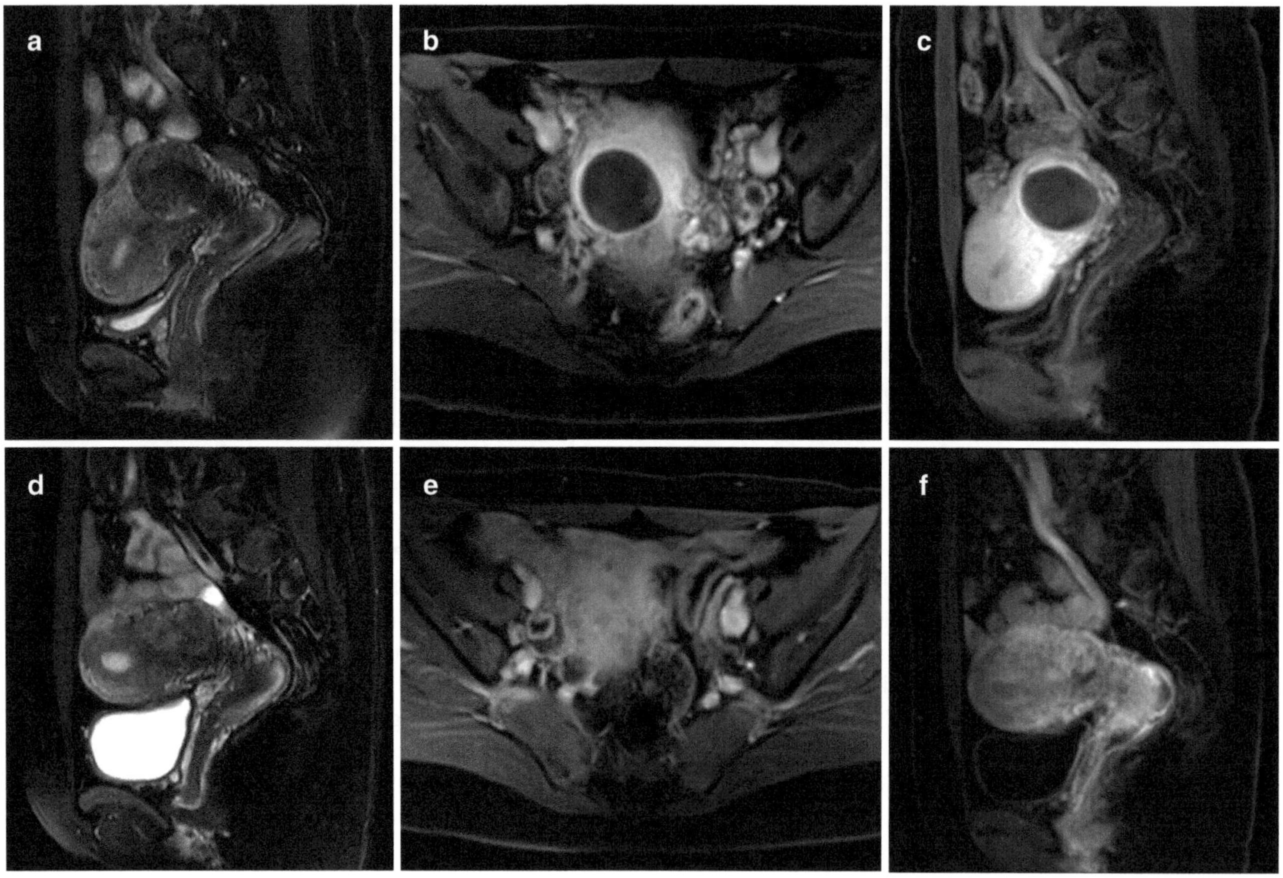

Fig. 4.85 MRI follow-up of type V intramural fibroids at 6 months (**a**–**c**) and 20 months (**d**–**f**) after treatment. (**a**) T2WI_FS sagittal, (**b**) T1WI_FS + C axial, (**c**) T1WI_FS + C sagittal, (**d**) T2WI_FS sagittal, (**e**) T1WI_FS + C axial, (**f**) T1WI_FS + C sagittal

4.2.22.5 Discussion

- For uterine fibroid adjacent to the vascular nerve plexus of the posterior pelvic wall, focused ultrasound ablation must be performed to obtain the best therapeutic effect on the premise of ensuring safety.
- This is a typical case that gives great consideration to safety and effectiveness. Long-term follow-up shows that the fibroid shrinks and tends to heal, and the uterine shape is restored.

4.2.23 Case 23 Type V Intramural Fibroid (5)

4.2.23.1 Case Description

The female patient was 46 years old. She had a uterine fibroid diagnosed for more than 1 year with symptoms of pelvic compression such as urinary frequency and back pain.

4.2.23.2 Pre-treatment Assessment

MRI showed a fibroid with a slightly low T2WI signal adjacent to the endometrium and serosa (Fig. 4.86a). The contrast-enhanced T1WI demonstrated that the fibroid had an abundant blood supply and a pseudocapsule (Fig. 4.86b, c). The fibroid was located in the anterior wall of the uterus and had a good acoustic pathway. Although it had an abundant blood supply, it was of hypointensity on T2WI. Therefore, it was predicted to be suitable for ultrasound ablation.

4.2.23.3 Treatment Techniques

1. **Focused ultrasound parameters.** Average acoustic power: 392 W, sonication time: 1122 s, duration of treatment: 117 min, total energy: 439,669 J.
2. **Focused ultrasound ablation techniques.** The acoustic pathway was satisfactory. A higher acoustic power was required for the treatment because the fibroid had an abundant blood supply.

4.2.23.4 Post-Treatment Assessment

1. **MRI evaluation after treatment.** The T2WI signal in the marginal area of the fibroid was significantly increased, and the fascia of the posterior pelvic wall was edematous. The contrast-enhanced T1WI showed that the fibroid was completely ablated, and the corresponding serosa and endometrium were intact (Fig. 4.87).
2. **MRI follow-up at 7 months after treatment.** The fascial edema of the posterior pelvic wall disappeared, and the fibroid volume was significantly reduced. The contrast-enhanced T1WI showed that the fibroid had no perfusion, with no signs of recurrence (Fig. 4.88).

4.2.23.5 Discussion

- In this case, the blood supply of the uterine fibroid was abundant, yet complete ablation was achieved after focused ultrasound ablation treatment. There was no edema in the abdominal wall. Still, the fascial edema of the posterior pelvic wall was significant, which may be related to the more energy of focused ultrasound far-field after using higher acoustic power (392 W). MRI follow-up showed that the edema had disappeared, indicating that the focused ultrasound ablation treatment is safe and the edema can be completely absorbed over time and restored. MRI is more sensitive to soft tissue edema and should be used as the main tool for follow-up.

4.2.24 Case 24 Type V Intramural Fibroid (6)

4.2.24.1 Case Description

The female patient was 48 years old with a uterine fibroid that was 89 mm in diameter. She presented with the abdominal distension and low back pain.

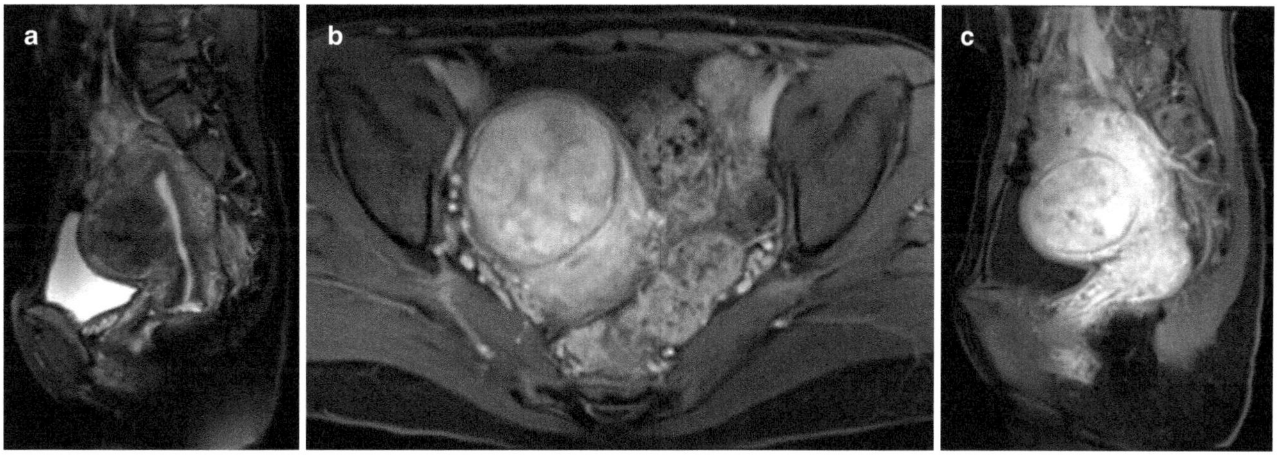

Fig. 4.86 Type V intramural fibroids before treatment. (**a**) T2WI_FS sagittal, (**b**) T1WI_FS + C axial, (**c**) T1WI_FS + C sagittal

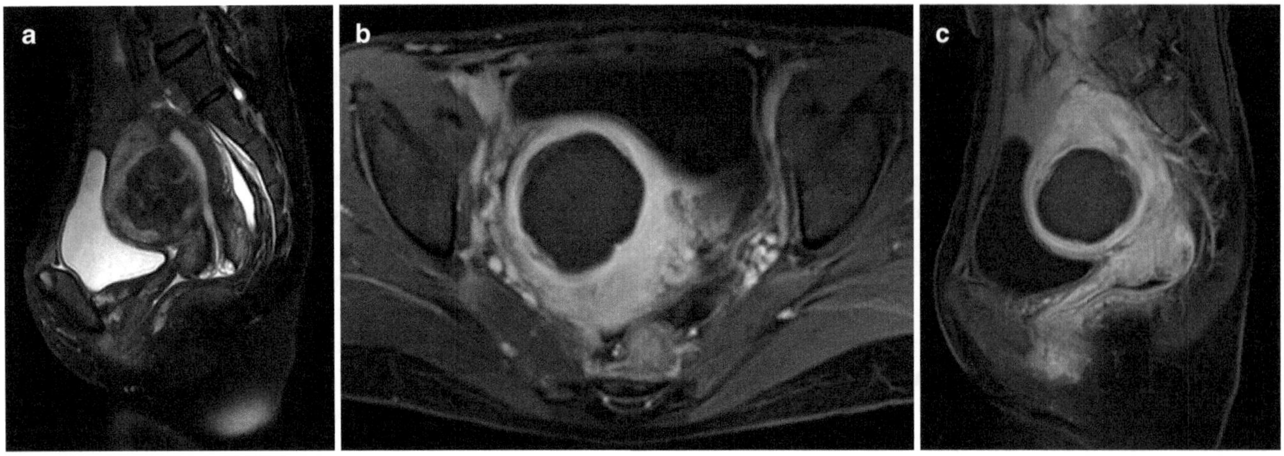

Fig. 4.87 MRI evaluation of type V intramural fibroids after treatment. (**a**) T2WI_FS sagittal, (**b**) T1WI_FS + C axial, (**c**) T1WI_FS + C sagittal

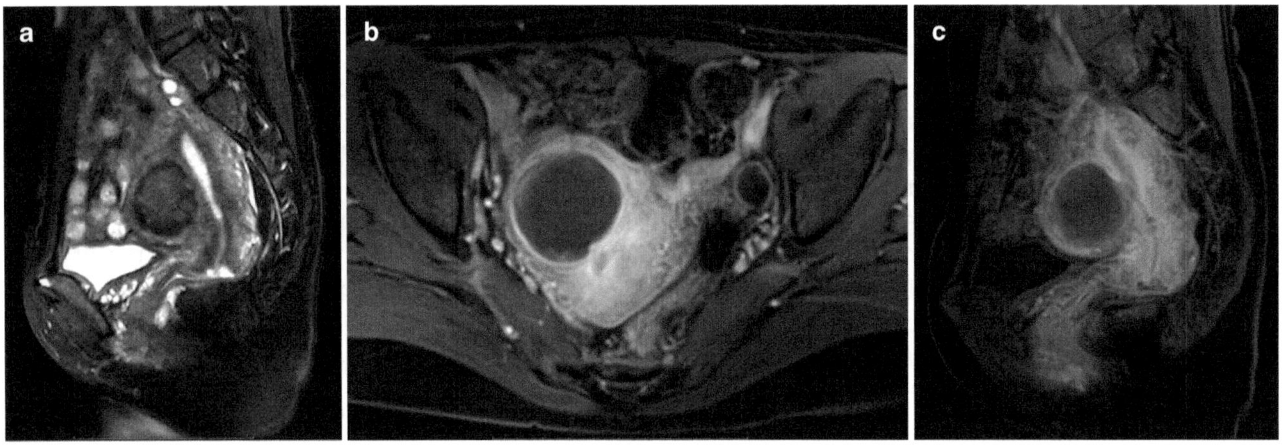

Fig. 4.88 MRI follow-up of type V intramural fibroids at 7 months after treatment. (**a**) T2WI_FS sagittal, (**b**) T1WI_FS + C axial, (**c**) T1WI_FS + C sagittal

4.2.24.2 Pre-Treatment Assessment

T2WI showed a fibroid with inhomogeneous hyperintensity on the uterus fundus (Fig. 4.89a). The contrast-enhanced T1WI showed that the fibroid had abundant blood supply with pseudocapsule (Fig. 4.89b, c). The acoustic pathway was clear, however, the fibroid with high T2 signal intensity and abundant blood supply would be predicted to be difficult to ablate with focused ultrasound treatment, therefore, the full communication with the patient was required.

4.2.24.3 Treatment Techniques

1. **Focused ultrasound parameters.** Average acoustic power: 240 W, sonication time: 3840 s, duration of treatment: 156 min, total energy: 1,096,330 J.
2. **Focused ultrasound ablation techniques.** With regard to the fibroids with T2WI hyperintensity and abundant blood supply, more acoustic energy needs to be delivered and the focal regions should be evenly distributed for complete ablation.

4.2.24.4 Post-Treatment Assessment

1. **MRI evaluation after treatment.** The contrast-enhanced MRI showed that the treated fibroid was completely ablated without any residual (Fig. 4.90a).
2. **MRI follow-up at 6 months after treatment.** The uterine fibroid, which presented with hyper- and hypointensity on T2WI (Fig. 4.90b), was significantly reduced in size without perfusion on the contrast-enhanced T1WI, and no recurrence was in the shrunken fibroid (Fig. 4.90c).

4.2.24.5 Discussion

- The heterogeneously hyperintense fibroids on T2WI can be considered as an indication of focused ultrasound ablation. Like this case, although it was hypervascular, 100% of the NPV ratio was achieved after focused ultrasound ablation with relatively higher energy, and there was no relapse in the follow-up.

4.2.25 Case 25 Type V Intramural Fibroid (7)

4.2.25.1 Case Description

The female patient was 38 years old. She had mild anemia associated with urinary frequency. She took traditional Chinese medicine to treat her uterine fibroid but failed.

4.2.25.2 Pre-Treatment Assessment

T2WI showed a uterine fibroid with heterogenous slight high signals (Fig. 4.91a). The contrast-enhanced MRI showed that the fibroid had an abundant blood supply and some

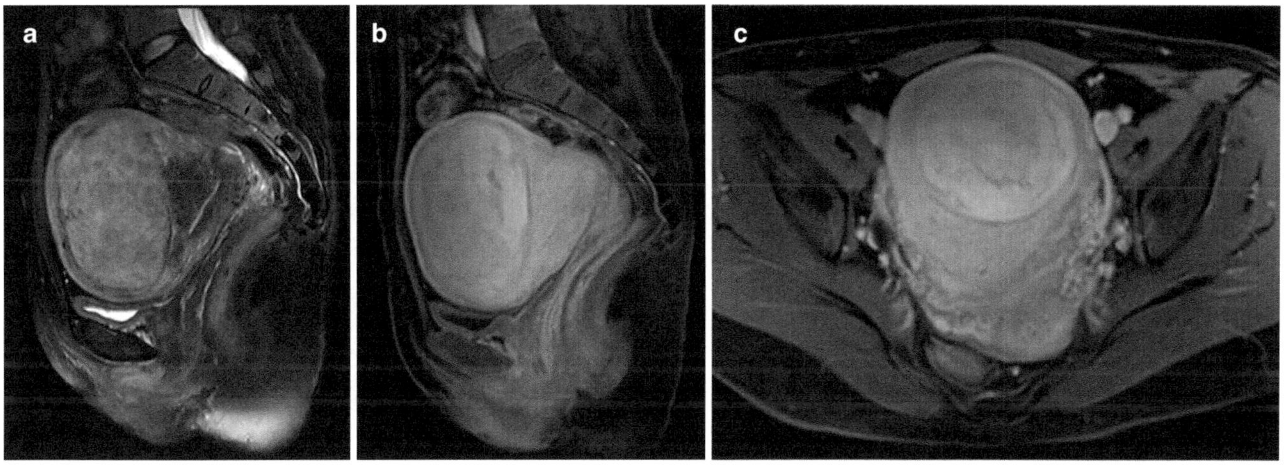

Fig. 4.89 Type V intramural fibroids before treatment. (**a**) T2WI_FS sagittal, (**b**) T1WI_FS + C sagittal, (**c**) T1WI_FS + C axial

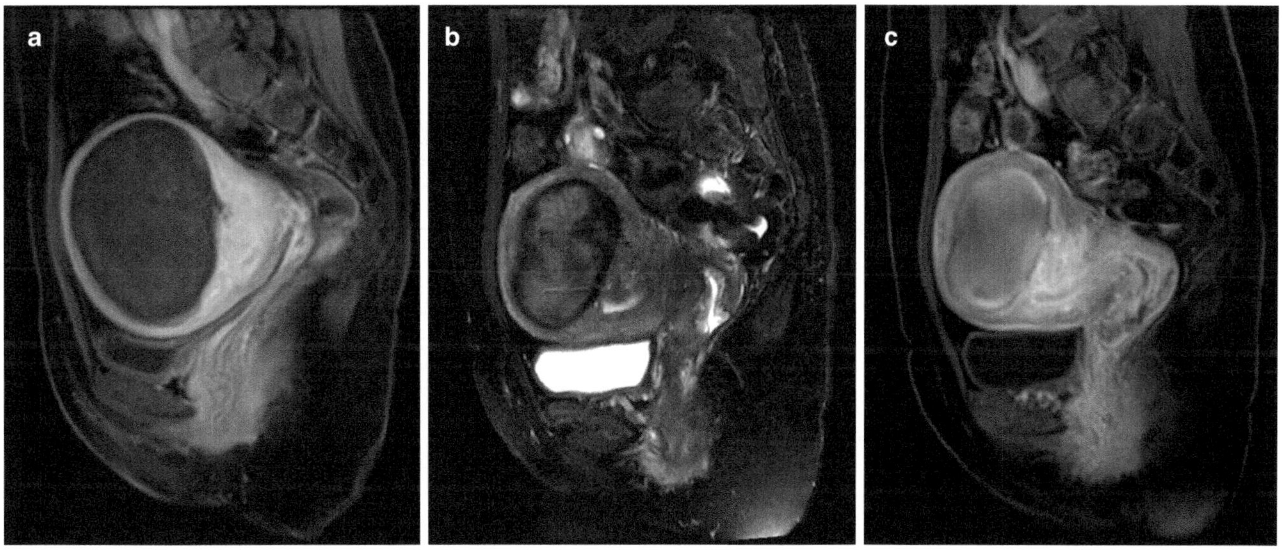

Fig. 4.90 MRI evaluation of type V intramural fibroids (**a**) and follow-up at 6 months (**b**, **c**) after treatment. (**a**) T1WI_FS + C sagittal, (**b**) T2WI_FS sagittal, (**c**) T1WI_FS + C sagittal

degenerations (Fig. 4.91b, c). The fibroid was located at the posterior wall of the uterus and adjacent to the sacrum and rectum, and some bowels lay in the acoustic pathway. Because of the above, it would not be easy for the fibroid to be ablated.

4.2.25.3 Treatment Techniques

1. **Focused ultrasound parameters.** Average acoustic power: 337 W, sonication time: 3301 s, duration of treatment: 181 min, total energy: 1,112,990 J.
2. **Focused ultrasound ablation techniques.** In order to improve the ablation efficacy of the fibroid, sonication with high acoustic power for a long time was required, and attention should be paid to avoiding damage to surrounding organs and tissues during the procedure.

4.2.25.4 Post-Treatment Assessment

1. **MRI evaluation after treatment.** The T2WI signal of the fibroid was significantly higher than that before treatment. The anterior abdominal wall was extensively edematous, and the edema was also seen in the posterior pelvic wall fascia (Fig. 4.92a). The contrast-enhanced T1WI showed that the NPV ratio of the fibroid was about 95%, with a small amount of residual fibroid on some edges (Fig. 4.92b, c).
2. **MRI follow-up at 6 months after treatment.** The fibroid volume was only slightly reduced, and the un-ablated residual fibroid significantly recurred, almost occupying the original ablation non-perfusion area. The soft tissue edema of the anterior abdominal wall and the posterior pelvic wall disappeared (Fig. 4.93). The patient received a second focused ultrasound ablation treatment after the fibroid recurrence.

4.2.25.5 Pre-Retreatment Assessment

In the follow-up after 9 months, T2WI showed that the fibroid had a mildly inhomogeneous high signal, and the fibroid had also enlarged in size. The contrast-enhanced T1WI showed a moderate blood supply, and a pseudocapsule could be seen at the edges (Fig. 4.94).

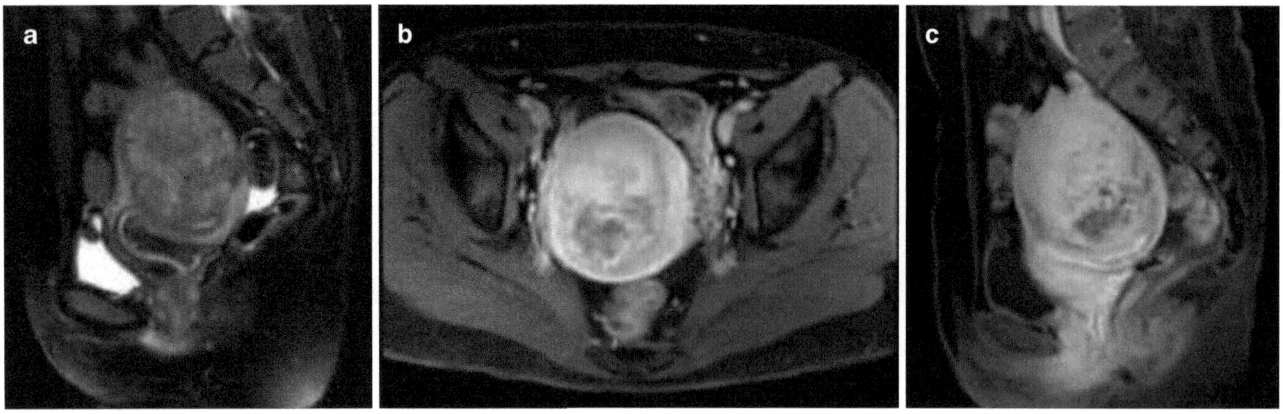

Fig. 4.91 Type V intramural fibroids before treatment. (**a**) T2WI_FS sagittal, (**b**) T1WI_FS + C axial, (**c**) T1WI_FS + C sagittal

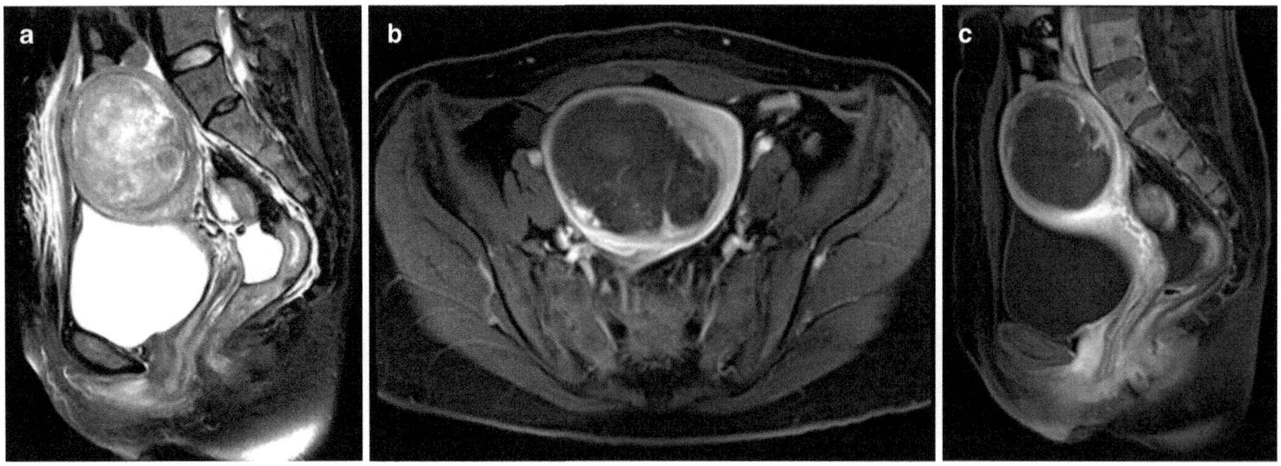

Fig. 4.92 MRI evaluation of type V intramural fibroids after treatment. (**a**) T1WI_FS sagittal, (**b**) T1WI_FS + C axial, (**c**) T1WI_FS + C sagittal

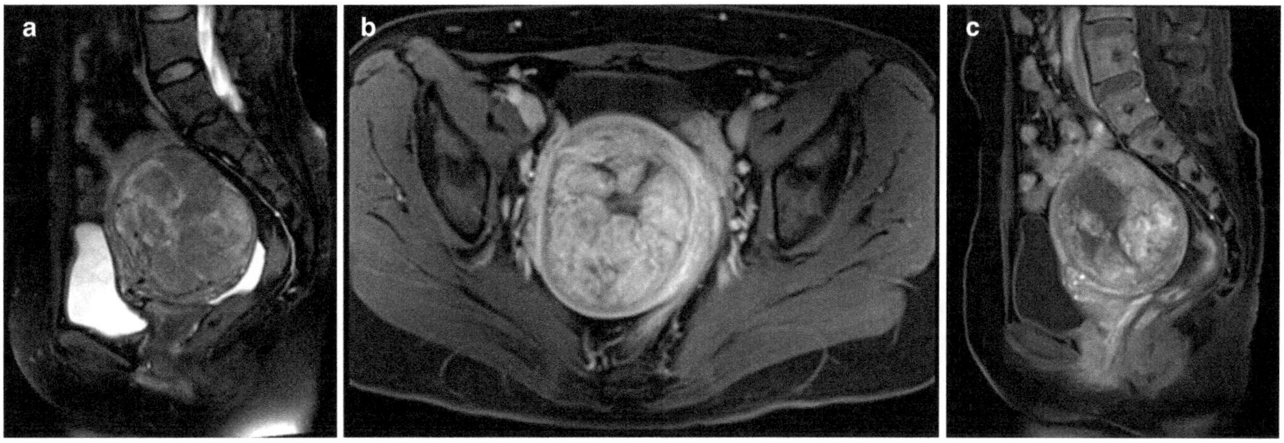

Fig. 4.93 MRI follow-up of type V intramural fibroids at 6 months after treatment. (**a**) T2WI_FS sagittal, (**b**) T1WI_FS + C axial, (**c**) T1WI_FS + C axial

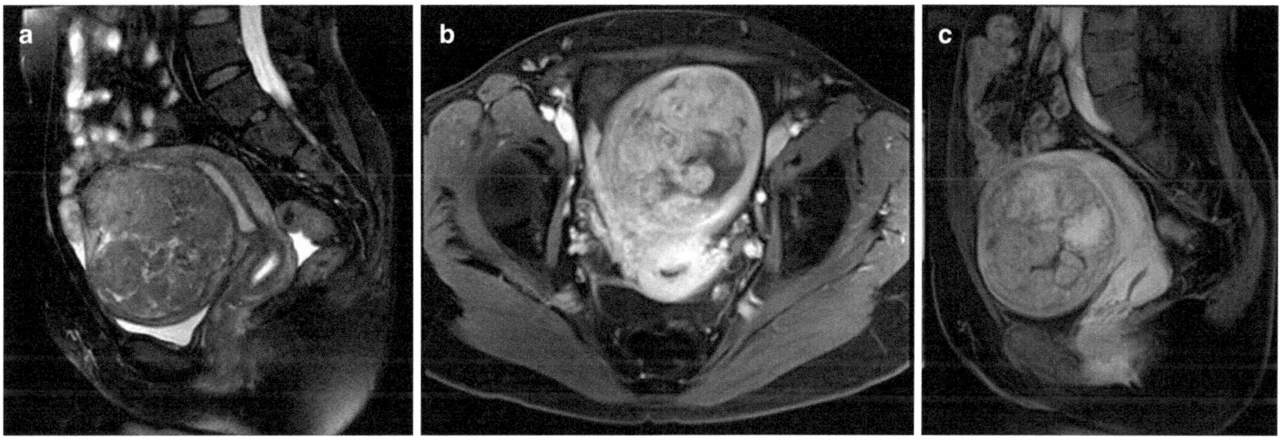

Fig. 4.94 Type V intramural fibroids before the retreatment. (**a**) T2WI_FS sagittal, (**b**) T1WI_FS + C axial, (**c**) T1WI_FS + C sagittal

4.2.25.6 Retreatment Technique

Focused Ultrasound Ablation Retreatment Parameters
Average acoustic power: 360 W, sonication time: 3890 ss, duration of treatment: 204 min, total energy: 1,463,330 J.

4.2.25.7 Post-Retreatment Assessment

MRI Evaluation after Retreatment The T2WI signal of myoma was significantly higher than that before treatment. There was obvious soft tissue edema of the abdominal wall (Fig. 4.95a). The contrast-enhanced T1WI showed partial fibroid ablation, and the NPV ratio was about 35% (Fig. 4.95b, c).

4.2.25.8 Discussion

- In this case, the efficacy of focused ultrasound ablation was still poor due to the long interval between two ultrasound ablations. After surgery, the uterine fibroids were removed. The pathological result revealed cell-rich uterine leiomyoma. For this kind of cell-rich uterine leiomyoma, even if the NPV ratio is about 95% after focused ultrasound ablation treatment, the remaining residual fibroid recurs and grows rapidly after half a year. The effect of focused ultrasound ablation treatment is poor.

4.2.26 Case 26 Type V Intramural Fibroid (8)

4.2.26.1 Case Description

The female patient was 46 years old. She presented with increased menstrual blood flow and shortened menstrual cycle, urinary frequency, and urgency in the past 6 months.

4.2.26.2 Pre-Treatment Assessment

T2WI showed a uterine fibroid with heterogenous hyperintensity located at the anterior wall of the uterus (Fig. 4.96a). The contrast-enhanced T1WI showed that the fibroid had a poor blood supply (Fig. 4.96b). According to its MRI signal characteristics and the good acoustic pathway, it is predicted that the fibroid could be treated by ultrasound ablation.

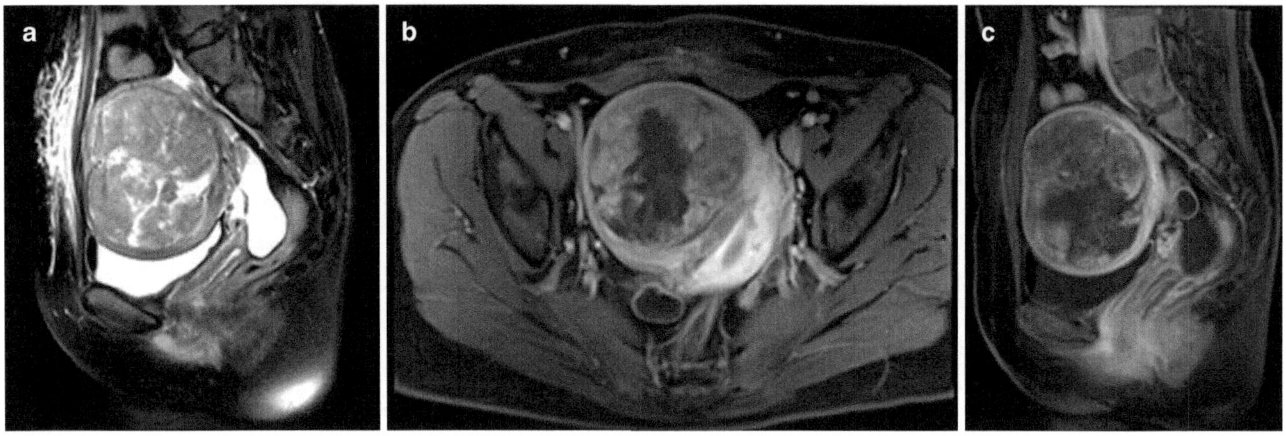

Fig. 4.95 MRI follow-up of the recurrent type V intramural fibroids immediately after retreatment. (**a**) T2WI_FS sagittal, (**b**) T1WI_FS + C axial, (**c**) T1WI_FS + C sagittal

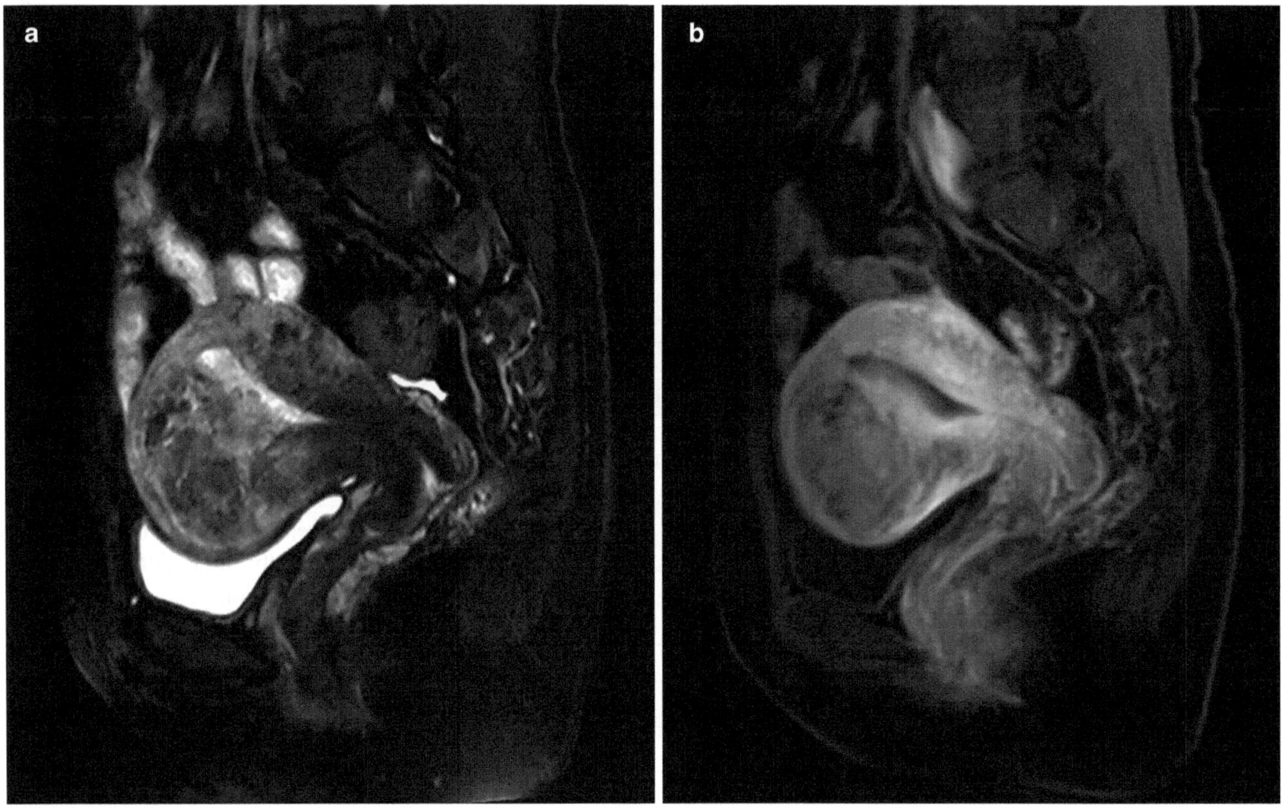

Fig. 4.96 Type V intramural fibroids before treatment. (**a**) T2WI_FS sagittal, (**b**) T1WI_FS + C sagittal

4.2.26.3 Treatment Techniques

1. **Focused ultrasound parameters.** Average acoustic power: 254 W, sonication time: 2560 s, total duration of treatment: 126 min, total energy: 649,570 J.
2. **Focused ultrasound ablation techniques.** The anterior part of the fibroid with markedly heterogenous hyperintense signal on T2WI indicated a higher water content in the tissue, so sufficient irradiation energy was needed to achieve better ablation results.

4.2.26.4 Post-Treatment Assessment

1. **MRI evaluation after treatment.** The muscle layer of the anterior abdominal wall was locally edematous, and the T2WI signal of myoma was significantly increased (Fig. 4.97a). The contrast-enhanced T1WI showed that the NPV ratio of the fibroid was about 87%, and residual tissue could be seen in the posterior area (Fig. 4.97b).
2. **MRI follow-up at 6 months after treatment.** The uterine fibroid was significantly reduced in size. No recurrence was in the residual fibroid (Fig. 4.98).

4.2.26.5 Discussion

- After focused ultrasound ablation treatment, in this case, the residual tissue in the posterior margin of the fibroid did not recur at 6 months follow-up. Whether it is related to the patient's older age or the significant increase in T2WI signal intensity of the residual fibroid after treatment is worthy of further study.

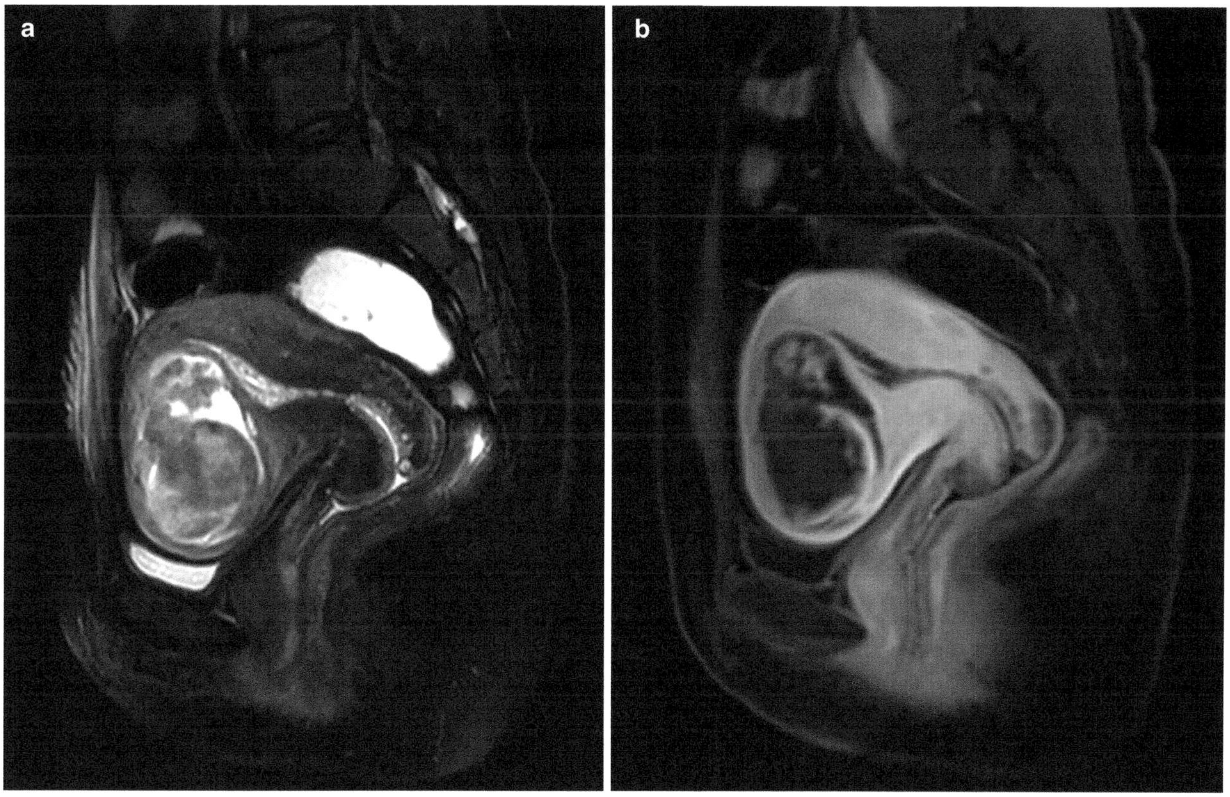

Fig. 4.97 MRI evaluation of type V intramural fibroids after treatment. (**a**) T2WI_FS sagittal, (**b**) T1WI_FS + C sagittal

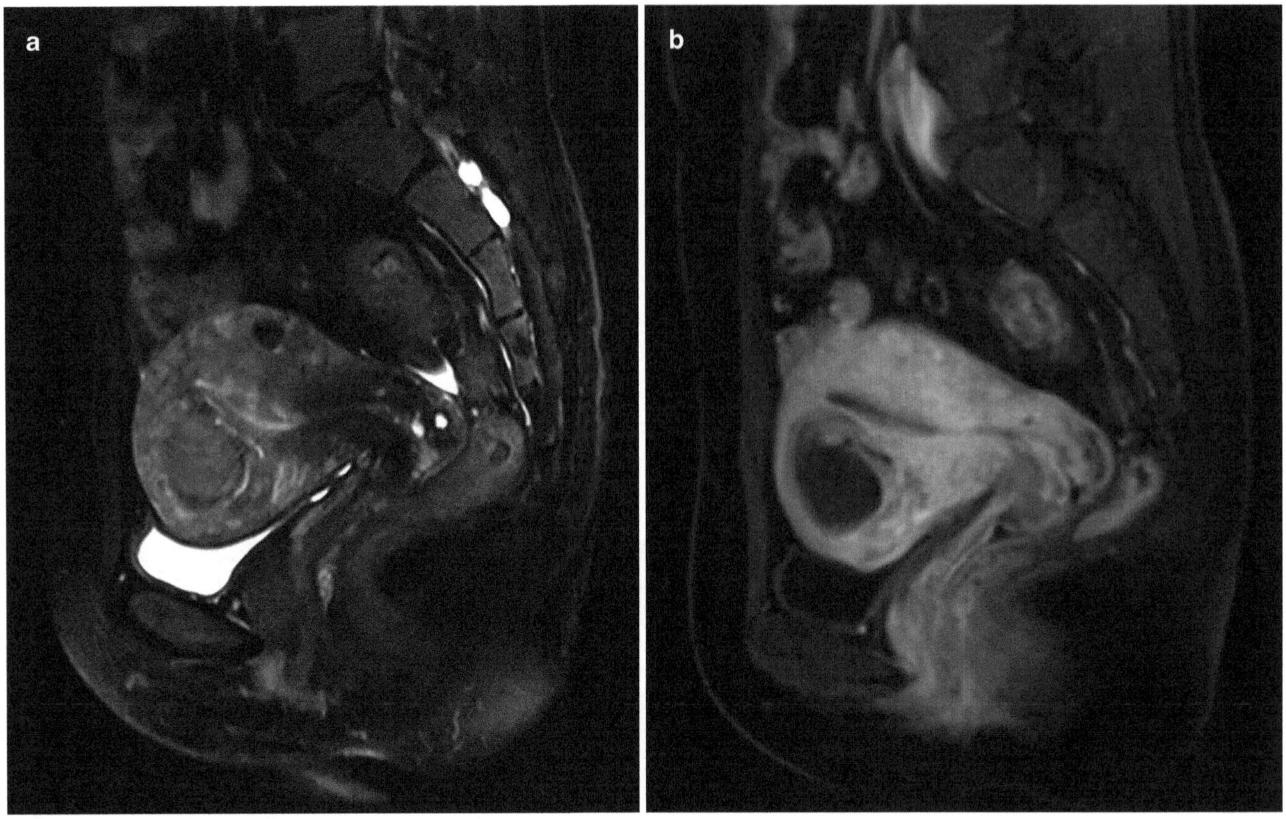

Fig. 4.98 MRI follow-up of type V intramural fibroids at 6 months after treatment. (**a**) T2WI_FS sagittal, (**b**) T1WI_FS + C sagittal

4.3 Focused Ultrasound Ablation for Subserosal Uterine Fibroids

4.3.1 Case 1 Type VI Subserosal Fibroid (1)

4.3.1.1 Case Description

A female patient was 38 years old. She had uterine fibroid, accompanied by symptoms of urinary frequency.

4.3.1.2 Pre-Treatment Assessment

T2WI showed a subserosal fibroid with hypointensity at the right anterior uterine wall, and the fibroid compressed the bladder downward (Fig. 4.99a). The contrast-enhanced T1WI showed that the fibroid was unevenly enhanced and had an abundant blood supply (Fig. 4.99b, c). There was a good acoustic pathway without bowels between the fibroid and the anterior abdominal wall, so it is predicted that focused ultrasound ablation can be performed.

4.3.1.3 Treatment Techniques

1. **Focused ultrasound parameters.** Average acoustic power: 254 W, sonication time: 2098 seconds, duration of treatment: 106 minutes, total energy: 532,640 J.
2. **Focused ultrasound ablation techniques.** The fibroid had homogeneous low intense signals on T2WI and was located at the anterior wall of the uterus, creating a good acoustic pathway. Reduced acoustic power should be used, especially at the junction between the fibroid and the uterine wall.

4.3.1.4 Post-Treatment Assessment

1. **MRI evaluation after treatment.** T2WI scan showed localized edema of the subcutaneous soft tissue of the anterior abdominal wall. The contrast-enhanced T1WI showed that the NPV ratio of the fibroid was about 98%, and there was only a small amount of residue fibroid at its left posterior edge and the junction of the uterine wall (Fig. 4.100).
2. **Medium- and long-term MRI follow-up after treatment.** T2WI showed that the edema of the subcutaneous soft tissue of the anterior abdominal wall gradually reduced. The contrast-enhanced T1WI showed no fibroid recurrence at 6, 18, and 26. After 26 months of treatment, T1WI follow-up found that the entire volume of the ablated fibroid gradually decreased. Follow-up at 38 months showed that the area of necrotic tissue continued to shrink. However, due to the increase in the area of fibroid recurrence, the fibroid volume was slightly larger than that at 26 months after treatment. Overall, the fibroid volume was reduced by about 30% compared with that

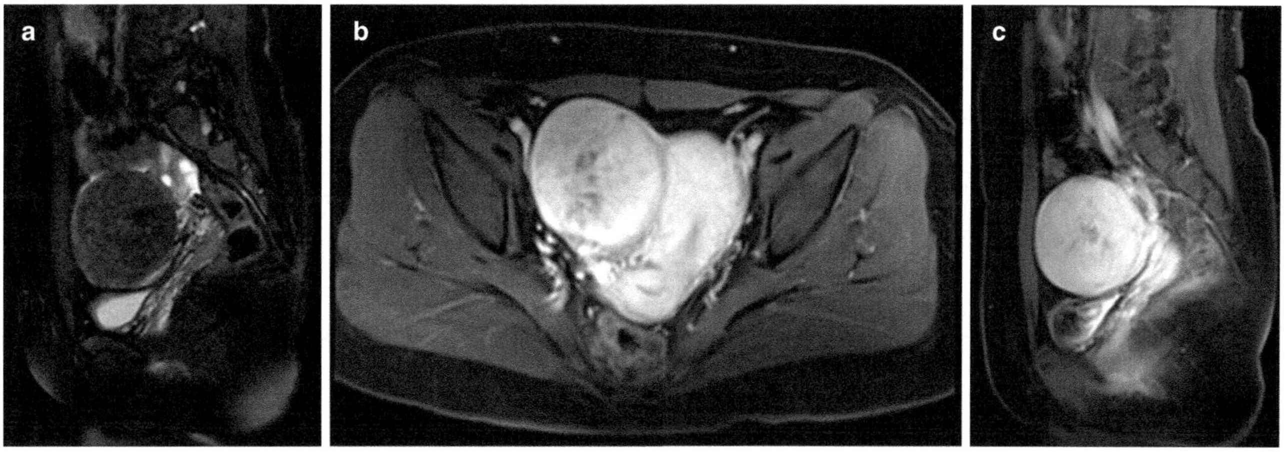

Fig. 4.99 Type VI subserosal fibroids before treatment. (**a**) T2WI_FS sagittal, (**b**) T1WI_FS + C axial, (**c**) T1WI_FS + C sagittal

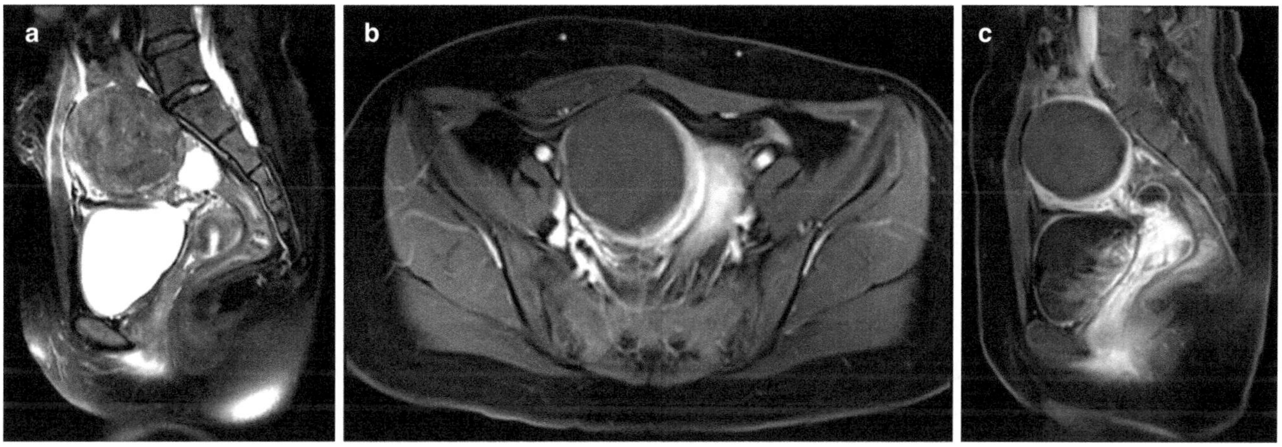

Fig. 4.100 MRI evaluation of type VI subserosal fibroids after treatment. (**a**) T2WI_FS sagittal, (**b**) T1WI_FS + C axial, (**c**) T1WI_FS + C sagittal

before focused ultrasound ablation treatment (Figs. 4.101, 4.102, 4.103, and 4.104).

4.3.1.5 Discussion

- Subserosal uterine fibroid has always been a contraindication for uterine artery embolization. The main concern is that necrotic fibroid may fall off and enter the abdominal and pelvic cavity. For patients unwilling to undergo surgical resection, focused ultrasound ablation therapy can take advantage of its precision and select the fibroid part connected to the uterine wall for ablation treatment.
- In this case, the width of the base between the subserous uterine fibroid and the edge of the uterus was more than 3 cm, and the whole fibroid was necrotic after focused ultrasound ablation treatment. While the ablation treatment at the base junction of the fibroid and the uterus is relatively un-ablated, resulting in a small amount of residue fibroid there. Despite reducing the fibroid size having achieved the purpose of treatment, the patient needs retreatment for the recurring residual fibroid with focused ultrasound ablation.

4.3.2 Case 2 Type VI Subserosal Fibroids (2)

4.3.2.1 Case Description

The female patient was 34 years old. She had reduced menstrual flow, accompanying lower abdomen distension and back pain.

4.3.2.2 Pre-Treatment Assessment

T2WI showed a uterine subserosal fibroid with low intense signals arising from the fundus of the uterus (Fig. 4.105a). The contrast-enhanced T1WI showed that the fibroid had an abundant blood supply (Fig. 4.105b, c). It was predicted that focused ultrasound ablation was feasible, but there might be difficulties in positioning during the procedure.

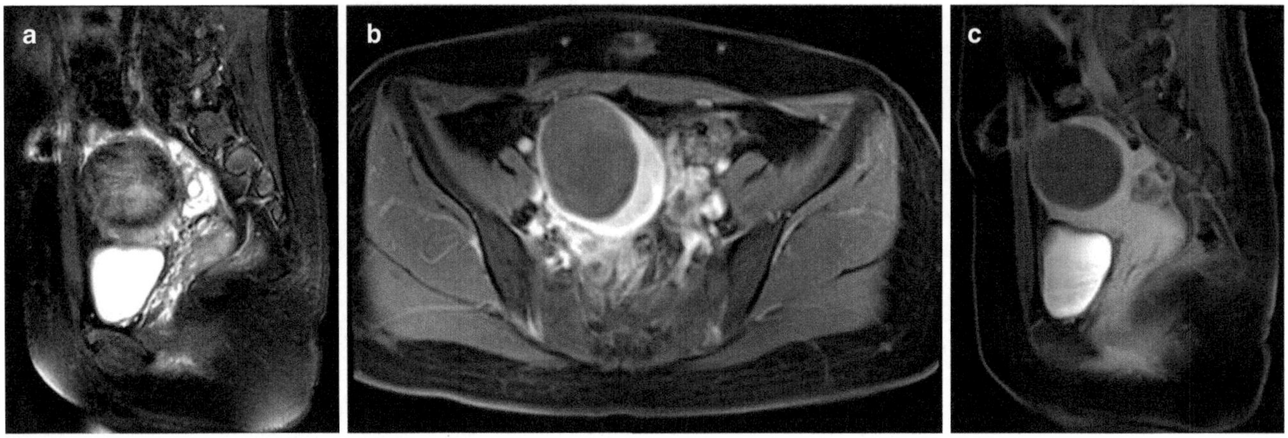

Fig. 4.101 MRI follow-up of type VI subserosal fibroids at 6 months after treatment. (**a**) T2WI_FS sagittal, (**b**) T1WI_FS + C axial, (**c**) T1WI_FS + C sagittal

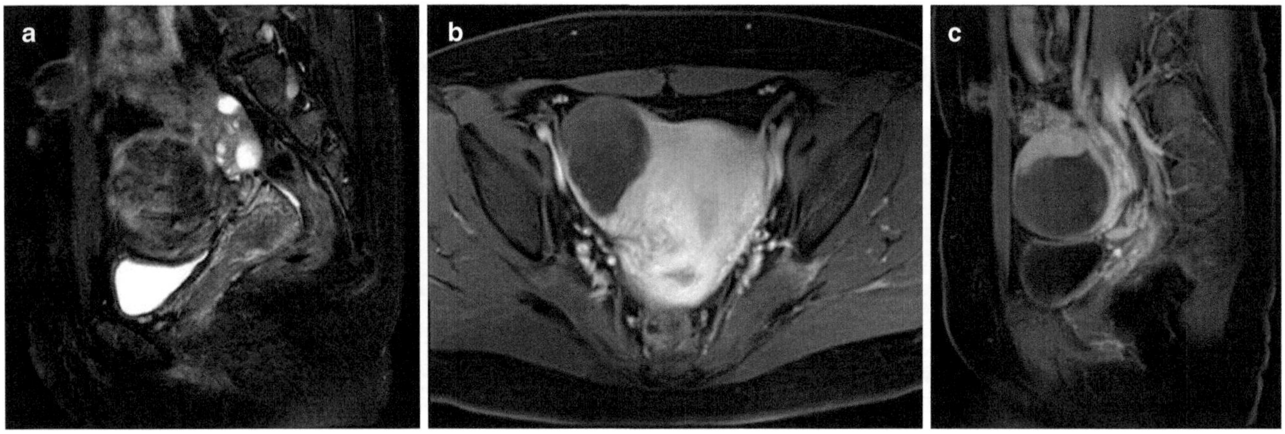

Fig. 4.102 MRI follow-up of type VI subserosal fibroids at 18 months after treatment. (**a**) T2WI_FS sagittal, (**b**) T1WI_FS + C axial, (**c**) T1WI_FS + C sagittal

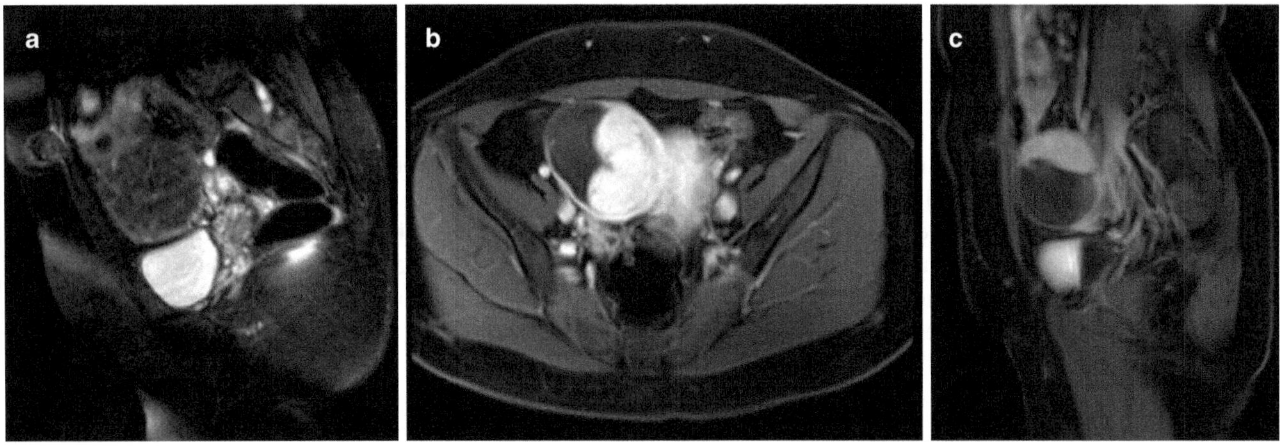

Fig. 4.103 MRI follow-up of type VI subserosal fibroids at 26 months after treatment. (**a**) T2WI_FS sagittal, (**b**) T1WI_FS + C axial, (**c**) T1WI_FS + C sagittal

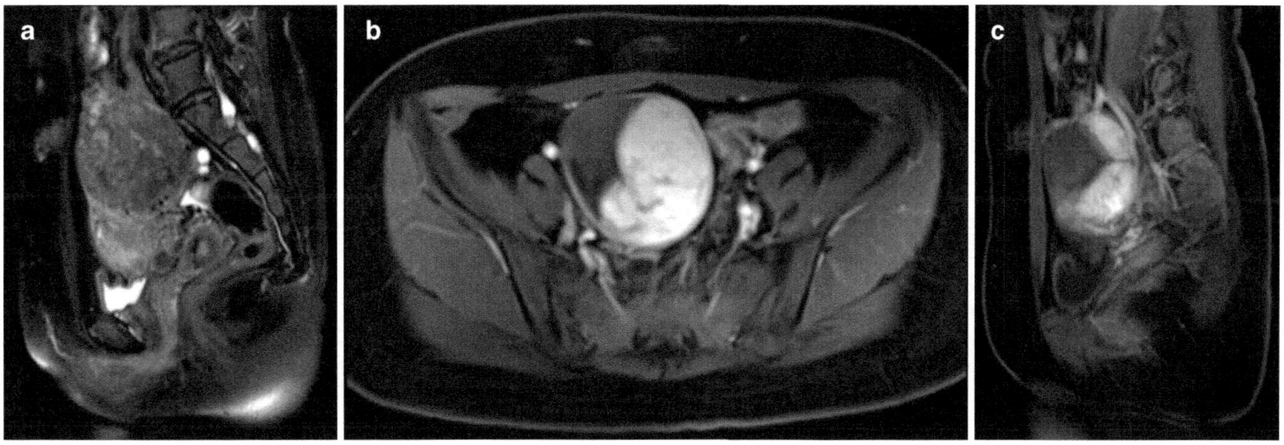

Fig. 4.104 MRI follow-up of type VI subserosal fibroids at 38 months after treatment. (**a**) T2WI_FS sagittal, (**b**) T1WI_FS + C axial, (**c**) T1WI_FS + C sagittal

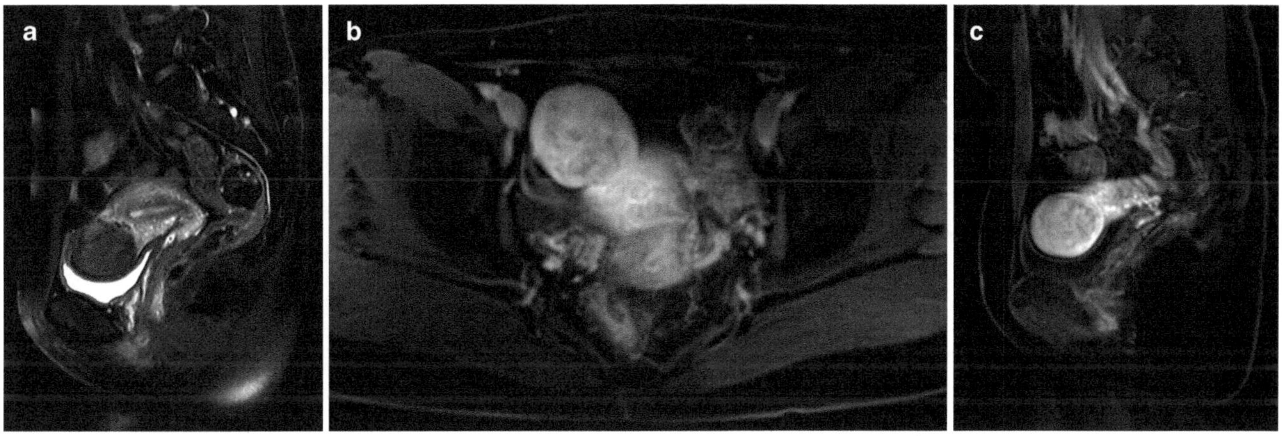

Fig. 4.105 Type VI subserosal fibroids before treatment. (**a**) T2WI_FS sagittal, (**b**) T1WI_FS + C axial, (**c**) T1WI_FS + C sagittal

4.3.2.3 Treatment Techniques

1. **Focused ultrasound parameters.** Average acoustic power: 209 W, sonication time: 1300 seconds, duration of treatment: 90 minutes, total energy: 271,850 J.
2. **Focused ultrasound ablation techniques.** The location of the subserosal fibroid at the fundus of the uterus is relatively special, with a wide range of motion. Take care not to damage the surrounding intestine and other tissue structures. Therefore, in addition to distending the bladder to fix the fibroid for accurate conformal ablation, it is also necessary to reduce the acoustic power to avoid serosal damage.

4.3.2.4 Post-Treatment Assessment

1. **MRI evaluation after treatment.** The position of the fibroid had changed, and the abdominal wall showed little edema on T2WI (Fig. 4.106a). The contrast-enhanced MRI showed that the NPV ratio of the fibroid was about 98%, and the serosal surface was intact (Fig. 4.106b, c).
2. **MRI follow-up at 6 months after treatment.** The fibroid volume had reduced by about 32%, without significant recurrence of the fibroid (Fig. 4.106d–f).

4.3.2.5 Discussion

- T2WI hypointense subserosal uterine fibroids should be irradiated with low acoustic power to avoid bowel damage or serosal breakthrough. By increasing the sonication time, sufficient ultrasound energy can be given to the fibroid, ablating the fibroid as much as possible and protecting the integrity of serosa. An intact uterine serosa ensures the safety of treatment.

4.3.3 Case 3 Type VI Subserosal Fibroid (3)

4.3.3.1 Case Description

The female patient was 39 years old. She consciously felt an enlarged abdomen and had urinary frequency.

4.3.3.2 Pre-Treatment Assessment

T2WI showed a subserosal uterine fibroid with homogeneous hypointensity and compressed the bladder downward (Fig. 4.107a). The contrast-enhanced T1WI showed that the fibroid had a moderate blood supply (Fig. 4.107b, c). The fibroid with a pseudocapsule was located at the right anterior wall of the uterus and close to the anterior sub-abdominal wall, which created a good acoustic pathway. Thus, it would be relatively easy for the focused ultrasound ablation procedure.

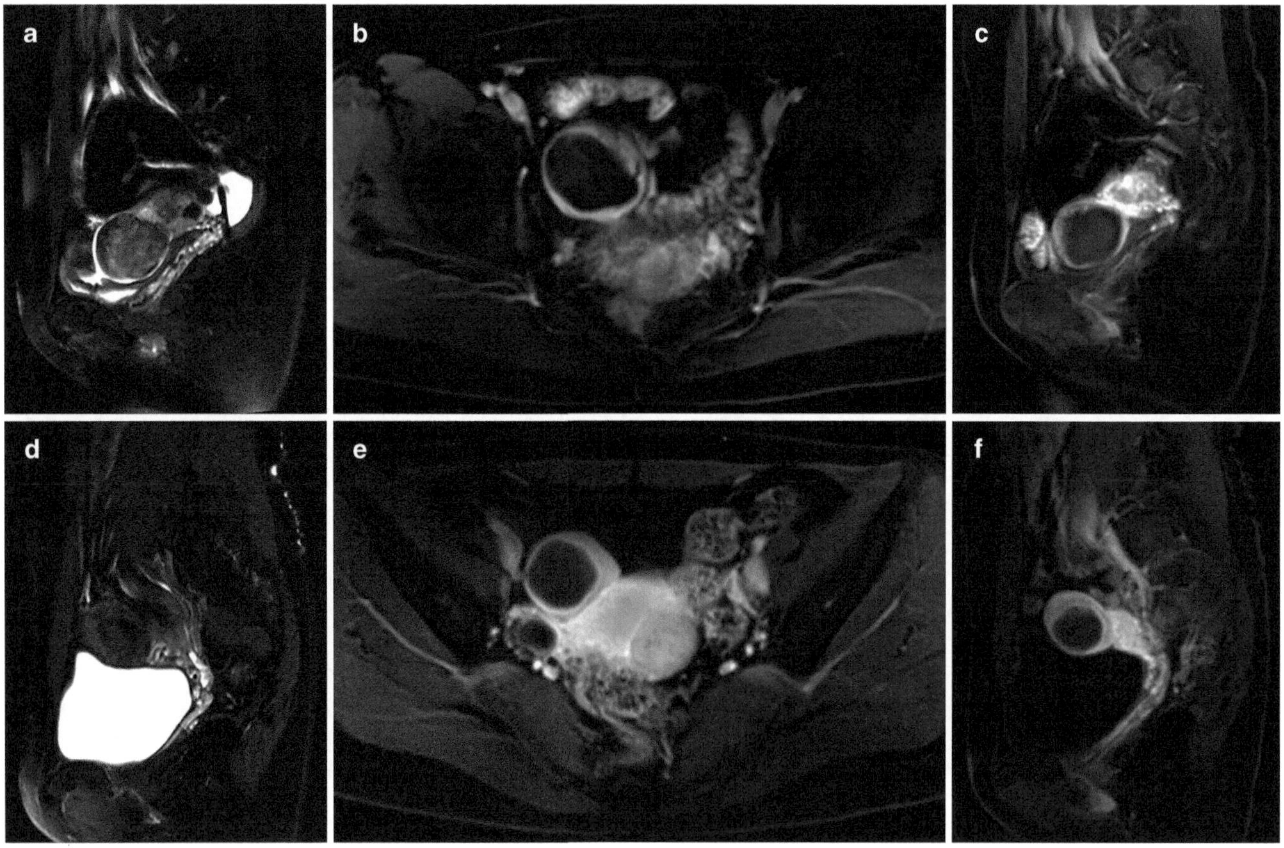

Fig. 4.106 MRI follow-up of type VI subserosal fibroids immediately (a-c) and at 6 months after treatment (d-f). (**a**) T2WI_FS sagittal, (**b**) T1WI_FS + C axial, (**c**) T1WI_FS + C sagittal, (**d**) T2WI_FS sagittal, (**e**) T1WI_FS + C axial, (**f**) T1WI_FS + C sagittal

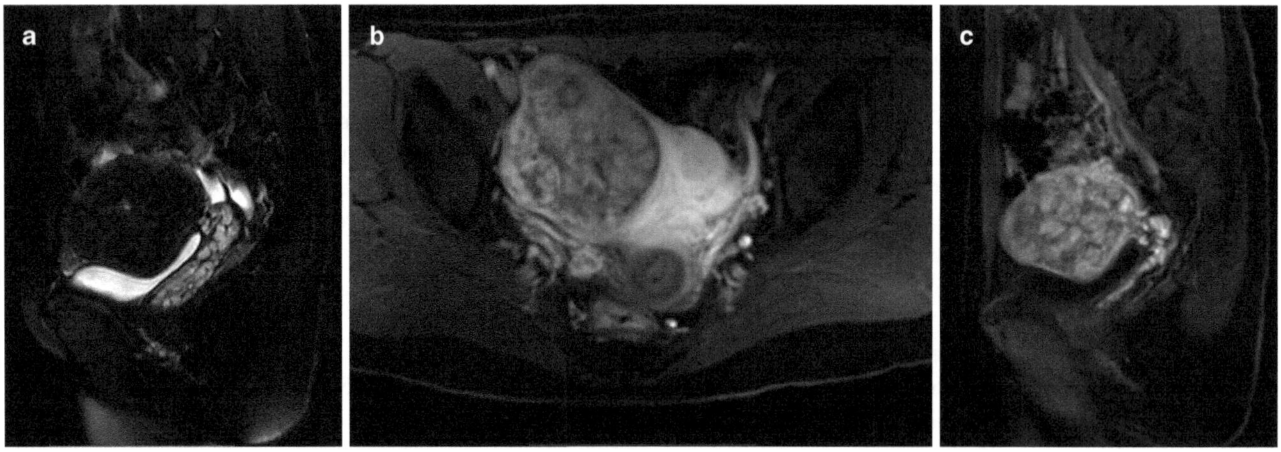

Fig. 4.107 Type VI subserosal fibroids before treatment. (**a**) T2WI_FS sagittal, (**b**) T1WI_FS + C axial, (**c**) T1WI_FS + C sagittal

4.3.3.3 Treatment Techniques

1. **Focused ultrasound parameters.** Average acoustic power: 209 W, sonication time: 1769 seconds, duration of treatment: 109 minutes, total energy: 370,320 J.
2. **Focused ultrasound ablation techniques.** The subserosal fibroid was large and occupied the whole right pelvic cavity. Avoid damaging its adjacent right ovary and peripheral vascular nerve plexus during ultrasound irradiation.

4.3.3.4 Post-Treatment Assessment

1. **MRI evaluation after treatment.** The T2WI showed edema of the soft tissue of the anterior abdominal wall. The contrast-enhanced T1WI showed that the NPV ratio of the fibroid exceeded 90%, and only a small part of the posterior edge of the fibroid remained un-ablated (Fig. 4.108).
2. **MRI follow-up at 6 months after treatment.** The fibroid volume was reduced by 56%, and the serosa was intact. The abdominal wall edema disappeared (Fig. 4.109).

4.3.3.5 Discussion

- Lower sonication power can be used for fibroid with low intense signals on T2WI and poor or moderate blood supply.
- After treatment, the serosa on the front edge of the fibroid is partially ablated, and most of the serosa is intact. Take care not to affect the uterine serosa during treatment.

4.3.4 Case 4 Type VI Subserosal Fibroid (4)

4.3.4.1 Case Description

The female patient was 30 years old. Five years ago, her physical examination revealed a uterine fibroid. She experienced frequent urination in recent years, accompanied by occasional pain in the lower abdomen.

4.3.4.2 Pre-Treatment Assessment

MRI showed an anterior subserosal uterine fibroid with inhomogeneous low signals on T2WI. The uterus was signifi-

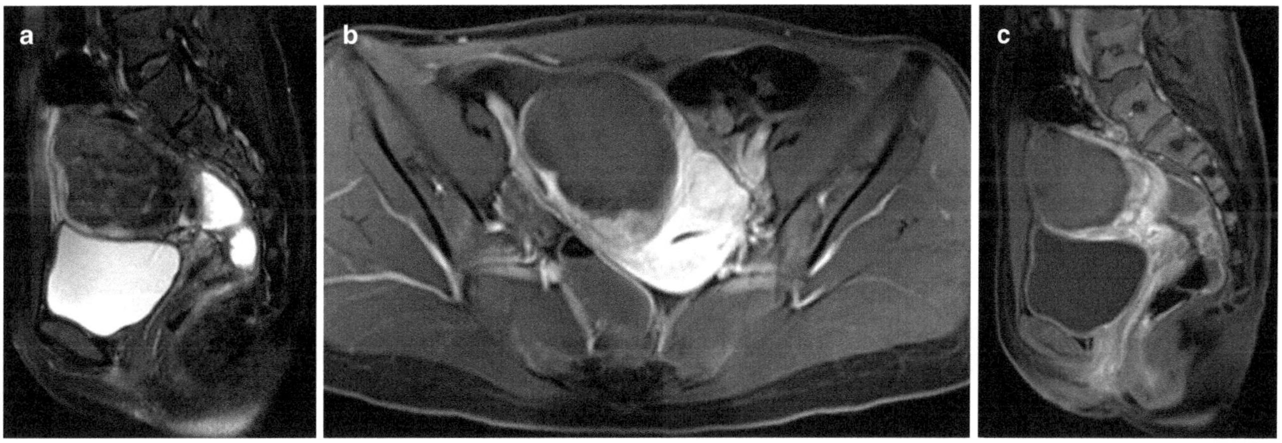

Fig. 4.108 MRI evaluation of type VI subserosal fibroids after treatment. (**a**) T2WI_FS sagittal, (**b**) T1WI_FS + C axial, (**c**) T1WI_FS + C sagittal

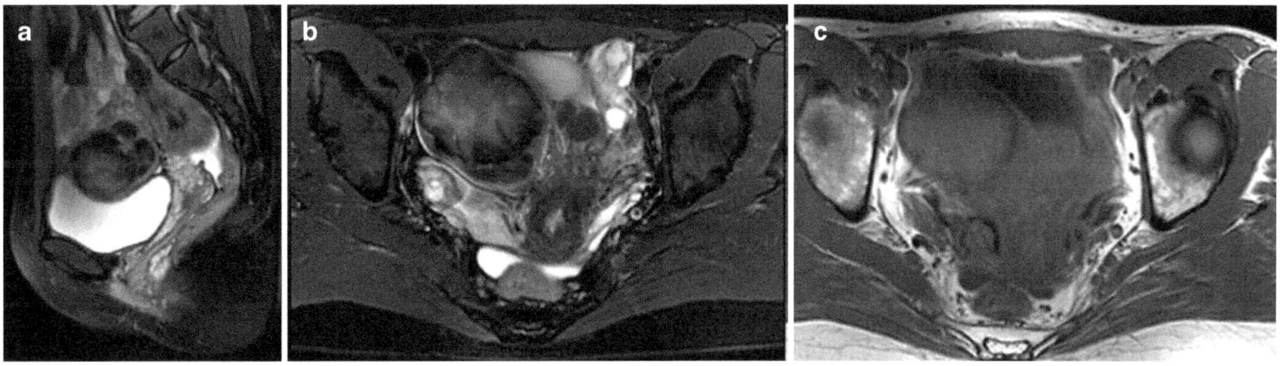

Fig. 4.109 MRI follow-up of Type VI subserosal fibroids at 6 months after treatment. (**a**) T2WI_FS sagittal, (**b**) T2WI_FS axial, (**c**) T1WI axial

cantly compressed down, leading to a backward tilt, with a significant space-occupying effect in the pelvic cavity (Fig. 4.110a). The contrast-enhanced T1WI showed that the fibroid had a poor blood supply with areas of degeneration or necrosis (Fig. 4.110b, c). This T2WI hypointense fibroid was located in the anterior wall of the retroverted uterus, with a good acoustic pathway and a clear boundary with the uterine wall. Therefore, this would be a suitable candidate for focused ultrasound ablation treatment.

4.3.4.3 Treatment Techniques

1. **Focused ultrasound parameters.** Average acoustic power: 250 W, sonication time: 1400 seconds, duration of treatment: 90 minutes, total energy: 349,760 J.
2. **Focused ultrasound ablation techniques.** This anterior subserosal fibroid with T2WI hypointense signal was larger and close to the abdominal wall. Therefore, low acoustic power should be used to avoid or reduce the soft tissue injury of the anterior abdominal wall.

4.3.4.4 Post-Treatment Assessment

MRI Evaluation after Treatment The T2WI showed no obvious edema occurred in the anterior abdominal wall, and the signal intensity of the fibroid increased. The contrast-enhanced T1WI showed that the NPV ratio of the fibroid exceeded 95%, and there was a small amount of residual tissue at the wide base of the posterior edge (Fig. 4.111).

4.3.4.5 Discussion

- For focused ultrasound ablation of uterine fibroids close to the anterior abdominal wall, the acoustic power should be reduced to avoid damage to the serosal layer as much as possible. In this case, there was no significant edema on the anterior abdominal wall after treatment.
- In order to avoid the necrotic subserosal fibroid from detaching from the uterus, a small amount of fibroid should be kept un-ablated at the base of the fibroid connected with the uterine wall during treatment.

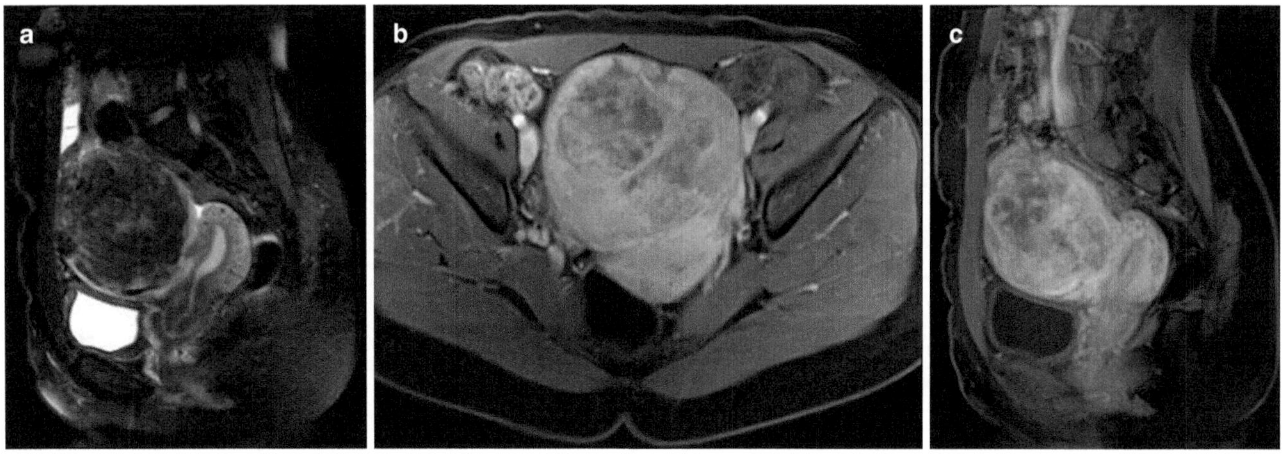

Fig. 4.110 Type VI subserosal fibroids before treatment. (**a**) T2WI_FS sagittal, (**b**) T1WI_FS + C axial, (**c**) T1WI_FS + C sagittal

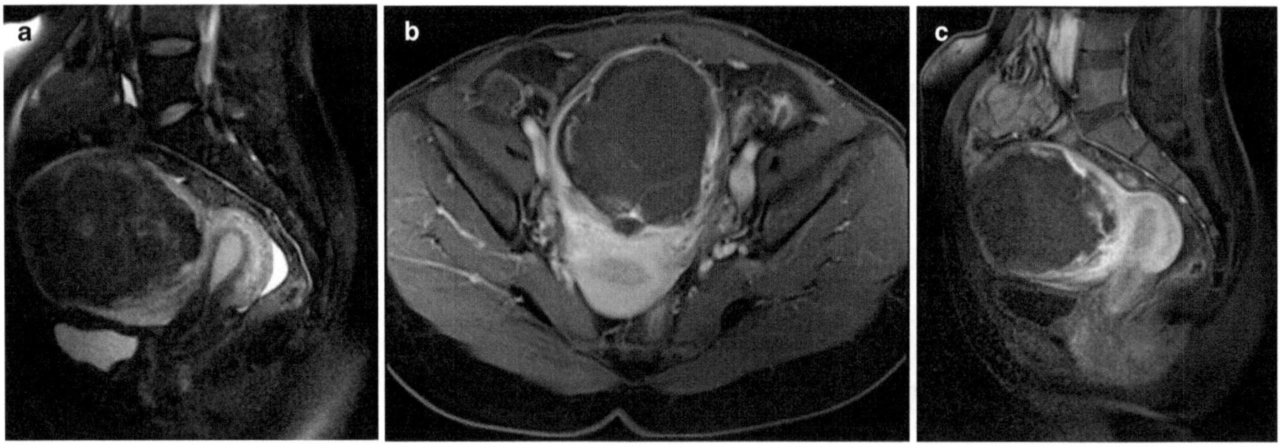

Fig. 4.111 MRI evaluation of type VI subserosal fibroids after treatment. (**a**) T2WI_FS sagittal, (**b**) T1WI_FS + C axial, (**c**) T1WI_FS + C sagittal

4.3.5 Case 5 Type VI Subserosal Fibroid (5)

4.3.5.1 Case Description

The female patient was 28 years old. Her uterine fibroid gradually increased in size with symptoms of urgency and urinary frequency. The recent menstrual period was also prolonged.

4.3.5.2 Pre-Treatment Assessment

MRI showed an anterior subserosal uterine fibroid with low signals on T2WI, mixed with a little high signal. It was connected to the uterine serosa with a wide pedicle (Fig. 4.112a). The position of a subserosal fibroid was easy to change, and there might be some difficulty in positioning the fibroid during ultrasound ablation.

4.3.5.3 Treatment Techniques

1. **Focused ultrasound parameters.** Average acoustic power: 195 W, sonication time: 1569 seconds, duration of treatment: 139 minutes, total energy: 306,090 J.
2. **The parameters. of ultrasound ablation.** Average acoustic power: 179 W, sonication time: 1500 seconds, duration of treatment: 92 minutes, total energy: 268,750 J.
3. **Focused ultrasound ablation techniques.** Filling the bladder to ensure the anterior subserosal fibroid was relatively fixed in position. The fibroid had low signals on T2WI; thus, the acoustic power should be reduced to avoid the breakthrough of the uterine serosa.

4.3.5.4 Post-Treatment Assessment

1. **MRI evaluation after treatment.** The subserosal fibroid showed high signals on T2WI, with their obvious margins. The sub-abdominal rectus abdominis was swollen and edematous. There was a small amount of pelvic fluid (Fig. 4.112b). The contrast-enhanced T1WI showed that the NPV ratio of the fibroid was about 96%, and the anterior superior serosal layer was not intact, which resulted from the partial ablation (Fig. 4.112c, d).
2. **MRI follow-up at 3 years after treatment.** The fibroid had a relapse except for a small non-perfusion area in its center. The fibroid volume was still 20% smaller than that 3 years ago (Fig. 4.113a–c), so a re-intervention was considered again.
3. **MRI evaluation after retreatment.** The abdominal wall soft tissue layer and muscle layer showed significant edema. The fibroid ablation was about 80%. There was a small amount of ablation breakthrough in the serosa of the left anterior margin, and residual fibroid tissue can still be seen on the left posterior margin of the fibroid (Fig. 4.113d–f).

4.3.5.5 Discussion

- In this case, the subserosal uterine fibroid had a higher ablation rate after ultrasound ablation, but the remaining residual fibroid tissue at the margin caused the fibroid recurrence after 3 years. Any ablation treatment should achieve complete ablation of the fibroid. But in this case, the treatment had to stop because of safety concerns when there was a small breakthrough in the serosa of the front edge of the fibroid.
- For retreatment of the recurring fibroid, focused ultrasound ablation has not been achieved completely, and small doses of mifepristone can be taken orally to reinforce the therapeutic effect.

4.3.6 Case 6 Type VI Subserosal Fibroid (6)

4.3.6.1 Case Description

The female patient was 31 years old. She felt a mass in her lower abdomen, accompanied by mild anemia.

4.3.6.2 Pre-Treatment Assessment

MRI showed a uterine fibroid with homogeneously low intense signals on T2WI, and it significantly compressed the bladder (Fig. 4.114a). The contrast-enhanced T1WI showed that the fibroid had a moderate blood supply (Fig. 4.114b). The fibroid was located at the anterior wall of the uterus; thus, it had a good acoustic pathway. It would be relatively easy to ablate.

4.3.6.3 Treatment Techniques

1. **Focused ultrasound parameters.** Average acoustic power: 151 W, sonication time: 1300 seconds, duration of treatment: 86 minutes, total energy: 196,080 J.
2. **Focused ultrasound ablation techniques.** The T2WI hypointense uterine fibroid was close to the bladder, and low acoustic power irradiation should be used.

4.3.6.4 Post-Treatment Assessment

MRI Evaluation after Treatment The T2WI showed no significant edema in the anterior abdominal wall, but there was edema on the edges of the uterine fibroid (Fig. 4.115a). The contrast-enhanced T1WI showed that the NPV ratio of the fibroid was about 75%, and only a small amount of thin residual layer remained on the fibroid margin adjacent to the uterine wall (Fig. 4.115b, c).

4.3.6.5 Discussion

● When treating T2WI hypointense fibroid with ultrasound ablation, low acoustic power irradiation should be used to

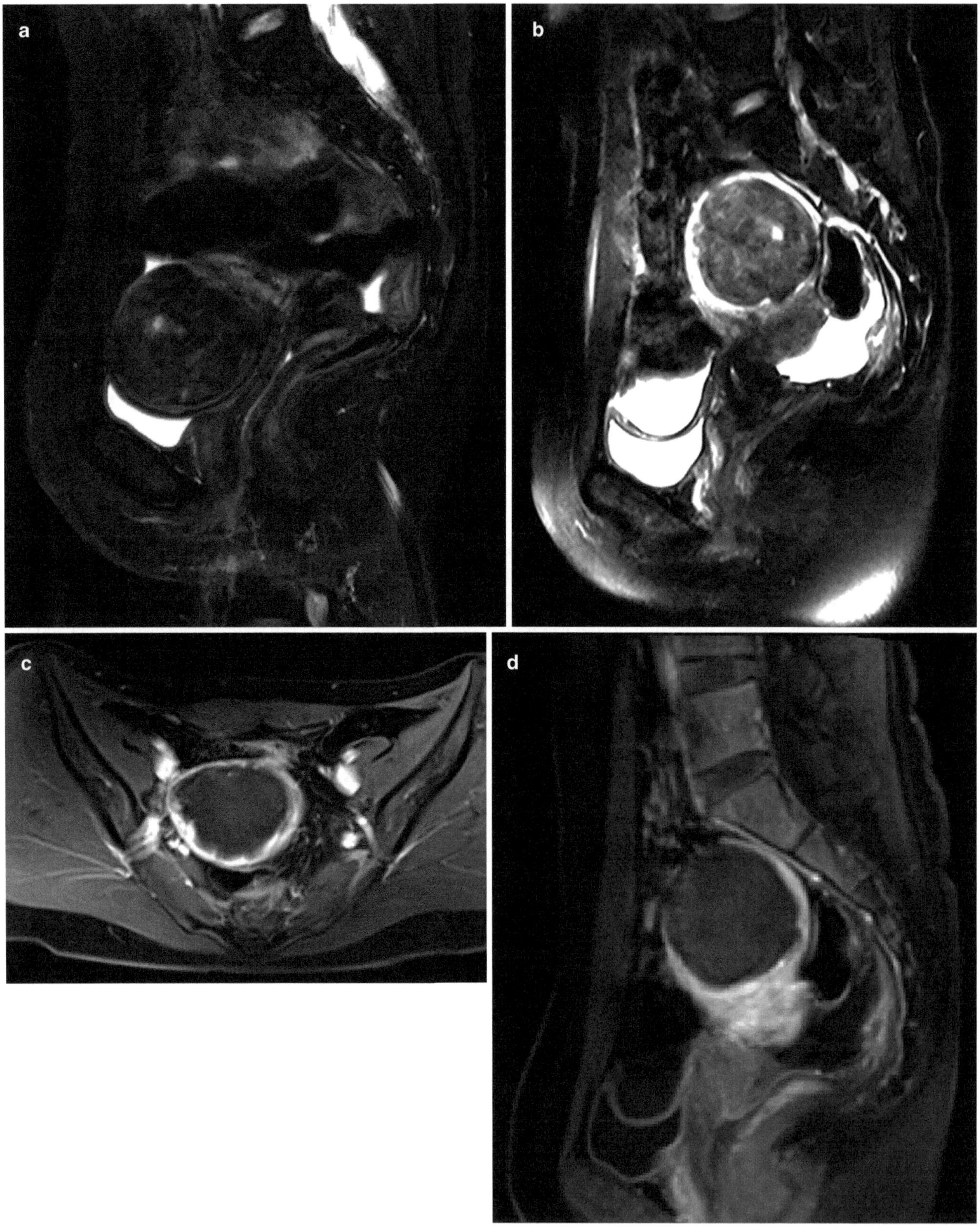

Fig. 4.112 MRI evaluation of type VI subserosal fibroids before treatment and after treatment. (**a**) T2WI_FS sagittal, (**b**) T2WI_FS sagittal, (**c**) T1WI_FS + C axial, (**d**) T1WI_FS + C sagittal

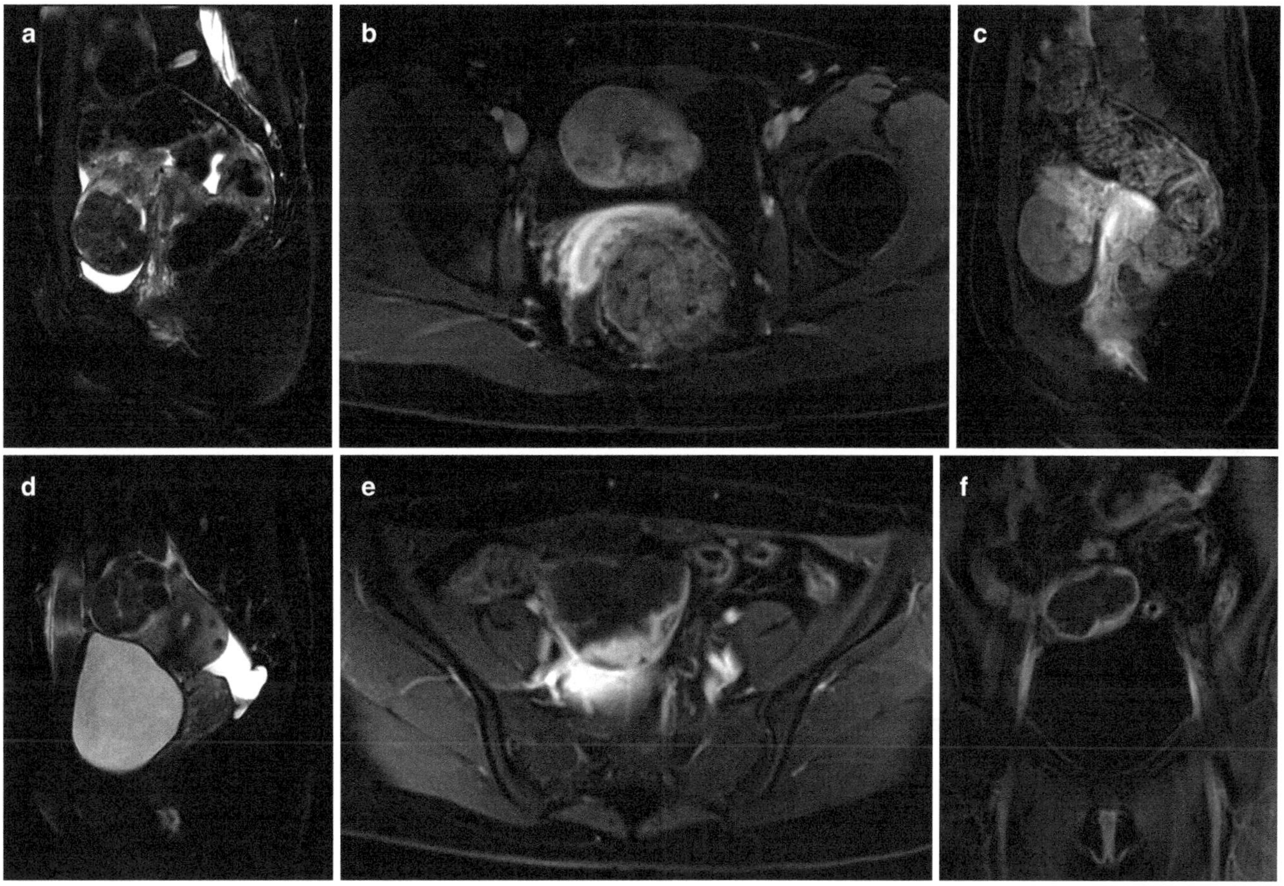

Fig. 4.113 MRI follow-up of type VI subserosal fibroids at 3 years after treatment and immediately after the second focused ultrasound ablation treatment. (**a**) T2WI_FS sagittal, (**b**) T1WI_FS + C axial, (**c**) T1WI_FS + C sagittal, (**d**) T2WI_FS sagittal, (**e**) T1WI_FS + C axial, (**f**) T1WI_FS + C coronal

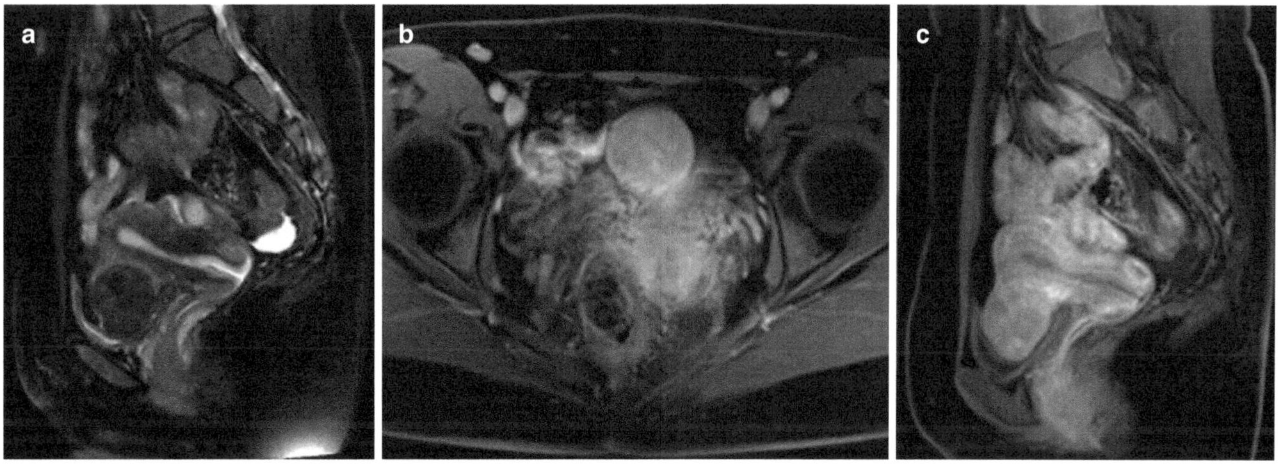

Fig. 4.114 Type VI subserosal fibroids before treatment. (**a**) T2WI_FS sagittal, (**b**) T1WI_FS + C axial, (**c**) T1WI_FS + C sagittal

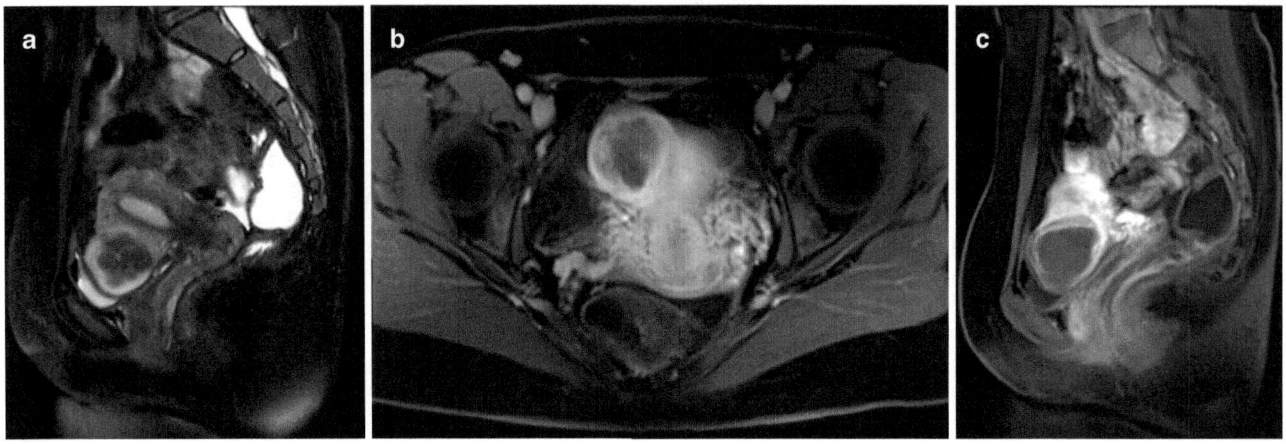

Fig. 4.115 MRI evaluation of type VI subserosal fibroids after treatment. (**a**) T2WI_FS sagittal, (**b**) T1WI_FS + C axial, (**c**) T1WI_FS + C sagittal

achieve a good result in ablating the fibroid. Still, the possibility of damage to surrounding organs is minimized.

4.3.7 Case 7 Type VI Subserosal Fibroid (7)

4.3.7.1 Case Description

The female patient was 29 years old. She presented with dysmenorrhea, accompanied by lower abdomen pain and back pain. Lately, there had been occasional pain in the right pubic bone radiating to the thigh during menstruation. The patient became pregnant 3 months after focused ultrasound ablation treatment and gave birth to a healthy baby at full term.

4.3.7.2 Pre-Treatment Assessment

MRI showed an anterior subserosal fibroid of the uterus with homogeneous low signals on T2WI (Fig. 4.116a). The contrast-enhanced T1WI showed that the fibroid had a moderate blood supply (Fig. 4.116b, c). The fibroid was compressed onto the bladder and was close to the pubic symphysis. The fibroid could be lifted away by filling the bladder to avoid bone injury. It was predicted that the fibroid was suitable to ablate after addressing the technical issue.

4.3.7.3 Treatment Techniques

1. **Focused ultrasound parameters.** Average acoustic power: 160 W, sonication time: 1232 seconds, duration of treatment: 82 minutes, total energy: 197,430 J.
2. **Focused ultrasound ablation techniques.** It is necessary to fill the bladder to keep the fibroid away from the pubic symphysis. During treatment, pay attention to avoid damage to the bowels around the fibroid.

4.3.7.4 Post-Treatment Assessment

MRI Evaluation after Treatment The bladder was full, the fibroid was pushed away from the pubic symphysis, and the abdominal wall had no edema on T2WI (Fig. 4.117a). The contrast-enhanced MRI showed the NPV ratio of the fibroid exceeded 90%, and there was only a small area of residual fibroid on both sides of the fibroid (Fig. 4.117b, c).

4.3.7.5 Discussion

- The bladder was distended with saline to displace the subserosal fibroid upwards and away from the pubic bone so that the pubic bone is outside the therapeutic acoustic pathway.
- Subserosal fibroid protruding from the uterus often has bowels around it. The treatment, in this case, should aim at the middle and inner layer of the fibroid. The fibroid's left and right margin layers rely mainly on heat diffusion to achieve the ablation effect. This approach can avoid any intestine lying within the conical acoustic pathway being irradiated to ensure treatment safety.

4.3.8 Case 8 Type VI Subserosal Fibroid (8)

4.3.8.1 Case Description

The female patient was 41 years old. The patient had increased menstrual flow, accompanied by dysmenorrhea for more than 1 year and frequent urinary symptoms.

4.3.8.2 Pre-Treatment Assessment

T2WI showed that two subserosal fibroids with hypointensity mixed with little hyperintensity were located at the anterior and posterior walls of the fundus of the uterus (Fig. 4.118a). The contrast-enhanced T1WI showed that both fibroids had moderate blood supply. A Type 0 small submucosal fibroid with a maximum diameter of about 17 mm was also seen in the uterine cavity (Fig. 4.118b, c). It was predicted that the two subserosal fibroids with good acoustic pathways were suitable to be ablated, whereas focused ultra-

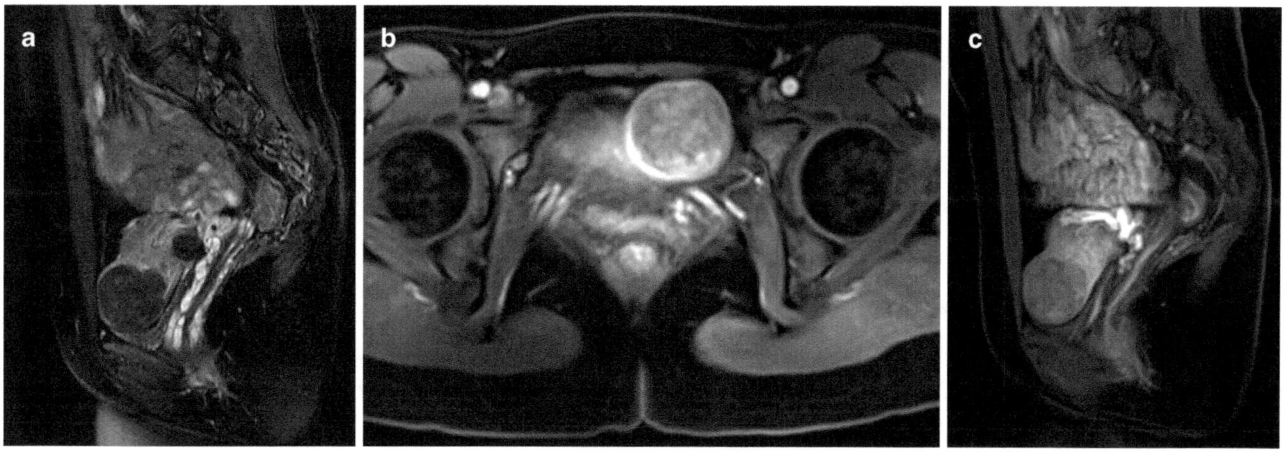

Fig. 4.116 Type VI subserosal fibroids before treatment. (**a**) T2WI_FS sagittal, (**b**) T1WI_FS + C axial, (**c**) T1WI_FS + C sagittal

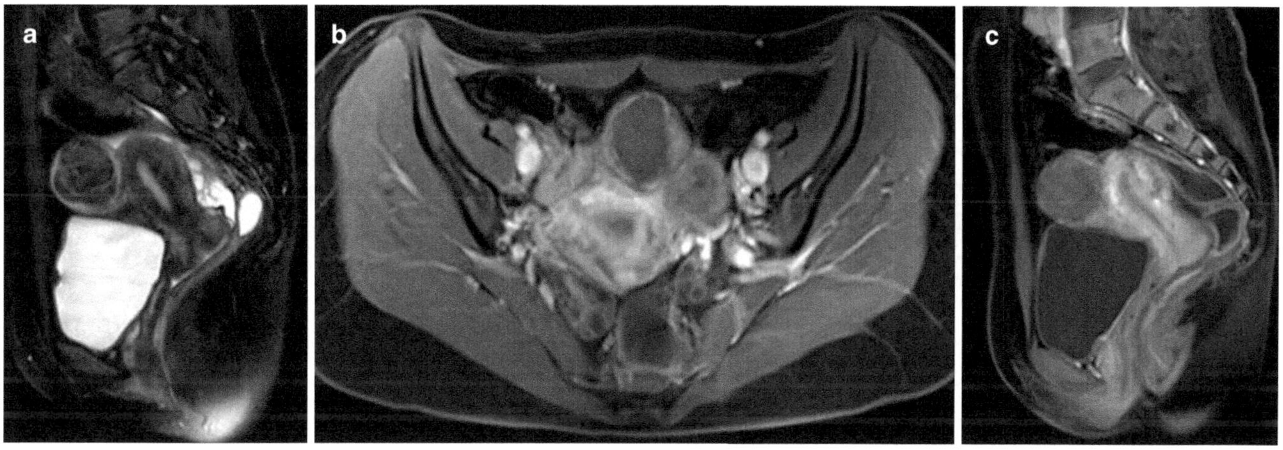

Fig. 4.117 MRI evaluation of type VI subserosal fibroids after treatment. (**a**) T2WI_FS sagittal, (**b**) T1WI_FS + C axial, (**c**) T1WI_FS + C sagittal

sound ablation of type 0 submucosal fibroid would be difficult.

4.3.8.3 Treatment Techniques

1. **Focused ultrasound parameters.** Average acoustic power: 294 W, sonication time: 3267 seconds, duration of treatment: 172 minutes, total energy: 960,300 J.
2. **Focused ultrasound ablation techniques.** The acoustic pathways of two subserosal uterine fibroids were safe. Even the posterior large fibroid was adjacent to the lumbosacral spine. Low back pain might occur during ablation treatment. According to the patient's response to the ultrasound ablation, the acoustic power could be adjusted appropriately during treatment. Pay attention to avoid damaging the endometrium when ablating the submucosal pedunculated fibroid.

4.3.8.4 Post-Treatment Assessment

1. **MRI evaluation after treatment.** There was little edema in the muscle layer of the abdominal wall on T2WI (Fig. 4.119a). The contrast-enhanced T1WI showed that the NPV ratios of the anterior and posterior subserosal fibroids were about 98% and 95%, respectively. The uterine serosa and the endometrium were intact (Fig. 4.119b, c).
2. **MRI follow-up at 6 months after treatment.** The abdominal wall edema disappeared, and the volumes of the two subserosal fibroids were reduced by about 53% and 55%, respectively (Fig. 4.120a). Thin layers of residual fibroids were seen on the posterior and both sides of the posterior subserosal fibroid and the lower margin of the anterior subserosal fibroids. They might lead to fibroid recurrence. The small submucosal fibroid appeared to be partially necrotic or about to fall off (Fig. 4.120b, c).

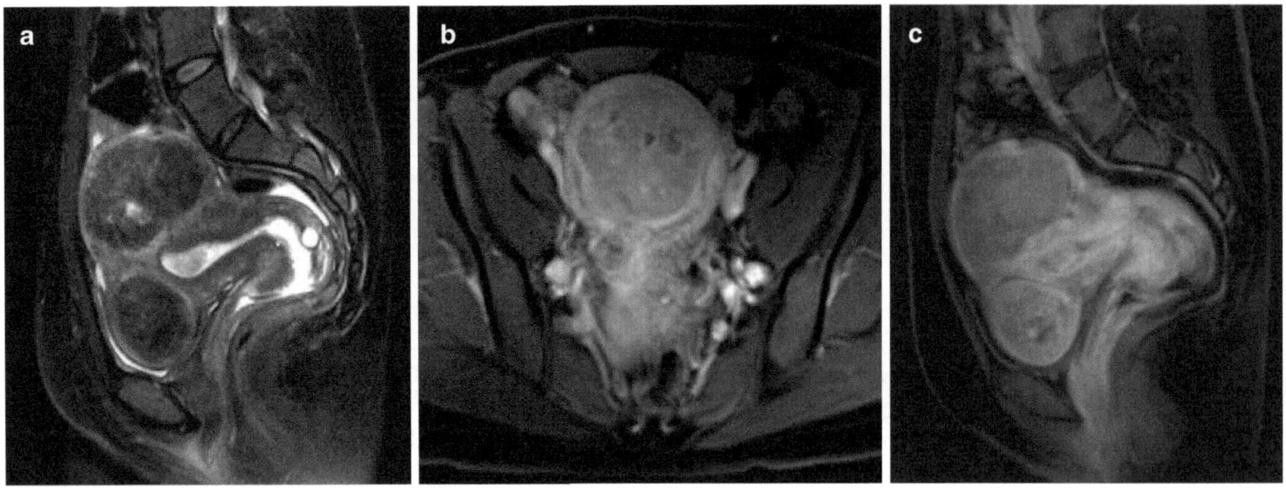

Fig. 4.118 Type VI subserosal fibroids before treatment. (**a**) T2WI_FS sagittal, (**b**) T1WI_FS + C axial, (**c**) T1WI_FS + C sagittal

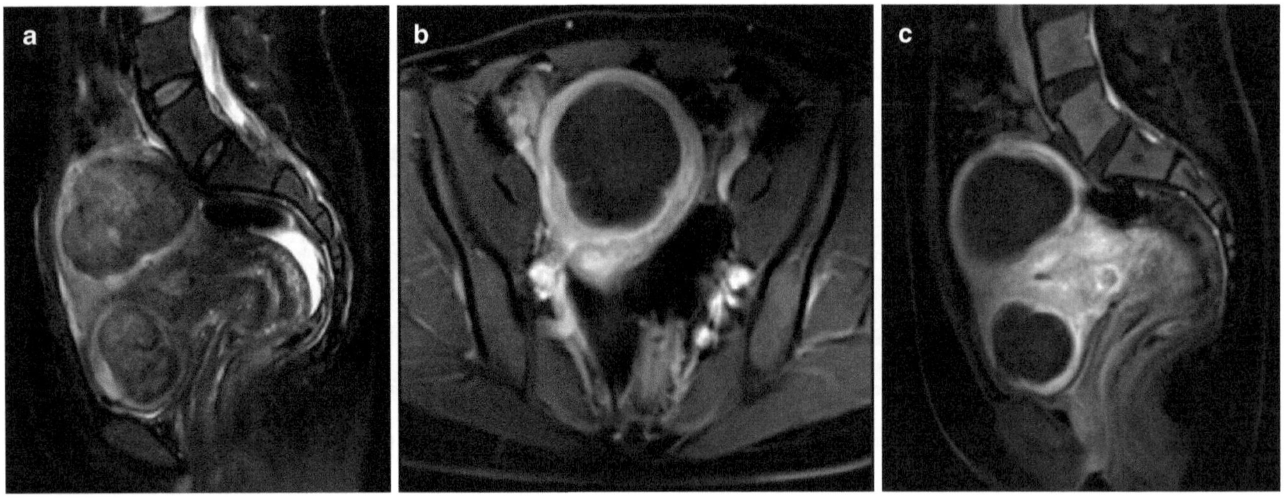

Fig. 4.119 MRI evaluation of type VI subserosal fibroids after treatment. (**a**) T2WI_FS sagittal, (**b**) T1WI_FS + C axial, (**c**) T1WI_FS + C sagittal

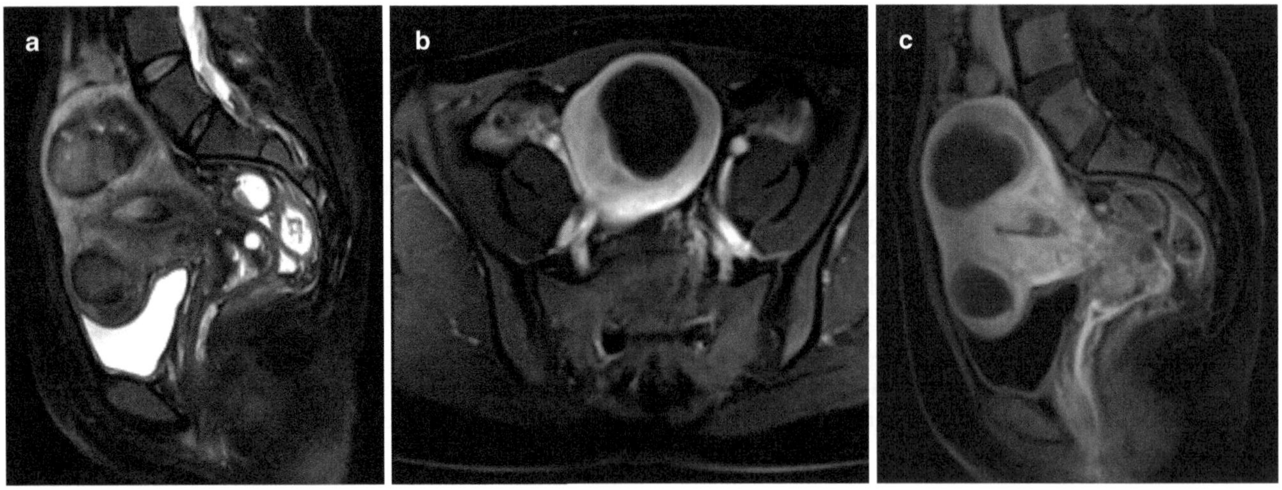

Fig. 4.120 MRI follow-up of type VI subserosal fibroids at 6 months after treatment. (**a**) T2WI_FS sagittal, (**b**) T1WI_FS + C axial, (**c**) T1WI_FS + C sagittal

4.3.8.5 Discussion

- During focused ultrasound ablation treatment of subserosal fibroids adjacent to the lumbosacral vertebrae, bowels, and bladder, the targeted focus region must be kept at a safe distance (≥15 mm) from its edge, and the corresponding edge area can be ablated by heat diffusion. However, the disadvantage of this operation strategy is that there may be residual fibroids in the peripheral areas. In this case, a small amount of residual fibroid recurrence can be seen at 6-month follow-up.
- Type 0 submucosal fibroid is not an indication for ultrasound ablation. Due to the patient's heavy menstrual flow, she was treated with focused ultrasound ablation after informed consent. The submucosal fibroid had avascular necrosis and partial shedding of the fibroid 6 months after treatment.

4.3.9 Case 9 Type VI Subserosal Fibroids (9)

4.3.9.1 Case Description

The female patient was 41 years old. She presented with heavy menstrual flow, accompanied by urinary frequency, urgency and back pain, and constipation before menstruation.

4.3.9.2 Pre-Treatment Assessment

T2WI showed a large anterior subserosal fibroid on the right side wall of the uterus, with low signals mixed with small cystic degeneration in the center. The space-occupying finding in the pelvic cavity was significant, and the bladder was compressed downward (Fig. 4.121a). The contrast-enhanced T1WI showed that the fibroid was of a moderate blood supply with a pseudocapsule (Fig. 4.121b, c). There was a clear acoustic pathway. It was anticipated that a good outcome would be achieved for focused ultrasound ablation of the fibroid.

4.3.9.3 Treatment Techniques

1. **Focused ultrasound parameters.** Average acoustic power: 258 W, sonication time: 2570 seconds, duration of treatment: 98 minutes, total energy: 664,100 J.
2. **Focused ultrasound ablation techniques.** The anterior subserosal uterine fibroid grew outwards, close to the anterior abdominal wall. The acoustic power was reduced to avoid thermal damage to the abdominal wall.

4.3.9.4 Post-Treatment Assessment

MRI Evaluation after Treatment The T2WI signal of the fibroid significantly increased, markedly in the marginal areas. There was no significant edema in the front abdominal wall (Fig. 4.122a). The contrast-enhanced T1WI showed that the fibroid was completely ablated, and the uterine serosa was intact (Fig. 4.122b, c).

4.3.9.5 Discussion

- For a uterine fibroid with a good acoustic pathway, focused ultrasound ablation can be used to irradiate the marginal area of the fibroid. Just like in this case, the sonication initially covers the marginal areas. By blocking the blood supply, the entire fibroid can become necrotic. It can double the effect with half the effort.

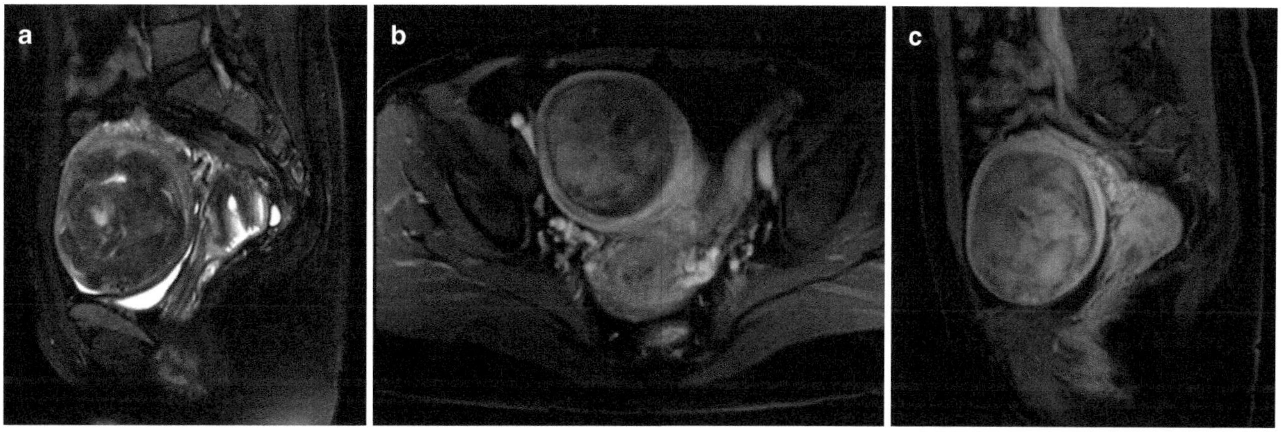

Fig. 4.121 Type VI subserosal fibroid before treatment. (**a**) T2WI_FS sagittal, (**b**) T1WI_FS + C axial, (**c**) T1WI_FS + C sagittal

4.3.10 Case 10 Type VI Subserosal Fibroid (10)

4.3.10.1 Case Description

The female patient was 45 years old. Her fibroid was diagnosed 3 years ago, and it increased in size year by year. There was a family history of uterine fibroids.

4.3.10.2 Pre-Treatment Assessment

MRI showed an anterior subserosal fibroid on the left side of the uterus with homogeneously low signals on T2WI. It compressed the bladder downward (Fig. 4.123a). The contrast-enhanced T1WI showed that the fibroid had a moderate blood supply (Fig. 4.123b, c). The near-field of the focal region for focused ultrasound to treat the fibroid was good.

4.3.10.3 Treatment Techniques

1. **Focused ultrasound parameters.** Average acoustic power: 393 W, sonication time: 1073 seconds, duration of treatment: 76 minutes, total energy: 421950 J.
2. **Focused ultrasound ablation techniques.** During treatment, the ultrasound focus point should irradiate the deep layer of the uterine fibroid using higher acoustic power. The ultrasound heat would diffuse laterally from the right to the left edge of the fibroid to avoid any direct irradiation damage to the nerves.

4.3.10.4 Post-Treatment Assessment

1. **MRI evaluation after treatment.** There was no edema in the anterior abdominal wall, and the signal intensity of the fibroid slightly increased on T2WI (Fig. 4.124a). The contrast-enhanced T1WI showed that the NPV ratio of the fibroid was 100%, with no residual fibroid tissue. The uterine serosa was intact (Fig. 4.124b, c).
2. **MRI follow-up at 6 months after treatment.** The volume of the fibroid was significantly reduced by about 60%, and the signal intensity of the fibroid significantly increased on T2WI. The contrast-enhanced T1WI showed complete fibroid necrosis, showing no recurrence (Fig. 4.125).

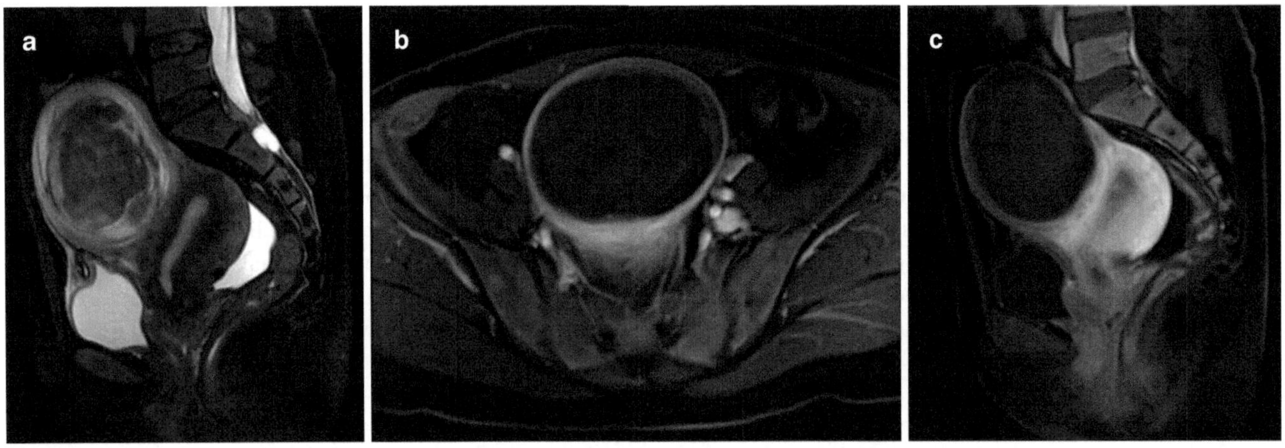

Fig. 4.122 MRI evaluation of type VI subserosal fibroids after treatment. (**a**) T2WI_FS sagittal, (**b**) T1WI_FS + C axial, (**c**) T1WI_FS + C sagittal

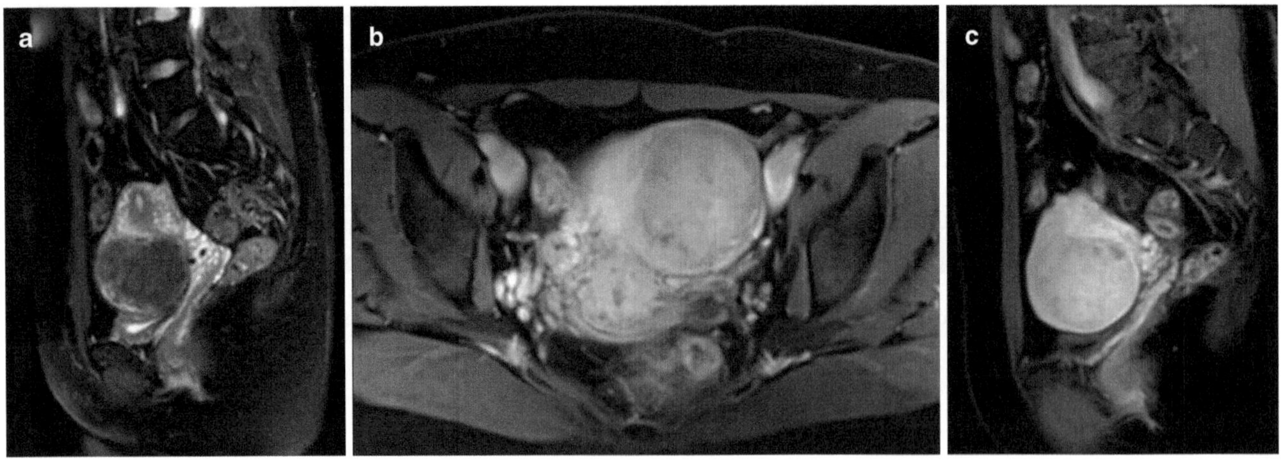

Fig. 4.123 Type VI subserosal fibroids before treatment. (**a**) T2WI_FS sagittal, (**b**) T1WI_FS + C axial, (**c**) T1WI_FS + C sagittal

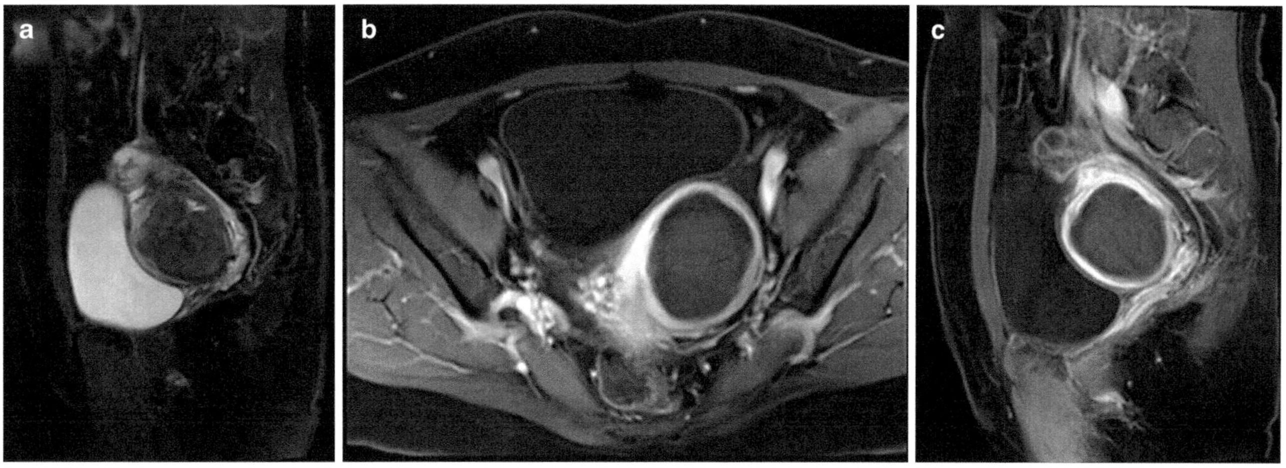

Fig. 4.124 MRI evaluation of type VI subserosal fibroids after treatment. (**a**) T1WI sagittal, (**b**) T1WI_FS + C axial, (**c**) T1WI_FS + C sagittal

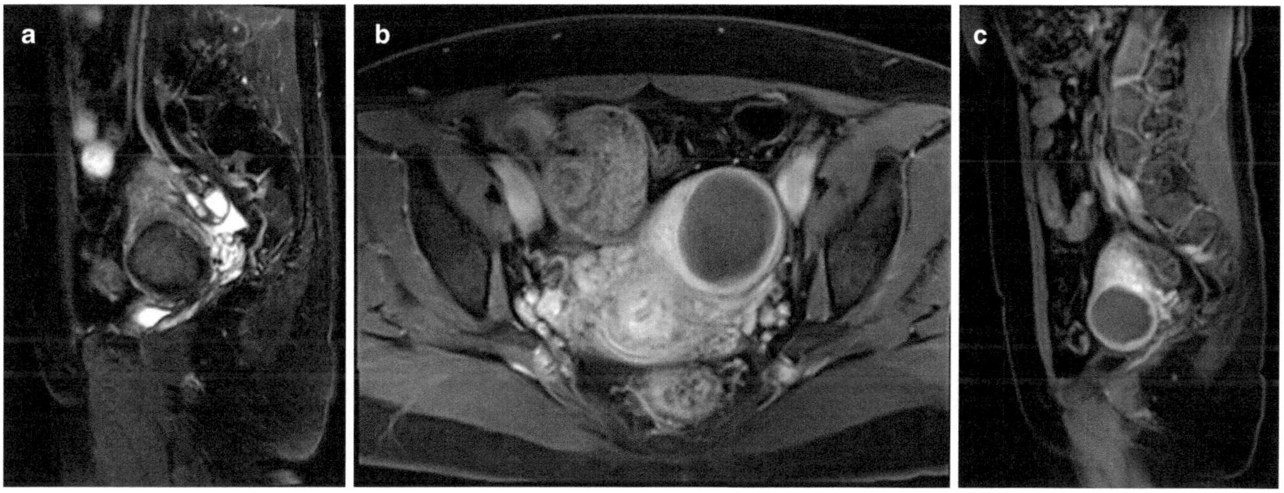

Fig. 4.125 MRI follow-up of type VI subserosal fibroids at 6 months after treatment. (**a**) T2WI_FS sagittal, (**b**) T1WI_FS + C axial, (**c**) T1WI_FS + C sagittal

4.3.10.5 Discussion

- In this case, the subserosal uterine fibroid was completely ablated after focused ultrasound ablation treatment. After 6 months of treatment, the fibroid had reduced in size with no recurrence.
- For the focused ultrasound ablation treatment of a subserosal fibroid, we can use increased acoustic power while ensuring the safety of the acoustic pathway and surroundings.

4.3.11 Case 11 Type VI Subserosal Fibroid (11)

4.3.11.1 Case Description

The female patient was 39 years old. She had increased menstrual flow, accompanied by dysmenorrhea. She also presented with occasional vomiting, diarrhea, and bladder compression symptoms for more than 1 year. These symptoms disappeared half a year after focused ultrasound ablation treatment.

4.3.11.2 Pre-Treatment Assessment

MRI showed two anterior subserosal fibroids located in the anterior wall (large fibroid) and fundus (small fibroid) of the uterus. The large fibroid had high and low confounding intense signals on T2WI, while the small fibroid had low signals (Fig. 4.126a). The contrast-enhanced T1WI showed that both fibroids had poor-moderate blood supply (Fig. 4.126b, c). According to the characteristics of fibroids and their good acoustic pathway, these fibroids were feasible to ablate.

4.3.11.3 Treatment Techniques

1. **Focused ultrasound parameters.** Average acoustic power: 238 W, sonication time: 3001 seconds, duration of treatment: 157 minutes, total energy: 714,540 J.
2. **Focused ultrasound ablation techniques.** The large subserosal fibroid rested on the anterior abdominal wall. Take care to avoid or reduce the irradiation damage to the anterior abdominal wall. The small subserosal fibroid at the fundus of the uterus was close to the lumbosacral spine. During treatment, reduced acoustic power was necessary to avoid damage to the lumbosacral bone and nerve in the back-field of the ultrasound focal region.

4.3.11.4 Post-Treatment Assessment

1. **MRI evaluation after treatment.** There was edema of the abdominal wall and the muscle layer (Fig. 4.127a). The contrast-enhanced T1WI showed the NPV ratio of the large subserosal fibroid exceeded 90%, and residual fibroid tissue was visible in the posterior layer of the large fibroid. The ablation of the small subserosal fibroids at the fundus of the uterus was about 65% (Fig. 4.127b, c).
2. **Short-term MRI follow-up after treatment.** The large subserosal fibroid was re-examined at 3 months (Fig. 4.128) and 6 months (Fig. 4.129) after treatment, and the fibroid volumes had reduced by 40% and 80%, respectively. The small fibroid shrank in size, but recurred in the un-ablated area (Fig. 4.128b, c).

4.3.11.5 Discussion

- Generally speaking, type VI subserosal fibroid shrinks more slowly than other types of fibroids after ultrasound ablation. Although the larger subserosal fibroid, in this case, was not completely ablated, the residual part of the posterior margin of the fibroid did not recur after 3 and 6 months of treatment. The volume of the fibroid was significantly reduced.

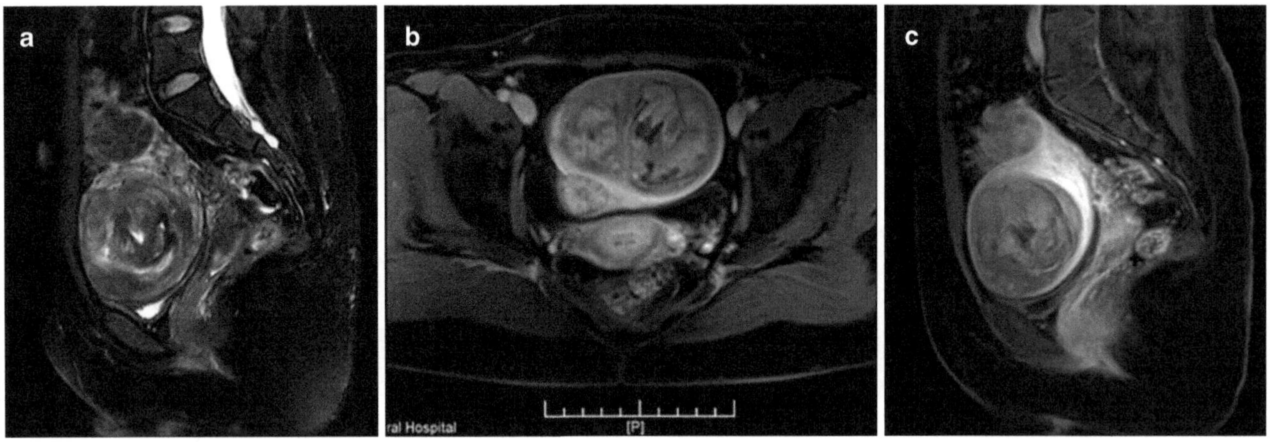

Fig. 4.126 Type VI subserosal fibroids before treatment. (**a**) T2WI_FS sagittal, (**b**) T1WI_FS + C axial, (**c**) T1WI_FS + C sagittal

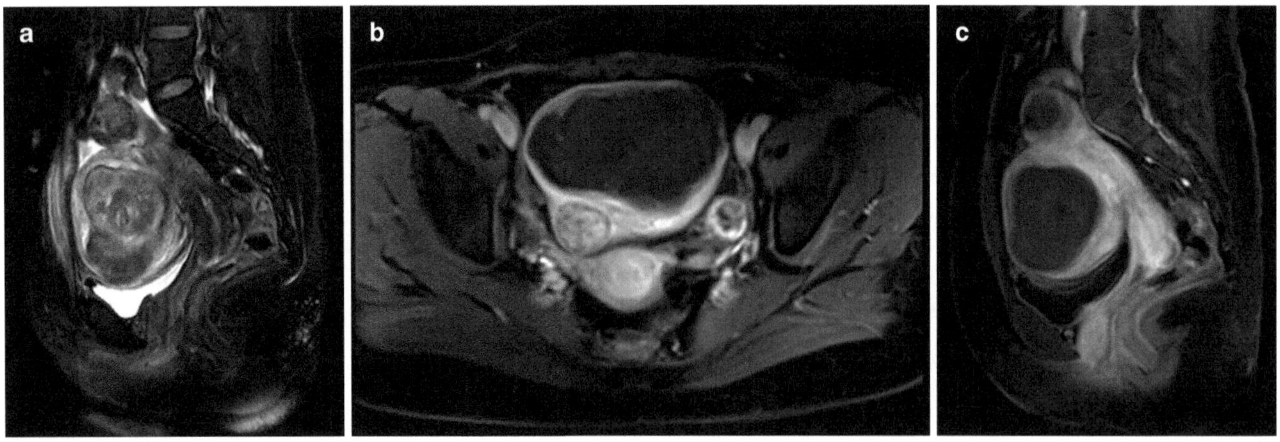

Fig. 4.127 MRI evaluation of type VI subserosal fibroids after treatment. (**a**) T2WI_FS sagittal, (**b**) T1WI_FS + C axial, (**c**) T1WI_FS + C sagittal

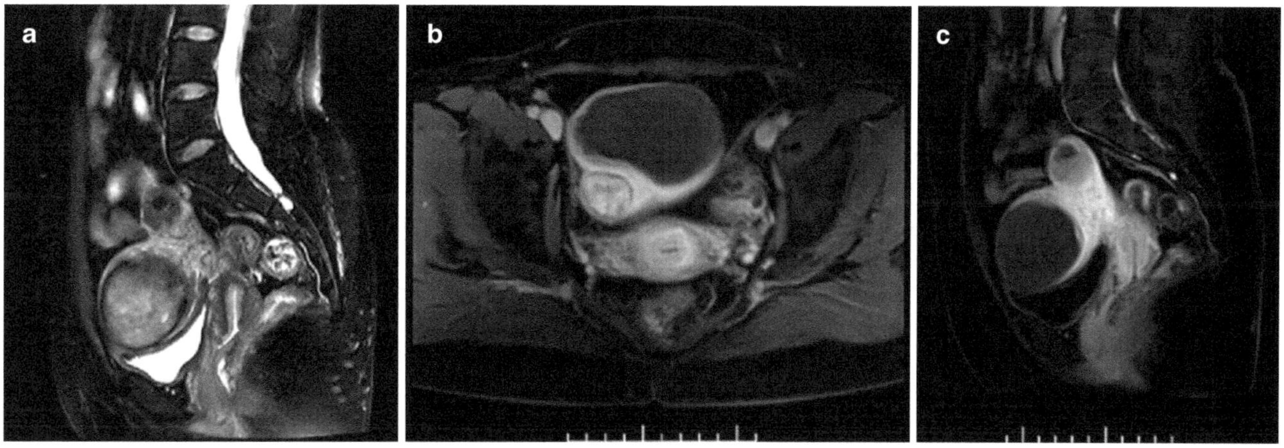

Fig. 4.128 MRI follow-up of type VI subserosal fibroids at 3 months after treatment. (**a**) T2WI_FS sagittal, (**b**) T1WI_FS + C axial, (**c**) T1WI_FS + C sagittal

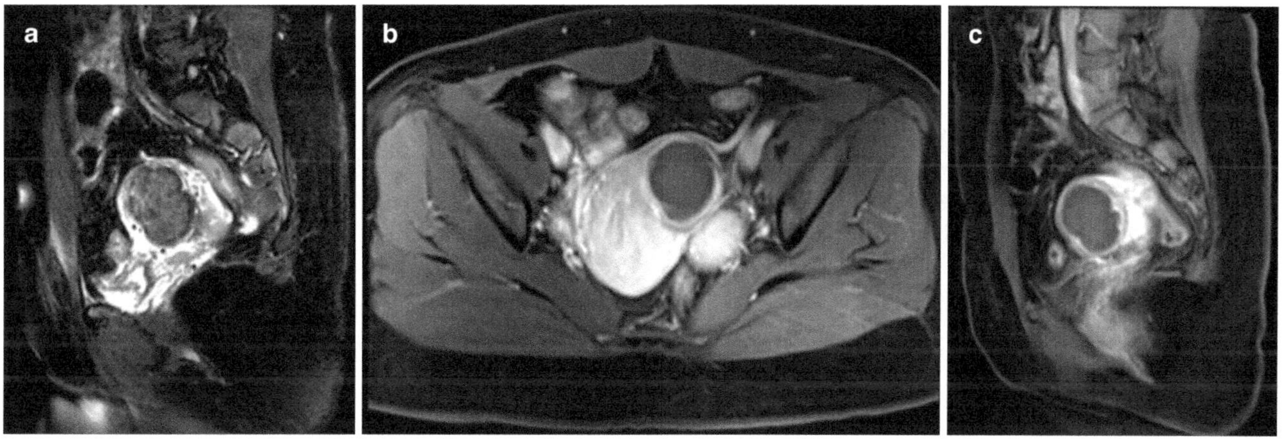

Fig. 4.129 MRI follow-up of type VI subserosal fibroids at 6 months after treatment. (**a**) T2WI_FS sagittal, (**b**) T1WI_FS + C axial, (**c**) T1WI_FS + C sagittal

4.3.12 Case 12 Type VI Subserosal Fibroids (12)

4.3.12.1 Case Description

The female patient was 42 years old. She had uterine fibroids for more than 3 years and suffered from frequent urination for more than 1 year. The urinary symptoms disappeared after focused ultrasound ablation treatment.

4.3.12.2 Pre-Treatment Assessment

MRI showed an anterior subserosal fibroid on the left side of the uterus, with homogeneous low intense signals on T2WI (Fig. 4.130a). The contrast-enhanced T1WI showed that the fibroid had a poor blood supply (Fig. 4.130b, c). This subserosal fibroid could have a good acoustic pathway, so they were relatively easy to ablate.

4.3.12.3 Treatment Techniques

1. **Focused ultrasound parameters.** Average acoustic power: 368 W, sonication time: 394 seconds, duration of treatment: 54 minutes, total energy: 145,000 J.
2. **Focused ultrasound ablation techniques.** When positioning a small subserosal fibroid, it was necessary to distend the bladder and push the bowels away together with an extracorporal water balloon to establish a good acoustic pathway.

4.3.12.4 Post-Treatment Assessment

1. **MRI evaluation after treatment.** There was no edema on the abdominal wall, but the signal of the fibroid markedly increased on T2WI. The contrast-enhanced T1WI showed that the NPV ratio of the fibroid was about 90%, and there was a small amount of residual fibroid in the

marginal area connected with the anterior wall of the uterus (Fig. 4.131).

2. **MRI follow-up at 6 months after treatment.** The fibroid volume was significantly reduced, and the contrast-enhanced T1WI showed that the residual fibroid tissue thickened and partially recurred (Fig. 4.132).

4.3.12.5 Discussion

- The purpose of focused ultrasound ablation to treat uterine fibroid is to relieve or eliminate the related symptoms of uterine fibroid.
- If the subserosal fibroid is small, focused ultrasound ablation treatment should aim at symptomatic treatment. The fibroid, in this case, shrank after treatment and the symptoms disappeared.

4.3.13 Case 13 Type VI Subserosal Fibroid (13)

4.3.13.1 Case Description

The female patient was 39 years old. She presented with dull pain in the lower abdomen.

4.3.13.2 Pre-Treatment Assessment

MRI showed an anterior subserosal fibroid on the right side of the uterus with high and low confounding signals on T2WI (Fig. 4.133a). The contrast-enhanced T1WI showed that the fibroid was inhomogeneously enhanced and had a moderate blood supply. The uterus was significantly pushed to the left by the fibroid (Fig. 4.133b, c). This subserosal fibroid had a good acoustic pathway and would be relatively easy to ablate.

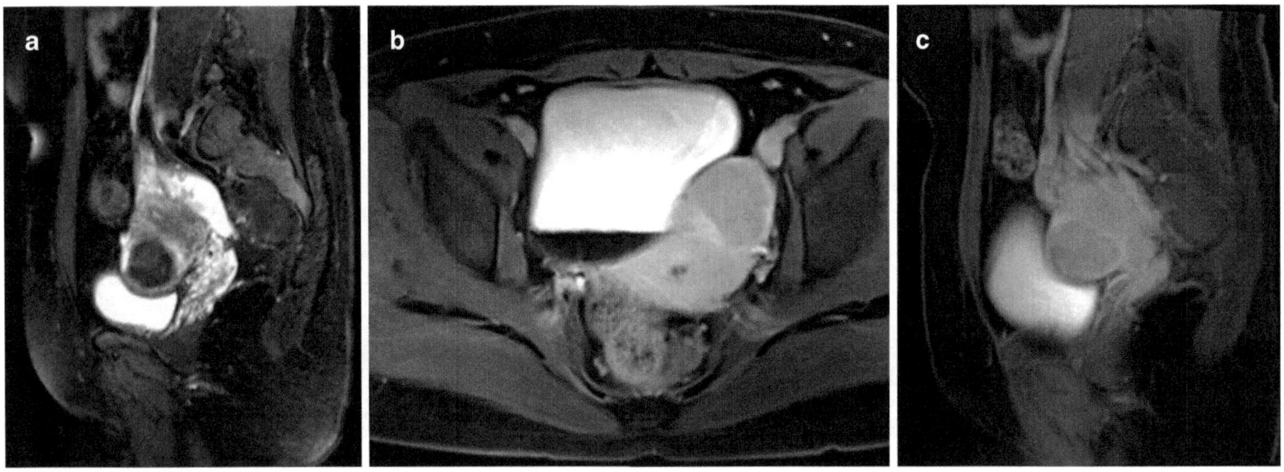

Fig. 4.130 Type VI subserosal fibroids before treatment. (**a**) T2WI_FS sagittal, (**b**) T1WI_FS + C axial, (**c**) T1WI_FS + C sagittal

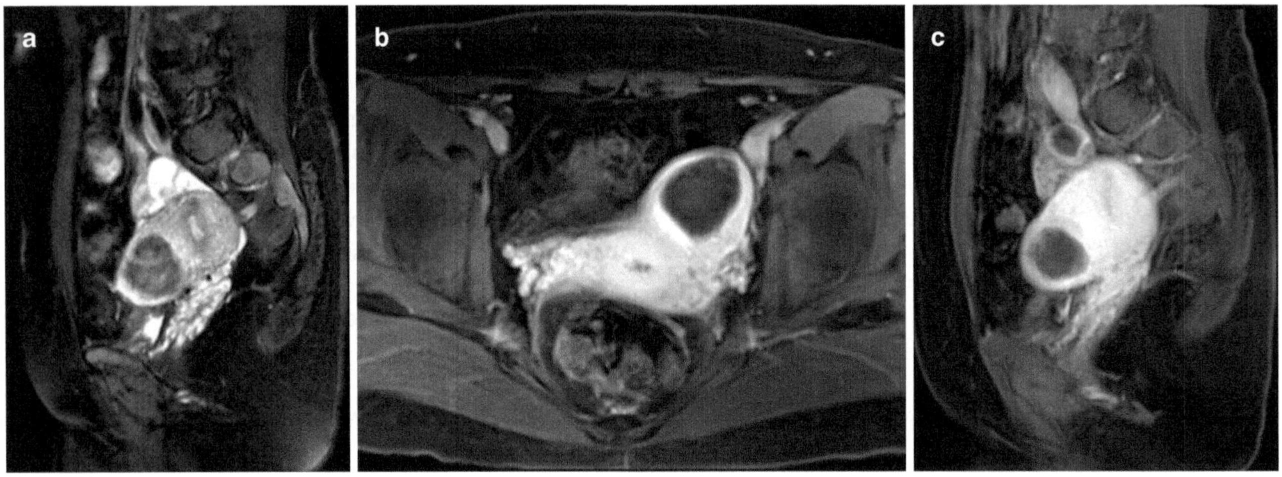

Fig. 4.131 MRI evaluation of type VI subserosal fibroids after treatment. (**a**) T2WI_FS sagittal, (**b**) T1WI_FS + C axial, (**c**) T1WI_FS + C sagittal

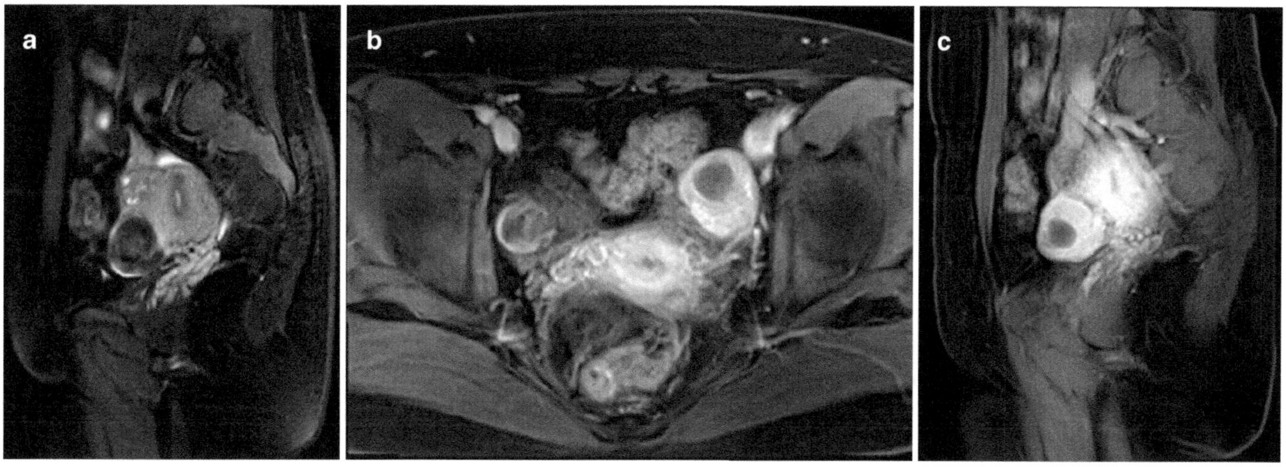

Fig. 4.132 MRI follow-up of type VI subserosal fibroids at 6 months after treatment. (**a**) T2WI_FS sagittal, (**b**) T1WI_FS + C axial, (**c**) T1WI_FS + C sagittal

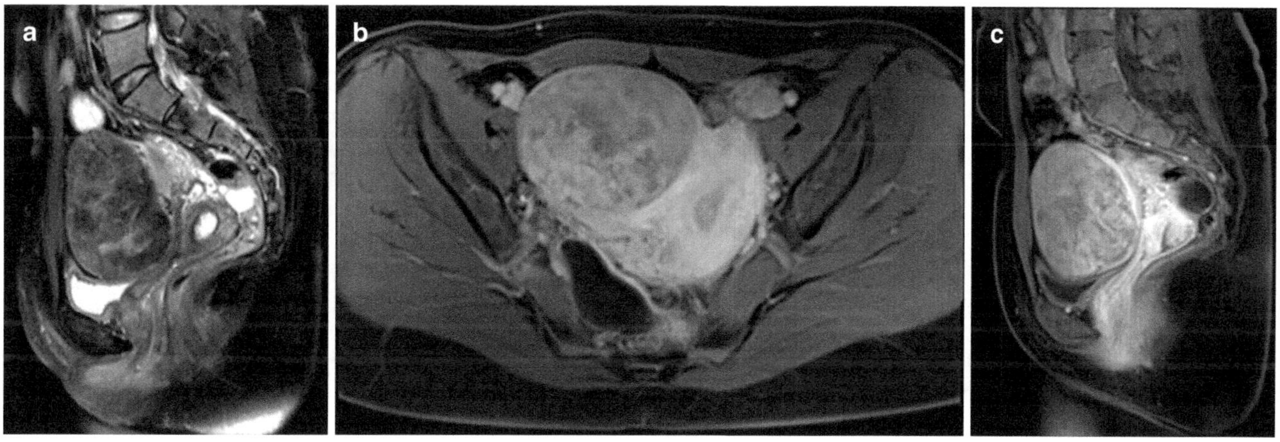

Fig. 4.133 Type VI subserosal fibroids before treatment. (**a**) T2WI_FS sagittal, (**b**) T1WI_FS + C axial, (**c**) T1WI_FS + C sagittal

4.3.13.3 Treatment Techniques

1. **Focused ultrasound parameters.** Average acoustic power: 158 W, sonication time: 2900 seconds, duration of treatment: 131 minutes, total energy: 458340 J.
2. **Focused ultrasound ablation techniques.** Since the right posterior margin of the fibroid was adjacent to the right pelvic vascular nerve plexus, the ultrasound focal regions should be kept at a certain distance, and the lower acoustic power would be used to avoid nerve injury.

4.3.13.4 Post-Treatment Assessment

1. **MRI evaluation after treatment.** The anterior abdominal wall's subcutaneous soft tissue and muscle layer showed significant edema on T2WI. The contrast-enhanced T1WI showed that the NPV ratio of the fibroid was about 95%, and there was a thin layer of residual fibroid at the posterior edge of the fibroid connected with the uterine wall (Fig. 4.134).
2. **MRI follow-up at 6 months after treatment.** The edema of the anterior abdominal wall disappeared, and the fibroid volume markedly decreased. The contrast-enhanced T1WI showed that the NPV ratio was 95%, with the fibroid becoming avascular and necrotic, and some residual fibroids at the posterior edge still existed (Fig. 4.135).

4.3.13.5 Discussion

- When the subserosal uterine fibroid is large and adjacent to the pelvic nerve plexus, apart from keeping a safe distance (≥15 mm) at the ultrasound focal regions, it is also necessary to reduce the acoustic power to avoid any damage to the nerves.

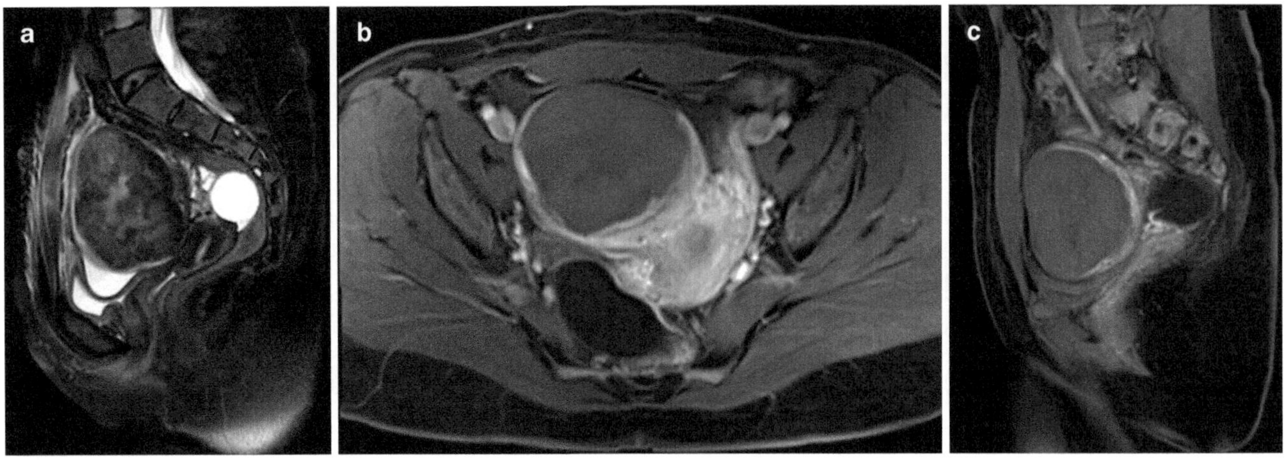

Fig. 4.134 MRI evaluation of type VI subserosal fibroids after treatment. (**a**) T2WI_FS sagittal, (**b**) T1WI_FS + C axial, (**c**) T1WI_FS + C sagittal

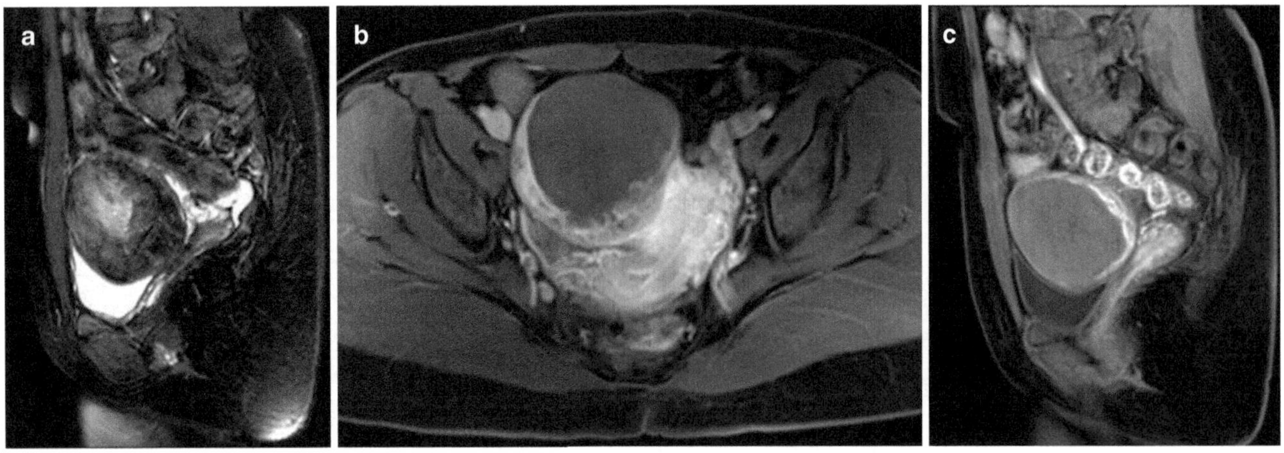

Fig. 4.135 MRI follow-up of type VI subserosal fibroids at 6 months after treatment. (**a**) T2WI_FS sagittal, (**b**) T1WI_FS + C axial, (**c**) T1WI_FS + C sagittal

- This is a typical case to ablate a fibroid with low acoustic power (150 W) irradiation, and it still can achieve more than a 95% fibroid ablation rate.

4.3.14 Case 14 Type VI Subserosal Fibroid (14)

4.3.14.1 Case Description

The female patient was 45 years old. She had increased menstrual flow, urinary frequency, and urgency for 3 years.

4.3.14.2 Pre-Treatment Assessment

MRI showed an anterior subserosal fibroid on the left side of the uterus, with homogeneous and slight hyperintensity on T2WI. It compressed the bladder downward (Fig. 4.136a). The contrast-enhanced T1WI showed that the fibroid had a poor blood supply (Fig. 4.136b, c). The acoustic pathway was good, and the blood supply was not abundant, so it was anticipated that focused ultrasound ablation could be performed with a better outcome.

4.3.14.3 Treatment Techniques

1. **Focused ultrasound parameters.** Average acoustic power: 248 W, sonication time: 3044 seconds, duration of treatment: 155 minutes, total energy: 754,130 J.
2. **Focused ultrasound ablation techniques.** The subserosal fibroid had slight hyperintensity on T2WI. Appropriate acoustic power was used together with increasing the irradiation time to achieve sufficient ablation energy to the fibroid while avoiding breakthrough of the uterine serosa.

4.3.14.4 Post-Treatment Assessment

MRI Evaluation after Treatment The T2WI showed a small amount of edema in the anterior abdominal wall and high intense signals in the peripheral area of the fibroid

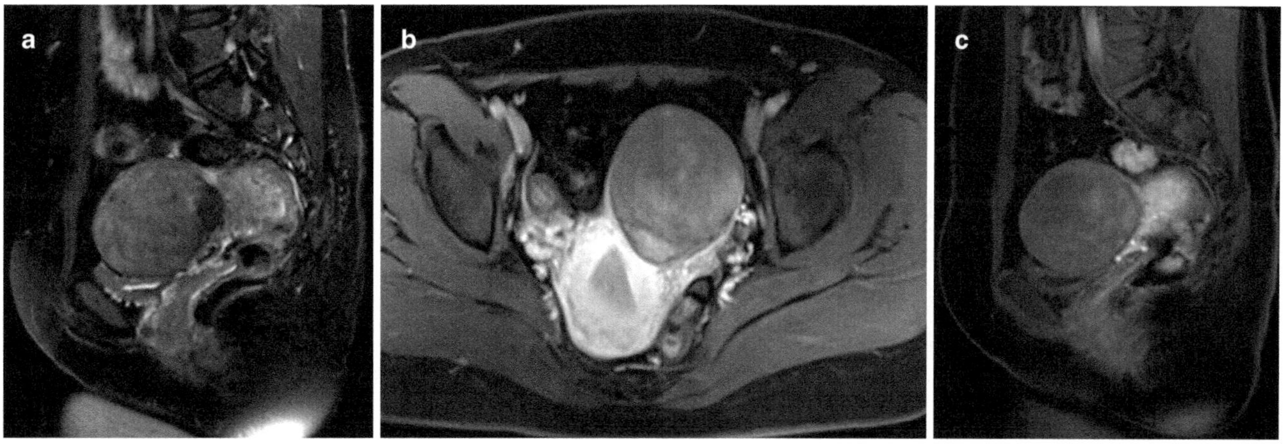

Fig. 4.136 Type VI subserosal fibroids before treatment. (**a**) T2WI_FS sagittal, (**b**) T1WI_FS + C axial, (**c**) T1WI_FS + C sagittal

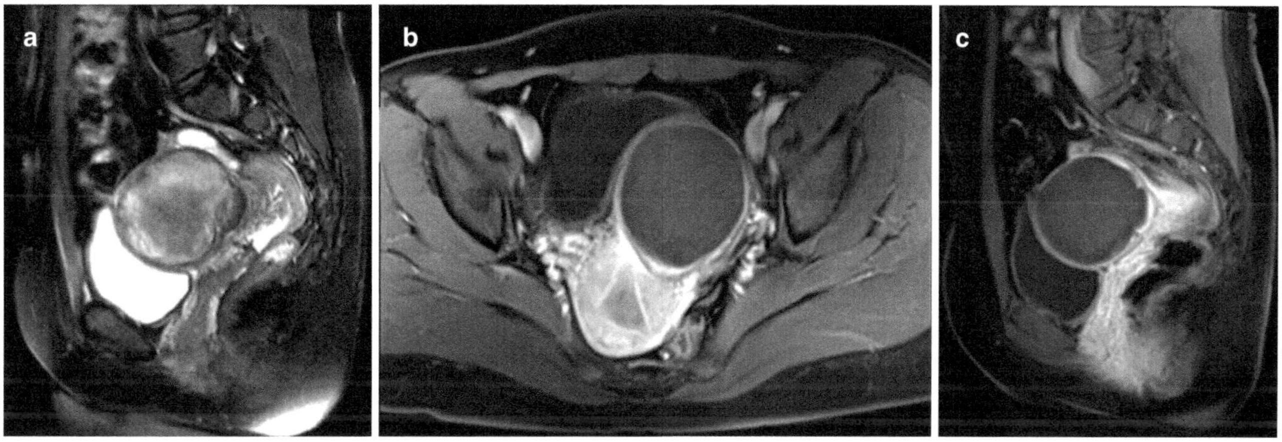

Fig. 4.137 MRI evaluation of type VI subserosal fibroids after treatment. (**a**) T2WI_FS sagittal, (**b**) T1WI_FS + C axial, (**c**) T1WI_FS + C sagittal

(Fig. 4.137a). The contrast-enhanced T1WI showed that the NPV ratio of the fibroid was about 98%, and the uterine serosa was intact (Fig. 4.137b, c).

4.3.14.5 Discussion

- Uterine fibroids with homogeneous and slight hyperintensity on T2WI are generally considered difficult to ablate by ultrasound ablation. In this case, the fibroid was of poor blood supply, which may be an important factor in achieving good ablation efficacy.
- For focused ultrasound ablation of large subserosal fibroids, the gray changes on ultrasonographic imaging that appear in the early stage of the treatment can rapidly expand toward the ultrasound source, blocking and reducing the radiation of ultrasound energy. Even though the ultrasound focal region is still at the deep layer of the fibroid, the grayscale echo extends rapidly to the shallow layer of the fibroid so that the subsequent ultrasound treatment to the other deep layers can be severely affected. The strategy of the initial focus placement in the deep layer of myoma can achieve the goal of conformal ablation.

4.3.15 Case 15 Type VI Subserosal Fibroid (15)

4.3.15.1 Case Description

The female patient was 43 years old. She complained of urinary frequency and severe nocturia. Her urinary symptoms disappeared half a year after focused ultrasound ablation treatment.

4.3.15.2 Pre-Treatment Assessment

MRI showed an anterior uterine fibroid on the left side of the uterus, with hypointensity mixed peripheral hyperintensity on T2WI (Fig. 4.138a). The contrast-enhanced T1WI showed that the fibroid had a moderate blood supply (Fig. 4.138b, c). The fibroid on the left anterior wall of the uterus had a good acoustic pathway. It is predicted that the fibroid was suitable for ultrasound ablation.

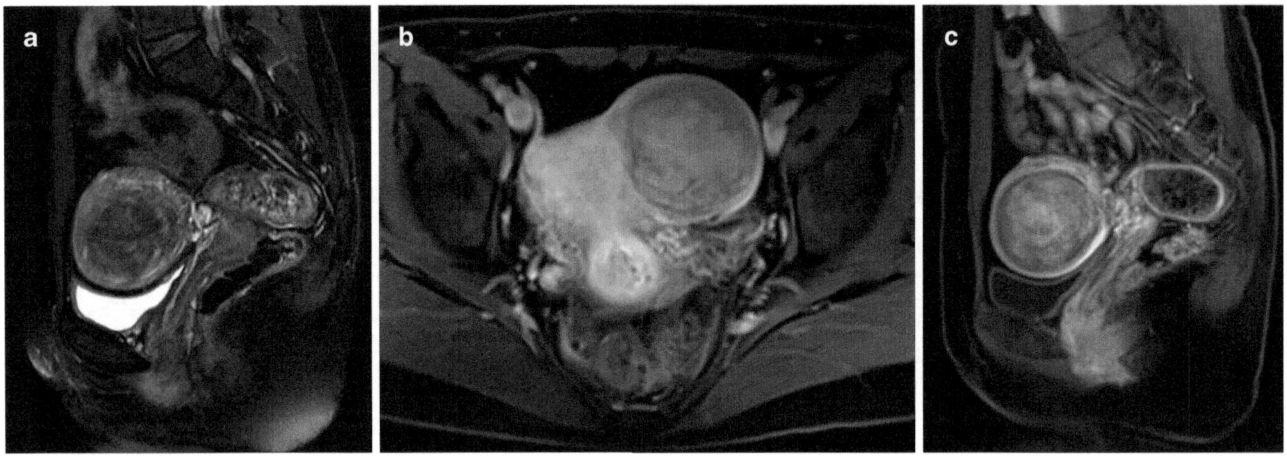

Fig. 4.138 Type VI subserosal fibroids before treatment. (**a**) T2WI_FS sagittal, (**b**) T1WI_FS + C axial, (**c**) T1WI_FS + C sagittal

4.3.15.3 Treatment Techniques

1. **Focused ultrasound parameters.** Average acoustic power: 335 W, sonication time: 1616 seconds, duration of treatment: 77 minutes, total energy: 541,250 J.
2. **Focused ultrasound ablation techniques.** This subserosal fibroid was located between the uterus and the left pelvic sidewall. High acoustic power was allowed because of the good acoustic pathway, but care should be taken to avoid irradiating the tissue structures of the left pelvic sidewall.

4.3.15.4 Post-Treatment Assessment

1. **MRI evaluation after treatment.** The T2WI signal in the peripheral area of the fibroid significantly increased, and a small amount of fluid was seen in the pelvic cavity (Fig. 4.139a). The contrast-enhanced T1WI showed that the NPV ratio of the fibroid was 88%. There was little un-ablated residual on the peripheral edges of the fibroid (Fig. 4.139b, c).
2. **MRI follow-up at 6 months after treatment.** The fibroid volume was reduced by about 66%, and there was no fluid accumulation in the pelvic cavity (Fig. 4.139d). The contrast-enhanced T1WI showed that the original residual part of the anterior and lateral edges of the fibroids did not recur. In contrast, the posterior edges of the fibroid showed signs of recurrence and slightly thickened (Fig. 4.139e, f).

4.3.15.5 Discussion

- Focused ultrasound ablation of subserosal uterine fibroids must master the extent of ablation. As a precise thermal ablation technique, it can be a one-time conformal ablation without damaging adjacent tissues or organs.
- Although the margin of the fibroid adjacent to the left pelvic wall was left after treatment, in this case, there was no significant abnormality in the structure of the pelvic wall. The safety of focused ultrasound ablation of subserosal fibroids is an important prerequisite.
- It is worth noting that the residual part of the anterior and lateral margins after focused ultrasound ablation shrank after 6 months, and did not recur. However, the posterior margin of the fibroid showed recurrence and thickening. Therefore, the ablation efficacy of uterine fibroid requires a period of follow-up examinations to determine its outcome.

4.3.16 Case 16 Type VII Subserosal Fibroid (1)

4.3.16.1 Case Description

The female patient was 45 years old. She complained of lower abdominal pain, abdominal distension, and heavy menstruation. At 6 months after the first focused ultrasound ablation treatment of the giant subserosal fibroid, GnRHa injections were given three times with an interval of 28 days. The second focused ultrasound ablation was performed for ablating her submucosal fibroid at 2-year follow-up after the first focused ultrasound ablation treatment.

4.3.16.2 Pre-Treatment Assessment

MRI showed a very large anterior subserosal uterine fibroid with mixed signals on T2WI. The fibroid was connected with a wide base to the uterus. The fibroid had a maximum axial diameter of about 155 mm. The effect of a pelvic space-occupying lesion was significant (Fig. 4.140a). The contrast-enhanced MRI showed that the fibroid had a moderate blood supply (Fig. 4.140b, c). Because the fibroid was huge, it was beyond the detection range of the ultrasound transducer in a position. At the same time, a submucosal fibroid of about 46 mm was seen in the uterine cavity. T2WI showed that the

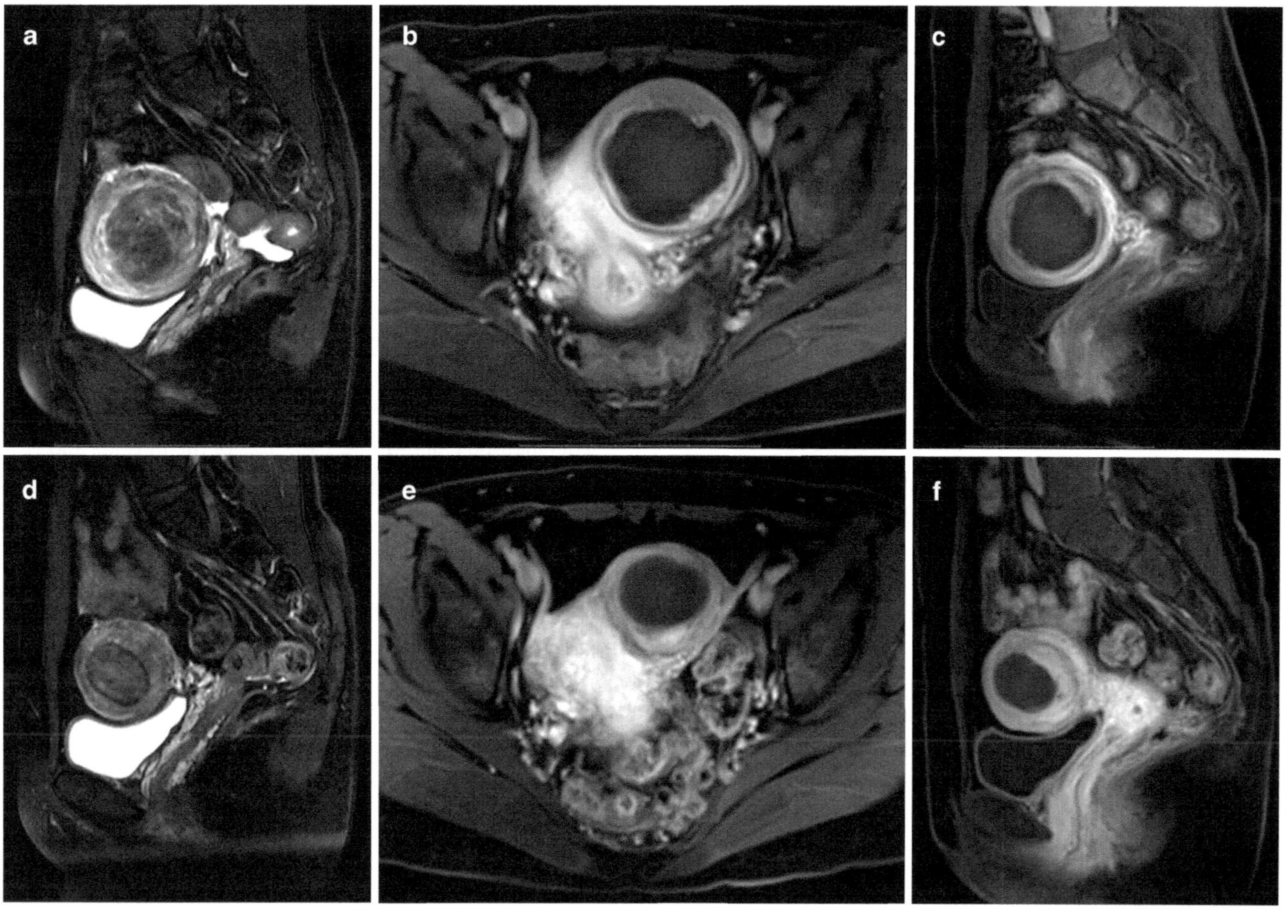

Fig. 4.139 MRI evaluation of type VI subserosal fibroids (**a**–**c**) and 6 months follow-up (**d**–**f**) after treatment. (**a**) T2WI_FS sagittal, (**b**) T1WI_FS + C axial, (**c**) T1WI_FS + C sagittal, (**d**) T2WI_FS sagittal, (**e**) T1WI_FS + C axial, (**f**) T1WI_FS + C Sagittal

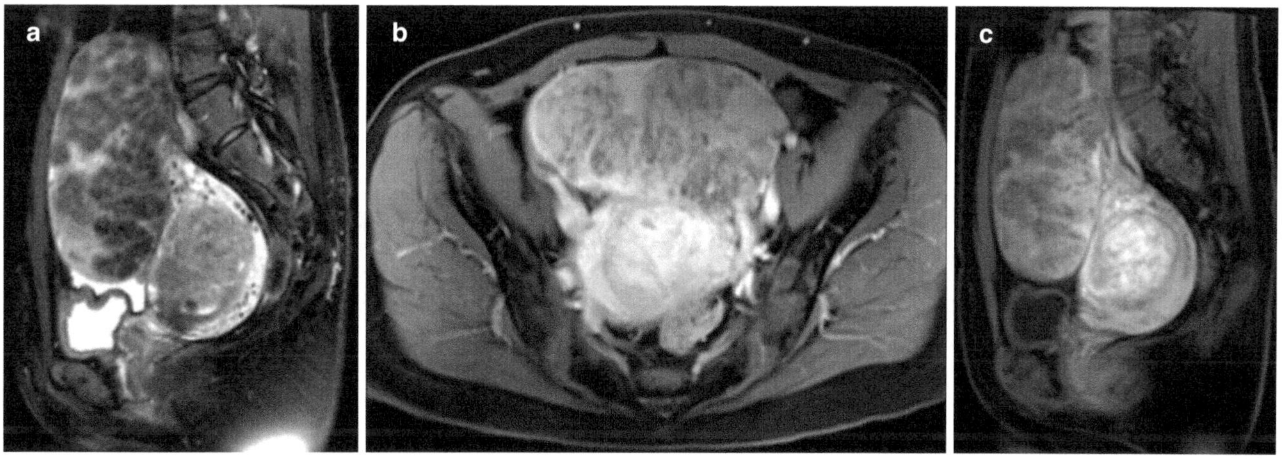

Fig. 4.140 Huge Type VII subserosal fibroids before treatment. (**a**) T2WI_FS sagittal, (**b**) T1WI_FS + C axial, (**c**) T1WI_FS + C sagittal

submucosal fibroid had homogeneous, slight hyperintensity on T2WI and abundant blood supply. It is predicted that a single focused ultrasound treatment was not easy to ablate.

4.3.16.3 Treatment Techniques

- **Focused ultrasound parameters.** Average acoustic power: 288 W, sonication time: 1000 seconds, duration of treatment: 57 minutes, total energy: 288,320 J.
- **Focused ultrasound ablation techniques.** The subserosal fibroid had a good acoustic pathway so that it could be treated with ultrasound ablation. Sonication can be performed on this fibroid first, and there was a chance to treat the type II submucosal fibroid as well.

4.3.16.4 Post-Treatment Assessment

- **MRI evaluation after the first treatment.** It showed edema of the abdominal wall muscle layer (Fig. 4.141a). The contrast-enhanced T1WI showed that most of the subserosal fibroids were non-perfusion areas. The submucosal fibroid was significantly enhanced, indicating that the fibroid was not ablated (Fig. 4.141b, c).
- **MRI follow-up at 6 months after the first treatment.** It showed that the subserosal fibroid's size was reduced, and the ablation fibroid remained non-perfusion, but the residual recurred, and its range increased on contrast-enhanced T1WI (Fig. 4.142a–c).
- **MRI follow-up at 2 years after the first treatment.** T2WI demonstrated that the subserosal fibroid's position was changed and its volume was reduced, and some hyperintense signals in the inner of the fibroid were shown, while the submucosal fibroid significantly increased in size (Fig. 4.142d, e).
- **MRI evaluation after the second treatment.** The contrast-enhanced T1WI showed that the NPV ratio of the subserosal fibroid was about 72% and the submucosal fibroid was completely ablated (Fig. 4.142f, g).
- **MRI follow-up at 3 months after the second treatment.** The subserosal fibroid was reduced in size, and the volume of the submucosal fibroid significantly decreased (Fig. 4.142h, i).

4.3.16.5 Discussion

- Huge fibroids (greater than 100 mm) occupy more than the pelvic cavity to the abdominal cavity and exceed the range irradiated when the transducer is positioned, resulting in residual unablated fundal part of the fibroid. Continuous use of GnRHa for 3 months after focused ultrasound ablation can inhibit the growth of residual fibroids and promote the absorption of the treated fibroids. This method can minimize the size of the fibroids and create a better condition for the second focused ultrasound ablation treatment or laparoscopic myomectomy. In principle: Fibroids below 100 mm are treated once; fibroids ranging from 100 to 200 mm may require to be treated one to two times; fibroids reaching 200 mm require to be subject to more than two divided treatments.
- For this kind of the huge fibroid, it is also recommended to pre-treat, first use GnRHa drugs to shrink a part of the fibroid, and then perform focused ultrasound ablation treatment. In the case of multiple ultrasound ablations, the interval between the two sessions is 3–6 months. Under safe conditions, the first focused ultrasound ablation treatment should ablate as much fibroid as possible. The basis of the entire treatment is to determine the difficulty of subsequent treatment and the ultimate efficacy.

4.3.17 Case 17 Type VII Subserosal Fibroids (2)

4.3.17.1 Case Description

The female patient was 43 years old. She had increased menstrual flow, shortened cycles, and moderate anemia.

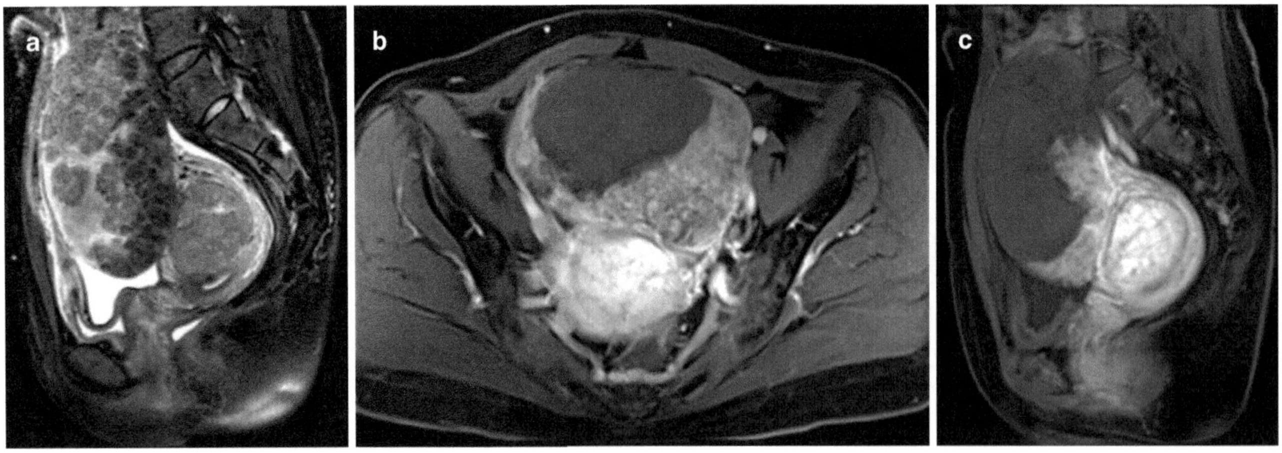

Fig. 4.141 MRI evaluation of a type VII subserosal fibroids after treatment. (**a**) T2WI_FS sagittal, (**b**) T1WI_FS + C axial, (**c**) T1WI_FS + C sagittal

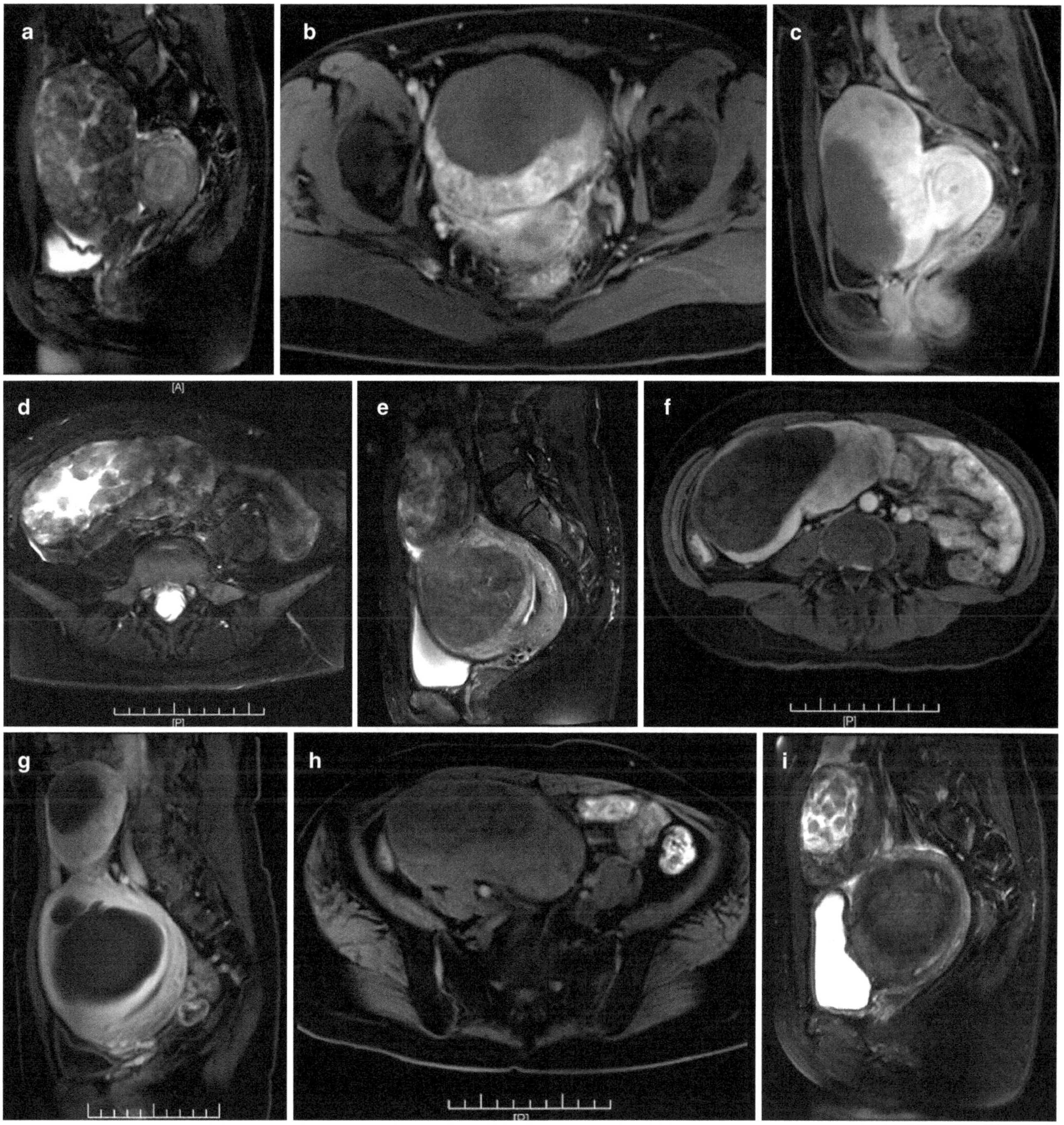

Fig. 4.142 MRI follow-up of type VII subserosal fibroids at 6 months(**a**–**c**) after the first FUAS treatment, 2 years(**d**, **e**) after the first FUAS treatment, immediately after the second HIFU treatment (**f**, **g**), 3 months (**h**, **i**) after the second FUUS treatment. (**a**) T2WI_FS sagittal, (**b**) T1WI_FS + C axial, (**c**) T1WI_FS + C sagittal, (**d**) T2WI_FS axial, (**e**) T2WI_FS sagittal, (**f**) T1WI_FS + C axial, (**g**) T1WI_FS + C sagittal, (**h**) T1WI axial, (**i**) T2WI_FS sagittal

4.3.17.2 Pre-Treatment Assessment

MRI showed multiple fibroids in the uterus. The left anterior subserosal fibroid showed mixed high and low signals on T2WI, connected to the uterine serosa with a wide pedicle base (Fig. 4.143a). The contrast-enhanced T1WI showed that this subserosal fibroid had a poor blood supply. Regarding the other two intramural fibroids, one had an abundant blood supply and the other had a poor supply (Fig. 4.143b, c). The subserosal fibroid would be easy to ablate, but it might not be easy to locate its position during ablation treatment.

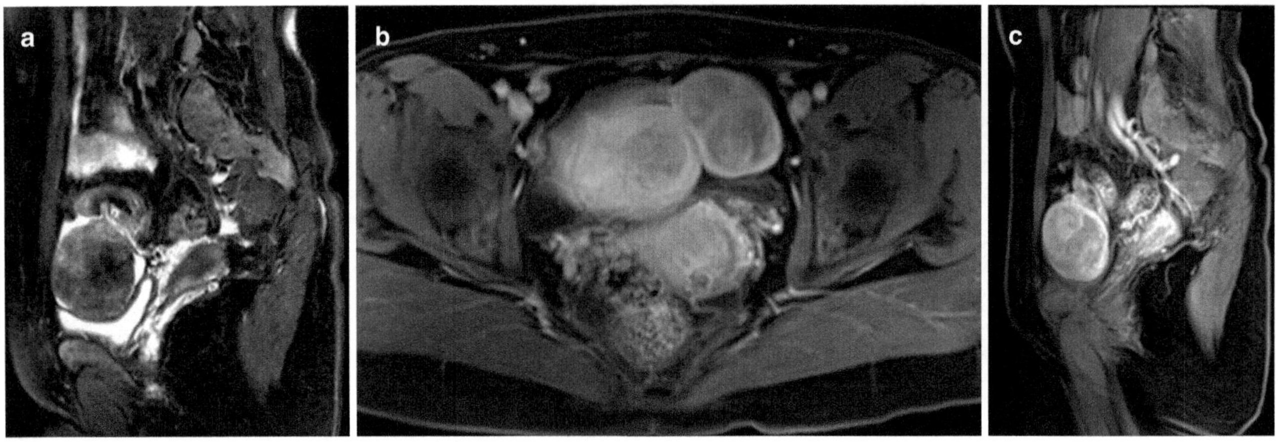

Fig. 4.143 Type VII subserosal fibroid before treatment. (**a**) T2WI_FS sagittal, (**b**) T1WI_FS + C axial, (**c**) T1WI_FS + C sagittal

4.3.17.3 Treatment Techniques

1. **Focused ultrasound parameters.** Average acoustic power: 249 W, sonication time: 3006 seconds, duration of treatment: 129 minutes, total energy: 747800 J.
2. **Focused ultrasound ablation techniques.** When focused ultrasound ablation was used to treat subserosal fibroids, the risk of intestinal injury was higher than that of submucosal and intramural fibroids. During ultrasound ablation, the bladder was fully distended, and an extracorporeal water balloon was used to push away the surrounding bowels to avoid injury. When treating pedicled subserosal fibroid, placing the ultrasound focal region at the center of the fibroid would be safer.

4.3.17.4 Post-Treatment Assessment

1. **MRI evaluation after treatment.** It showed no edema in the anterior abdominal wall, and the fibroid signal intensity had increased on T2WI. There was a small amount of pelvic fluid around (Fig. 4.144a). The contrast-enhanced T1WI showed that the NPV ratio of the fibroid was about 95%, and there was a small amount of residual fibroid remaining at the base of the uterus and on the side of the fundus. The two intramural fibroids were completely ablated (Fig. 4.144b, c).
2. **MRI follow-up at 6 months after treatment.** The residual un-ablated part of the subserosal fibroid at the base with the uterus and the fundal area recurred. Yet the overall size was reduced by about 50%, and the uterine serosa was intact (Fig. 4.144d–f).

4.3.17.5 Discussion

- In this case, the subserosal fibroid was treated simultaneously with focused ultrasound ablation of the two intramural fibroids. A safe acoustic pathway was established by filling the bladder and using a water balloon to push away the intestine. It is a prerequisite for a safe treatment.
- If there is only a pedicled subserosal fibroid, laparoscopic myomectomy is generally preferred. This patient has multiple uterine fibroids. The pedicled subserosal fibroid and the two intramural fibroids can simultaneously be treated with ultrasound ablation.

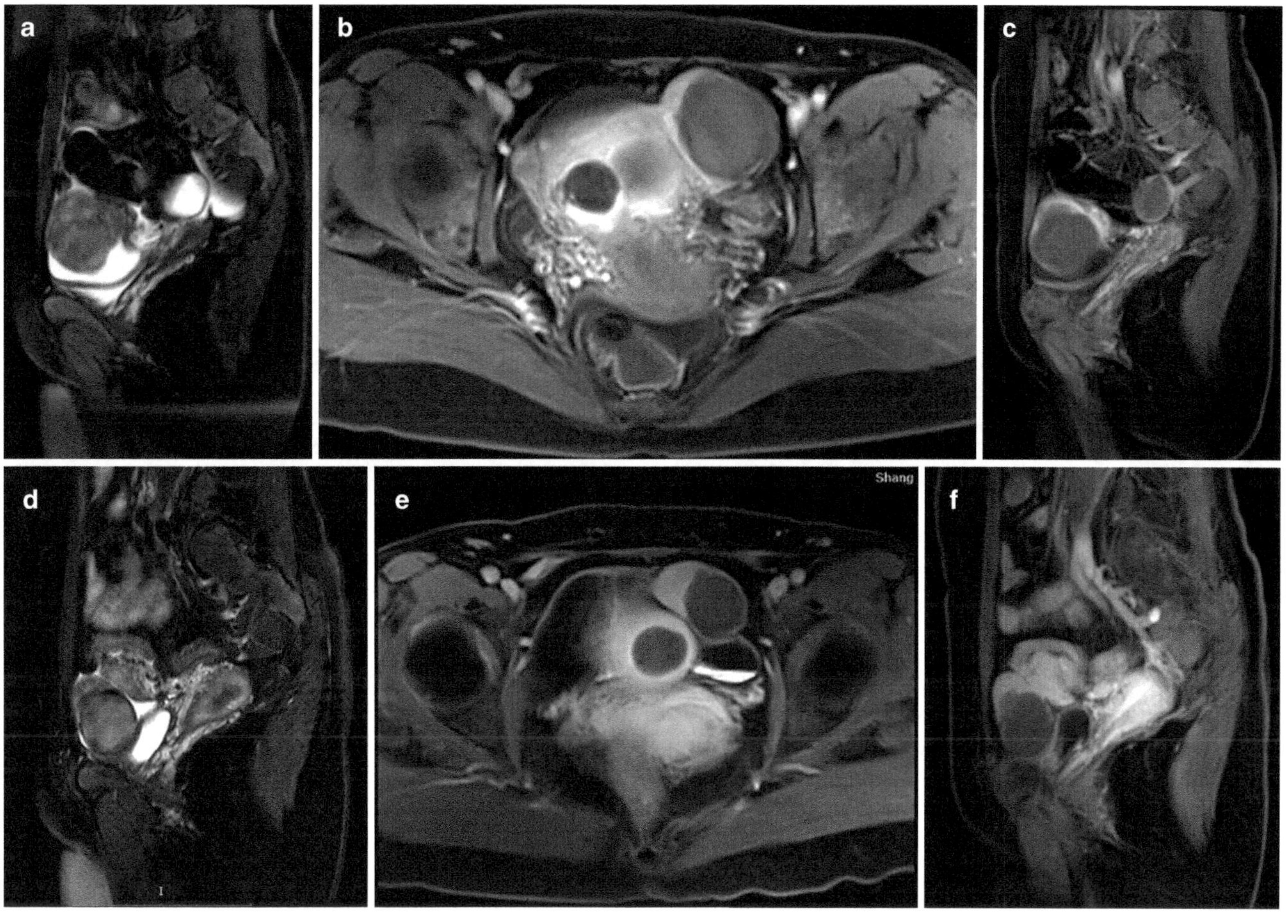

Fig. 4.144 MRI evaluation of type VII subserosal fibroids immediately (**a**–**c**) and 6 months follow-up (**d**–**f**) after treatment. (**a**) T2WI_FS sagittal, (**b**) T1WI_FS + C axial, (**c**) T1WI_FS + C sagittal, (**d**) T2WI_FS sagittal, (**e**) T1WI_FS + C axial, (**f**) T1WI_FS + C sagittal

4.4 Focused Ultrasound Ablation for Special Types of Uterine Fibroids (Type VIII Uterine Fibroid)

4.4.1 Focused Ultrasound Ablation Treatment of Cervical Uterine Fibroids

4.4.1.1 Case 1

Case Description

The female patient was 42 years old. She had a uterine fibroid for 8 years, accompanied by frequent urination and perineal distension for more than 1 year.

Pre-Treatment Assessment

MRI showed a cervical fibroid with low signals and some high signals on T2WI (Fig. 4.145a). The contrast-enhanced MRI showed that the fibroid had an abundant blood supply, and the vascular flow void effect was visible (Fig. 4.145b). Larger cervical fibroids were mainly low signals on T2WI, which was predicted to be relatively easy to ablate. The bladder, however, needed to be distended to create a good acoustic pathway.

Treatment Techniques

- **Focused ultrasound parameters.** Average acoustic power: 232 W, sonication time: 2317 seconds, duration of treatment: 141 minutes, total energy: 526,482 J.
- **Focused ultrasound ablation techniques.** Use the full bladder to lift the cervical fibroid as much as possible while pushing the bowels between the uterus and the abdominal wall away to form a safe acoustic pathway. Changing the incident direction of focused ultrasound, that is, tilting from the head side to the foot side, can avoid the barrier of the pubic symphysis to the ultrasound energy waves.

Post-Treatment Assessment

MRI Evaluation after Treatment It showed that the NPV ratio of the cervical fibroids was 98%, and the adjacent serosal membrane was intact (Fig. 4.145c).

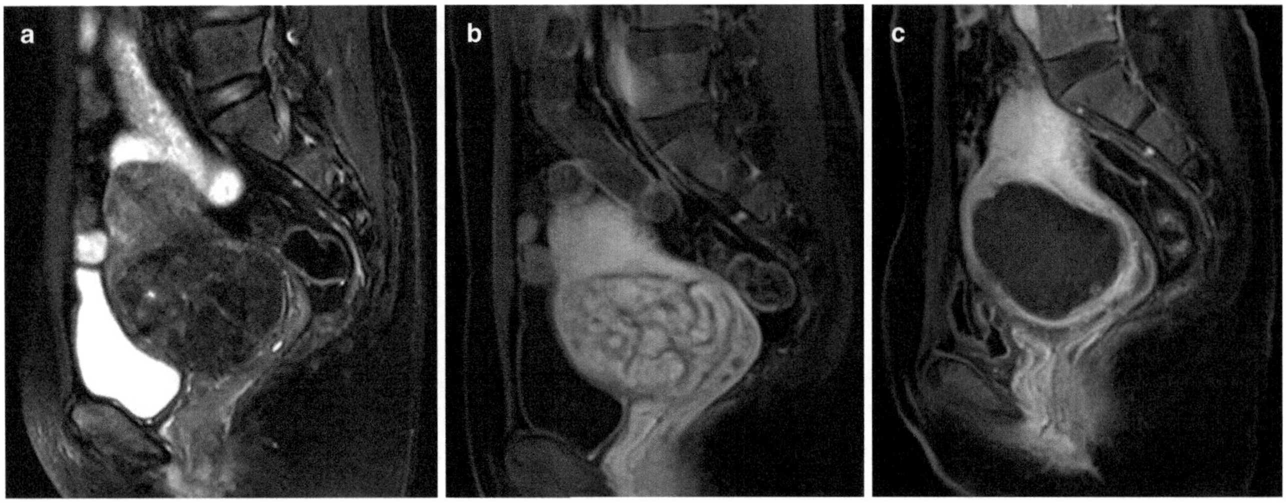

Fig. 4.145 MRI evaluation of uterine cervical fibroids before and after treatment. (**a**) T2WI_FS sagittal before treatment, (**b**) T1WI_FS + C sagittal before treatment, (**c**) T1WI_FS + C sagittal after treatment

Discussion

- The cervical fibroid is located in the cervix of the uterus and has an abundant blood supply. There is a high risk of postoperative bleeding when the cervical fibroid is surgically removed. Focused ultrasound ablation treatment avoids the risk of bleeding after ablation of the fibroid in the uterus.
- Due to its relatively low position, the ultrasound energy can get more attenuated when the cervical fibroid is behind the pubic symphysis. Improved treatment skills and experience can overcome it.

4.4.1.2 Case 2

Case Description

The female patient was 42 years old. She was diagnosed with a fast-growing fibroid and lower back pain.

Pre-Treatment Assessment

MRI showed a subserous cervical fibroid with low signals on T2WI, compressing on the bladder and adjacent to the pubic symphysis (Fig. 4.146a). The contrast-enhanced T1WI showed that the fibroid had an abundant blood supply (Fig. 4.146b, c). Subserous cervical fibroid with low signals on T2WI and located on the anterior uterine wall would have a good acoustic pathway available to ultrasound ablation.

Treatment Techniques

1. **Focused ultrasound parameters.** Average acoustic power: 242 W, sonication time: 2043 seconds, duration of treatment: 107 minutes, total energy: 493,470 J.
2. **Focused ultrasound ablation techniques.** The acoustic power should be reduced because the subserous fibroid was adjacent to the left pelvic sacral plexus. The bladder should be distended to push the cervical fibroid away from pubic symphysis, which can block the ultrasound energy waves.

Post-Treatment Assessment

MRI Evaluation after Treatment It showed no significant edema in the subcutaneous soft tissue of the anterior abdominal wall (Fig. 4.147a). The contrast-enhanced T1WI showed that the NPV ratio of the cervical fibroid was 98% (Fig. 4.147b, c).

Discussion

- Since this fibroid is adjacent to the pelvic sacral plexus, the ultrasound focal region should be ≥15 mm from the posterior edge of the fibroid during ultrasound ablation. The deep layer of the fibroid not irradiated can still be thermally damaged through the indirect heat diffusion beyond the focal region. However, this method may have residual fibroid un-ablated, and there may be a risk of recurrence in the future. Therefore, lower acoustic power can be used together with a longer sonication time for the complete ablation, avoiding damage to the sacral plexus and achieving a more satisfactory ablation effect.
- Aseptic inflammation caused by necrosis of cervical fibroid may cause bladder irritation after ablation. Most urine tests are normal, and the antibiotics can be ineffective. The symptoms can be relieved with non-steroidal anti-inflammatory drugs and smooth muscle relaxants.

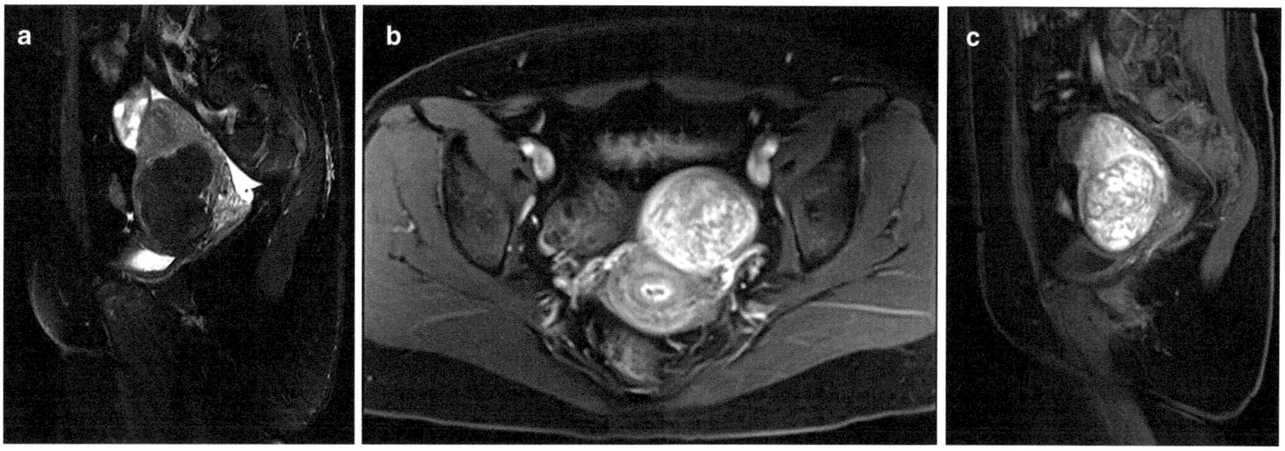

Fig. 4.146 A cervical fibroid before treatment. (**a**) T2WI_FS sagittal, (**b**) T1WI_FS + C axial, (**c**) T1WI_FS + C sagittal

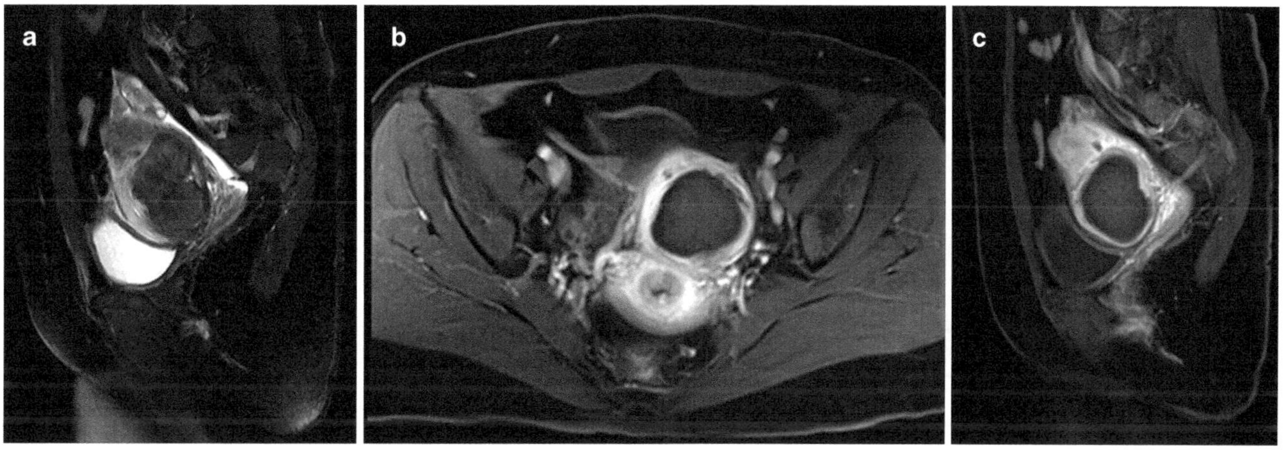

Fig. 4.147 MRI evaluation after treatment of cervical fibroids. (**a**) T2WI_FS sagittal, (**b**) T1WI_FS + C axial, (**c**) T1WI_FS + C sagittal

4.4.1.3 Case 3

Case Description

The female patient was 46 years old. She had uterine fibroids gradually increasing in size during follow-up visits in recent months.

Pre-Treatment Assessment

T2WI showed a cervical fibroid with heterogenous hyperintensity (Fig. 4.148). The cervical fibroid was large at the lower uterine position. It would be relatively difficult for ultrasound ablation. In addition, another small subserosal fibroid on the right anterior uterine wall had a low signal on T2WI.

Treatment Techniques

1. **Focused ultrasound parameters.** Average acoustic power: 369 W, sonication time: 2929 seconds, duration of treatment: 157 minutes, total energy: 1,020,500 J.
2. **Focused ultrasound ablation techniques.** This cervical fibroid showed high signals in many areas on T2WI. Increasing the acoustic power and energy was needed, so pay attention to avoiding injury to the pubic symphysis.

Post-Treatment Assessment

MRI Evaluation after Treatment T2WI showed significant edema of the anterior abdominal wall's subcutaneous soft tissue and muscle layer but no abnormal findings in the pubic symphysis (Fig. 4.149a). The NPV ratio of the cervical fibroid was about 98%, and the smaller right anterior subserosal fibroid of the uterus was almost completely ablated (Fig. 4.149b, c).

Discussion

- Due to the location of cervical fibroids, a total hysterectomy is generally recommended. During surgical procedures, postoperative bleeding may occur, associated with possible damage to the surrounding organs.

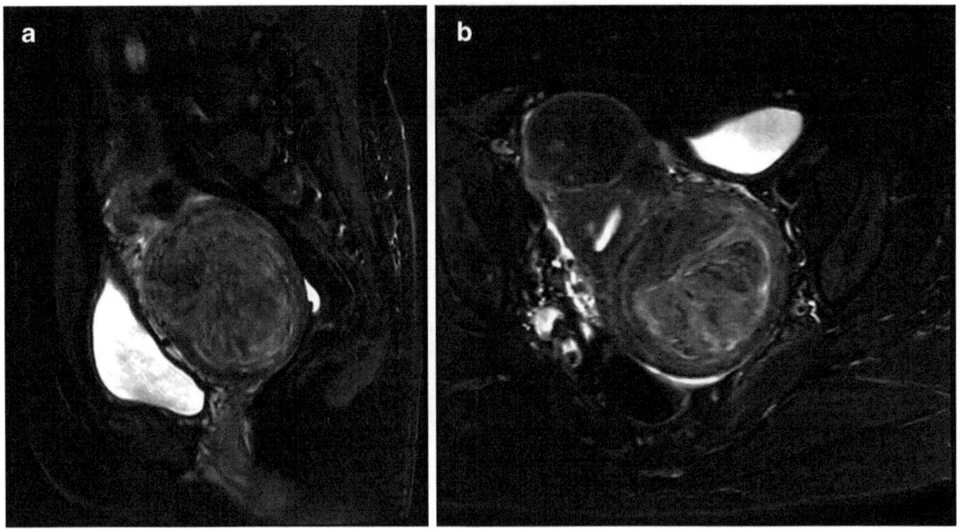

Fig. 4.148 A cervical fibroid before treatment. (**a**) T2WI_FS sagittal, (**b**) T2WI_FS axial

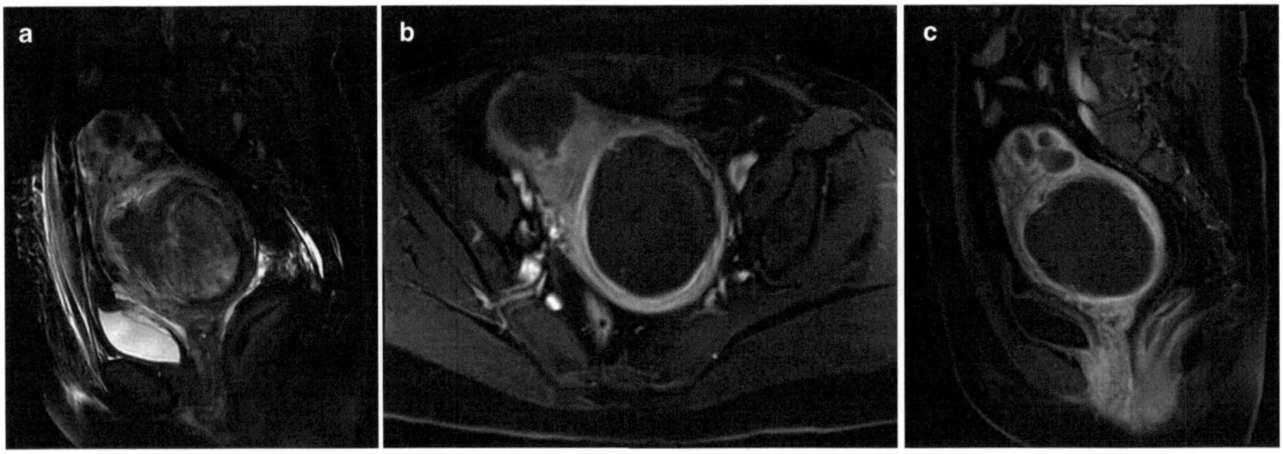

Fig. 4.149 MRI evaluation after treatment of the cervical fibroid. (**a**) T2WI_FS sagittal, (**b**) T1WI_FS + C axial, (**c**) T1WI_FS + C sagittal

- While non-invasive ablation treatment is performed, focused ultrasound ablation can preserve the normal function of the uterus without damaging the surrounding organs or tissues adjacent to the cervical fibroid. It should be a recommended method for the treatment of cervical fibroids.

4.4.1.4 Case 4

Case Description
The female patient was 47 years old. She had recurrent fibroids after a previous laparoscopic myomectomy. She also suffered from mild anemia.

Pre-Treatment Assessment
MRI showed a cervical fibroid with inhomogeneously and markedly hyperintensity on T2WI and slightly low signals on T1WI (Fig. 4.150). It is predicted that it would be difficult to ablate, and higher ultrasound energy and power were required.

Treatment Techniques
1. **Focused ultrasound parameters.** Average acoustic power: 384 W, sonication time: 3802 seconds, duration of treatment: 165 minutes, total energy: 1,460,140 J.
2. **Focused ultrasound ablation techniques.** Because this fibroid was located in the cervix and close to the uterine

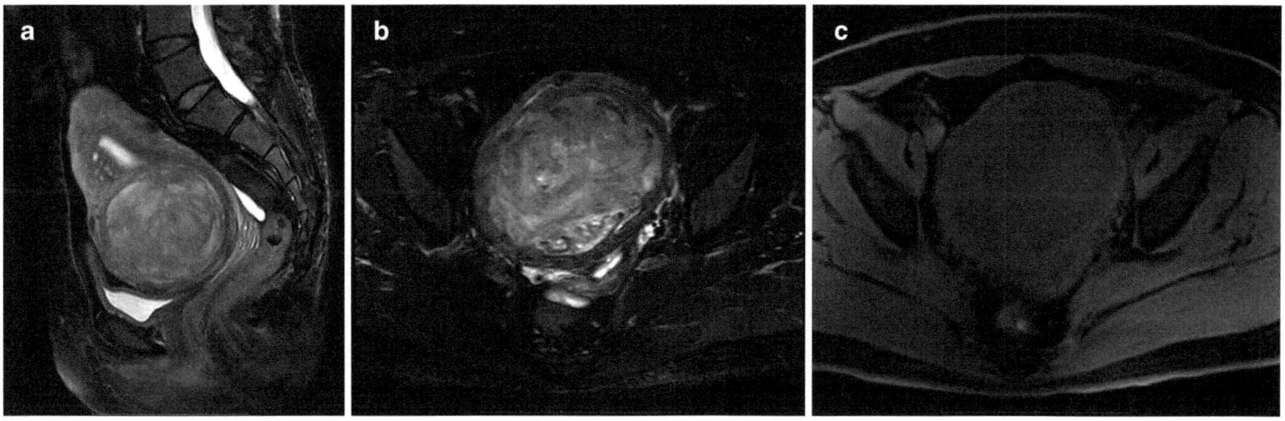

Fig. 4.150 A cervical fibroid before treatment. (**a**) T2WI_FS sagittal, (**b**) T2WI_FS axial, (**c**) T1WI axial

serosa, this location was special. During treatment, the closer the ultrasound focal region was to the uterine body, the safer it should be, and the distance from the ultrasound focal region to the endometrium should be ≥10 mm.

Post-Treatment Assessment

MRI Evaluation after Treatment T2WI showed that the subcutaneous soft tissue of the anterior abdominal wall was slightly edematous, the symphysis pubis remained unchanged, and the signal intensity of fibroids significantly increased, especially at its periphery (Fig. 4.151a). The contrast-enhanced T1WI showed the NPV ratio of the fibroid was about 96%, and the serosa and endometrium layers were fully protected and intact (Fig. 4.151b, c).

Discussion

- The aseptic inflammation caused by focused ultrasound ablation and necrosis of the cervical fibroid adjacent to the bladder may lead to bladder irritation.
- Although higher acoustic power and more accumulated energy were used in this case, the soft tissue of the anterior abdominal wall was only slightly edematous, which was related to the treatment technique and the patient's body's tolerance to thermal ablation.

4.4.2 Focused Ultrasound Ablation for the Treatment of Broad Ligament Uterine Fibroids

4.4.2.1 Case 1

Case Description

The female patient was 31 years old and had a uterine fibroid 5 years ago. The size of the fibroid increased to 8 cm in the ultrasound examination without changes in menstrual volume and menstrual cycle recently.

Pre-Treatment Assessment

MRI showed a left broad ligament uterine fibroid of 84 mm in size, and it presented mainly with low signals mixed with some hyperintensity on T2WI (Fig. 4.152a). The contrast-enhanced T1WI showed that the fibroid mostly had contrast perfusion with a central partial lack of blood supply (Fig. 4.152b, c). The fibroid mostly had low signals on T2WI, which was relatively suitable for ultrasound ablation; and the acoustic pathway was clear for sonication when the bladder was full and enlarged.

Treatment Techniques

1. **Focused ultrasound parameters.** Average acoustic power: 253 W, sonication time: 1331 seconds, duration of treatment: 70 minutes, total energy: 336,890 J.
2. **Focused ultrasound ablation techniques.** The broad ligament uterine fibroid is easy to be moved in its position. It could be relatively fixed in position by filling up the bladder and compressed by an extracorporal water balloon, which helped to improve the ablation effectiveness and treatment safety.

Post-Treatment Assessment

MRI Evaluation after Treatment There was a small amount of fluid in the pelvic cavity, and the signal intensity of the treated fibroid slightly increased on T2WI (Fig. 4.153a). The contrast-enhanced MRI showed that the NPV ratio was almost 100%. The corresponding fibroid capsule was intact (Fig. 4.153b, c).

Discussion

- Because the broad ligament fibroid was larger and connected to the uterus with a connecting basal part, it might

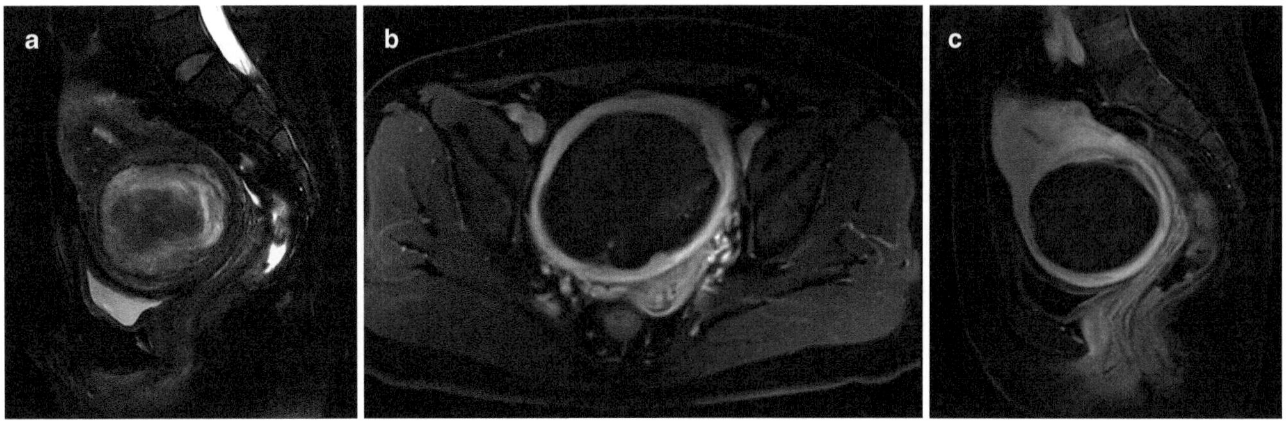

Fig. 4.151 MRI evaluation after treatment of the cervical fibroid. (**a**) T2WI_FS sagittal, (**b**) T1WI_FS + C axial, (**c**) T1WI_FS + C sagittal

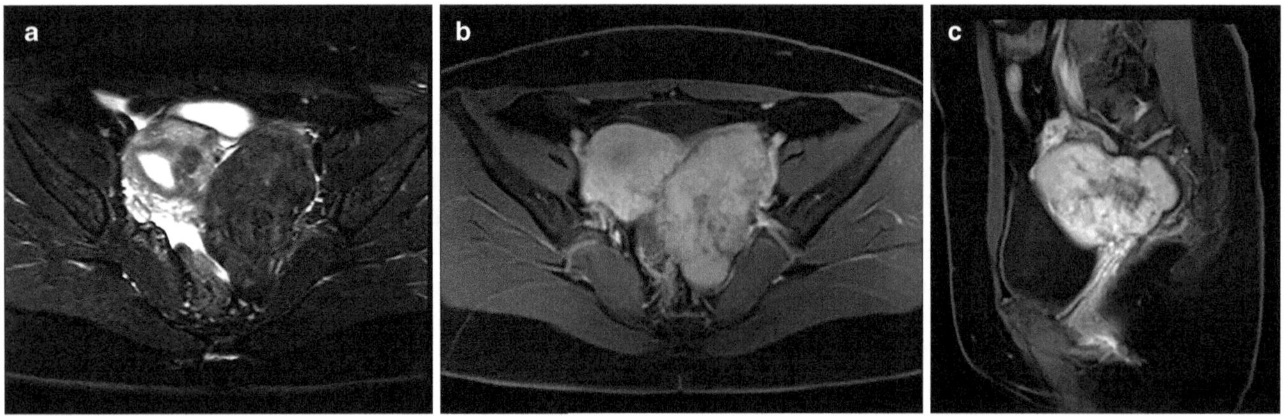

Fig. 4.152 A left broad ligament uterine fibroid before treatment. (**a**) T2WI_FS axial, (**b**) T1WI_FS + C axial, (**c**) T1WI_FS + C sagittal

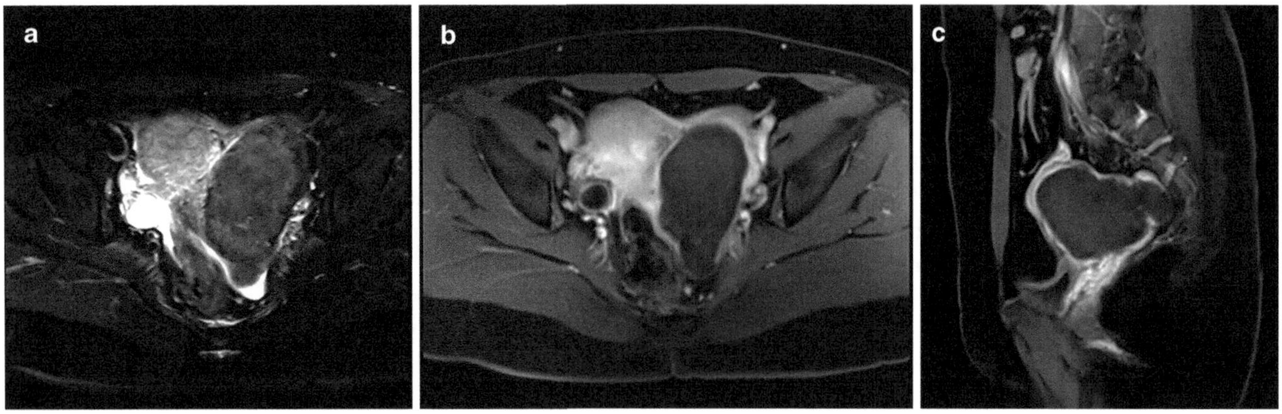

Fig. 4.153 MRI evaluation after the treatment of the left broad ligament uterine fibroids. (**a**) T2WI_FS axial, (**b**) T1WI_FS + C axial, (**c**) T1WI_FS + C sagittal

move when the body position changed during treatment. To improve the effectiveness and safety of the ablation treatment, it was necessary to use special measures to ensure it is relatively fixed. Thus, the precise treatment of focused ultrasound ablation would be achieved, especially for the broad ligament fibroid with irregular shape.

- Basically, it was challenging to use the high-intensity focused ultrasound procedure to ablate broad ligament fibroids. The therapeutic strategy was that the initial focal regions should target the fibroid's deeper layer with lower acoustic power to produce the coagulation necrosis, then, sonication with higher acoustic power was moved from sub-deep to the shallow layer of the tumor. This was carried out to reduce the ultrasonic energy diffusing through the focal area to the far-field, in order to avoid injuries of the organs and tissues surrounding the fibroid.

4.4.2.2 Case 2

Case Description

The female patient was 38 years old. She had menstrual disorders with reduced menstrual flow, backache, and occasional frequent urination. Ultrasonography revealed a right broad ligament uterine fibroid.

Pre-Treatment Assessment

MRI showed a right broad ligament uterine fibroid with mixed high and low signals on T2WI (Fig. 4.154a). The contrast-enhanced T1WI showed that the fibroid was of an abundant blood supply (Fig. 4.154b, c). The fibroid was large and close to the right pelvic sidewall and was relatively fixed. It is predicted that the fibroids could be ablated.

Treatment Techniques

1. **Focused ultrasound parameters.** Average acoustic power: 276 W, sonication time: 2604 seconds, duration of treatment: 117 minutes, total energy: 718,280 J.
2. **Focused ultrasound ablation techniques.** The position of the broad ligament fibroid was fixed by filling the bladder, which could provide a good acoustic pathway. Because the fibroid was close to the fallopian tubes, ureters, ovaries, and so on, it was necessary to set the ultrasound focal region ≥15 mm away from the fibroid edges while controlling the accumulating ultrasound energy to avoid heat diffusion damaging surrounding tissues or organs.

Post-Treatment Assessment

MRI Evaluation after Treatment There was no edema in the subcutaneous tissue of the abdominal wall (Fig. 4.155a). The contrast-enhanced MRI showed that the NPV ratio of the fibroid reached 95%, with only a small amount of residual fibroid layer at the margins (Fig. 4.155b, c).

Discussion

- Broad ligament uterine fibroid generally has no clinical symptoms when they are small. When they enlarge, they can cause pelvic compression symptoms.
- In this case, the right broad ligament uterine fibroid was large in size so that more ultrasound energy could be accumulated during the ablation treatment. Be careful that the focused ultrasound ablation should not break through the fibroid's boundary to avoid the heat diffusion from damaging the adjacent vessels, ureter, nerves, ovaries, and other soft tissues.

4.4.2.3 Case 3

Case Description

The female patient was 34 years old. Her uterine fibroid enlarged yearly, and she required treatment because of her psychological stress.

Pre-Treatment Assessment

MRI showed a right broad ligament uterine fibroid with hypointensity on T2WI (Fig. 4.156a). The contrast-enhanced

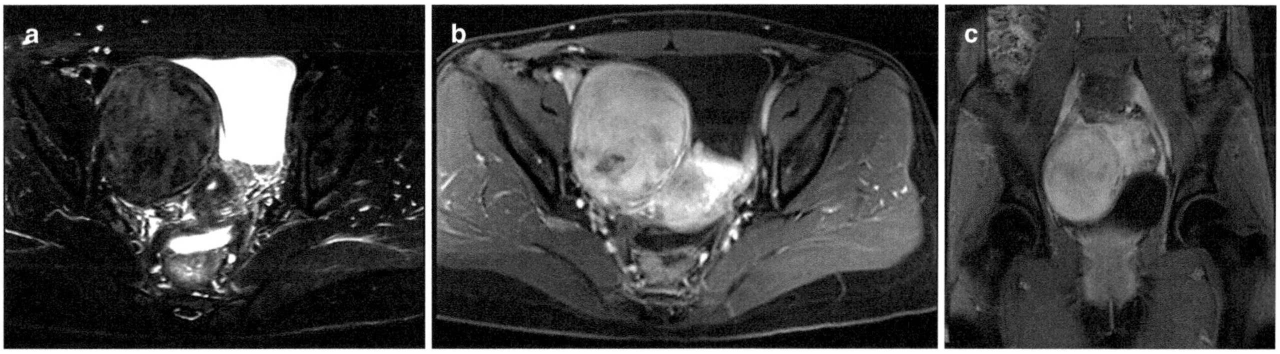

Fig. 4.154 A right broad ligament uterine fibroid before treatment. (**a**) T2WI_FS axial, (**b**) T1WI_FS + C axial, (**c**) T1WI_FS + C coronal

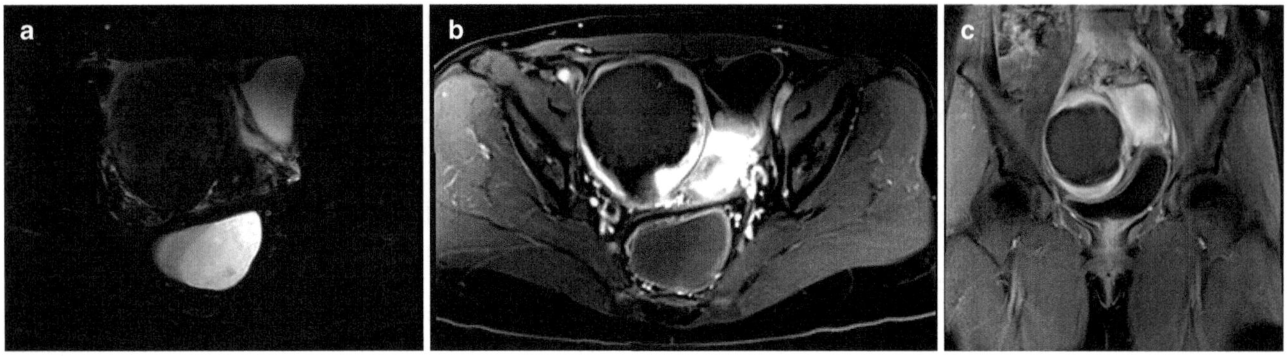

Fig. 4.155 MRI evaluation after the treatment of right broad ligament uterine fibroids. (**a**) T2WI_FS axial, (**b**) T1WI_FS + C axial, (**c**) T1WI_FS + C coronal

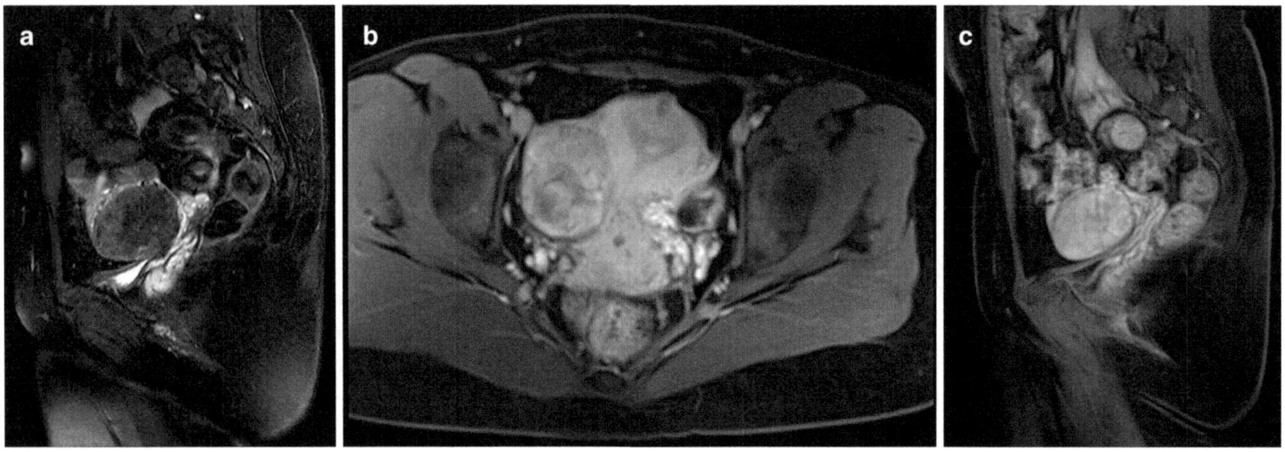

Fig. 4.156 A right broad ligament uterine fibroid before treatment. (**a**) T2WI_FS sagittal, (**b**) T1WI_FS + C axial, (**c**) T1WI_FS + C sagittal

T1WI showed the fibroid had an abundant blood supply (Fig. 4.156b, c). Because the fibroid was located between the right wall of the uterus and the lateral pelvic wall, its mobility was relatively small and fixed during treatment. This fibroid had low intense signals on T2WI. Thus, it was predicted that the fibroid would be relatively easy to be ablated.

Treatment Techniques

1. **Focused ultrasound parameters.** Average acoustic power: 208 W, sonication time: 1500 seconds, duration of treatment: 75 minutes, total energy: 312,600 J.
2. **Focused ultrasound ablation techniques.** This broad ligament fibroid had less mobility. During treatment, the bladder distension and extracorporeal water balloon were used to push the bowels away from the acoustic pathway. The ultrasound waves incident path needed to be adjusted at an appropriate entry angle by position.

Post-Treatment Assessment

MRI Evaluation after Treatment T2WI showed no edema in the soft tissue of the anterior abdominal wall, and the signal intensity of the fibroid markedly increased (Fig. 4.157a). The contrast-enhanced T1WI showed that the broad ligament fibroid was completely ablated, and its capsule was intact (Fig. 4.157b, c).

Discussion

- Focused ultrasound ablation treatment of broad ligament uterine fibroid is an in-situ ablation inside the treated fibroid. Unlike traditional surgery or laparoscopic surgery, a fibroid can be removed. The fibroid capsule has to be intact to ensure the safety of treatment.

4.4.2.4 Case 4

Case Description

The female patient was 35 years old. She presented with irregular menstrual cycles, lower back soreness, and frequent urination.

Pre-Treatment Assessment

MRI showed a right broad ligament uterine fibroid with homogeneous low signals on T2WI (Fig. 4.158a). The contrast-enhanced MRI showed that the fibroid had a poor blood supply

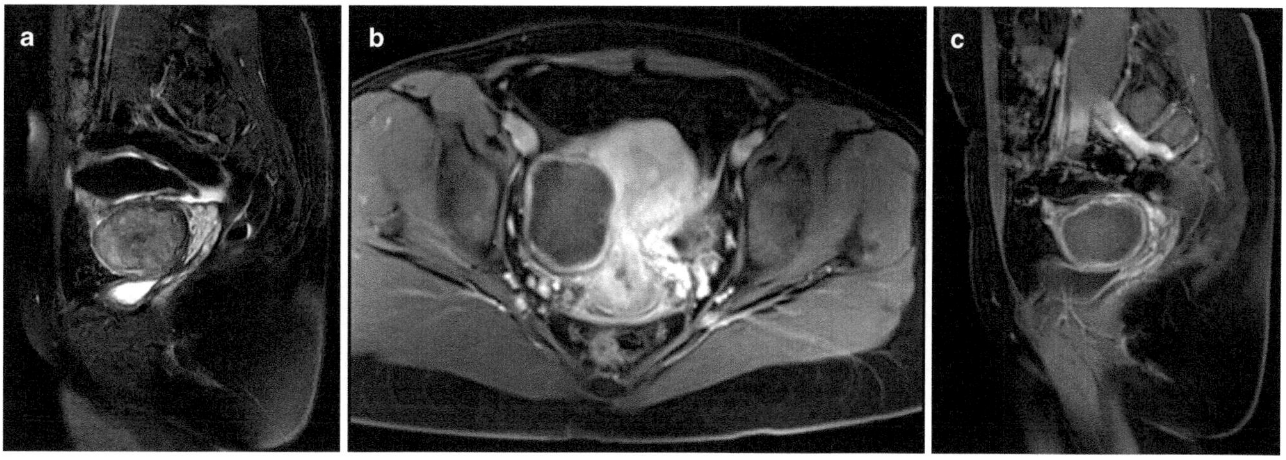

Fig. 4.157 MRI evaluation after the treatment of right broad ligament uterine fibroids. (**a**) T2WI_FS sagittal, (**b**) T1WI_FS + C axial, (**c**) T1WI_FS + C sagittal

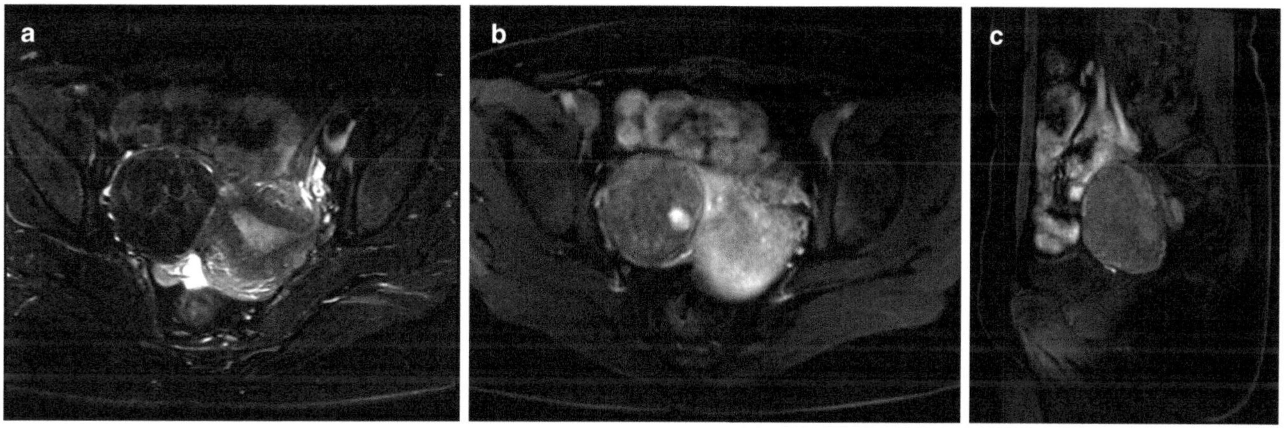

Fig. 4.158 A right broad ligament uterine fibroid before treatment. (**a**) T2WI_FS axial, (**b**) T1WI_FS + C axial, (**c**) T1WI_FS + C sagittal

(Fig. 4.158b). It was predicted that the fibroid would be relatively easy to ablate. However, there were bowels, blood vessels, ovaries, and fallopian tubes around the fibroid, and the right posterior edge of the fibroid was closely adjacent to the pelvic nerve and vascular plexus. Care should be taken to protect the tissues or organs around the fibroid during treatment.

Treatment Techniques

1. **Focused ultrasound parameters.** Average acoustic power: 285 W, sonication time: 2200 seconds, duration of treatment: 121 minutes, total energy: 626,880 J.
2. **Focused ultrasound ablation techniques.** Fill the bladder and use an extracorporeal water balloon to push the bowels away to form a good acoustic pathway. The acoustic power can be reduced to ablate this type of fibroid. Pay close attention to the patient's response to avoid nerve damage.

Post-Treatment Assessment

MRI Evaluation after Treatment The T2WI showed mild edema around the fibroid and its capsule (Fig. 4.159a). The contrast-enhanced T1WI showed that the fibroid was completely ablated with the intact capsule (Fig. 4.159b, c).

Discussion

- Broad ligament uterine fibroid always has been a contraindication for interventional therapy (including uterine artery embolization, radiofrequency ablation, etc.).
- Because the broad ligament uterine fibroid is close to surrounding tissues and organs like the fallopian tubes, iliac vessels, ovaries, ureters, bowels, and other tissues, even routine surgical resection is difficult and prone to postoperative complications. Therefore, focused ultrasound ablation for treating broad ligament uterine fibroid is an alternative treatment.

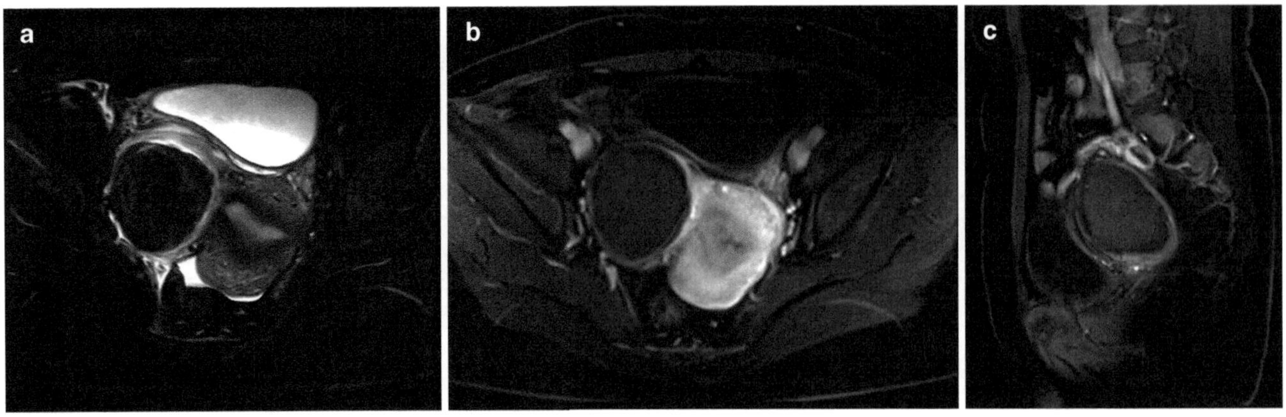

Fig. 4.159 MRI evaluation after the treatment of right broad ligament uterine fibroids. (**a**) T2WI_FS axial, (**b**) T1WI_FS + C axial, (**c**) T1WI_FS + C sagittal

4.4.3 Focused Ultrasound Ablation for Multiple Uterine Fibroids

4.4.3.1 Case 1

Case Description

The female patient was 35 years old. She complained of backache sometimes.

Pre-Treatment Assessment

T2WI showed the multiple fibroids were mainly located on the anterior wall and fundus of the uterus, and most fibroids showed low intense signals while some showed homogeneous slight hyperintensity (Fig. 4.160a). The contrast-enhanced T1WI showed that these fibroids had poor blood supply (Fig. 4.160b, c). It was predicted that focused ultrasound ablation was feasible for these fibroids.

Treatment Techniques

1. **Focused ultrasound parameters.** Average acoustic power: 301 W, sonication time: 3434 seconds, duration of treatment: 180 minutes, total energy: 1,034,130 J.
2. **Focused ultrasound ablation techniques.** Because the fibroids at the posterior wall of the uterus were small, with more bowels nearby, the therapeutic strategy was to mainly treat larger fibroids in the anterior wall and the fundus of the uterus.

Post-Treatment Assessment

1. **MRI evaluation after treatment.** Mild edema was found in the muscle layer of the anterior abdominal wall adjacent to the fibroids on T2WI (Fig. 4.161a). The contrast-enhanced T1WI showed that the NPV ratios of the three larger fibroids in the anterior wall and fundus of the uterus exceeded 95%, the smaller fibroids in the posterior wall were not treated, and the uterine serosa and endometrium were intact (Fig. 4.161b, c).
2. **MRI follow-up at 10 months after treatment.** The fibroids of the anterior wall and fundus of the uterus were significantly reduced in size. The uterine cavity was restored to normal shape, but the small fibroids of the posterior wall of the uterus increased slightly in size (Fig. 4.162).

Discussion

- Even if all multiple uterine fibroids are removed surgically, not only will the myometrium be severely damaged, the fibroid recurrence rate will remain high.
- Focused ultrasound ablation treatment can reduce fibroid volume, improve the environment of the uterine cavity, and protect the uterine serosa and endometrium. Even if the fibroids recur or enlarge, they can be treated repeatedly.

4.4.3.2 Case 2

Case Description

The female patient was 42 years old and underwent a cesarean section 14 years ago. Ultrasound examination showed multiple uterine fibroids, the larger one of which was about 6.4 cm in diameter 1 year ago. The patient presented with constipation and pelvic distension. She has been treated with traditional Chinese medicine orally and the efficacy is poor; she then seeks non-invasive treatment.

Pre-Treatment Assessment

MRI revealed multiple subserosal and intramural fibroids of the uterus, and the largest one of them was 6.7 cm in diameter. They were mainly subserosal fibroids with low signals on T2WI (Fig. 4.163a, b). The contrast-enhanced T1WI showed that fibroids were mostly of moderate blood supply (Fig. 4.163c, d). It was predicted that those fibroids with low intense signals would be easy to ablate, but the subserosal fibroid close to the sacral coccyx should be cautious of nerve injury.

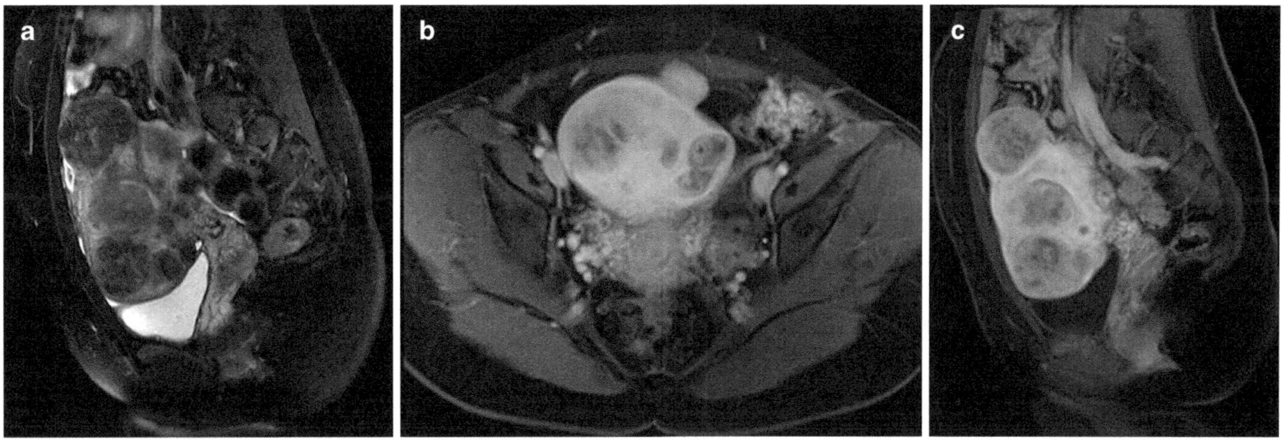

Fig. 4.160 Multiple uterine fibroids before treatment. (**a**) T2WI_FS sagittal, (**b**) T1WI_FS + C axial, (**c**) T1WI_FS + C sagittal

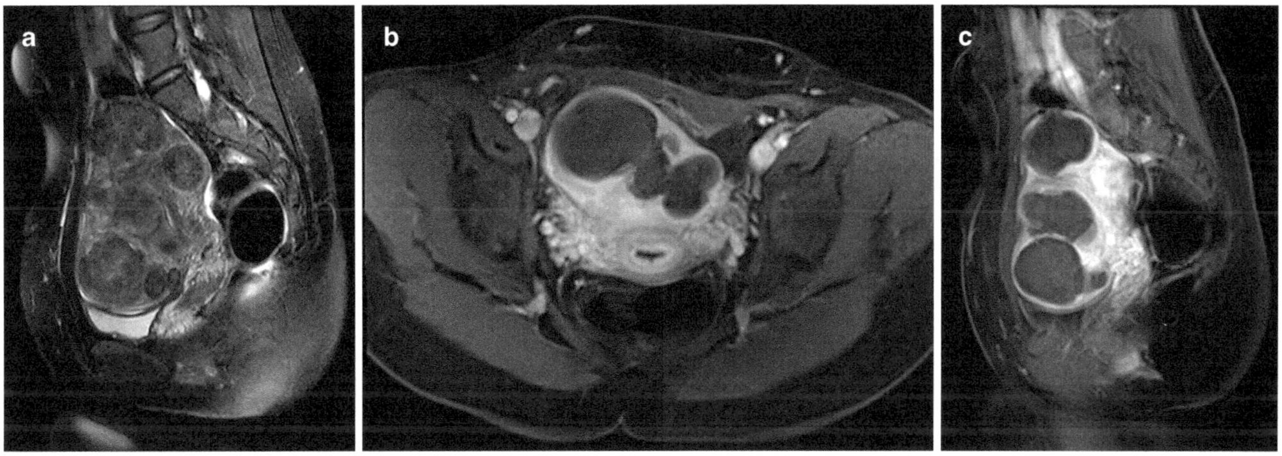

Fig. 4.161 MRI evaluation after the treatment of multiple uterine fibroids. (**a**) T2WI_FS sagittal, (**b**) T1WI_FS + C axial, (**c**) T1WI_FS + C sagittal

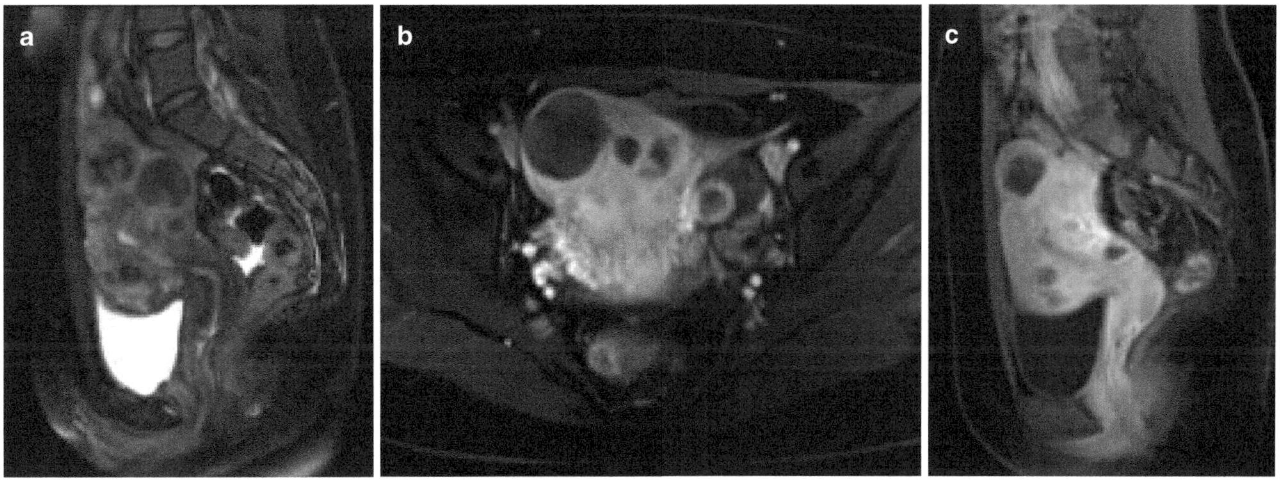

Fig. 4.162 MRI follow-up of multiple uterine fibroids at 10 months after treatment. (**a**) T2WI_FS sagittal, (**b**) T1WI_FS + C axial, (**c**) T1WI_FS + C sagittal

Treatment Techniques

1. **Focused ultrasound parameters.** Average acoustic power: 293 W, sonication time: 3242 seconds, duration of treatment: 160 minutes, total energy: 948,700 J.
2. **Focused ultrasound ablation techniques.** Because the subserosal fibroids were mainly causing the symptoms in this patient, the ablation was mainly for treating these fibroids. It is necessary to distend the bladder to push away the bowel between the anterior abdominal wall and uterus, which could create a good acoustic pathway.

Post-Treatment Assessment

1. **MRI evaluation after treatment.** There was slight swelling of the rectus abdominis of the abdominal wall. The contrast-enhanced T1WI showed that the majority of the subserosal and intramural fibroids were non-perfused, and the largest subserosal fibroid located in the left posterior wall of the uterus was completely ablated with its intact capsule (Fig. 4.164a, b).
2. **MRI follow-up at 6 months after treatment.** The ablated fibroids significantly shrank, and the left posterior subserosal fibroid still was completely not perfused without any recurrence.

Discussion

- This patient had multiple uterine fibroids in different sizes. Traditional open surgery and laparoscopic surgery find it difficult to remove so many fibroids apart from a hysterectomy, and even then, the uterus is more traumatized.
- Focused ultrasound ablation was employed to treat the fibroids that caused the clinical symptoms. These were mainly subserosal fibroids located at the posterior wall of the uterus, which was close to the sacrococcygeal region. Attention should be paid to the sensory activities of the patients' lower limbs during treatment to avoid nerve damages.

4.4.3.3 Case 3

Case Description

The female patient was 52 years old. She had heavy menstrual flow and prolonged menstrual period, with moderate anemia.

Pre-Treatment Assessment

MRI showed multiple uterine fibroids of various sizes. The intramural fibroids in the posterior uterine wall were the main ones, and some small subserosal and submucosal fibroids were also seen. Most fibroids showed low signals on T2WI (Fig. 4.165a). The contrast-enhanced T1WI showed that these fibroids were of abundant blood supply (Fig. 4.165b, c). It was predicted that the focused ultrasound ablation of intramural fibroids was relatively easy to ablate.

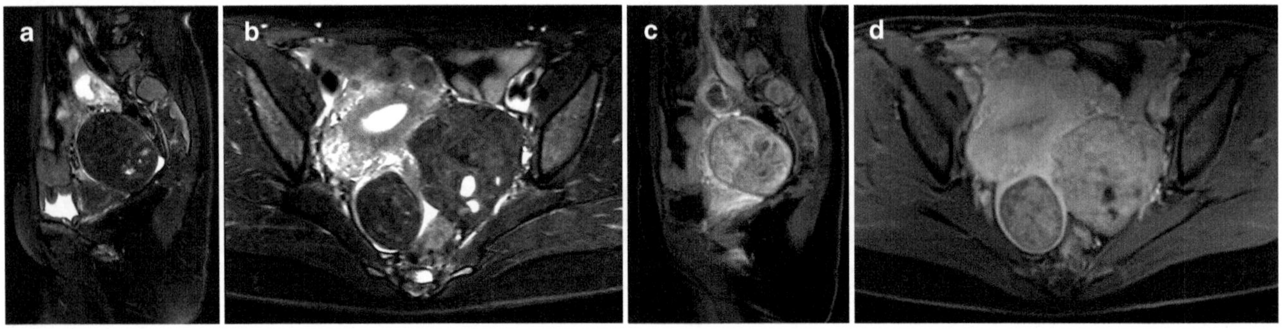

Fig. 4.163 Multiple uterine fibroids before treatment. (**a**) T2WI_FS sagittal, (**b**) T2WI_FS axial, (**c**) T1WI_FS + C sagittal, (**d**) T1WI_FS + C axial

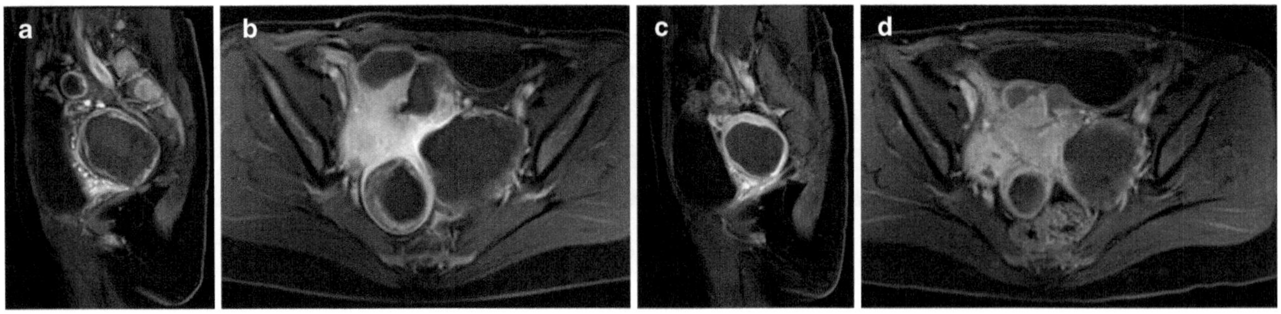

Fig. 4.164 MRI evaluation (**a**, **b**) and 6 month follow-up (**c**, **d**) after the treatment of multiple uterine fibroids. (**a**) T1WI_FS + C sagittal, (**b**) T1WI_FS + C axial, (**c**) T1WI_FS + C sagittal, (**d**) T1WI_FS + C axial

But it might be difficult to treat the small type 0 submucosal fibroids because it would be hard to identify and position them.

Treatment Techniques

1. **Focused ultrasound parameters.** Average acoustic power: 298 W, sonication time: 3100 seconds, duration of treatment: 190 minutes, total energy: 1,185,310 J.
2. **Focused ultrasound ablation techniques.** The therapeutic plan was mainly for treating intramural fibroids. Small Type 0 submucosal and posterior subserosal fibroids were not considered for ultrasound ablation. Treating the small submucosal fibroids might damage the endometrium, and treating the subserosal fibroids might cause injury to the sacral plexus and intestine because of their proximity.

Post-Treatment Assessment

1. **MRI evaluation after treatment.** There was no edema in the subcutaneous soft tissue of the anterior abdominal wall (Fig. 4.166a). The contrast-enhanced T1WI showed that the majority of the intramural fibroids had been ablated with no perfusion, especially the largest fibroid was completely ablated (Fig. 4.166b, c).
2. **MRI follow-up at 3 years after treatment.** The volume of the uterus was significantly reduced. The small fibroids in the anterior and posterior walls had been absorbed and disappeared. The volumes of larger fibroids were significantly reduced, yet the small submucosal and the posterior subserosal fibroids did not change significantly (Fig. 4.167).

Discussion

- For the focused ultrasound ablation treatment of subserosal uterine fibroids close to the posterior wall of the pelvis, it is necessary to avoid damage to the adjacent bowels and the sacral plexus at the posterior pelvic wall.
- In this case of multiple uterine fibroids, the intramural fibroids can be treated to reduce the size of the entire

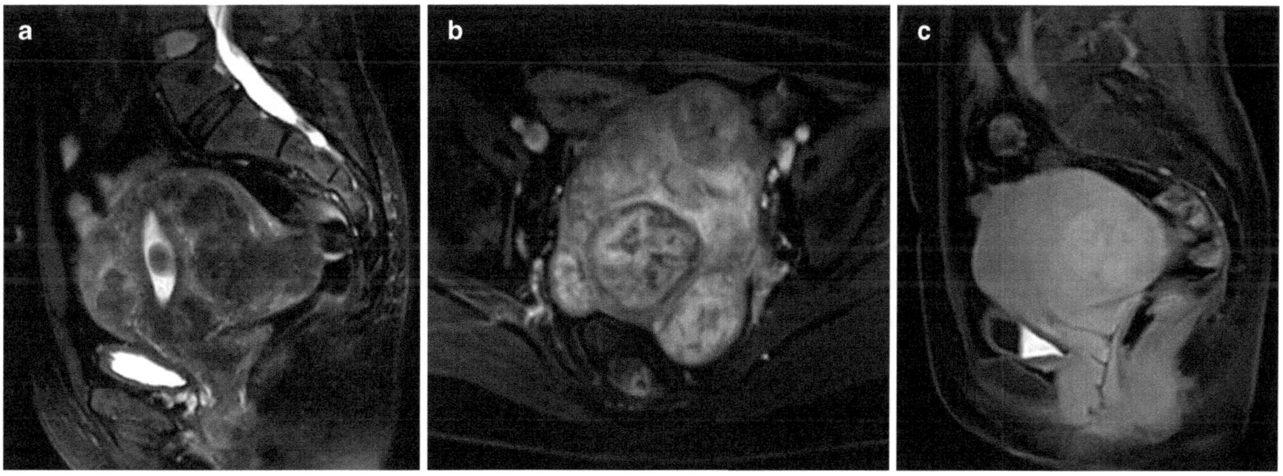

Fig. 4.165 Multiple uterine fibroids before treatment. (**a**) T2WI_FS sagittal, (**b**) T1WI_FS + C axial, (**c**) T1WI_FS + C sagittal

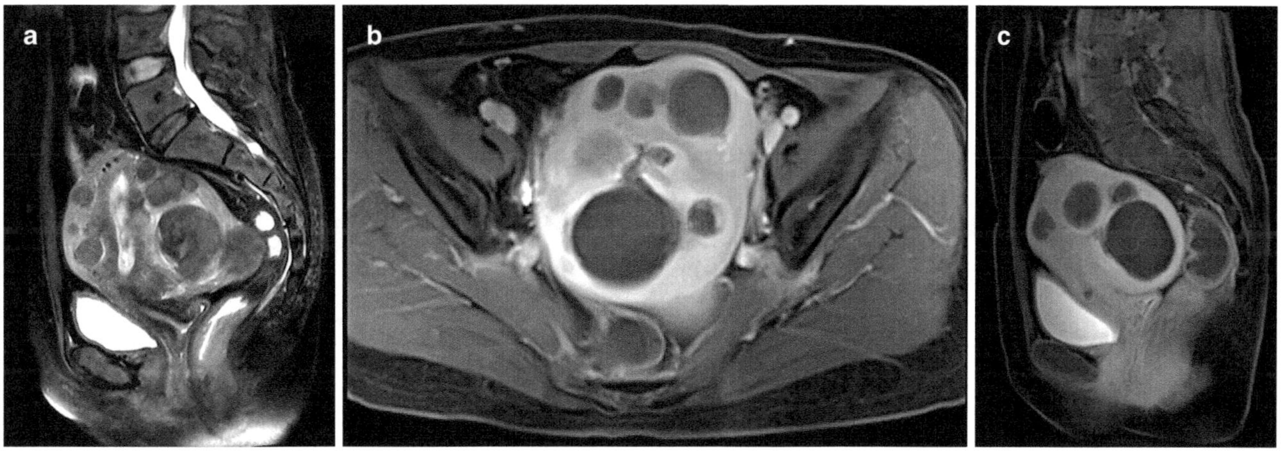

Fig. 4.166 MRI evaluation after the treatment of multiple uterine fibroids. (**a**) T2WI_FS sagittal, (**b**) T1WI_FS + C axial, (**c**) T1WI_FS + C sagittal

uterus so that the symptoms of pelvic compression caused by uterine fibroids can be relieved or even disappear.
- In this case, the small type 0 submucosal fibroids should not be treated by focused ultrasound ablation due to their size, difficult treatment, and risks of damaging the endometrium.

4.4.3.4 Case 4

Case Description

The female patient was 44 years old. She had lower abdominal distension, low back pain, and urinary frequency and urgency.

Pre-Treatment Assessment

MRI showed a significantly enlarged uterus, and the entire uterine wall was occupied by fibroids of various sizes, showing low signals mixed with a little hyperintensity on T2WI (Fig. 4.168a). The contrast-enhanced T1WI showed that the fibroids were of poor-moderate blood supply (Fig. 4.168b, c). It was predicted that focused ultrasound ablation would not be difficult to be performed but take time to finish. Still, the uterine size was too large, and the fibroids beyond the moving range of the transducer might not be treated with ultrasound ablation.

Treatment Techniques

1. **Focused ultrasound parameters.** Average acoustic power: 347 W, sonication time: 3600 seconds, duration of treatment: 210 minutes, total energy: 1,249,210 J.
2. **Focused ultrasound ablation techniques.** The patient's body position could be changed during treatment so that the therapeutic transducer should cover the entire uterus. When moving the ultrasound transducer head, attention

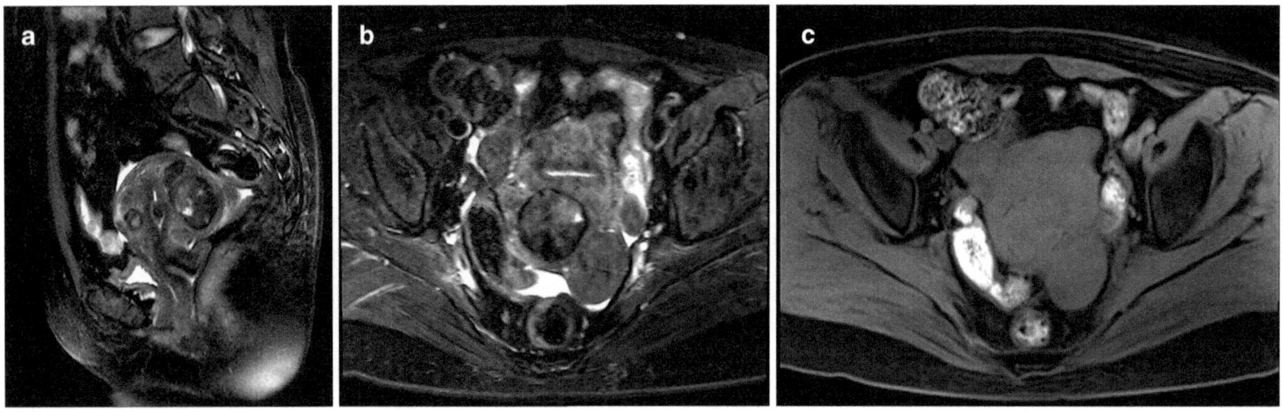

Fig. 4.167 MRI follow-up of multiple uterine fibroids at 3 years after treatment. (**a**) T2WI_FS sagittal, (**b**) T2WI_FS axial, (**c**) T1WI axial

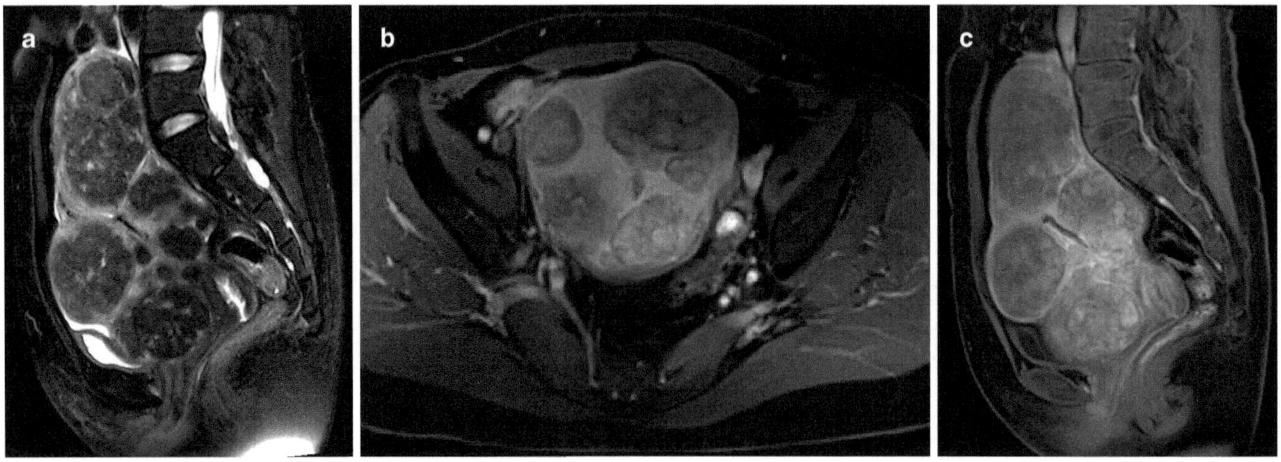

Fig. 4.168 Multiple uterine fibroids before treatment. (**a**) T2WI_FS sagittal, (**b**) T1WI_FS + C axial, (**c**) T1WI_FS + C sagittal

should be paid to avoid crushing the skin of the abdominal wall.

Post-Treatment Assessment

1. **MRI evaluation after treatment.** T2WI showed slight edema in the muscular layer of the anterior abdominal wall around the umbilical area. The signal intensities of the anterior uterine wall and the treated fibroids also increased (Fig. 4.169a). The contrast-enhanced T1WI showed that most fibroids were ablated without perfusion, and the uterine serosa and endometrium were intact (Fig. 4.169b, c).
2. **MRI follow-up at 1 year after treatment.** The volume of the uterus was slightly smaller than that before the treatment, and the larger fibroids in the anterior wall of the uterus were significantly reduced. Still, the residual fibroid tissue in the posterior layer of the fibroids recurred (Fig. 4.170).

Discussion

- A huge uterus caused by multiple fibroids is often clinically treated by hysterectomy as the first choice. Focused ultrasound ablation may become an alternative treatment for uterine preservation.

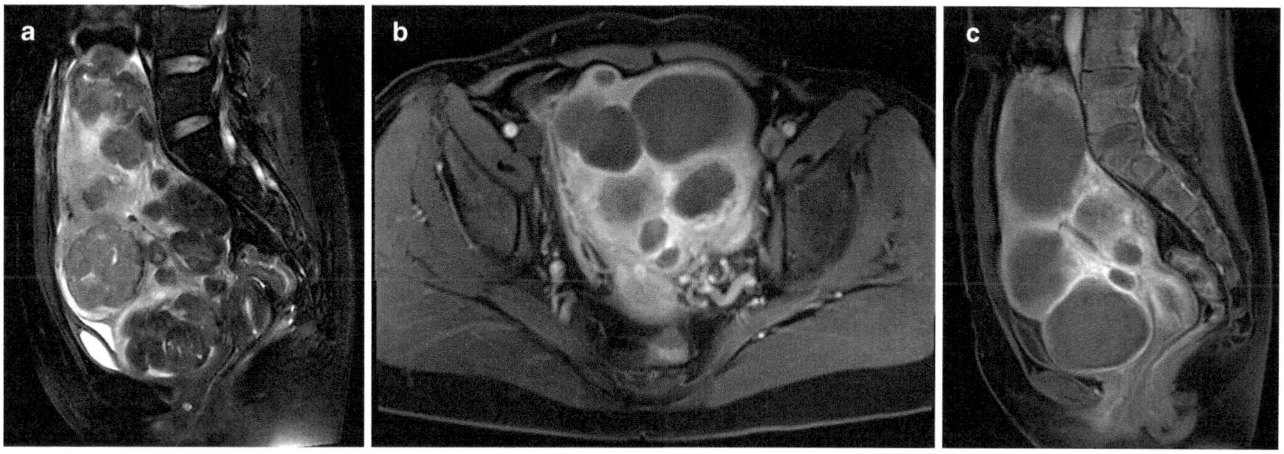

Fig. 4.169 MRI evaluation of multiple uterine fibroids after treatment. (**a**) T2WI_FS sagittal, (**b**) T1WI_FS + C axial, (**c**) T1WI_FS + C sagittal

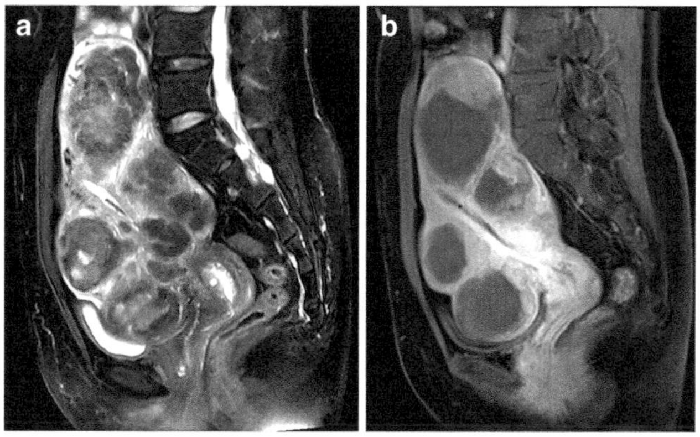

Fig. 4.170 MRI follow-up of multiple uterine fibroids at 12 months after treatment. (**a**) T2WI_FS sagittal, (**b**) T1WI_FS + C sagittal

- The patient, in this case, was followed up 1 year later, and the anterior uterine fibroids were shrunken, thereby reducing the size of the uterus to relieve the symptoms of bladder compression. If the residual fibroid part in the posterior layer of fibroids recurs, focused ultrasound ablation can be performed again.

4.4.3.5 Case 5

Case Description

The female patient was 43 years old. She had heavy menstrual flow, dysmenorrhea with low back pain, and symptoms of pelvic compression.

Pre-Treatment Assessment

MRI showed multiple fibroids in the uterus. The largest fibroid, located in the anterior wall of the uterus, showed high signals on T2WI. The other smaller fibroids of anterior and posterior uterine walls showed isointense and hyperintense signals on T2WI, respectively (Fig. 4.171a). The contrast-enhanced T1WI showed that all these fibroids had an abundant blood supply (Fig. 4.171b). It was predicted that focused ultrasound ablation would be difficult.

Treatment Techniques

1. **Focused ultrasound parameters.** Average acoustic power: 370 W, sonication time: 4107 seconds, duration of treatment: 180 minutes, total energy: 1,520,650 J.
2. **Focused ultrasound ablation techniques.** The abdominal wall was thin with a good acoustic pathway for treatment. However, the fibroids with hyperintensity on T2WI were of abundant blood supply. Focused ultrasound ablation could be difficult to ablate these fibroids. If the patient can tolerate it, the acoustic power and the therapeutic radiation energy should be increased.

Post-Treatment Assessment

MRI Evaluation after Treatment The subcutaneous tissue and muscle layer of the anterior abdominal wall were significantly edematous. The skin was intact with no burn injury (Fig. 4.172a). The contrast-enhanced T1WI showed that the NPV ratios of these three fibroids exceeded 90% (Fig. 4.172b).

Discussion

- Uterine fibroids with hyperintensity on T2WI and abundant blood supply are more difficult to be ablated by

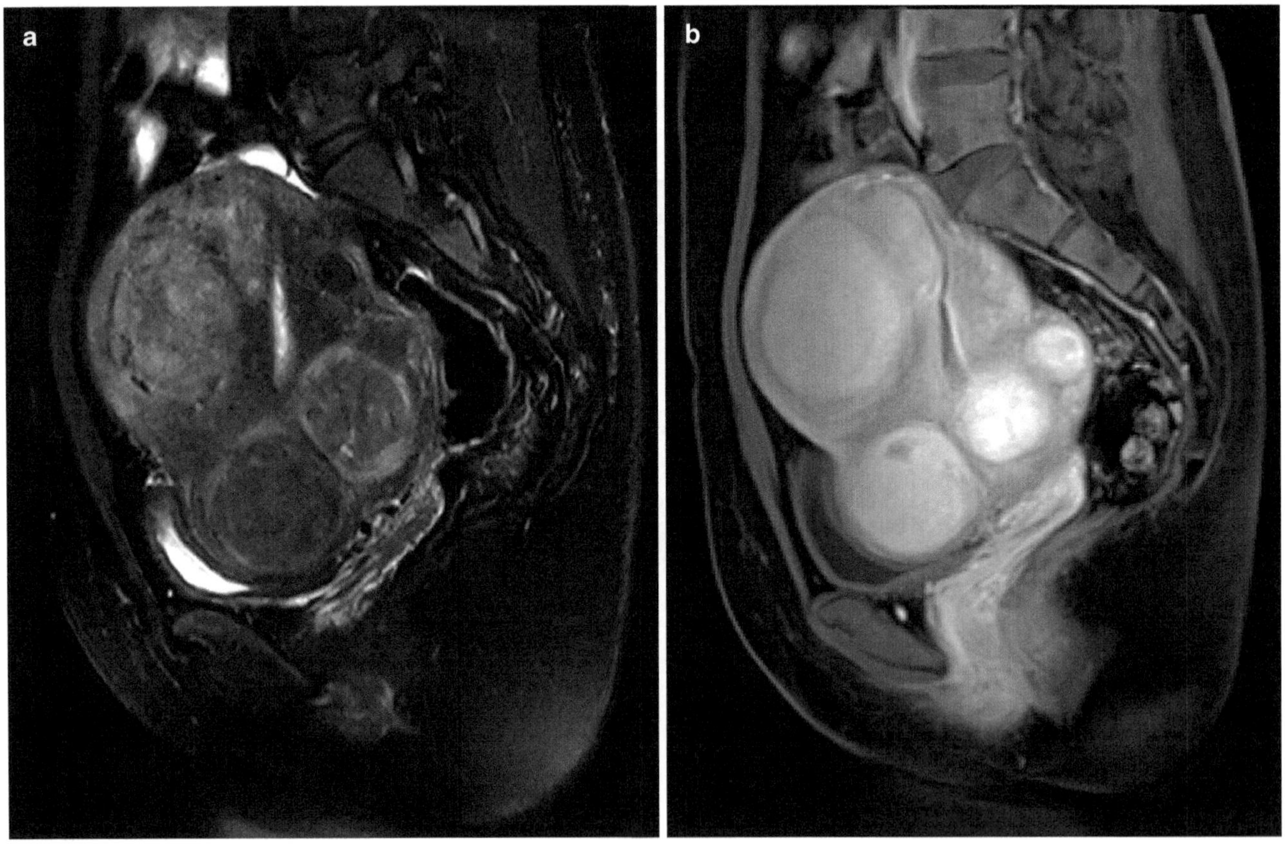

Fig. 4.171 Multiple uterine fibroids before treatment. (**a**) T2WI_FS sagittal, (**b**) T1WI_FS + C sagittal

focused ultrasound. Yet, in this case, the fibroids have achieved good ablation results.

- During treatment, the total energy of local irradiation (1520 650 J) was large, and the anterior abdominal wall edema was significant. At the end of the treatment, 4–10 °C cold normal saline is used to fill the bladder together and an ice pack is used for external application to cool the local abdominal skin temperature and to avoid the high temperature from these fibroids causing thermal damage to the surrounding tissues, especially the anterior abdominal wall.

4.4.3.6 Case 6

Case Description

The female patient was 46 years old. She had increased menstrual flow, dysmenorrhea, and mild anemia.

Pre-Treatment Assessment

MRI showed multiple uterine fibroids with homogeneous low signals on T2WI (Fig. 4.173a). The contrast-enhanced T1WI showed that fibroids were mostly of moderate blood supply (Fig. 4.173b, c). Because these fibroids had a good

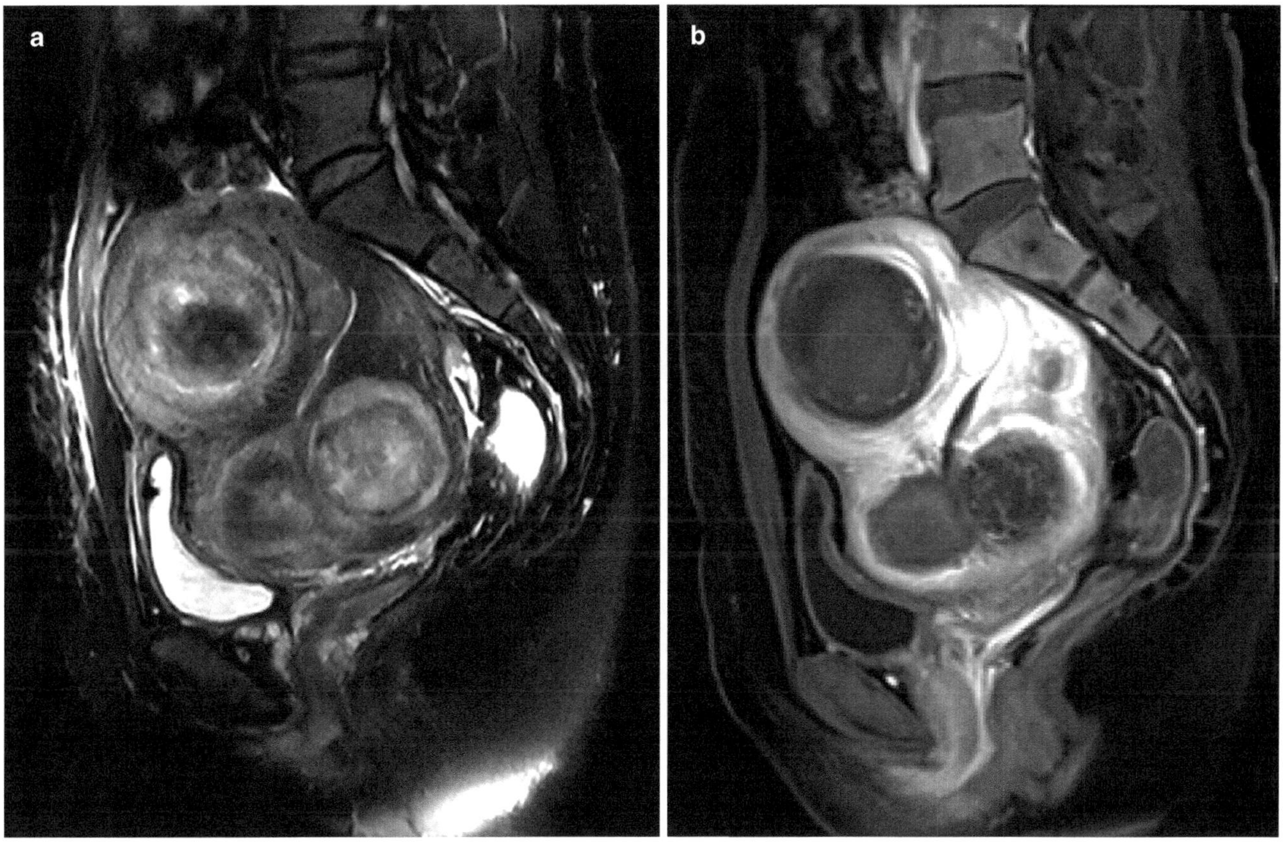

Fig. 4.172 MRI evaluation of multiple uterine fibroids after treatment. (**a**) T2WI_FS sagittal, (**b**) T1WI_FS + C sagittal

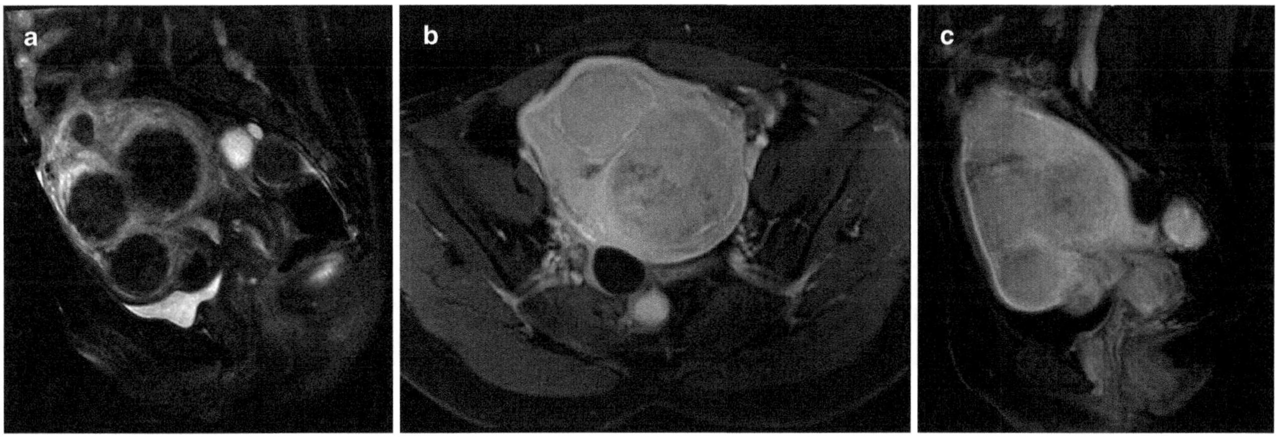

Fig. 4.173 Multiple uterine fibroids before treatment. (**a**) T2WI_FS sagittal, (**b**) T1WI_FS + C axial, (**c**) T1WI_FS + C sagittal

acoustic pathway, it was predicted that they were relatively easy to ablate.

Treatment Techniques

1. **Focused ultrasound parameters.** Average acoustic power: 314 W, sonication time: 2100 seconds, duration of treatment: 128 minutes, total energy: 68,390 J.
2. **Focused ultrasound ablation techniques.** The uterus was anteriorly inclined and large. The majority of multiple fibroids were intramural with a good acoustic pathway. The fibroid on the left uterine wall was the largest and was adjacent to the sacral plexus. Take care to avoid nerve damage.

Post-Treatment Assessment

1. **MRI evaluation after treatment.** There is no significant edema in the subcutaneous tissue of the anterior abdominal wall (Fig. 4.174a). The contrast-enhanced T1WI showed that the NPV ratio of the fibroids exceeded 95%, and the uterine serosa and endometrium were intact (Fig. 4.174b, c).
2. **MRI follow-up at 6 months after treatment.** The volumes of these uterine fibroids were significantly reduced, and they showed no perfusion and no recurrence. The uterine cavity returned to normal shape (Fig. 4.175).

Discussion

- Even if many uterine fibroids exist, focused ultrasound ablation can achieve better therapeutic effects if the fibroids have low intense signals on T2WI.
- Whether uterine fibroids can be ablated by focused ultrasound is mainly determined by the MRI signal characteristics, not by the number and size of fibroids.

4.4.3.7 Case 7

Case Description

The female patient was 41 years old. She had increased menstrual flow and prolonged menstrual cycles, accompanied by pressure symptoms such as frequent urination and low backache.

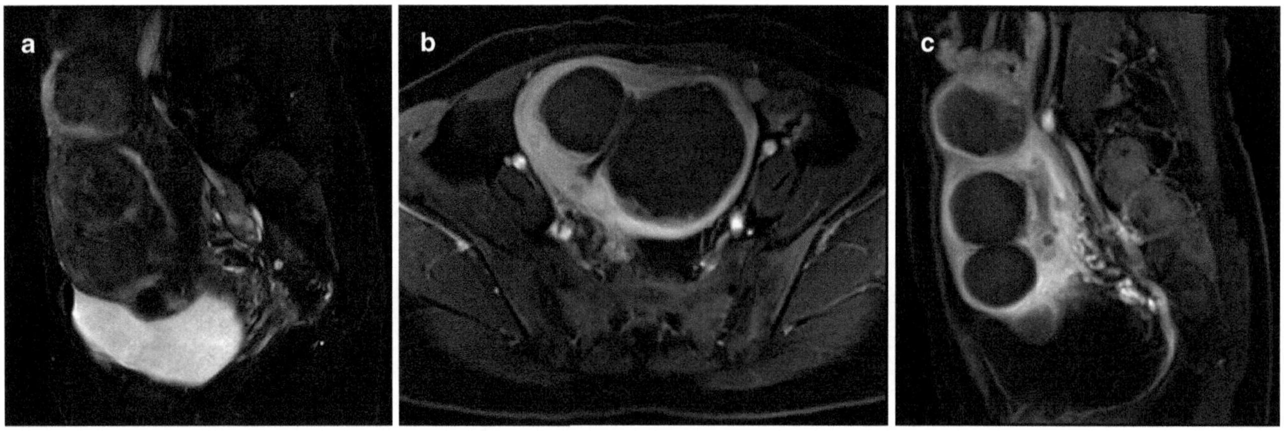

Fig. 4.174 MRI evaluation of multiple uterine fibroids after treatment. (**a**) T2WI_FS sagittal, (**b**) T1WI_FS + C axial, (**c**) T1WI_FS + C sagittal

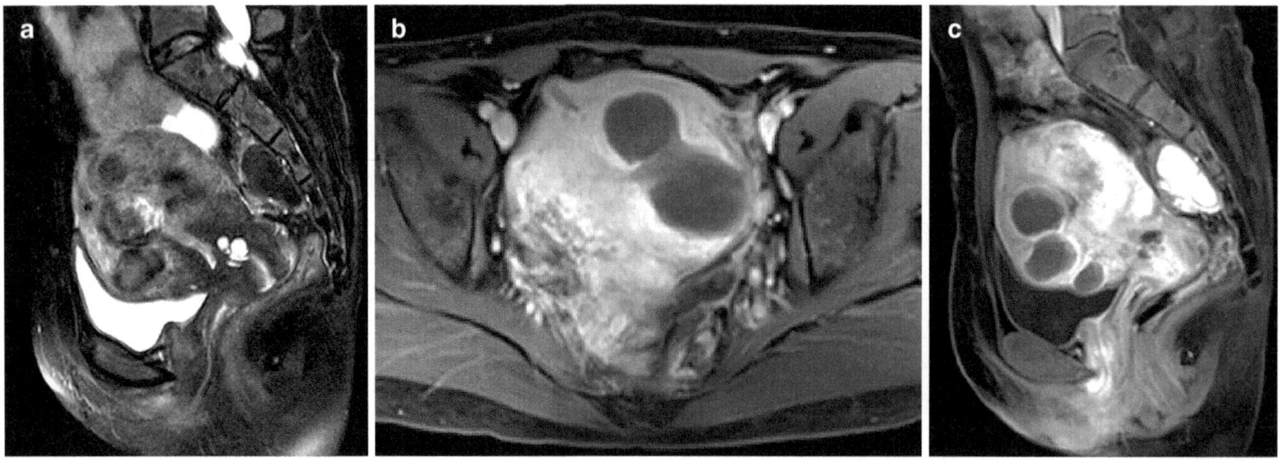

Fig. 4.175 MRI follow-up of multiple uterine fibroids at 6 months after treatment. (**a**) T2WI_FS sagittal, (**b**) T1WI_FS + C axial, (**c**) T1WI_FS + C sagittal

Pre-Treatment Assessment

MRI showed five fibroids of the uterus, of which a posterior fibroid was the largest, with low signal on T2WI (Fig. 4.176a). The contrast-enhanced T1WI showed that these fibroids had moderate blood supply (Fig. 4.176b, c). It was evaluated that these fibroids were suitable for ultrasound ablation.

Treatment Techniques

1. **Focused ultrasound parameters.** Average acoustic power: 400 W, sonication time: 1754 seconds, duration of treatment: 105 minutes, total energy: 700,820 J.
2. **Focused ultrasound ablation techniques.** The posterior uterine fibroid was adjacent to the coccyx and sacral plexus. The ultrasound focal region should be more than 15 mm away from the posterior edge of the fibroid.

Post-Treatment Assessment

1. **MRI evaluation after treatment.** Significant edema was found in the subcutaneous soft tissue and muscle layer of the anterior abdominal wall (Fig. 4.177a). The contrast-enhanced T1WI showed that the NPV ratio of the multiple fibroids was about 98%, and the uterine serosa and endometrium were intact (Fig. 4.177b, c).
2. **MRI follow-up at 6 months after treatment.** The subcutaneous soft tissue and muscular layer edema of the anterior abdominal wall disappeared completely. The five fibroids treated were significantly reduced in size, and the original compressed and deformed uterine cavity basically returned to its normal shape (Fig. 4.178a). The contrast-enhanced T1WI showed that these fibroids still had the sign of ablation and necrosis without perfusion, and no recurrence was seen (Fig. 4.178b, c).

Discussion

- Focused ultrasound ablation for multiple uterine fibroids can achieve the best ablation treatment effect for fibroids with low signals on T2WI.

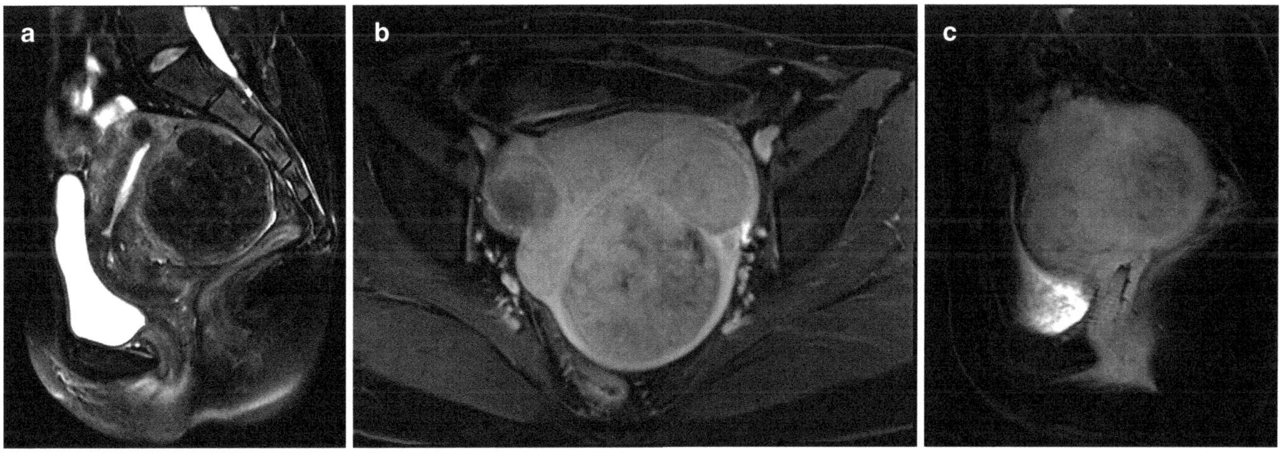

Fig. 4.176 Multiple uterine fibroids before treatment. (**a**) T2WI_FS sagittal, (**b**) T1WI_FS + C axial, (**c**) T1WI_FS + C sagittal

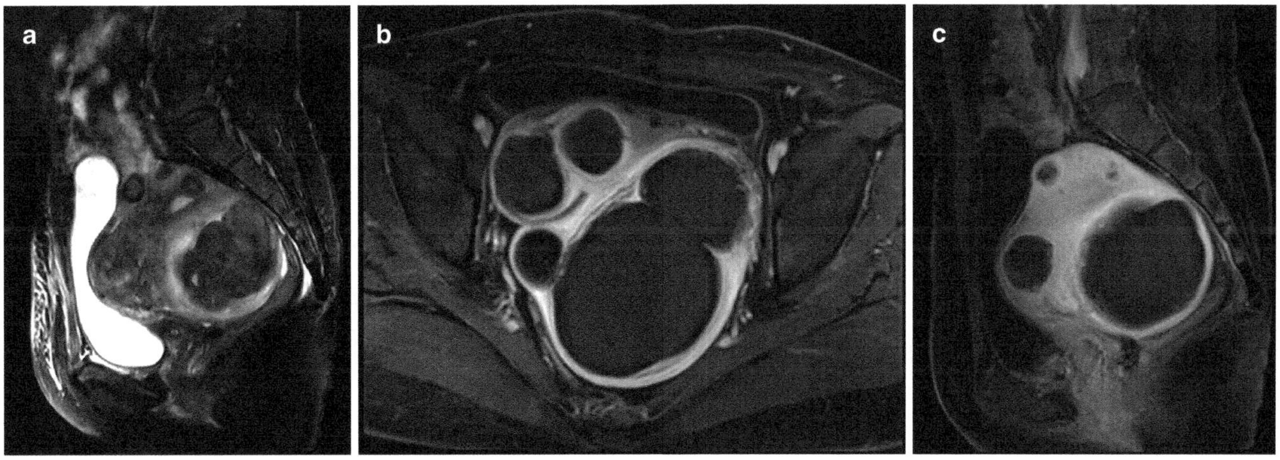

Fig. 4.177 MRI evaluation of multiple uterine fibroids after treatment. (**a**) T2WI_FS sagittal, (**b**) T1WI_FS + C axial, (**c**) T1WI_FS + C sagittal

4.4.3.8 Case 8

Case Description

The female patient was 47 years old. She had fibroid recurrence after surgical removal of uterine fibroids. She presented with heavy menstrual flow, accompanied by moderate anemia.

Pre-Treatment Assessment

MRI showed multiple intramural and submucosal fibroids with low signals on T2WI (Fig. 4.179a). The contrast-enhanced T1WI showed that these fibroids were of poor blood supply (Fig. 4.179b, c) with a good acoustic pathway for treatment. It was predicted that the majority of the fibroids were relatively easy to ablate, but some small submucosal fibroids were difficult to ablate completely.

Treatment Techniques

1. **Focused ultrasound parameters.** Average acoustic power: 297 W, sonication time: 3145 seconds, duration of treatment: 140 minutes, total energy: 934,030 J.
2. **Focused ultrasound ablation techniques.** The acoustic power could be appropriately reduced to treat the intramural fibroids with T2WI hypointensity, and type I submucosal fibroids could be ablated simultaneously.

Post-Treatment Assessment

1. **MRI evaluation after treatment.** The muscle layer of the abdominal wall was significantly edematous, and the signal intensity of the majority of treated fibroids heterogeneously increased on T2WI (Fig. 4.180a). The contrast-enhanced T1WI showed that the NPV ratios of the multiple uterine fibroids exceeded 90%. Only a small amount of the marginal area of the fibroids remained, and the endometrium was undamaged and intact (Fig. 4.180a).
2. **MRI follow-up at 3 months after treatment.** The size of the uterus was significantly reduced. While the volumes of intramural fibroids were significantly reduced, the submucosal fibroids were not clearly displayed. The uterine cavity and endometrium returned to normal shapes, and the muscle layer edema of the anterior abdominal wall disappeared (Fig. 4.181).

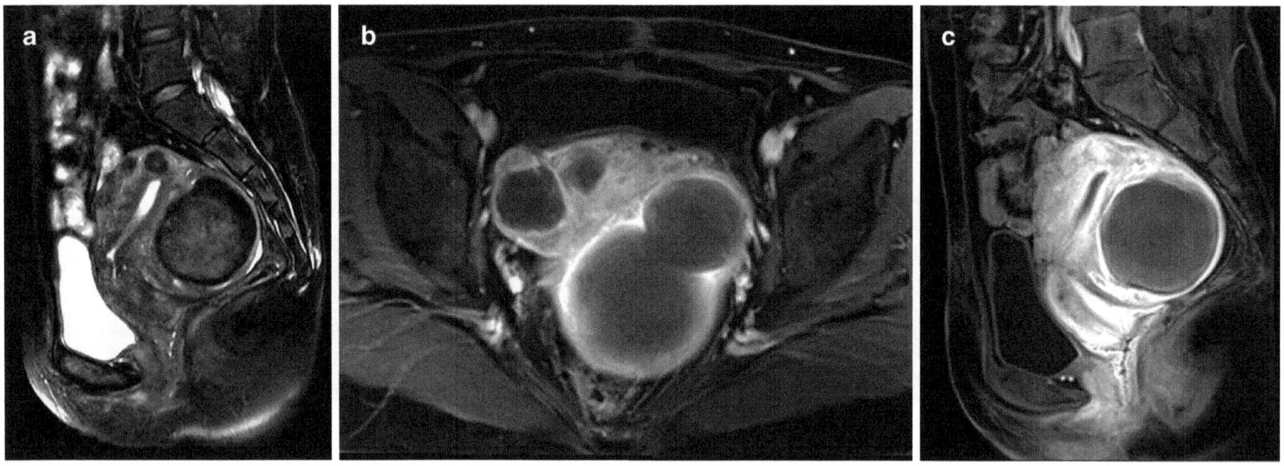

Fig. 4.178 MRI follow-up of multiple uterine fibroids at 6 months after treatment. (**a**) T2WI_FS sagittal, (**b**) T1WI_FS + C axial, (**c**) T1WI_FS + C sagittal

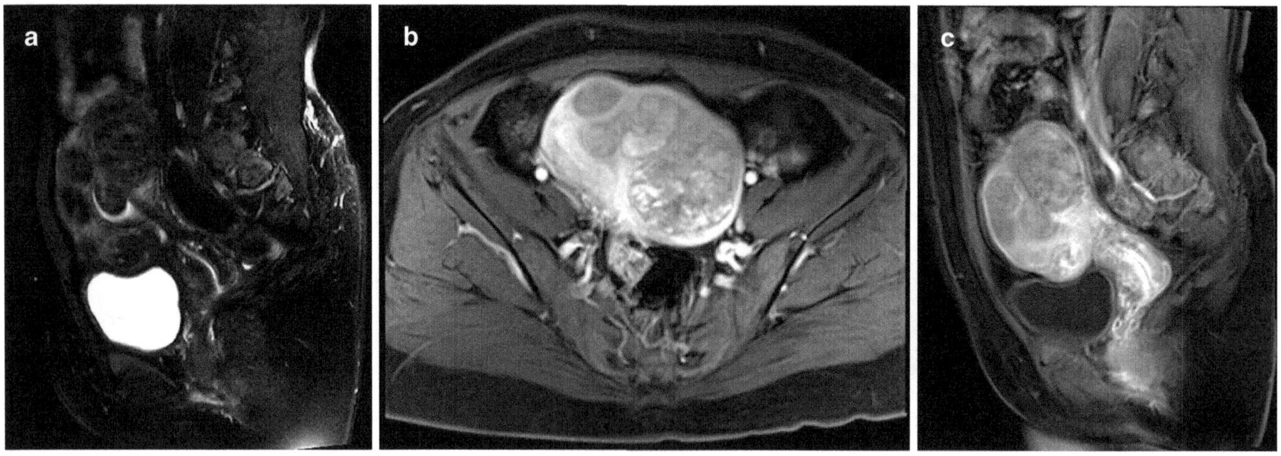

Fig. 4.179 Multiple uterine fibroids before treatment. (**a**) T2WI_FS sagittal, (**b**) T1WI_FS + C axial, (**c**) T1WI_FS + C sagittal

Discussion

- After ultrasound ablation, the treated fibroids showed coagulative necrosis. For intramural fibroids, the outcome is mainly absorption and reduction in size. The ablated submucosal fibroids may fall off and be discharged through the uterine cavity and vagina.

4.4.3.9 Case 9

Case Description

The female patient was 44 years old. Recently, she had increased menstrual flow, accompanied by mild anemia and frequent urination.

Pre-Treatment Assessment

MRI showed multiple fibroids of various sizes (more than 100 fibroids), and they had low signals on T2WI (Fig. 4.182a). The contrast-enhanced T1WI showed that most of the larger fibroids were of moderate-rich blood supply, and a few of them had poor blood supply (Fig. 4.182b, c). It was predicted that larger fibroids would be relatively easy to ablate, but it was difficult to achieve a complete ablation for all lesions due to the large numbers of small fibroids.

Treatment Techniques

1. **Focused ultrasound parameters.** Average acoustic power: 328 W, sonication time: 2479 seconds, duration of treatment: 130 minutes, total energy: 812,700 J.
2. **Focused ultrasound ablation techniques.** There were a large number of uterine fibroids. The aim was to ablate as many fibroids as possible. The posterior fibroids were preferentially treated first in order.

Post-Treatment Assessment

MRI Evaluation after Treatment It showed no edema in the anterior abdominal wall, but the anterior uterine wall around the treated fibroids was edematous, and the signals of fibroids increased on T2WI (Fig. 4.183a). The contrast-enhanced T1WI showed that most fibroids had been completely ablated with no perfusion, and only very few fibroids had some residues at the edge (Fig. 4.183b, c).

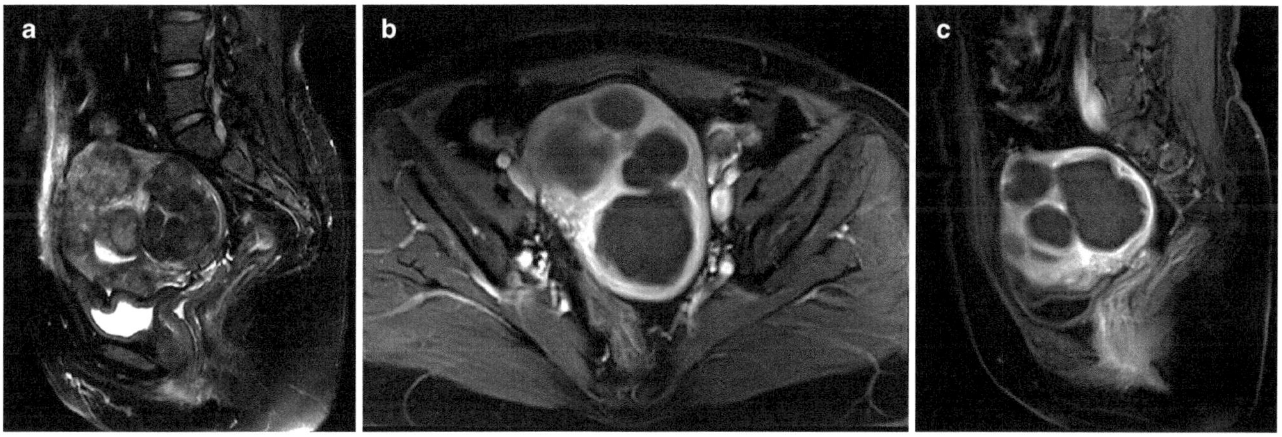

Fig. 4.180 MRI evaluation of multiple uterine fibroids after treatment. (**a**) T2WI_FS sagittal, (**b**) T1WI_FS + C axial, (**c**) T1WI_FS + C sagittal

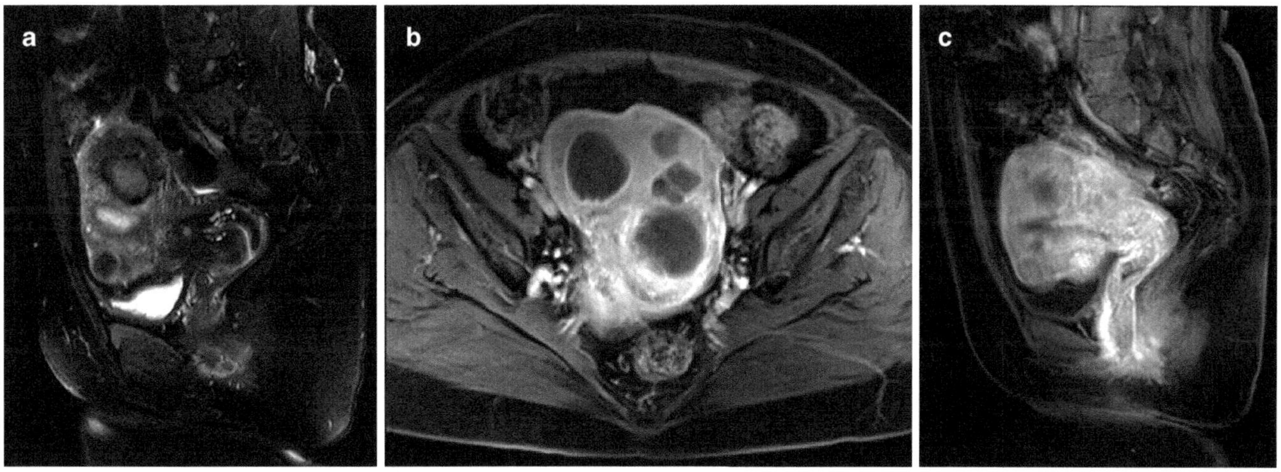

Fig. 4.181 MRI follow-up of multiple uterine fibroids at 3 months after treatment. (**a**) T2WI_FS sagittal, (**b**) T1WI_FS + C axial, (**c**) T1WI_FS + C sagittal

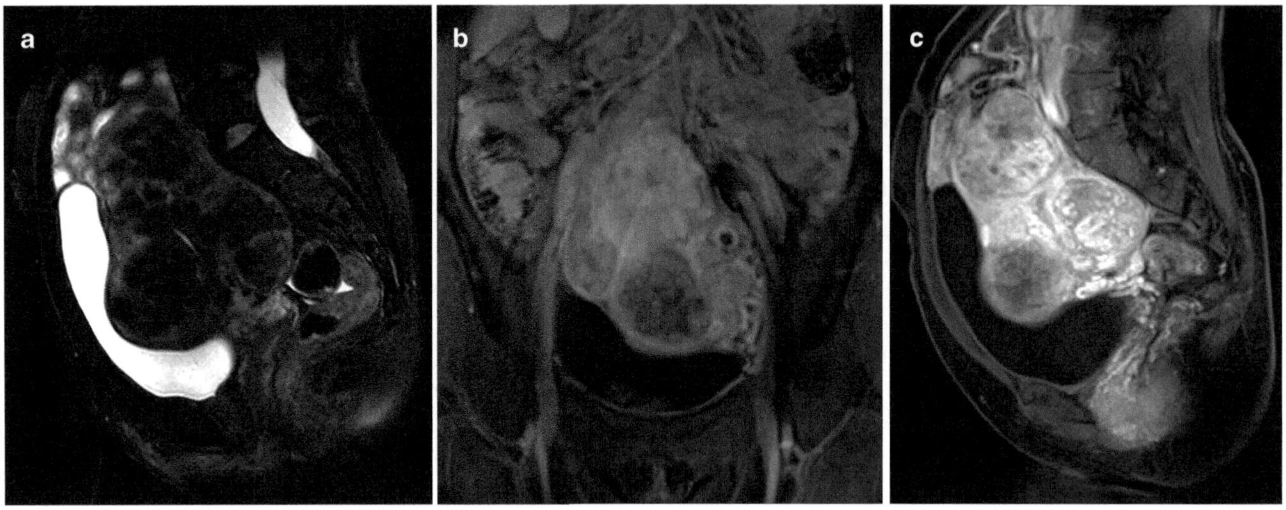

Fig. 4.182 Multiple uterine fibroids before treatment. (**a**) T2WI_FS sagittal, (**b**) T1WI_FS + C coronal, (**c**) T1WI_FS + C sagittal

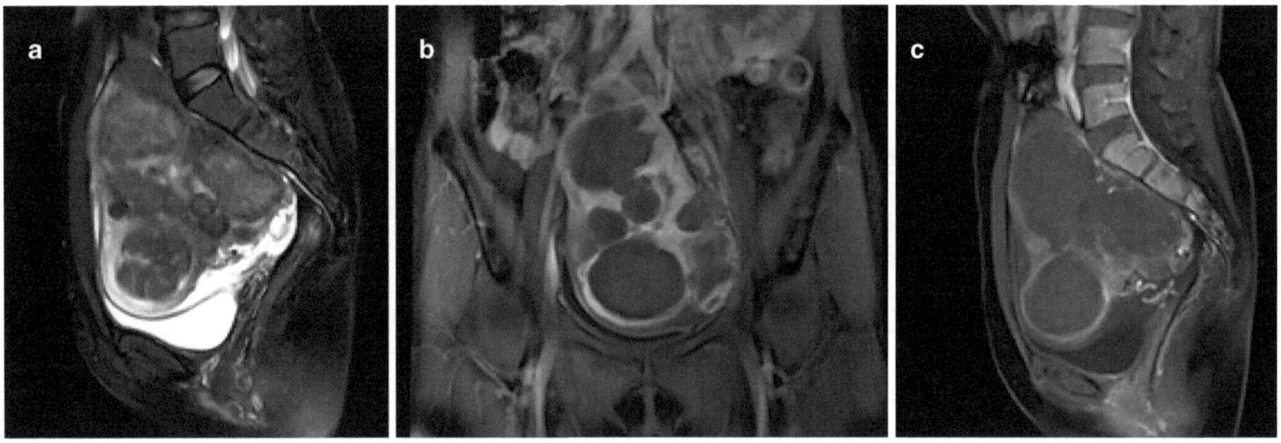

Fig. 4.183 MRI evaluation of multiple uterine fibroids after treatment. (**a**) T2WI_FS sagittal, (**b**) T1WI_FS + C coronal, (**c**) T1WI_FS + C sagittal

Discussion

- This patient had so many fibroids, but they had the low intense signals on T2WI either with moderate-rich or with poor blood supply. Most fibroids had achieved complete ablation, which meant the overall ablation treatment effect was ideal.
- The strategy of focused ultrasound ablation to multiple uterine fibroids is to first treat those posterior fibroids in the far-field of the ultrasound source. This will avoid the interference of the ablation energy by the ablated necrotic fibroids in the near-field of the ultrasound focal region, thus affecting the treatment effect.

4.4.3.10 Case 10

Case Description

The female patient was 42 years old. She had a significant increase in menstrual flow, and the self-administration of Chinese herb medicine did not improve it. The patient had scar diathesis with a wide longitudinal cesarean section scar on the anterior abdominal wall. In the follow-up after focused ultrasound ablation treatment, her menstruation returned to normal.

Pre-Treatment Assessment

MRI showed that a type 0 submucosal fibroid protruded into the uterine cavity and another anterior subserosal fibroid on the left anterior wall of the uterus. They had low signals on T2WI (Fig. 4.184a, b). The contrast-enhanced T1WI showed that these fibroids were of abundant blood supply (Fig. 4.184c–f). The positions of the two fibroids were variable, and their positioning might be difficult to fix during treatment. The subserosal fibroid had a good acoustic pathway, and the positioning of the submucosal fibroid required the intestine to be pushed away. It was predicted that focused ultrasound ablation was feasible.

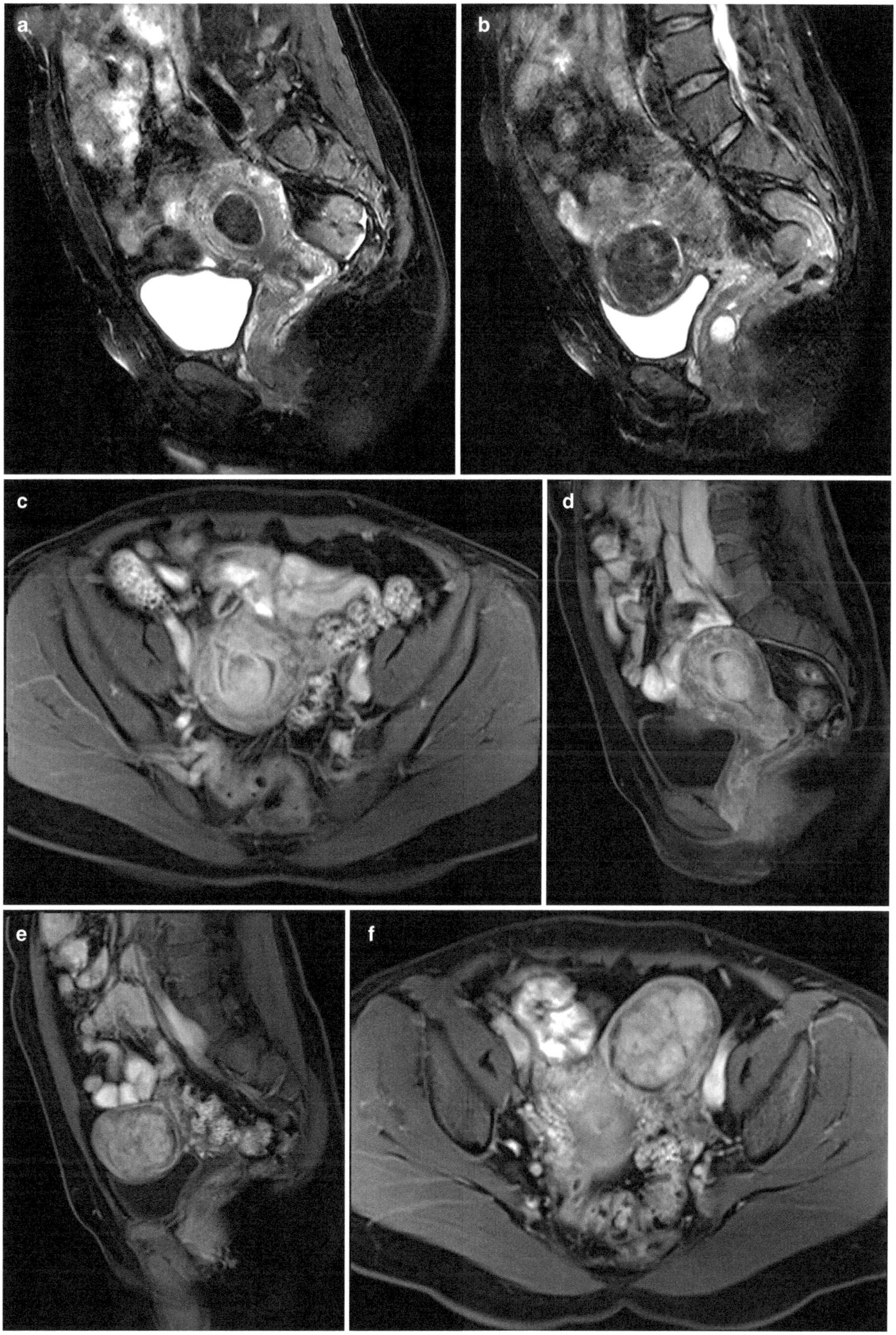

Fig. 4.184 Multiple uterine fibroids before treatment. (**a**, **b**) T2WI_FS sagittal, (**c**) T1WI_FS + C axial, (**d**, **e**) T1WI_FS + C sagittal, (**f**) T1WI_FS + C axial

Treatment Techniques

1. **Focused ultrasound parameters.** Average acoustic power: 277 W, sonication time: 2300 seconds, duration of treatment: 50 minutes, total energy: 659,600 J.
2. **Focused ultrasound ablation techniques.** The submucosal fibroid was treated by focused ultrasound ablation first to improve heavy menstrual flow symptoms. If there were a fertility requirement, it would be necessary to reduce the acoustic power to minimize the damage to the endometrium. During treatment, pay close attention to the patient's reaction to the skin at the scar to avoid skin burns. The treatment of subserosal fibroid needs to fill the bladder and compression with the water balloon to fix the subserosal fibroid's position from movement during the procedure.

Post-Treatment Assessment

1. **MRI evaluation after treatment.** It showed significant edema of the subcutaneous soft tissue and muscle layer at the scar of the anterior abdominal wall (Fig. 4.185a, b). The contrast-enhanced T1WI showed that the NPV ratio of the submucosal and subserosal fibroids exceeded 95% (Fig. 4.185c–f).
2. **MRI follow-up at 6 months after treatment.** The area of subcutaneous soft-tissue edema in the scar of the anterior abdominal wall was significantly reduced. Both submucosal and subserosal fibroids were significantly reduced in size; only some recurrent fibroids were noticed in the residual fibroid edge (Fig. 4.186).

Discussion

- Submucosal fibroids and subserosal fibroids can exist together, while the patient might not be suitable for surgery due to scars. Then the focused ultrasound ablation treatment can be an alternative instead. In focused ultrasound ablation treatment, close attention should be paid to the irradiation interval for skin cooling so that the abdominal wall surface should be cooled in time to avoid skin burns.
- The patient's menstruation returned to normal after the focused ultrasound ablation treatment. Therefore, for patients with scar diathesis, this treatment provides an alternative and non-invasive treatment for subserosal and submucosal fibroids.

4.4.3.11 Case 11

Case Description

The female patient was 49 years old. She had multiple uterine fibroids and increased menstrual flow accompanied by severe anemia.

Pre-Treatment Assessment

MRI showed three uterine fibroids, two intramural fibroids with hypointensity at the anterior and right walls of the uterus, and one larger type II submucosal fibroid with heterogenous hyperintensity at the anterior wall of the uterus on T2WI (Fig. 4.187a). The contrast-enhanced T1WI showed that the two intramural fibroids were of abundant blood supply, and the submucosal fibroid was of moderate blood supply (Fig. 4.187b, c). It was predicted that the submucosal fibroid would be difficult to ablate, and the two intramural fibroids were easy to ablate.

Treatment Techniques

1. **Focused ultrasound parameters.** Average acoustic power: 370 W, sonication time: 2600 seconds, duration of treatment: 157 minutes, total energy: 962,400 J.
2. **Focused ultrasound ablation techniques.** Due to the good acoustic pathway, the acoustic power could be increased to treat the submucosal fibroid while protecting the endometrium.

Post-Treatment Assessment

1. **MRI evaluation after treatment.** The muscle layer of the anterior abdominal wall was significantly edematous (Fig. 4.188a). The contrast-enhanced T1WI showed that the NPV ratio of the multiple fibroids exceeded 90%, and a small amount of residual fibroid remained at the posterior edge of the submucosal fibroid (Fig. 4.188b, c).
2. **MRI follow-up at 1 year after treatment.** All the fibroids shrank significantly in size; especially the submucosal fibroids shrank the most. The remaining part showed some thickening and recurrence with the blood supply restored. The uterus basically returned to normal size (Fig. 4.189).

Discussion

- For the submucosal fibroids with hyperintense signal on T2WI, the acoustic power needs to be increased to achieve a better ablation effect. The follow-up can confirm a positive result.
- Although the NPV ratio of the submucosal fibroid after treatment was greater than 90%, and its volume was reduced after half a year, the fibroid is easy to recur with an abundant blood supply; re-intervention should be recommended.

4.4.3.12 Case 12

Case Description

The female patient was 47 years old. She had multiple uterine fibroids and recently suffered from increased menstrual flow, shortened menstrual cycles, and moderate anemia.

Pre-Treatment Assessment

MRI showed multiple intramural fibroids on the fundus, anterior and right side wall of the uterus with low signals on T2WI (Fig. 4.190a, b), and isointense signals on T1WI (Fig. 4.190c). It was predicted that the fibroids would be relatively easy to ablate.

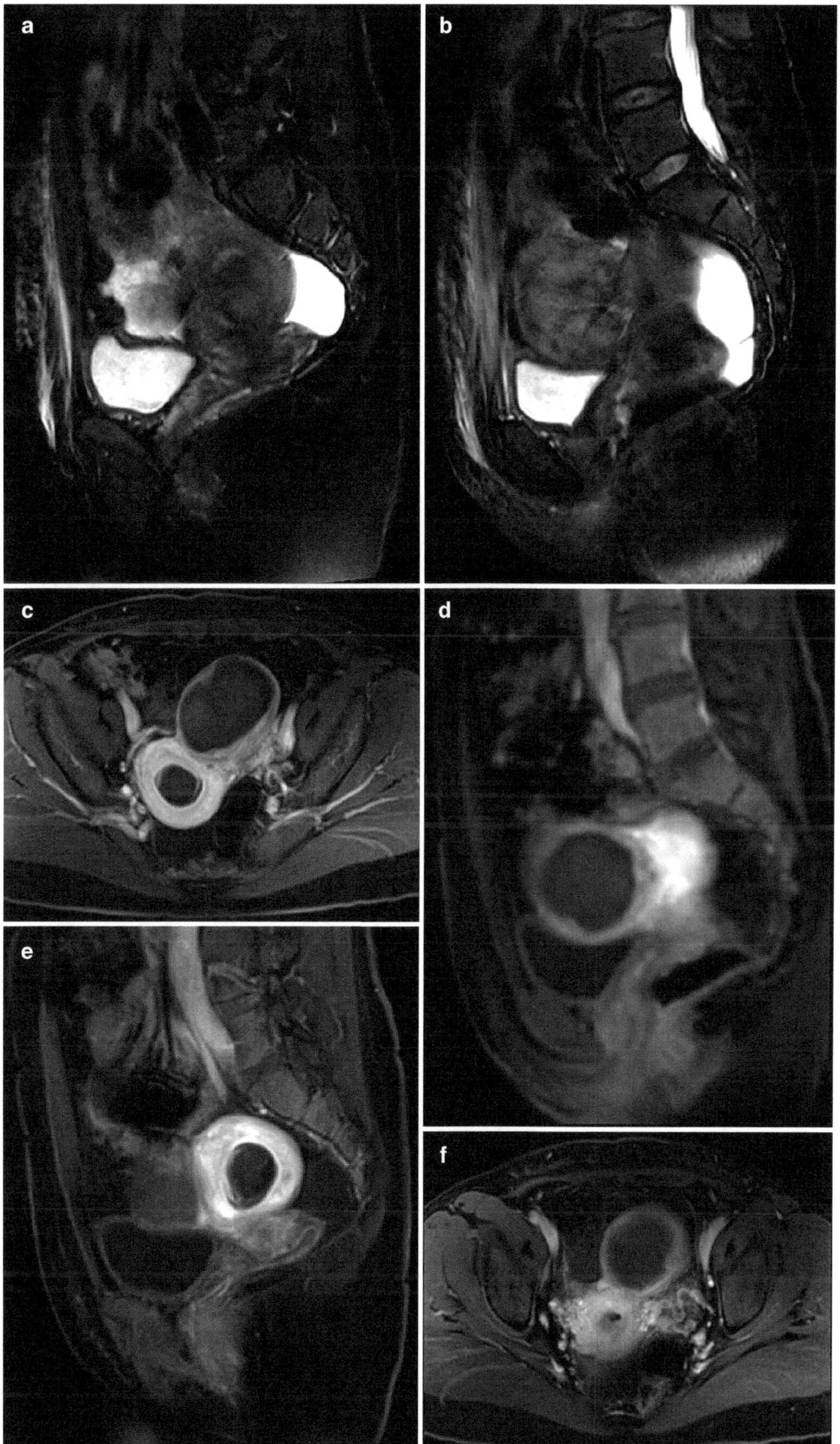

Fig. 4.185 MRI evaluation of multiple uterine fibroids after treatment. (**a**, **b**) T2WI_FS sagittal, (**c**) T1WI_FS + C axial, (**d**, **e**) T1WI_FS + C sagittal, (**f**) T1WI_FS + C axial

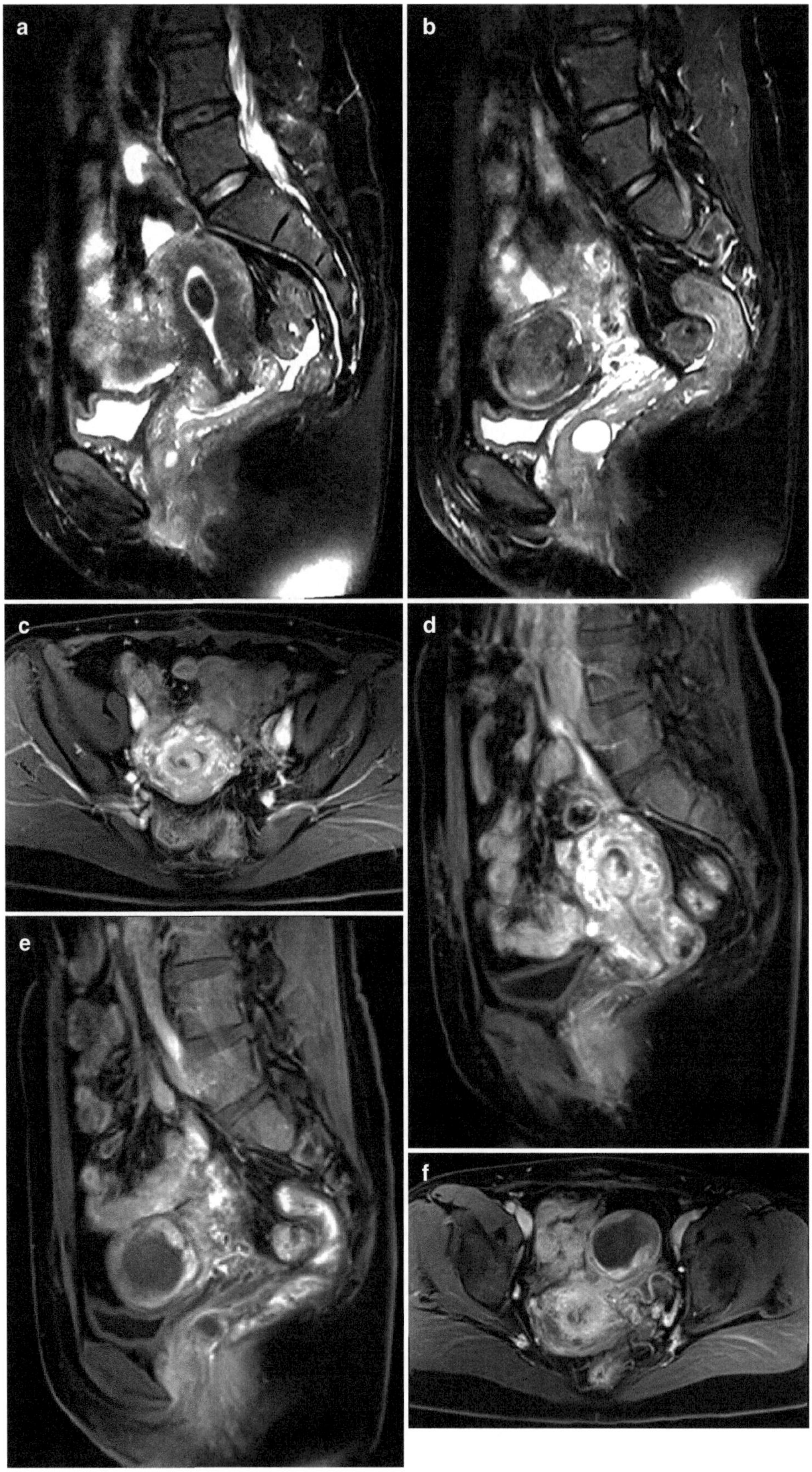

Fig. 4.186 MRI follow-up of multiple uterine fibroids at 6 months after treatment. (**a**, **b**) T2WI_FS sagittal, (**c**) T1WI_FS + C axial, (**d**, **e**) T1WI_FS + C sagittal, (**f**) T1WI_FS + C axial

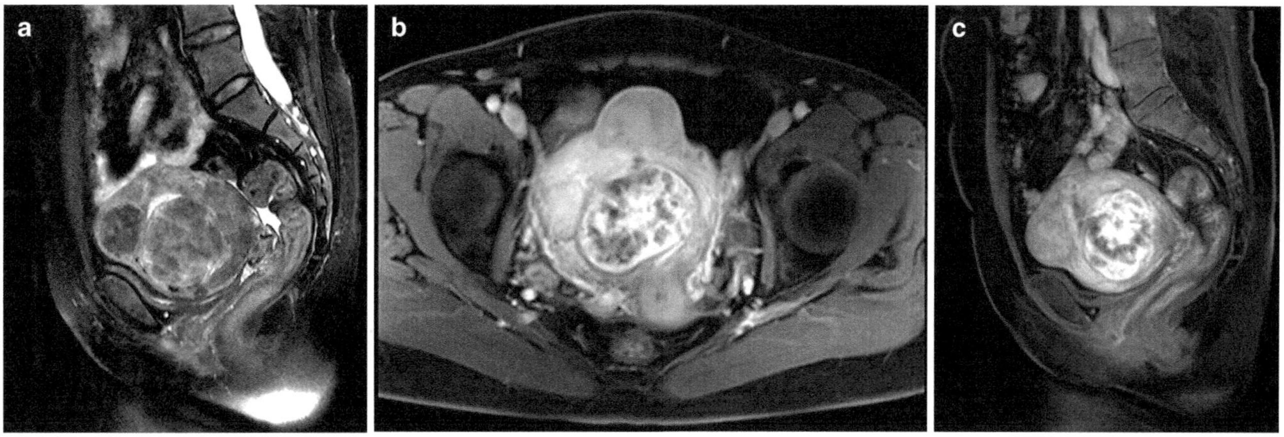

Fig. 4.187 Multiple uterine fibroids before treatment. (**a**) T2WI_FS sagittal, (**b**) T1WI_FS + C axial, (**c**) T1WI_FS + C sagittal

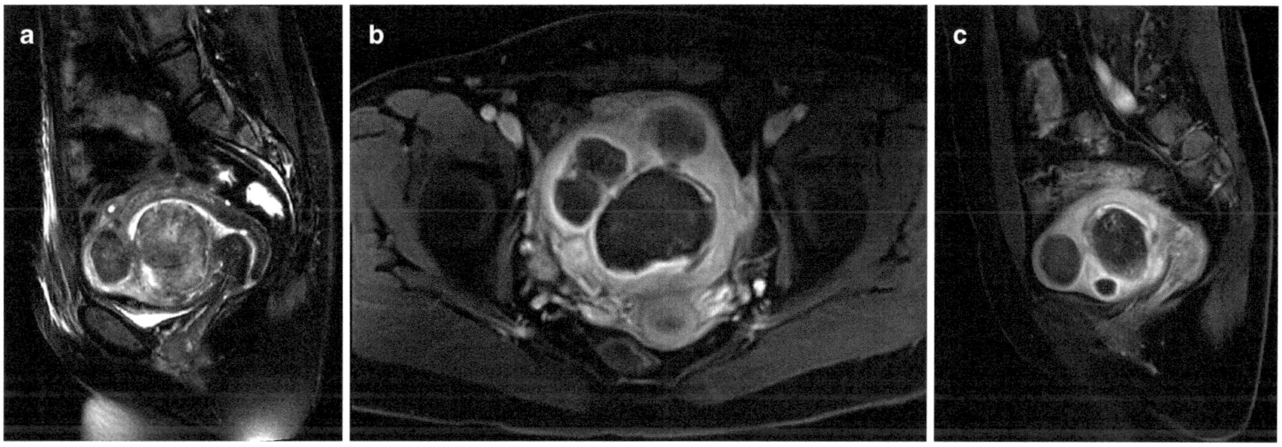

Fig. 4.188 MRI evaluation of multiple uterine fibroids after treatment. (**a**) T2WI_FS sagittal, (**b**) T1WI_FS + C axial, (**c**) T1WI_FS + C sagittal

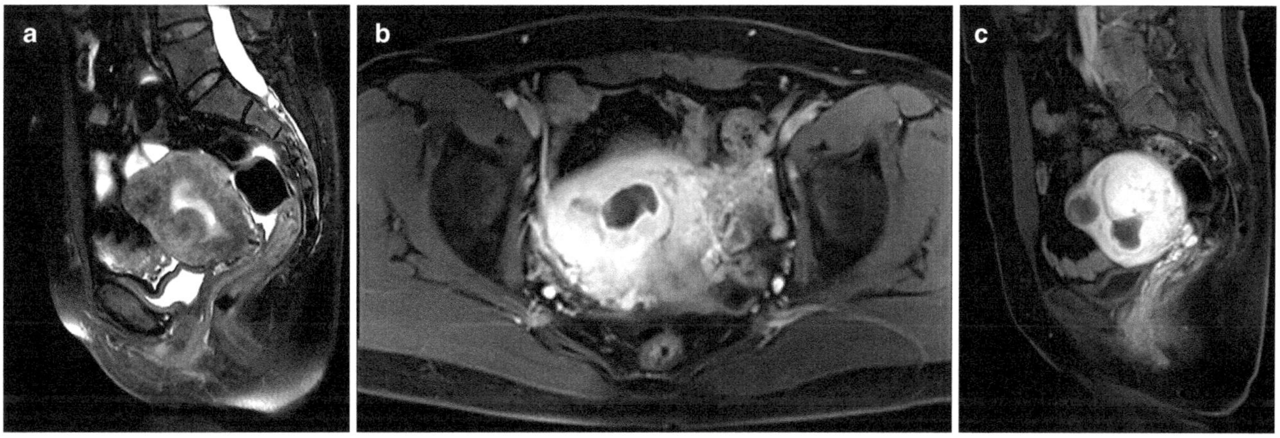

Fig. 4.189 MRI follow-up of multiple uterine fibroids at 1 year after treatment. (**a**) T2WI_FS sagittal, (**b**) T1WI_FS + C axial, (**c**) T1WI_FS + C sagittal

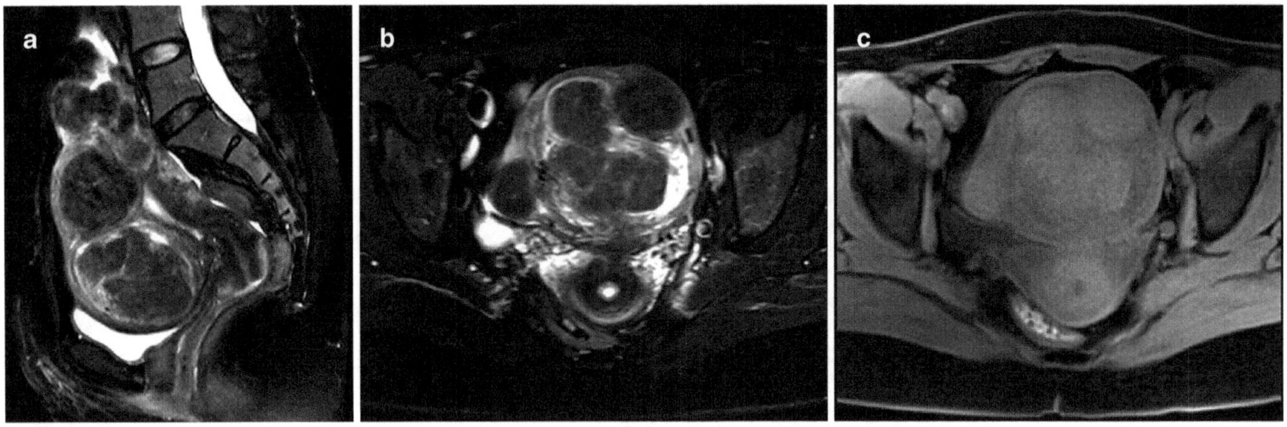

Fig. 4.190 Multiple uterine fibroids before treatment. (**a**) T2WI_FS sagittal, (**b**) T2WI_FS axial, (**c**) T1WI axial

Treatment Techniques

1. **Focused ultrasound parameters.** Average acoustic power: 297 W, sonication time: 3768 seconds, duration of treatment: 167 minutes, total energy: 1119850 J.
2. **Focused ultrasound ablation techniques.** The anterior uterine fibroids are close to the abdominal wall, and the acoustic pathway is good. In contrast, there might be increasing risks of thermal damage to the anterior abdominal wall, paying attention to the cooling time between the ultrasound irradiation.

Post-Treatment Assessment

MRI Evaluation after Treatment The subcutaneous tissue and muscle layer of the periumbilical region of the anterior abdominal wall showed significant edema (Fig. 4.191a). The contrast-enhanced MRI showed that the NPV ratios of these fibroids exceeded 95%. The endometrium and serosa of the uterus were intact (Fig. 4.191b, c).

Discussion

- Fibroids with low signals on T2WI can achieve a good focused ultrasound ablation result.
- For anterior uterine fibroids close to the anterior abdominal wall, it is necessary to pay attention to the diffusion of the heat from the fibroids to cause thermal damage to the abdominal wall.
- In this case, there was severe edema in the subcutaneous soft tissues after treatment because the ultrasonic waves difficultly penetrated the fold umbilicus, resulting in thermal energy deposit. Yet, it was still within a controllable range.

4.4.3.13 Case 13

Case Description

The female patient was 37 years old. She had multiple recurrent fibroids after uterine artery embolization. Her menstruation was prolonged. She felt a dull pain in the right lower abdomen in the past year.

Pre-Treatment Assessment

MRI showed multiple fibroids with low signals were located at the uterus's anterior and right side walls on T2WI (Fig. 4.192). The contrast-enhanced MRI showed that they had poor blood supply from the other clinic. It was predicted that these fibroids would be relatively easy to ablate.

Treatment Techniques

1. **Focused ultrasound parameters.** Average acoustic power: 277 W, sonication time: 3200 seconds, duration of treatment: 134 minutes, total energy: 886,040 J.
2. **Focused ultrasound ablation techniques.** The fibroids were with low intense signals on T2WI. They were adjacent to the left and right ovaries. We should reduce the acoustic power and increase the irradiation time during treatment. The center of the ultrasound focal region should be more than 15 mm away from the edge of the fibroids. The bladder should be fully distended to push the bowel away from the acoustic pathway to avoid damage to the tissue or organs around the fibroids.

Post-Treatment Assessment

MRI Evaluation after Treatment There was mild edema of the muscle layer of the anterior left abdominal wall (Fig. 4.193a, b), and the contrast-enhanced MRI showed that two fibroids had completely ablated and their capsules were intact (Fig. 4.193c–e).

Discussion

- Uterine fibroids recurring after uterine artery embolization are generally unsuitable for re-arterial embolization. Focused ultrasound ablation is the treatment of choice and can avoid affecting ovarian function.

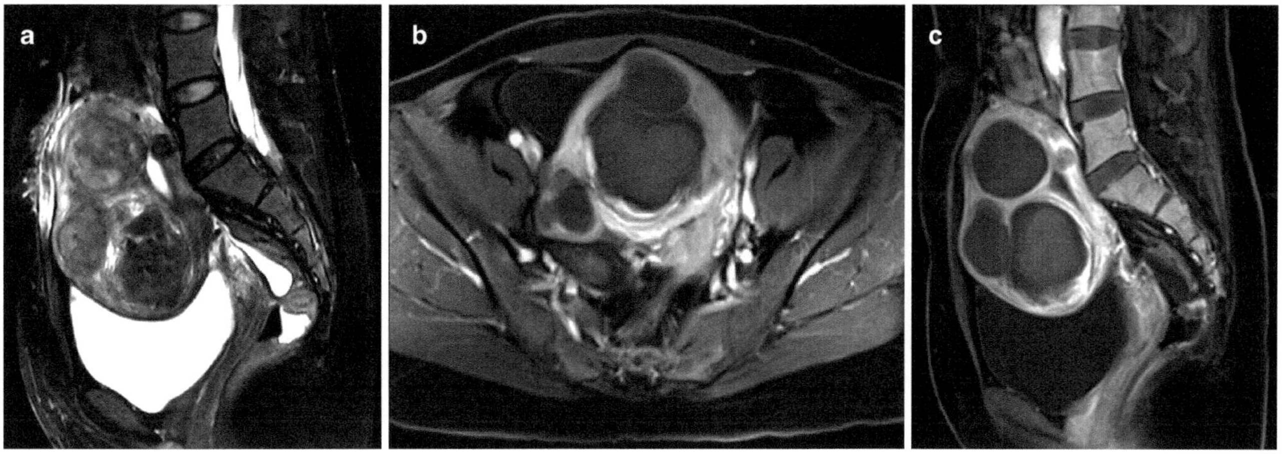

Fig. 4.191 MRI evaluation of multiple uterine fibroids after treatment. (**a**) T2WI_FS sagittal, (**b**) T1WI_FS + C axial, (**c**) T1WI_FS + C sagittal

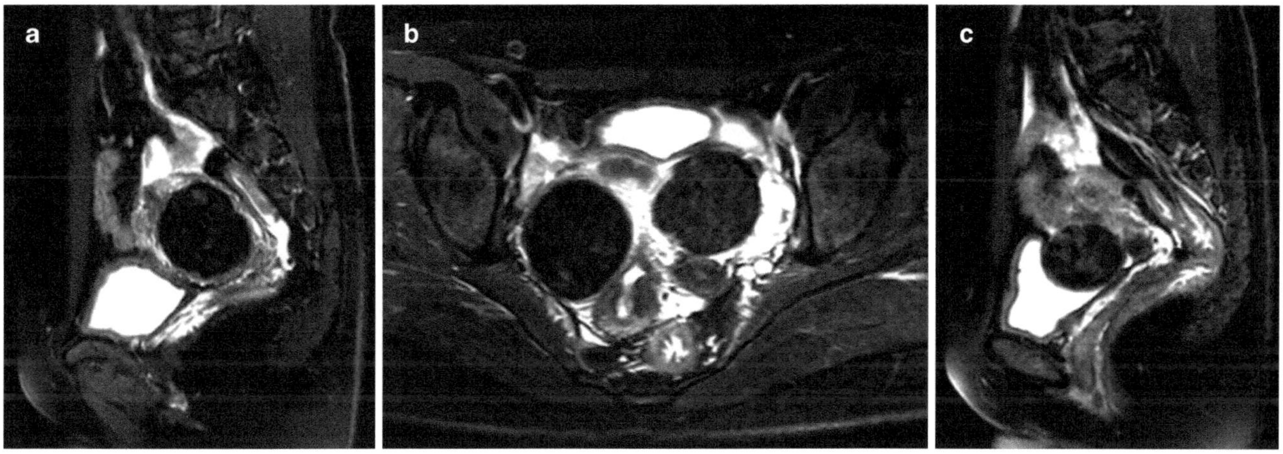

Fig. 4.192 Multiple uterine fibroids before treatment. (**a**) T2WI_FS sagittal, (**b**) T2WI_FS axial, (**c**) T2WI_FS sagittal

4.4.4 Focused Ultrasound Ablation for Treatment of Diffuse Uterine Leiomyomatosis (DUL)

4.4.4.1 Case 1

Case Description

The female patient was 42 years old. She had laparoscopic myomectomy twice. Her menstrual periods were prolonged in the past 2 years, with heavy menstrual flow and blood clots, accompanied by lower abdominal pain, lower back pain, urinary frequency, and anemia. The corresponding symptoms disappeared after the focused ultrasound ablation treatment.

Pre-Treatment Assessment

MRI showed that multiple fibroids of varying sizes spread all over the entire uterus, resulting in a huge uterine volume. The larger fibroids had low signals, and most of the smaller fibroids had isointense signals on T2WI (Fig. 4.194a). The contrast-enhanced MRI showed that most fibroids had abundant blood supply (Fig. 4.194b, c). It was predicted that these fibroids were difficult to ablate. It was planned for the patient to have two times of focused ultrasound ablation treatments 3 months apart.

Treatment Techniques

1. Focused ultrasound parameters
   (a) **The first treatment parameters.** Average acoustic power: 355 W, sonication time: 4438 seconds, duration of treatment: 202 minutes, total energy: 1,573,890 J.
   (b) **The second treatment parameter.** Average acoustic power: 347 W, sonication time: 4020 seconds, duration of treatment: 192 minutes, total energy: 1,393,270 J.
2. **Focused ultrasound ablation techniques.** Two times of the focused ultrasound ablation treatments with an interval of 3 months were used, during which gonadotropin-releasing hormone agonist (GnRH-a) was given three times with an interval of 28 days.

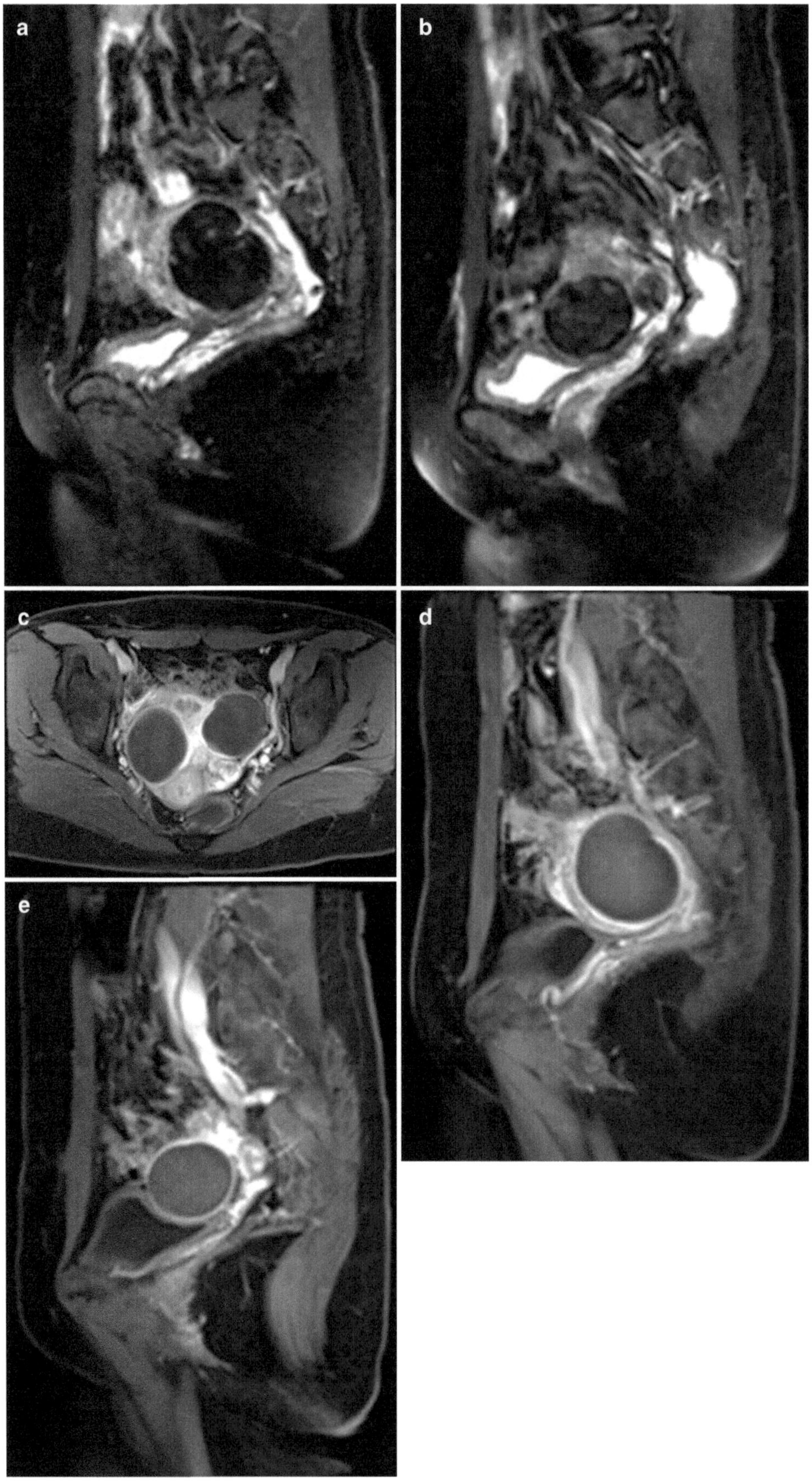

Fig. 4.193 MRI evaluation of multiple uterine fibroids after treatment. (**a**, **b**) T2WI_FS sagittal, (**c**) T1WI_FS + C axial, (**d**, **e**) T1WI_FS + C sagittal

Post-Treatment Assessment

1. **MRI evaluation after the first treatment** It showed edema of the subcutaneous soft tissue and muscle layer of the anterior abdominal wall. The contrast-enhanced MRI showed that some parts of the fibroids were ablated (Fig. 4.195).
2. **MRI evaluation after the second treatment.** Compared with the first treatment, the uterine size was significantly reduced. The anterior abdominal wall had significant edema (Fig. 4.196a). The contrast-enhanced MRI showed that only small parts of the fibroids were ablated (Fig. 4.196b, c).

Discussion

- If the first focused ultrasound ablation is ineffective, GnRH-a can be given as adjuvant treatment, and focused ultrasound ablation can be performed again after 3 months. After treatment, take low-dose mifepristone (2.5 mg/d) for 3–6 months. The principle of palliative treatment is to improve the symptoms of anemia and reduce the size of the uterus and fibroids.

4.4.4.2 Case 2

Case Description

The female patient was 31 years old. She had multiple uterine fibroids which had undergone laparoscopic and hysteroscopic removal, respectively, and they recurred quickly after surgery. She complained of increased menstrual flow with significant dysmenorrhea and moderate anemia. Two months after the MRI diagnosis of diffuse uterine leiomyomatosis, she underwent focused ultrasound ablation, then took oral low-dose (2.5 mg/d) mifepristone for 6 months. Nine months later, she got pregnant with twins. One of the fetuses stopped at the third month of pregnancy, and she eventually gave birth to a healthy full-term girl. At the 4-year follow-up after ultrasound ablation, the ultrasound examination demon-

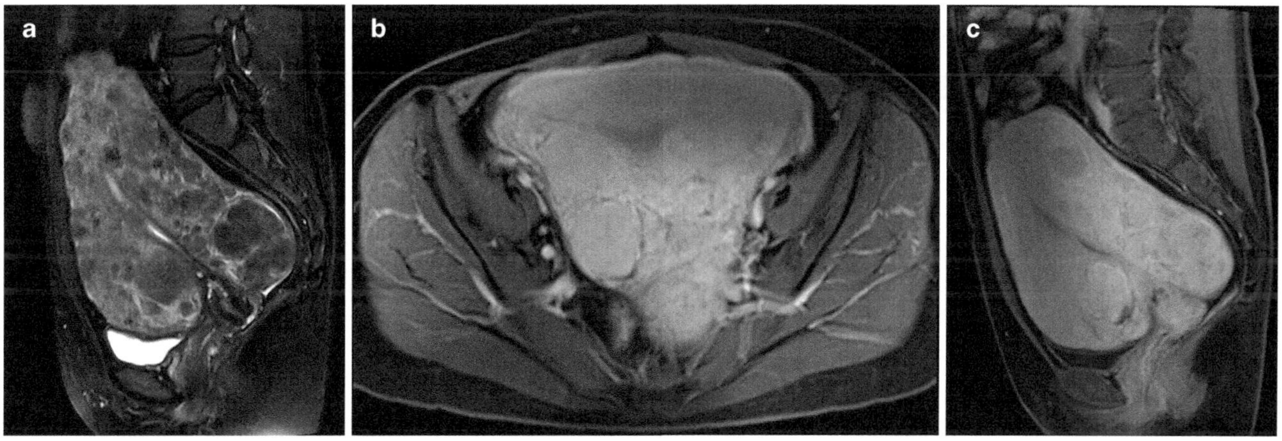

Fig. 4.194 Diffuse uterine leiomyomatosis before treatment. (**a**) T2WI_FS sagittal, (**b**) T1WI_FS + C axial, (**c**) T1WI_FS + C sagittal

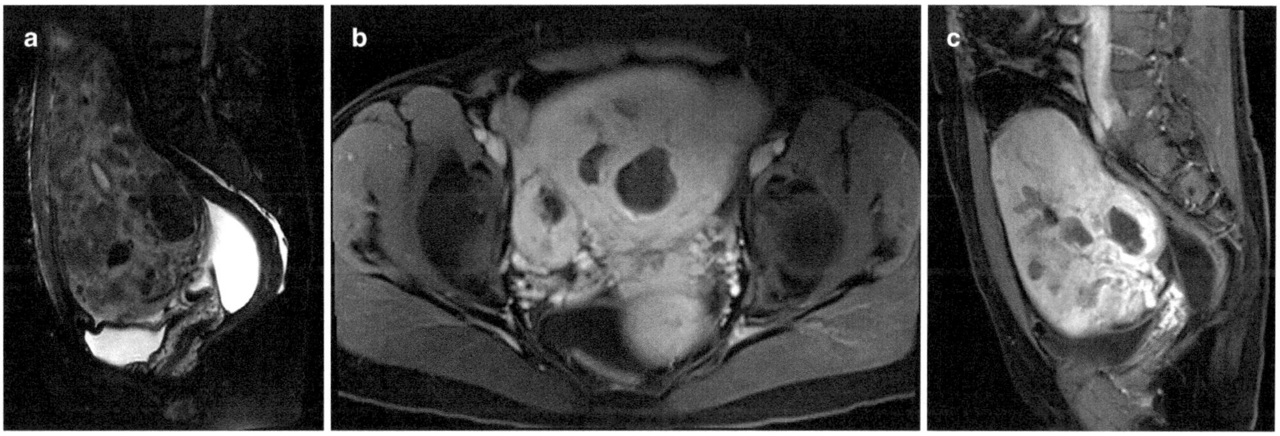

Fig. 4.195 MRI evaluation of diffuse uterine leiomyomatosis after the first treatment. (**a**) T2WI_FS sagittal, (**b**) T1WI_FS + C axial, (**c**) T1WI_FS + C sagittal

strated the uterus volume was 58 mm × 48 mm × 50 mm in normal size.

Pre-Treatment Assessment

MRI showed diffuse fibroids throughout the whole uterus; they are of diameter ≤ 30 mm. Some fibroids showed low signals, and others showed hyperintense signals on T2WI (Fig. 4.197a). The contrast-enhanced MRI showed the coexistence of moderate and poor blood. The latter were mainly small fibroids in the anterior uterine wall (Fig. 4.197b, c). Since the uterine volume significantly increased compared to that 2 months ago, these anterior wall fibroids of the giant uterus were relatively easy to ablate, which would be a therapeutic priority.

Treatment Techniques

1. **Focused ultrasound parameters.** Average acoustic power: 210 W, sonication time: 5196 seconds, duration of treatment: 165 minutes, total energy: 1, 090,080 J.
2. **Focused ultrasound ablation techniques.** In this case, there were widespread small fibroids in the uterus. We used lower acoustic power and long sonication time to increase the effect by increasing the irradiation energy per unit volume during treatment.

Post-Treatment Assessment

1. **MRI evaluation after treatment.** There was obvious edema in the anterior abdominal wall's subcutaneous tissue and muscle, and the signal intensity of the majority of fibroids slightly increased on T2WI (Fig. 4.198a). The contrast-enhanced MRI showed that most of the fibroids were ablated as non-perfusion areas, mainly in the anterior wall of the uterus (Fig. 4.198b, c).
2. **MRI follow-up at 6 months after treatment.** The size of the uterus was significantly reduced, and the volumes and number of the anterior fibroids were reduced (Fig. 4.199).

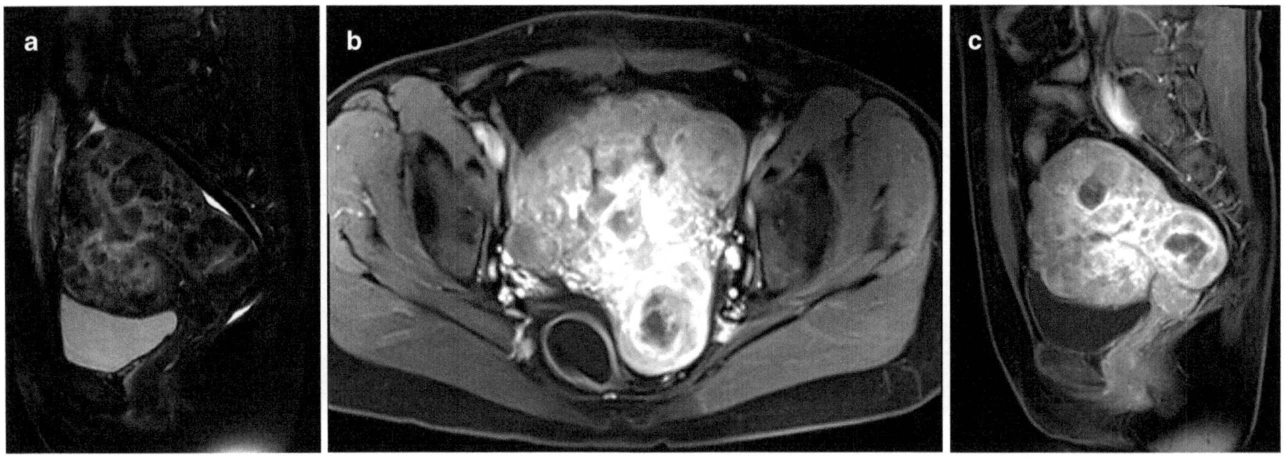

Fig. 4.196 MRI evaluation of diffuse uterine leiomyomatosis after the second treatment. (**a**) T2WI_FS sagittal, (**b**) T1WI_FS + C axial, (**c**) T1WI_FS + C sagittal

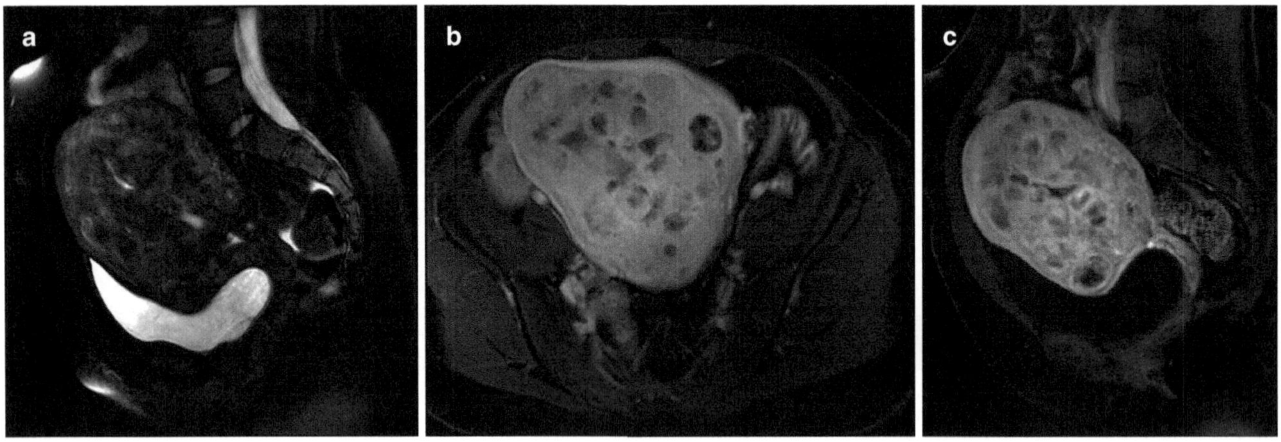

Fig. 4.197 Diffuse uterine leiomyomatosis before treatment. (**a**) T2WI_FS sagittal, (**b**) T1WI_FS + C axial, (**c**) T1WI_FS + C sagittal

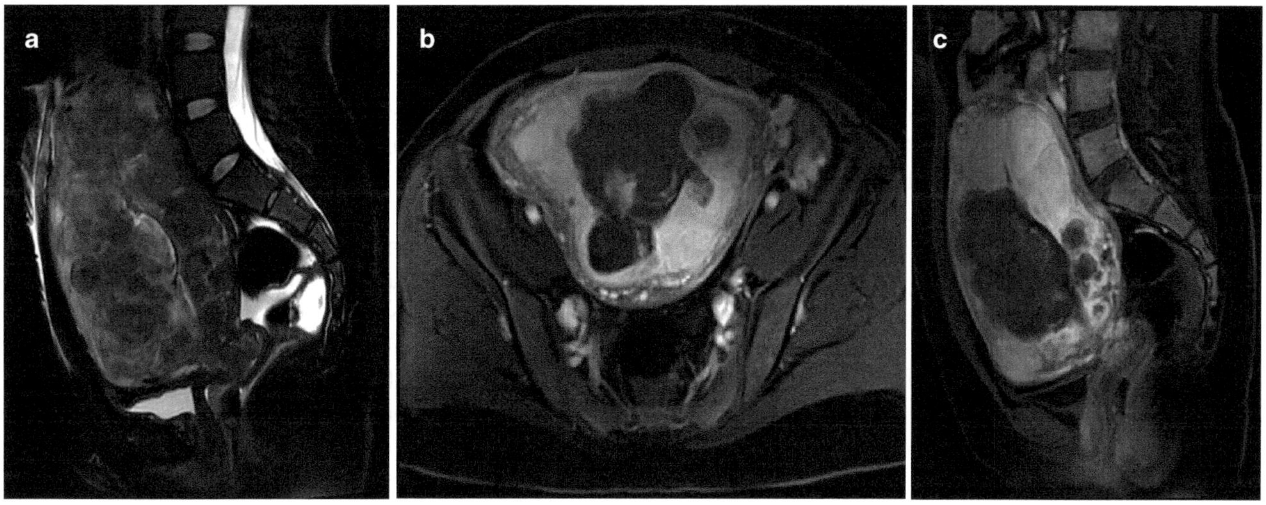

Fig. 4.198 MRI evaluation of diffuse uterine leiomyomatosis after treatment. (**a**) T2WI_FS sagittal, (**b**) T1WI_FS + C axial, (**c**) T1WI_FS + C sagittal

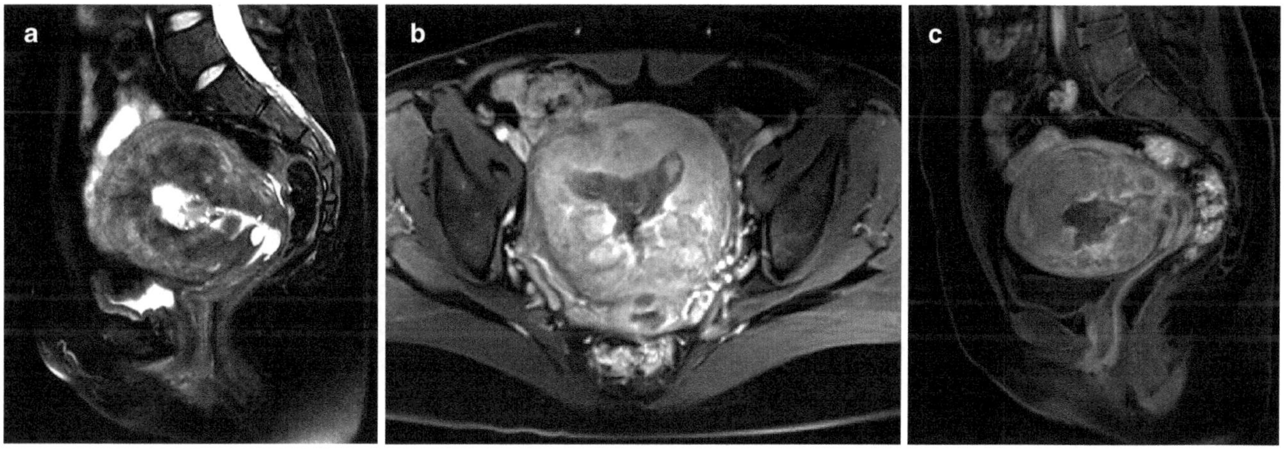

Fig. 4.199 MRI follow-up of diffuse uterine leiomyomatosis at 6 months after treatment. (**a**) T2WI_FS sagittal, (**b**) T1WI_FS + C axial, (**c**) T1WI_FS + C sagittal

3. **MRI follow-up 9 months after treatment.** The uterus gradually returned to normal looking, and the diffuse distribution of fibroids was significantly reduced. There appeared to have small submucosal fibroids with pedicles on the anterior uterine wall; they should be removed by hysteroscopic resection (Fig. 4.200).

Discussion

- After focused ultrasound ablation treatment, this patient took low-dose mifepristone (1.25–2.5 mg/d) orally for 6 months, and the symptoms of anemia were significantly improved. After mifepristone was stopped for 3 months, menstruation returned to normal, and at that time, an MRI examination showed that the uterus returned to normal size and shape (Fig. 4.200). Basically, focused ultrasound ablation therapy can be used with oral low-dose mifepristone to treat diffuse uterine leiomyomatosis.
- In the case of diffuse uterine leiomyomatosis, hundreds of fibroids were spread all over the uterus, inducing its anatomical and endometrial receptivity changes, which could cause infertility or miscarriage. The focused ultrasound ablation might be a therapeutic method to cure diffuse uterine leiomyomatosis to improve fertility and pregnancy.

4.4.4.3 Case 3

Case Description

The female patient was 34 years old. She had dysmenorrhea, heavy and inexhaustible menstruation, backache, frequent urination, and anemia. A laparoscopic myomectomy was performed 2 years ago, and fibroids recurred. The dysmenorrhea was relieved after focused ultrasound ablation treatment, in addition, the menstrual flow returned to normal, and anemia improved.

Pre-Treatment Assessment

MRI showed that the uterus had diffused multiple fibroids of varying sizes, partially fused, with unclear borders. Most fibroids showed inhomogeneous low signals on T2WI and isointense signals on T1WI (Fig. 4.201). There was a clear acoustic pathway. It was predicted that these fibroids could be suitable for focused ultrasound ablation.

Treatment Techniques

1. **Focused ultrasound parameters.** Average acoustic power: 400 W, sonication time: 4005 seconds, duration of treatment: 145 minutes, total energy: 1,600,900 J.
2. **Focused ultrasound ablation techniques.** The uterus had diffuse multiple fibroids, and the response to focused ultrasound ablation treatment would vary greatly. The treatment was mainly for fibroids that respond quickly to ablation. High acoustic power and irradiation energy were required to ablate these fibroids. GnRH-a (every 4 weeks) was given for the first 3 months after treatment, and low-dose mifepristone (2.5 mg/d) was given for the last 3 months.

Post-Treatment Assessment

1. **MRI evaluation after treatment.** The subcutaneous tissue and muscle layer of the anterior abdominal wall were significantly edematous (Fig. 4.202a). The contrast-enhanced T1WI showed that the majority of the uterine fibroids were completely ablated. The anterior wall fibroids had a better ablation effect. The endometrium at the anterior wall was partially ablated (Fig. 4.202b, c).

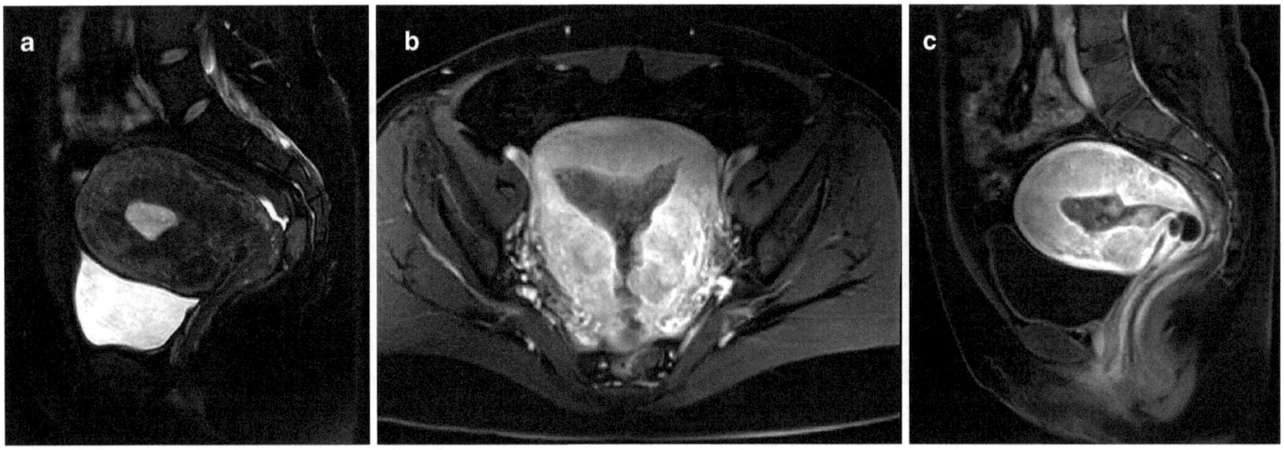

Fig. 4.200 MRI follow-up of diffuse uterine leiomyomatosis at 9 months after treatment. (**a**) T2WI_FS sagittal, (**b**) T1WI_FS + C axial, (**c**) T1WI_FS + C sagittal

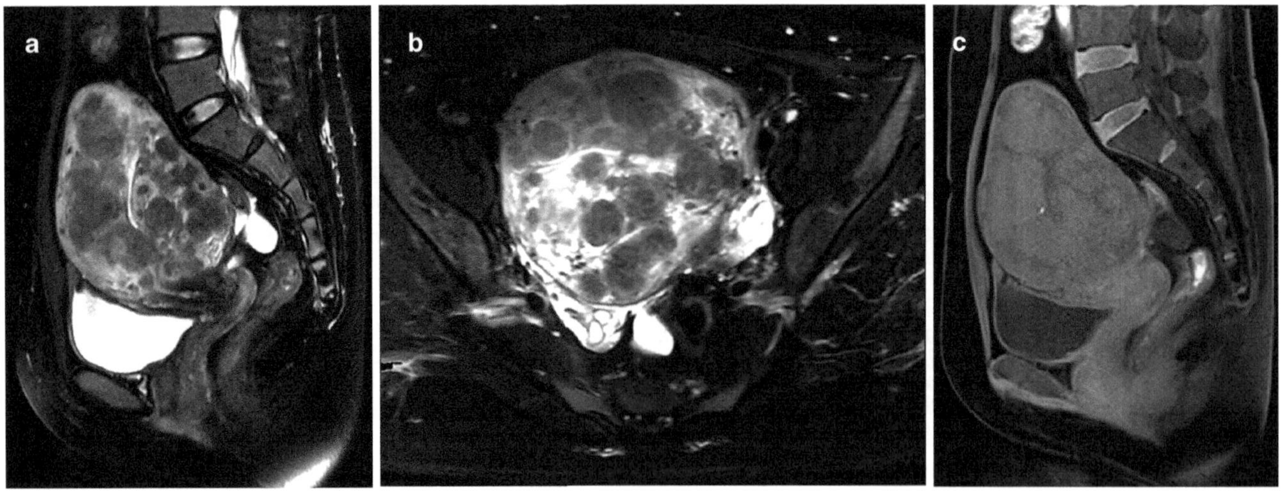

Fig. 4.201 Diffuse uterine leiomyomatosis before the first treatment. (**a**) T2WI_FS sagittal, (**b**) T2WI_FS axial, (**c**) T1WI axial

2. **MRI follow-up at 3 months after treatment.** The size of the uterus was significantly reduced. Some fibroids of the anterior wall were partially discharged. The edema of the anterior abdominal wall disappeared (Fig. 4.203).
3. **MRI follow-up at 6 months after treatment.** Most fibroids shrank or disappeared. The uterus shrank significantly, and its shape returned to normal (Fig. 4.204).

Discussion

- The focused ultrasound ablation treatment strategy for uterine myomatosis is to cover the fibroids of the whole uterus with ultrasound irradiation. Although some leiomyomas did not reach non-perfusion, representing coagulative necrosis, better therapeutic efficacy can be achieved by supplemented therapy with anti-estrogen drugs.
- In the follow-up of this case, MRI showed that some uterine fibroids were significantly reduced or disappeared, and the uterine shape gradually returned to normal. On the whole, the long-term efficacy for treating uterine myomatosis needs further observation.

4.4.5 Focused Ultrasound Ablation for Treatment of Uterine Giant Fibroids

4.4.5.1 Case 1

Case Description

The female patient was 35 years old. In the past 2–3 months, the menstrual cycle was prolonged, with a reduced amount of menstruation. The abdomen was enlarged as if it was about 7 months of pregnancy.

Pre-Treatment Assessment

MRI showed a huge fibroid with a length of about 198 mm on the right anterior wall of the uterus. It showed low signals

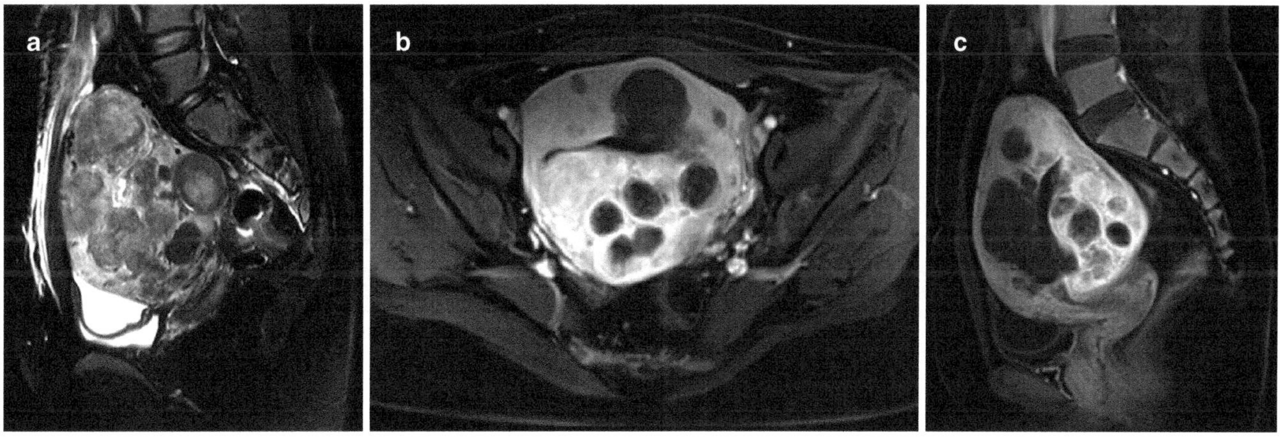

Fig. 4.202 MRI evaluation of diffuse uterine leiomyomatosis after the first treatment. (**a**) T2WI_FS sagittal, (**b**) T1WI_FS + C axial, (**c**) T1WI_FS + C sagittal

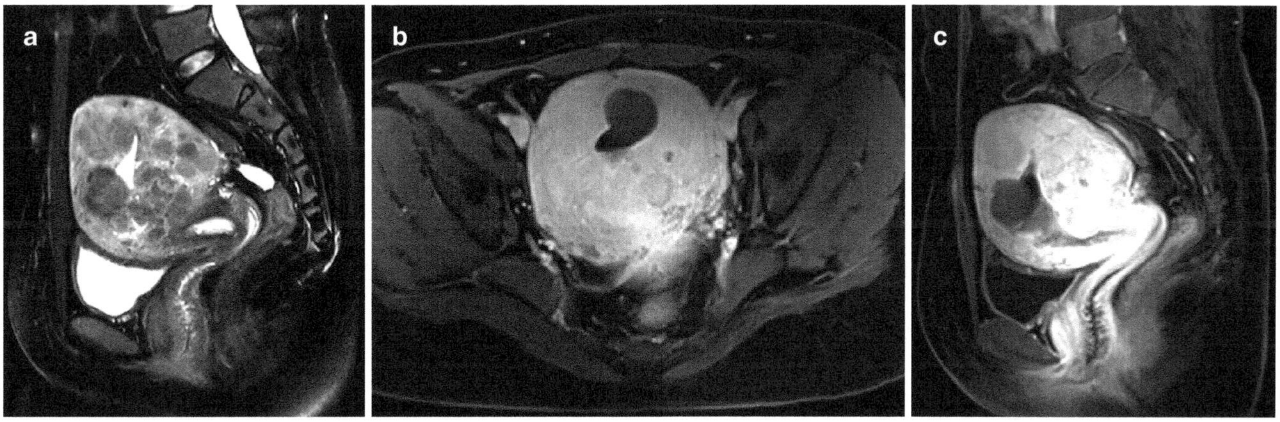

Fig. 4.203 MRI follow-up of diffuse uterine leiomyomatosis at 3 months after the first treatment. (**a**) T2WI_FS sagittal, (**b**) T1WI_FS + C axial, (**c**) T1WI_FS + C sagittal

mixed with a few hyperintense signals on T2WI (Fig. 4.205a). The contrast-enhanced T1WI showed that the fibroid was of moderate blood supply (Fig. 4.205b, c), and they had a good acoustic pathway. It was predicted that the fibroid could be ablated.

Treatment Techniques

1. **Focused ultrasound parameters.** Average acoustic power: 398 W, sonication time: 2614 seconds, duration of treatment: 168 minutes, total energy: 1,040,800 J.
2. **Focused ultrasound ablation techniques.** The posterior edge of the fibroid was close to the lumbosacral spine, and the front was adjacent to the abdominal wall. During the ablation treatment, care must be taken to prevent damage to the lumbar-sacral nerves and bones, anterior abdominal wall, and pelvic soft tissues. At the same time, allow sufficient cooling time in between the irradiation interval to avoid heat accumulation.

Post-Treatment Assessment

MRI Evaluation after Treatment MRI showed visible edema in the anterior abdominal wall and muscle layer (Fig. 4.206a). The contrast-enhanced T1WI showed that the NPV ratio of the fibroids was about 98%. The pseudocapsule of the fibroid was intact, with only a few residuals at its margins (Fig. 4.206b, c).

Discussion

- The normal uterine wall surrounding a huge uterine fibroid is squeezed. Therefore, the effect of focused ultrasound ablation of a giant fibroid does not depend on the size but on its tissue characteristics and texture. The supplying blood vessels to the fibroid are also squeezed or stretched by the large fibroid, which makes their blood supply relatively poor.
- During or after treatment, its heat dissipation capacity is relatively poor. Therefore, precautions must allow the treated fibroid to cool down after ablation.

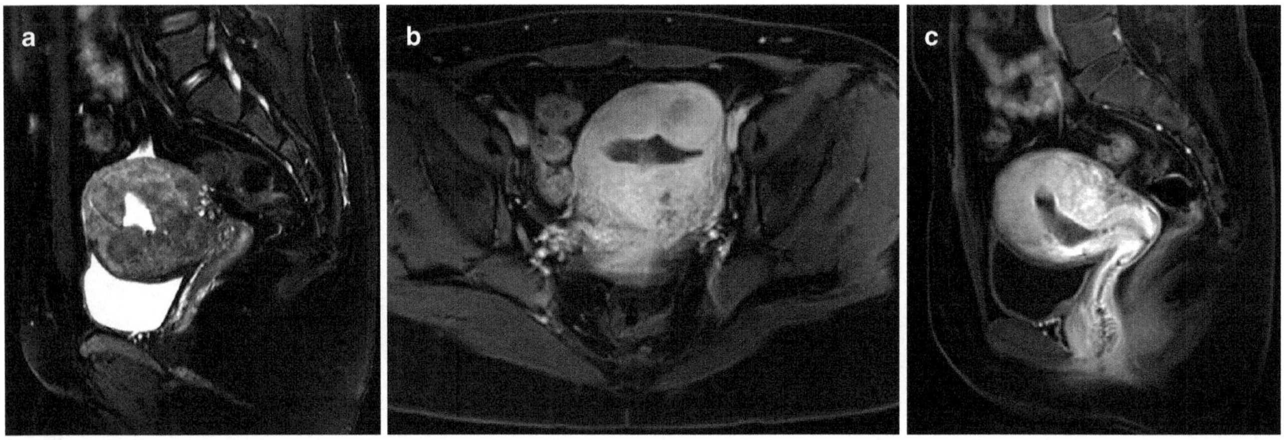

Fig. 4.204 MRI follow-up of diffuse uterine leiomyomatosis at 6 months after the second treatment. (**a**) T2WI_FS sagittal, (**b**) T1WI_FS + C axial, (**c**) T1WI_FS + C sagittal

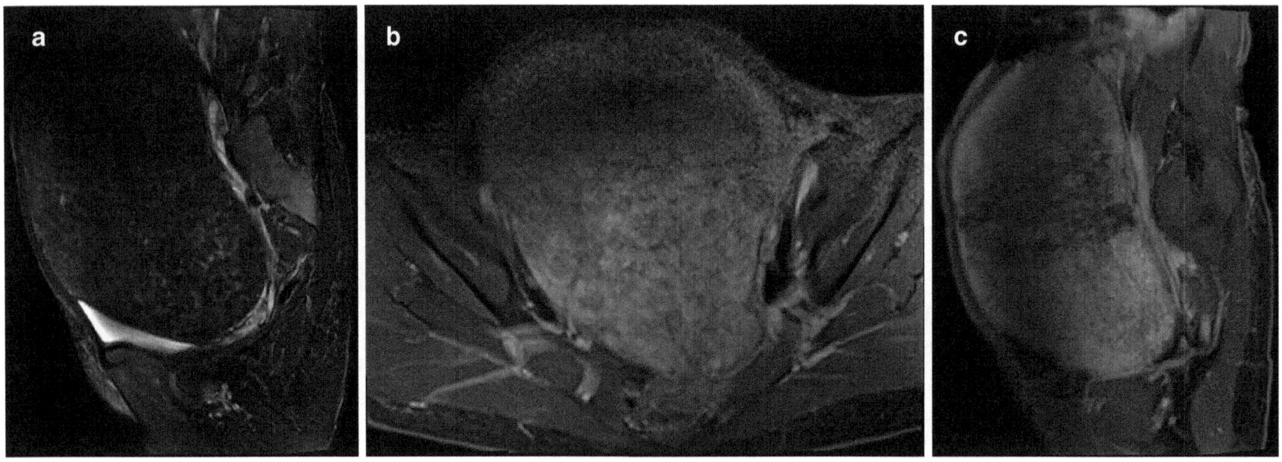

Fig. 4.205 Uterine giant fibroids before treatment. (**a**) T2WI_FS sagittal, (**b**) T1WI_FS + C axial, (**c**) T1WI_FS + C sagittal

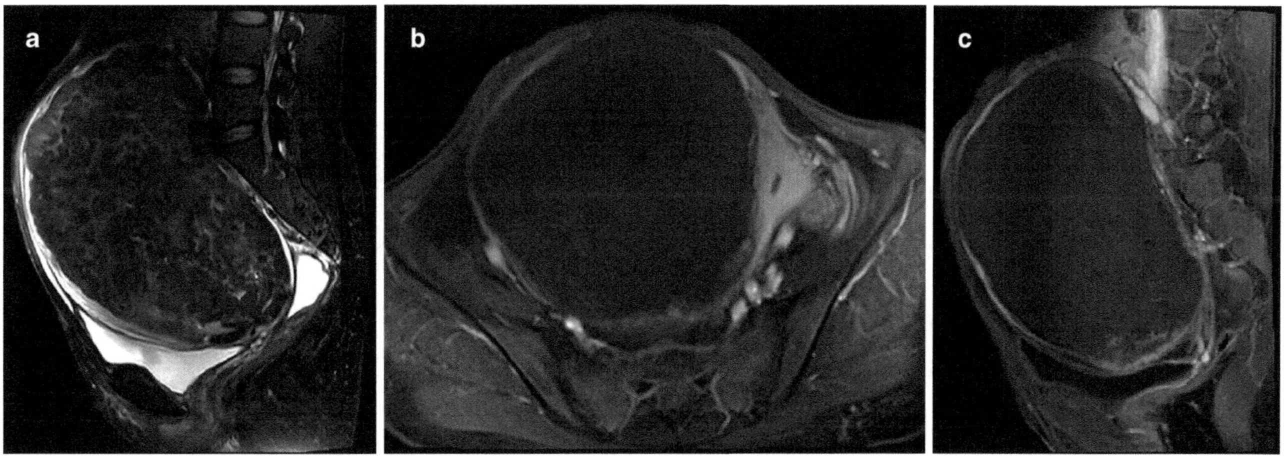

Fig. 4.206 MRI evaluation of uterine giant fibroids immediately after treatment. (**a**) T2WI_FS sagittal, (**b**) T1WI_FS + C axial, (**c**) T1WI_FS + C sagittal

- Encourage patients to change their positions after treatment to avoid prolonged supine positions causing compression and heat damage to the sacral nerve plexus.

4.4.5.2 Case 2

Case Description

The female patient was 37 years old. She had heavy menstrual flow, blood clots, and moderate anemia accompanied by urinary frequency and urgency. A previous cesarean section was performed with an axial scar on the lower abdominal wall. After focused ultrasound ablation treatment, she took low-dose mifepristone (2.5 mg/d) orally for 3 months.

Pre-Treatment Assessment

MRI showed that a huge fibroid with a length of about 179 mm in the anterior wall of the uterus had heterogenous hyperintense signals on T2WI and the isointense signals on T1WI (Fig. 4.207a, b). The contrast-enhanced T1WI showed that the fibroid had a poor blood supply, and its boundary with the surrounding tissues was clear (Fig. 4.207c, d). It was predicted that the fibroid could be ablated with focused ultrasound.

Treatment Techniques

1. **Focused ultrasound parameters.** Average acoustic power: 351 W, sonication time: 3270 seconds, duration of treatment: 188 minutes, total energy: 1,147,620 J.
2. **Focused ultrasound ablation techniques.** The giant fibroids of the anterior uterine wall had a good acoustic pathway. The completion of ablation treatment in one session required more acoustic energy, but there was a cesarean section scar on the lower abdominal wall. In order to avoid or reduce thermal damage to the skin and subcutaneous soft tissue of the anterior abdominal wall, a sufficient cooling interval was required during the procedure.

Post-Treatment Assessment

1. **MRI evaluation after treatment.** It showed significant edema of the subcutaneous tissue and muscle layer of the abdominal wall (Fig. 4.208a). The contrast-enhanced T1WI showed that the NPV ratio of the fibroids was about 95%, with a little residue on the edge (Fig. 4.208b, c). The T1WI scan showed high signals of hemorrhagic necrosis in the ablation focal area (Fig. 4.208d).
2. **MRI follow-up at 8 months after treatment.** The volume of the huge uterine fibroid was significantly reduced without the residual recurrence, and the edema of the anterior abdominal wall disappeared (Fig. 4.209).

Discussion

- The indications for focused ultrasound ablation treatment of uterine fibroids are the same as surgical treatment, so in this case, the patient with huge uterine fibroids can complete the focused ultrasound ablation treatment.
- The contraindications of focused ultrasound ablation for the treatment of uterine fibroids are as follows: (1) fibroids without a safe acoustic pathway or without an effective acoustic pathway; (2) fibroids that the ultrasound focal regions cannot effectively cover; (3) fibroids combined with a history of collagen connective tissue diseases; (4) acute or subacute infection in the pelvic or reproductive tract; (5) combined with non-benign lesions of the uterus and appendages; (6) patients who cannot lie prone for 1 h; (7) when there is skin ulceration or infection over the treatment area; (8) patients who have received more than 45 Gy of radiation therapy on the skin of the relevant area; (9) patients with vital organ failure; (10) patients with severe coagulopathy.

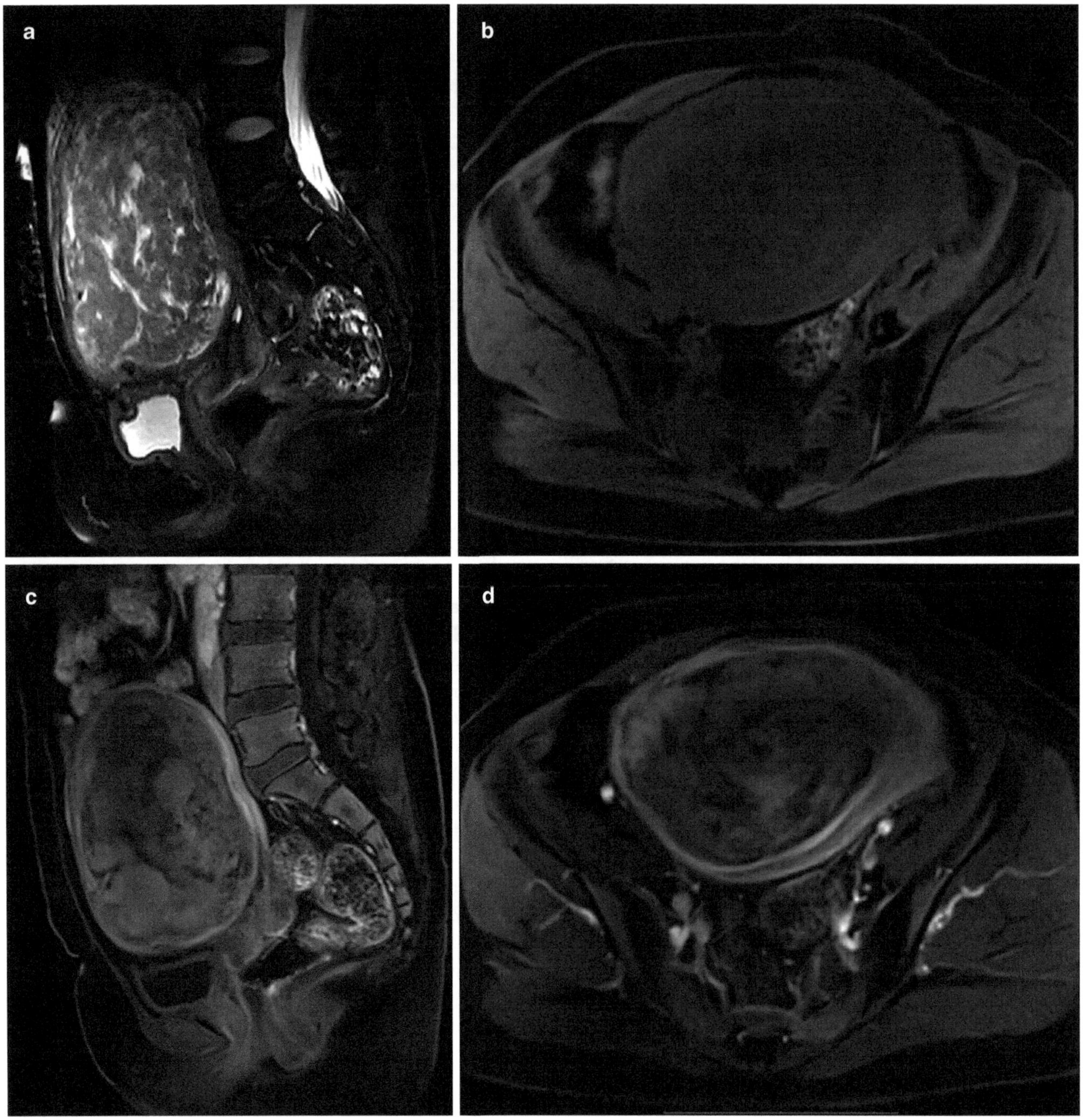

Fig. 4.207 Uterine giant fibroid before treatment. (**a**) T2WI_FS sagittal, (**b**) T1WI axial, (**c**) T1WI_FS + C sagittal, (**d**) T1WI_FS + C axial

4.4.5.3 Case 3

Case Description

The female patient was 49 years old. She had a huge uterine fibroid as large as 5 months of pregnancy. She presented with symptoms of pelvic compression for more than 5 years. On follow-up after focused ultrasound ablation treatment, the patient's uterine size had significantly reduced, and her clinical symptoms improved significantly.

Pre-Treatment Assessment

MRI showed a giant fibroid with a length of about 189 mm in the anterior wall of the uterus, and the fibroid had slightly homogenous hyperintensity on T2WI (Fig. 4.210a). The contrast-enhanced T1WI showed that the fibroid had an abundant blood supply (Fig. 4.210b). Due to MRI characteristics and the huge size of the fibroid, focused ultrasound ablation treatment was planned to perform twice, with an interval of 3 months.

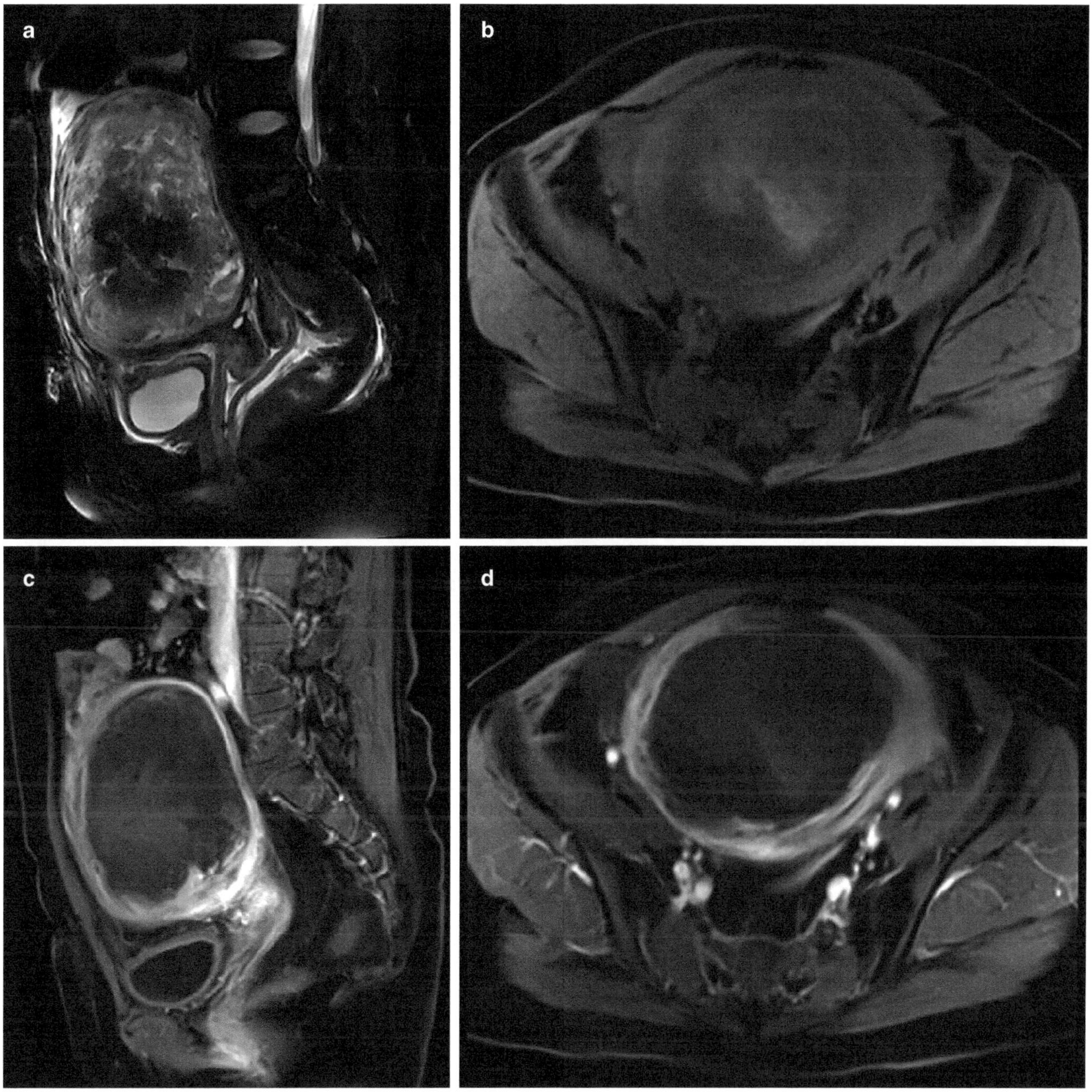

Fig. 4.208 MRI evaluation of uterine giant fibroids after treatment. (**a**) T2WI_FS sagittal, (**b**) T1WI axial, (**c**) T1WI_FS + C sagittal, (**d**) T1WI_FS + C axial

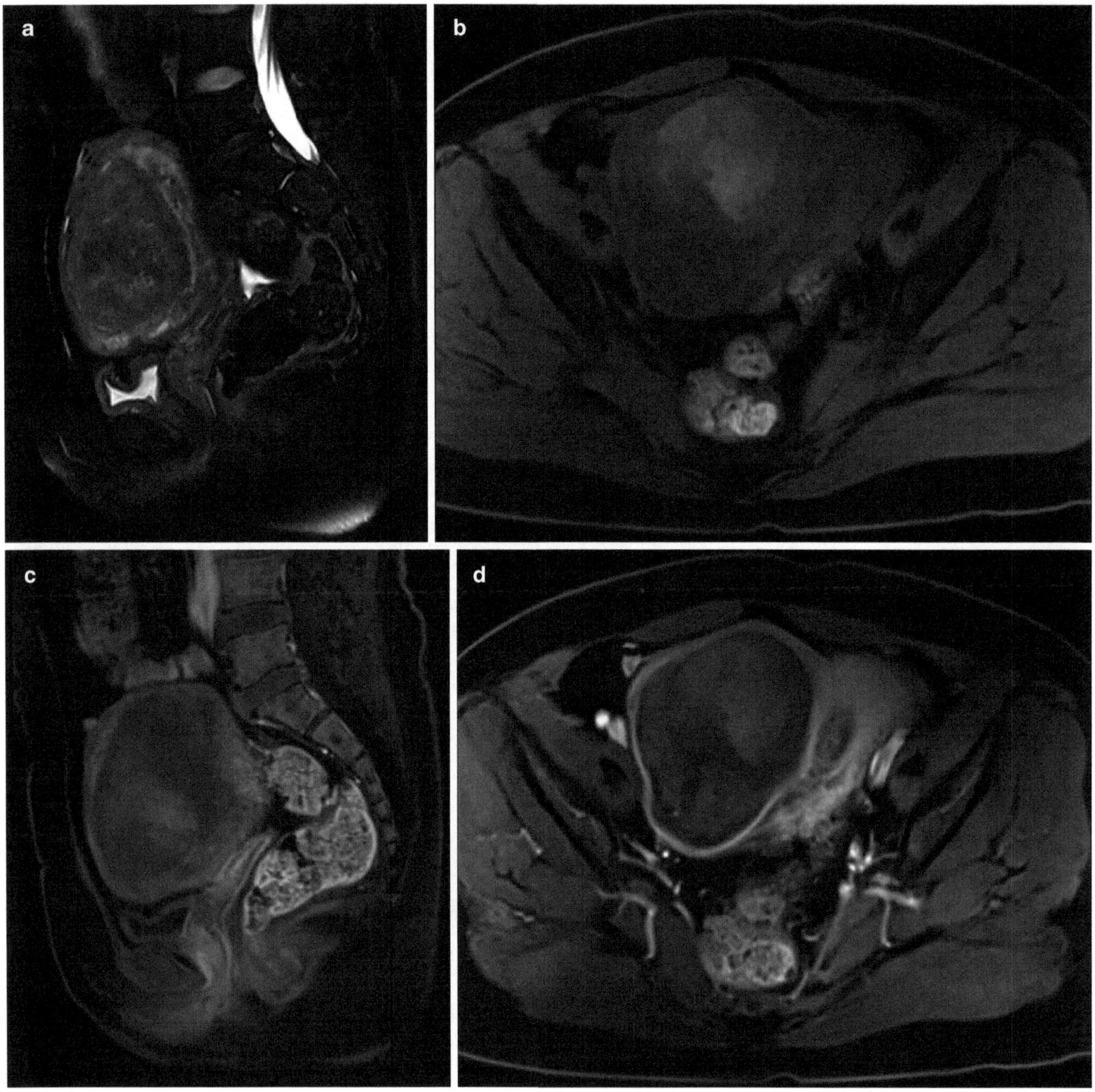

Fig. 4.209 MRI follow-up of uterine giant fibroids at 8 months after treatment. (**a**) T2WI_FS axial, (**b**) T1WI axial, (**c**) T1WI_FS + C sagittal, (**d**) T1WI_FS + C axial

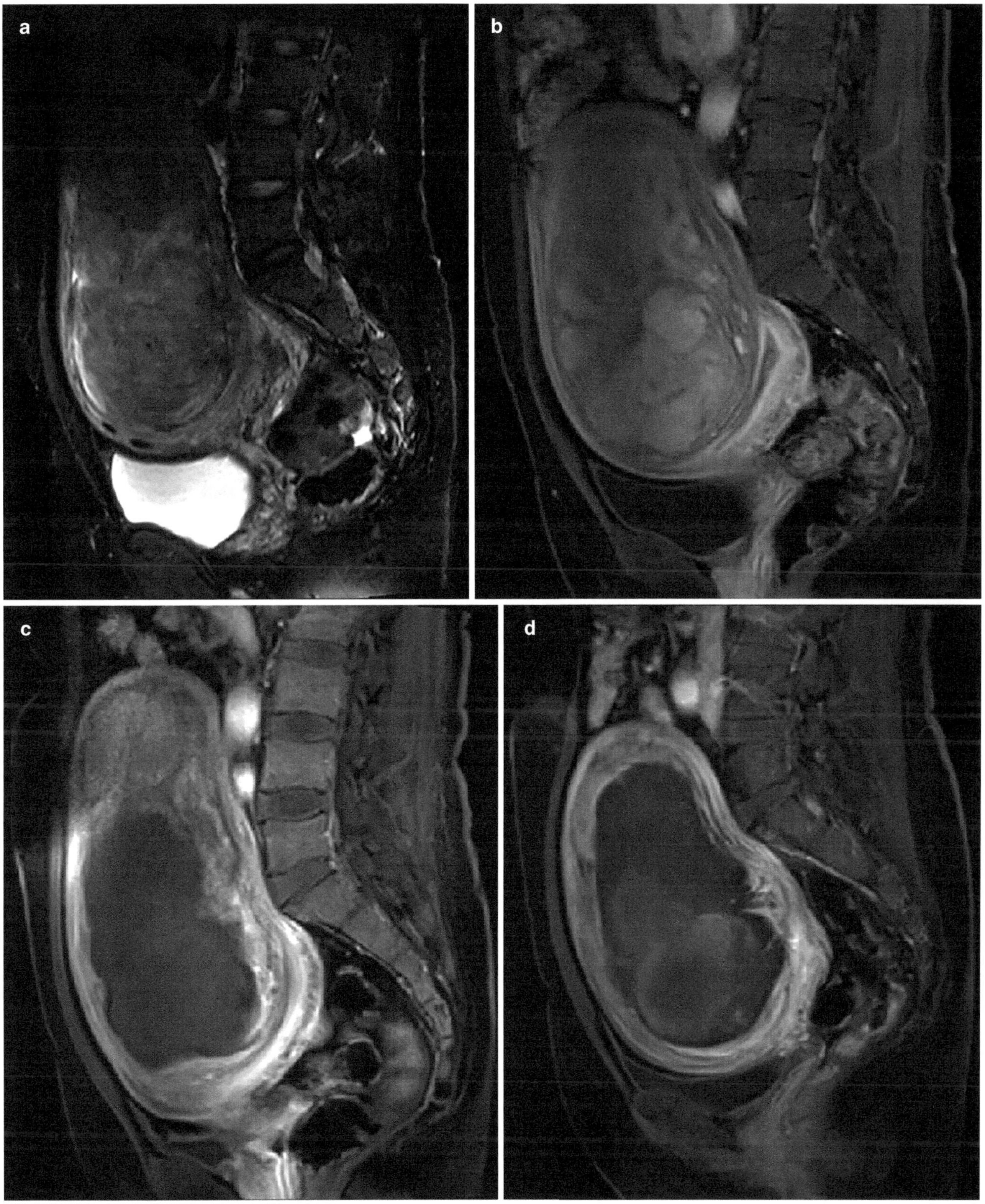

Fig. 4.210 Uterine giant fibroid MRI follow-up before and after treatment. (**a**) Sagittal T2WI imaging before treatment, (**b**) sagittal T1WI_FS + C imaging before treatment, (**c**) sagittal T1WI_FS + C imaging after the first treatment, (**d**) T1WI_FS + C sagittal imaging after the second treatment 3 months later

Treatment Techniques

1. **Focused ultrasound parameters.** (1) The first treatment parameters: Average acoustic power: 320 W, sonication time: 3720 seconds, duration of treatment: 135 minutes, total energy: 1,125,200 J. (2) The second treatment parameters.: Average acoustic power: 280 W, sonication time: 1843 seconds, duration of treatment: 84 minutes, total energy: 592,310 J.
2. **Focused ultrasound ablation techniques.** For a giant uterine fibroid, we treated the caudal (lower) end of the fibroid first. When the fibroid underwent necrosis and reduced in size, the fibroid's residual cephalic (upper) end was treated at the second ablation treatment.

Post-Treatment Assessment

1. **MRI evaluation after the first treatment.** The contrast-enhanced T1WI showed that the NPV ratio of the fibroid was about 70%, but the cephalic part of the fibroid was not fully covered as planned (Fig. 4.210c).
2. **3 months later, MRI evaluation after the second treatment.** There was no significant swelling of the anterior abdominal wall. The uterine fibroid in the anterior wall was significantly reduced from 189 mm to 135 mm in length. The contrast-enhanced T1WI showed that the residual fibroid on the cephalic end was completely ablated. At this time, the NPV ratio of the entire fibroid was about 99%. There was only a small amount of residual in the posterior lower edge of the fibroid (Fig. 4.210d).

Discussion

- For a giant uterine fibroid with slightly homogenous hyperintensity on T2WI and abundant blood supply, two focused ultrasound ablation treatments can be performed at an interval of 3 months. GnRH-a (Norad) is given monthly for 3 months after the first focused ultrasound ablation treatment to prevent recurrence from the remaining residual.
- A 3 months interval between the two focused ultrasound ablation treatments is to allow the complete absorption of the edema at the abdominal wall. It ensures that the acoustic pathway is not disturbed for the second treatment.

Focused Ultrasound Ablation for Adenomyosis

5

Yonghua Xu, Lixia Yang, Yu Cheng, and Felix Wong

Abstract

MRI assessments of focal adenomyosis (adenomyoma) and diffuse adenomyosis before and after focused ultrasound ablation are described. The therapeutic techniques, focused ultrasound parameters, and treatment outcomes are demonstrated, while the key issues to pay attention are mentioned.

Keywords

MRI · High-intensity focused ultrasound · Ablation · Adenomyoma · Adenomyosis

Adenomyosis is caused by benign invasion of the ectopic endometrium (glands and stroma) into the normal myometrium. According to the location and scope of the lesion, it can be divided into two types: focal type (also known as adenomyoma) and diffuse type. The main treatment methods include drug therapy, surgical treatment, minimally invasive treatment, and so on. However, it is difficult, at present, to cure adenomyosis, and individualized integrative treatment should be carried out in combination with clinical symptoms, imaging changes, age, and fertility requirements. Focused ultrasound ablation is more advantageous for young patients with adenomyosis who are willing to preserve the uterus and have fertility requirements since it can accurately locate and focus the ultrasonic energy on the ultrasound focal area in the myometrium so that the lesion will produce coagulated necrosis. The treating physician can adjust the treatment area and parameters during the whole treatment process in real time, based on the shape, size, range of the lesion, and individual differences of each patient. Provided the safety and effectiveness are ensured, individualized treatment can be maximized. Focused ultrasound ablation has its unique advantages for different types of adenomyosis. This chapter attempts to elaborate on the treatment of many clinical cases and the related factors.

5.1 Focused Ultrasound Ablation for Focal Adenomyosis (Adenomyoma)

5.1.1 Case 1

5.1.1.1 Case Description

The female patient was 48 years old. She suffered from adenomyosis with heavy menstrual blood flow, dysmenorrhea, and anemia. After focused ultrasound ablation treatment, follow-up visits showed that her menstrual blood flow had decreased, and her dysmenorrhea was significantly relieved.

5.1.1.2 Pre-Treatment Assessment

MRI showed the focal adenomyosis of the left posterior wall of the uterus with a single round hypointense area and multiple scattered hyperintense spots within the lesion, lying adjacent to the rectum posteriorly on T2WI (Fig. 5.1a). The contrast-enhanced T1WI showed that the adenomyoma had an abundant blood supply without a clear boundary (Fig. 5.1b, c). The adenomyoma was located in the posterior wall of the retroverted uterus, so it might be difficult to locate the lesion during ultrasound ablation.

5.1.1.3 Treatment Techniques

1. **Focused ultrasound parameters.** Average acoustic power: 245 W, sonication time: 3052 s, duration of treatment: 111 mins, total energy: 792,000 J.

Y. Xu (✉) · L. Yang · Y. Cheng
Zhongshan-Xuhui Hospital, Fudan University, Shanghai, China

F. Wong
The University of New South Wales, Sydney, NSW, Australia

Y. Xu et al. (eds.), *Surgical Techniques of Focused Ultrasound Ablation in Benign Uterine Diseases*,
https://doi.org/10.1007/978-981-19-7180-8_5

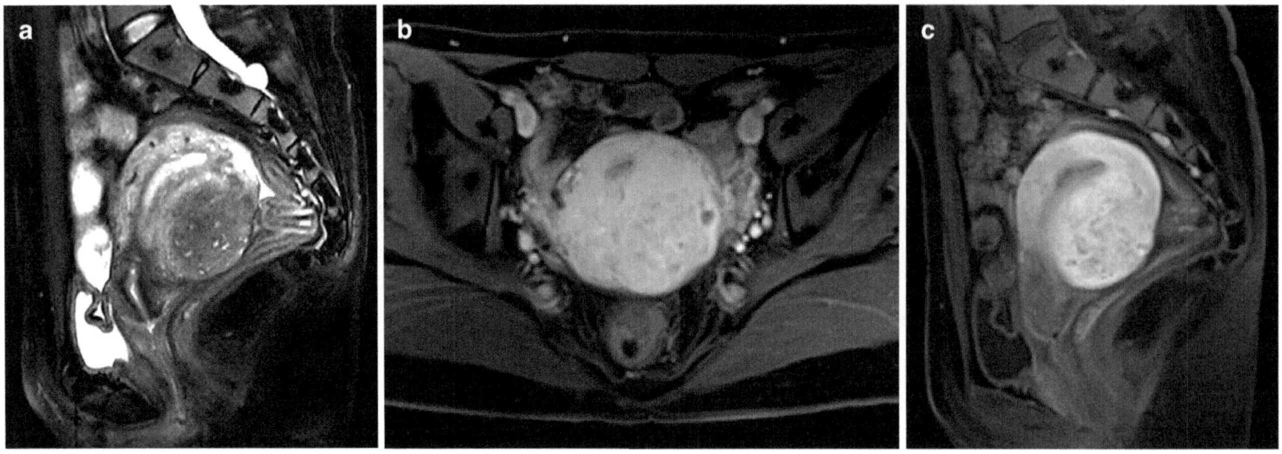

Fig. 5.1 Adenomyoma before treatment. (**a**) T2WI_FS sagittal, (**b**) T1WI_FS + C axial, (**c**) T1WI_FS + C sagittal

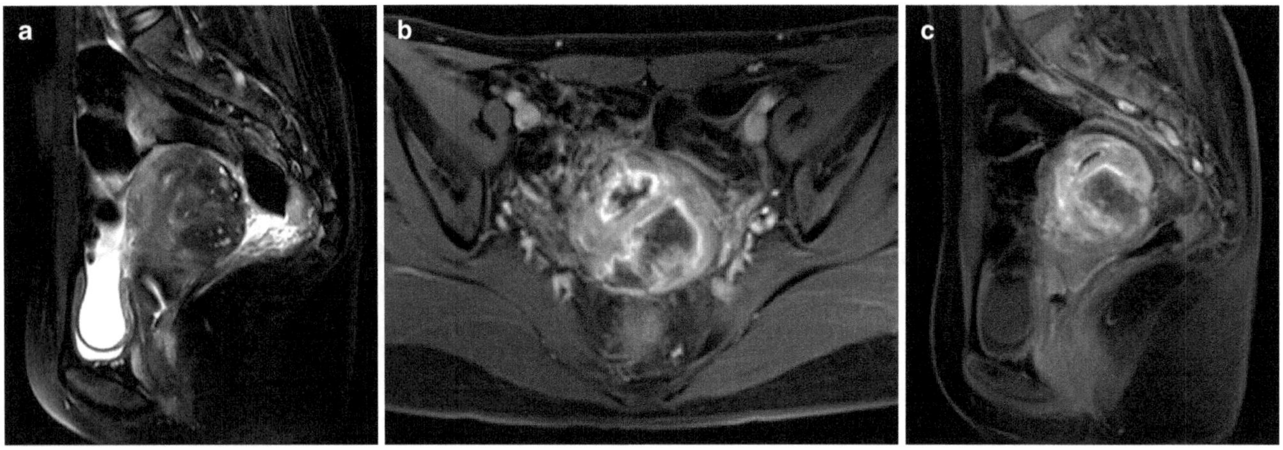

Fig. 5.2 MRI evaluation of adenomyoma after treatment. (**a**) T2WI_FS sagittal, (**b**) T1WI_FS + C axial, (**c**) T1WI_FS + C sagittal

2. **Focused ultrasound ablation techniques.** By distending the bladder, the bowels were moved away from the acoustic pathway. Also, the focused ultrasound ablation power should be reduced to avoid damage to the adjacent rectum and sacral plexus.

5.1.1.4 Post-Treatment Assessment

MRI Evaluation after Treatment There was no edema in the subcutaneous soft tissue of the anterior abdominal wall (Fig. 5.2a). The contrast-enhanced T1WI showed that the adenomyoma became a heterogonous non-perfusion area. The NPV ratio of the adenomyosis was about 75%. The posterior serosal layer of the uterus was still present, but there was a small discontinuity at the posterior margin (Fig. 5.2b, c).

5.1.1.5 Discussion

- A distended bladder and a water balloon can be used to compress and push the bowels away to establish a safe acoustic pathway for treating a posterior uterine wall lesion. But the addition of an extracorporeal water balloon may sometimes cause the ultrasound focal regions failing to cover the whole lesion.
- Focal adenomyosis has no capsule, and the ultrasound heat is easy to diffuse. The posterior serosal layer of this lesion has a small breakthrough area, yet the patient has no discomfort after treatment. It might be because the ablation treatment is still within a safe range.

5.1.2 Case 2

5.1.2.1 Case Description

The female patient was 54 years old. She had amenorrhea for more than 1 year. Her menstruation returned 13 days ago, accompanied by lower abdominal pain, urinary frequency, and urgency. The clinical diagnosis was adenomyosis, and surgical hysterectomy was recommended, which was refused by this patient. After focused ultrasound ablation treatment, her menstruation was still present, but dysmenorrhea, urinary, and other clinical symptoms disappeared.

5.1.2.2 Pre-Treatment Assessment

MRI showed a 57 mm × 58 mm adenomyoma in the anterior uterine wall, with mixed iso- and hyperintense signals on T2WI (Fig. 5.3a). The contrast-enhanced T1WI showed that the lesion had a moderate-abundant blood supply (Fig. 5.3b, c). The lesion was located on the anterior uterine wall, compressing down on the bladder with a good acoustic pathway. It was predicted that focused ultrasound ablation was feasible.

5.1.2.3 Treatment Techniques

1. **Focused ultrasound parameters.** Average acoustic power: 180 W, sonication time: 4, 543 s, duration of treatment: 92 mins, total energy: 788000 J.
2. **Focused ultrasound ablation techniques.** The uterine adenomyosis was located in the anterior wall. The lesion was localized, but the boundary was not clear. The focused ultrasound ablation should be performed at low acoustic power with extended sonication time, thus avoiding damage to the anterior wall and the endometrium.

5.1.2.4 Post-treatment Assessment

1. **MRI evaluation after treatment.** The subcutaneous muscular layer of the anterior abdominal wall showed edema, and the signal intensity of the treated lesion increased on T2WI (Fig. 5.4a). The contrast-enhanced T1WI revealed a non-perfusion ablation area with the serosal layer and endometrium fully protected and intact (Fig. 5.4b, c).
2. **MRI follow-up at 12 months after treatment.** The uterine size and the anterior wall adenomyoma decreased, with homogeneous hypointensity on T2WI (Fig. 5.5a). The contrast-enhanced T1WI showed that the non-perfused ablation area was also reduced to almost invisible (Fig.5.5b).

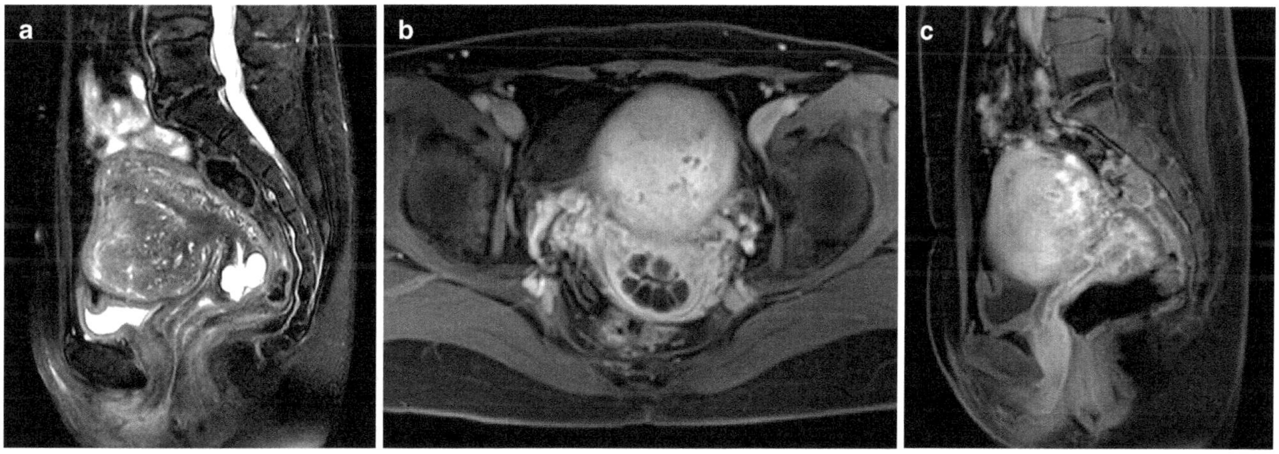

Fig. 5.3 Adenomyoma before treatment. (**a**) T2WI_FS sagittal, (**b**) T1WI_FS + C axial, (**c**) T1WI_FS + C sagittal

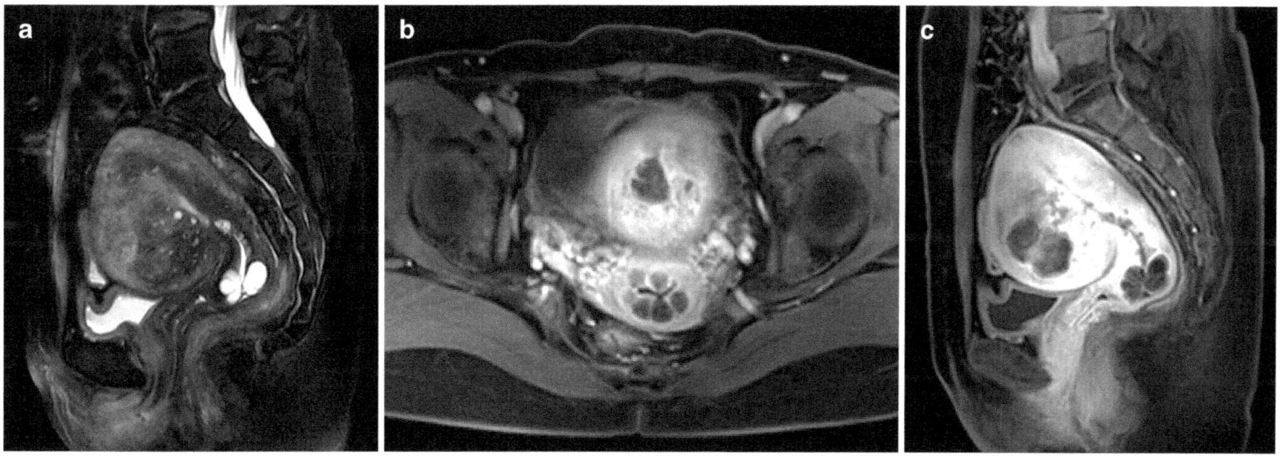

Fig. 5.4 MRI evaluation of adenomyoma after treatment. (**a**) T2WI_FS sagittal, (**b**) T1WI_FS + C axial, (**c**) T1WI_FS + C sagittal

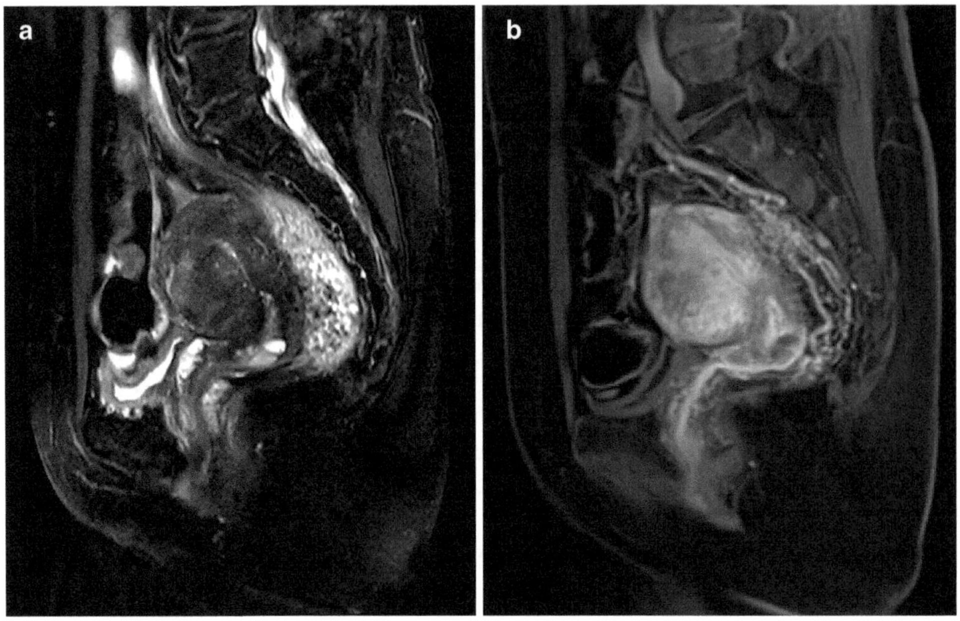

Fig. 5.5 MRI follow-up of uterine adenomyoma at 12 months after treatment. (**a**) T2WI_FS sagittal, (**b**) T1WI_FS + C sagittal

5.1.2.5 Discussion

- The symptoms associated with adenomyosis usually disappear after menopause. Although the patient was over 50 years old but not completely menopausal, she still had symptoms of dysmenorrhea, urinary frequency, and urgency, so intervention was needed. The purpose of focused ultrasound ablation therapy is to improve the clinical symptoms.

5.1.3 Case 3

5.1.3.1 Case Description

The female patient was 42 years old. She had dysmenorrhea accompanied by increased menstrual blood flow and sometimes thigh pain during the non-menstrual period. She often had abdominal pain, bowel colicky pain, and mild anemia. Two years after focused ultrasound ablation treatment, her menstrual blood flow returned to normal, and the dysmenorrhea was significantly relieved.

5.1.3.2 Pre-Treatment Assessment

MRI showed that an adenomyoma was located at the posterior wall of the uterus. It showed a hypointense area of 58 mm × 71 mm × 83 mm, with speckled hyperintense shadows on T2WI (Fig. 5.6a). The contrast-enhanced T1WI revealed the adenomyoma was of an abundant blood supply with a small area of depleted blood supply (Fig. 5.6b). Although the adenomyoma was located in the posterior wall of the uterus, it is a large anteverted uterus, and the acoustic pathway was good. Low intense signals on T2WI mainly characterized the lesions, and it would be easy to ablate.

5.1.3.3 Treatment Techniques

1. **Focused ultrasound parameters.** Average acoustic power: 291 W, sonication time: 3000 s, duration of treatment: 134 mins, total energy: 874,500 J.
2. **Focused ultrasound ablation techniques.** The adenomyoma was located in the posterior wall of the uterus, and it was adjacent to the rectum. Pay attention to the grayscale changes of the ultrasound image in the lesion during the treatment to avoid serosal breakthrough of the posterior uterine wall.

5.1.3.4 Post-Treatment Assessment

MRI Evaluation After Treatment MRI showed the edema of rectus abdominis in the anterior abdominal wall, and the signal intensity of the treated area of the posterior uterine wall increased on T2WI (Fig. 5.7a). The contrast-enhanced T1WI showed that most of the lesion area was ablated to the posterior serosal layer. The serosal and endometrium of the uterus were fully protected and intact (Fig. 5.7b).

5.1.3.5 Discussion

- The effect of focused ultrasound ablation of adenomyoma, in this case, is satisfactory. Although the serosa of

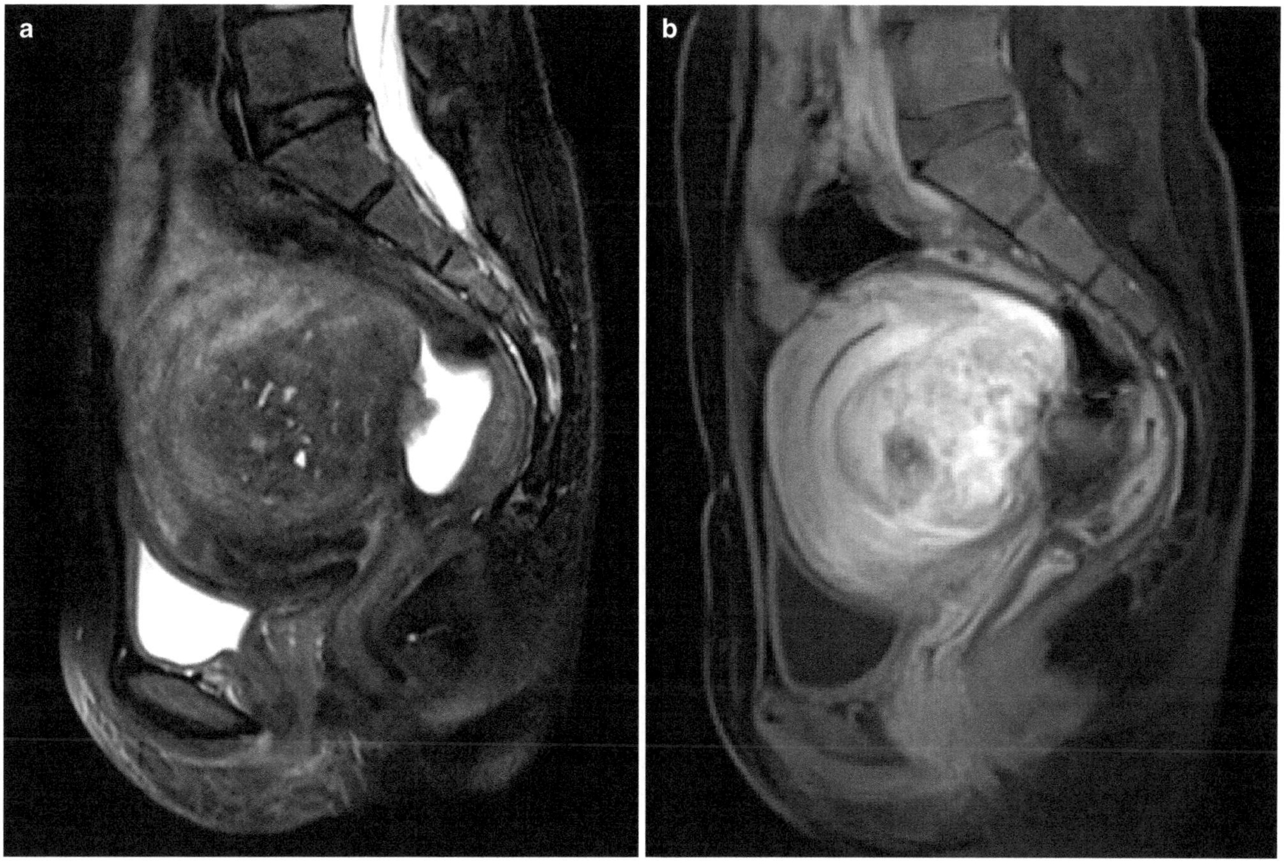

Fig. 5.6 Adenomyoma before treatment. (**a**) T2WI_FS sagittal, (**b**) T1WI_FS + C sagittal

the posterior wall of the uterus did not break, and a thin uterine layer remained, the average acoustic power was about 290 W (still high), which can be appropriately reduced to ensure treatment safety.

5.1.4 Case 4

5.1.4.1 Case Description

The female patient was 35 years old. She was clinically diagnosed with adenomyosis, presenting with dysmenorrhea, increased menstrual blood flow, and moderate anemia for nearly a decade. After two focused ultrasound ablation treatments, the patient's symptoms, such as dysmenorrhea and increased menstrual blood flow, completely disappeared.

5.1.4.2 Pre-Treatment Assessment

MRI showed localized thickening of the posterior uterine wall. It had low signals with scattered speckled hyperintensity on T2WI (Fig. 5.8a). The contrast-enhanced T1WI demonstrated that it had a moderate blood supply with a poorly defined boundary (Fig. 5.8b, c). Despite its deep location in the posterior wall of the uterus, the focused ultrasound ablation could achieve a good effect due to its low intense signals on T2WI.

5.1.4.3 Treatment Techniques

1. **The first Focused ultrasound parameters.** Average acoustic power: 250 W, sonication time: 3255 s, duration of treatment: 148 mins, total energy: 715,000 J.
2. **The second Focused ultrasound parameters.** Average acoustic power: 201 W, sonication time: 2500 s, duration of treatment: 120 mins, total energy: 414,100 J.
3. **Focused ultrasound ablation techniques.** Uterine adenomyosis did not have a pseudocapsule, and attention should be paid to controlling the sonication dose during treatment. By appropriately reducing the acoustic power, it was to avoid excessive expansion of the necrotic area outside the lesion and injury to sacrococcygeal fascia and bone.

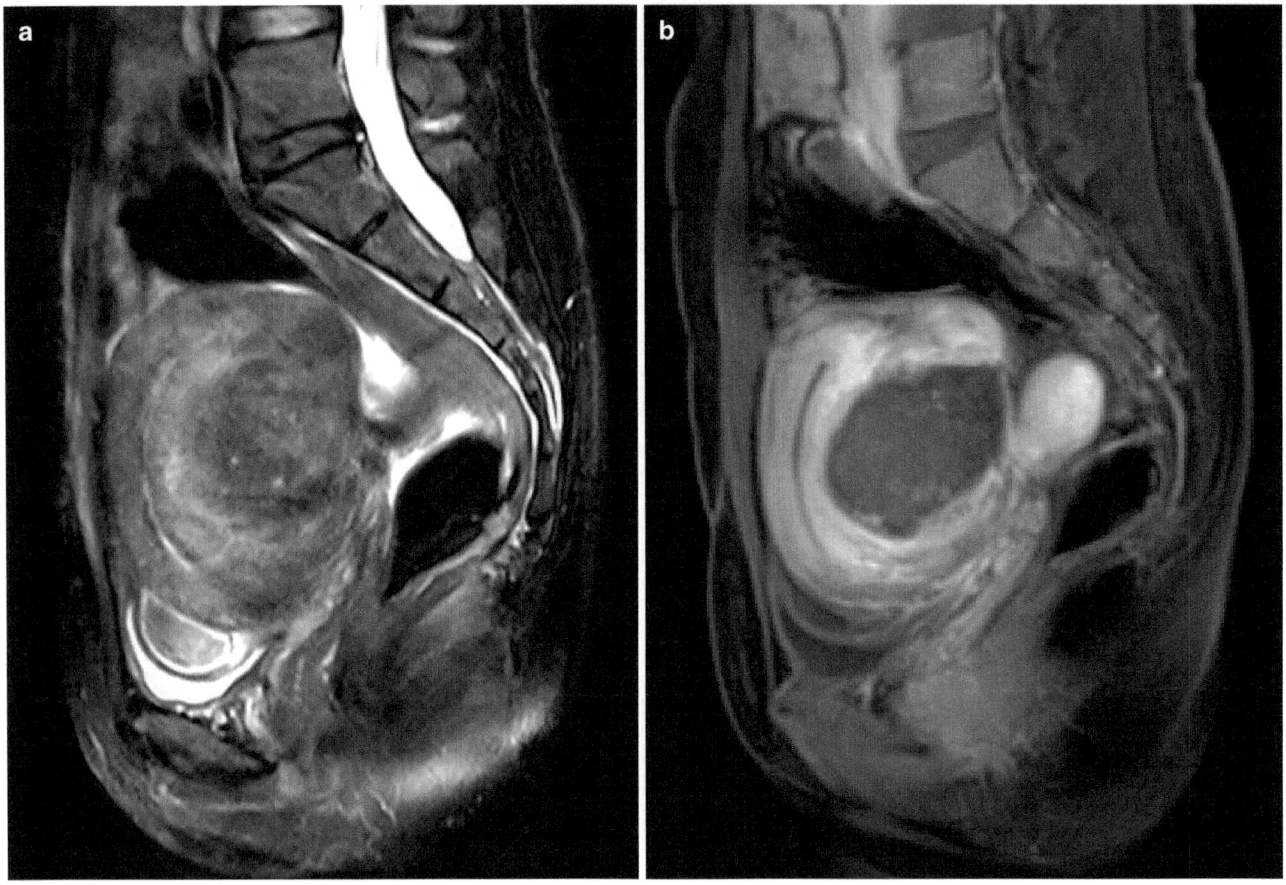

Fig. 5.7 MRI evaluation of adenomyoma immediately of treatment. (**a**) T2WI_FS sagittal, (**b**) T1WI_FS + C sagittal

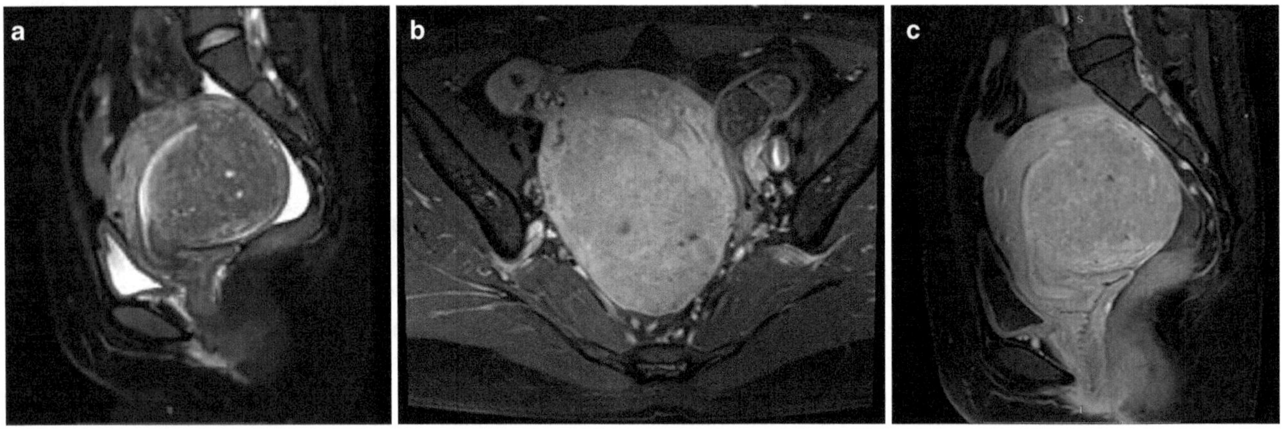

Fig. 5.8 Adenomyoma before the first treatment. (**a**) T2WI_FS sagittal, (**b**) T1WI_FS + C axial, (**c**) T1WI_FS + C sagittal

5.1.4.4 First Post-Treatment Assessment

1. **MRI evaluation after treatment.** The subcutaneous soft tissue of the anterior abdominal wall was slightly edematous, and the signal intensity of the peripheral lesion significantly increased on T2WI (Fig. 5.9a). The contrast-enhanced T1WI showed that most of the adenomyomas were ablated; only a small residual remained in some marginal areas. The endometrium had a small area of breakthrough (Fig. 5.9b, c).
2. **MRI follow-up at 5 months after treatment.** The non-perfusion area of adenomyoma was significantly smaller, and the endometrium was partially repaired. There was increased recurrence in the residual lesion of the adenomyoma. The shape and size of the uterus were similar to

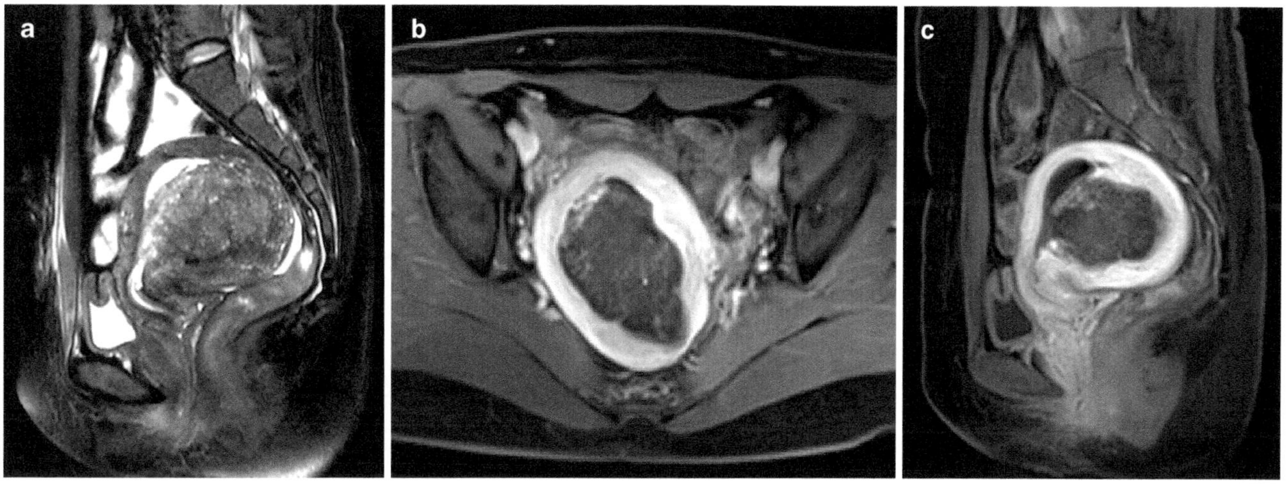

Fig. 5.9 MRI evaluation of adenomyoma after the first treatment. (**a**) T2WI_FS sagittal, (**b**) T1WI_FS + C axial, (**c**) T1WI_FS + C sagittal

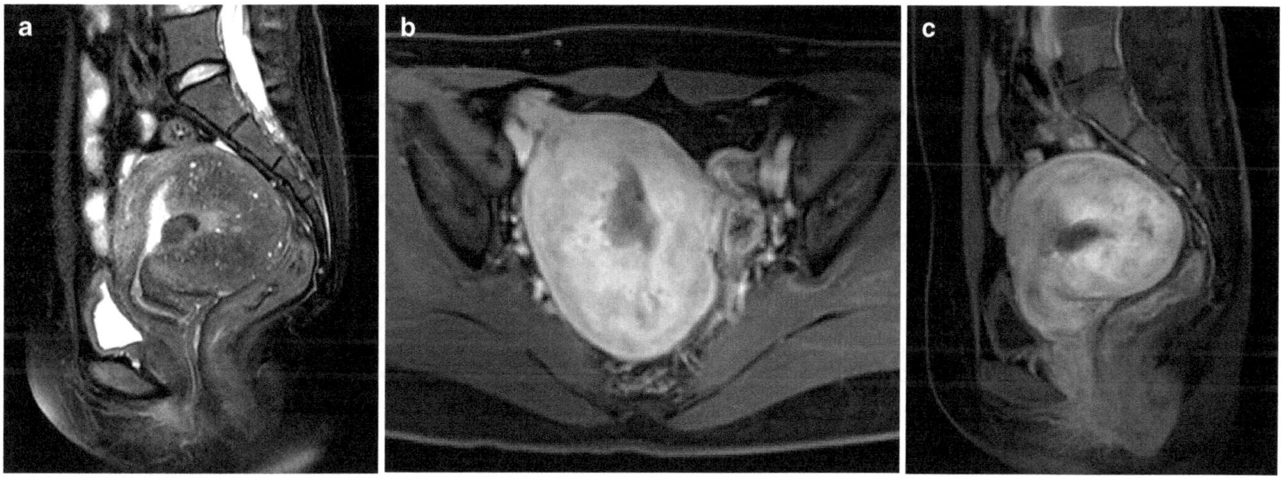

Fig. 5.10 MRI follow-up of adenomyoma at 5 months after the first treatment. (**a**) T2WI_FS sagittal, (**b**) T1WI_FS axial, (**c**) T1WI_FS sagittal

those before treatment (Fig. 5.10). Focused ultrasound ablation was recommended again.

5.1.4.5 Second Post-Treatment Assessment

1. **MRI evaluation after treatment.** There is no edema in the anterior abdominal wall, and the signal intensity in the treated area of adenomyoma was significantly increased on T2WI (Fig. 5.11a). The contrast-enhanced T1WI showed that the NPV ratio of the posterior wall was more than 95%, and the adjacent endometrium and serosal layer were fully protected and intact (Fig. 5.11b, c).
2. **MRI follow-up at 3 months and 5 months after the second treatment.** After 3 months, the shape and size of the uterus returned to normal, the size of adenomyoma was significantly reduced, and only the posterior wall of the uterus was still thicker (Fig. 5.12a); after 5 months, the posterior wall of the uterus was thicker than before. The size of the uterus was slightly larger than that before, and the contrast-enhanced T1WI showed that the non-perfusion area had disappeared (Fig. 5.12b, c).

5.1.4.6 Discussion

- Although the lesion is localized, there may still be residual lesions after treatment. Unlike fibroids, adenomyosis can grow rapidly and relapse in a short period, even if a good ablation rate is achieved. Therefore, focused ultrasound ablation therapy can be considered again.
- During focused ultrasound ablation of adenomyoma adjacent to the endometrium, the endometrium in the near acoustic field in the ultrasound focal area is prone to damage due to high temperature and heat diffusion. In this case, some endometrial linings can be broken, followed by an outflow of necrotic tissues after treatment. Therefore, 5 months after treatment, contrast-enhanced

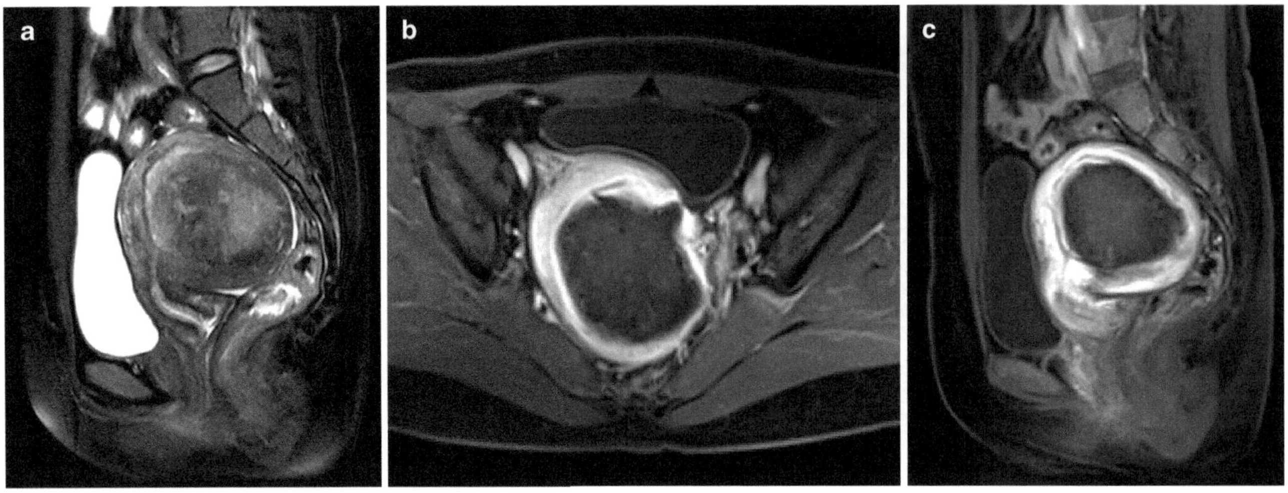

Fig. 5.11 MRI evaluation of adenomyoma after the second treatment. (**a**) T2WI_FS sagittal, (**b**) T1WI_FS + C axial, (**c**) T1WI_FS + C sagittal

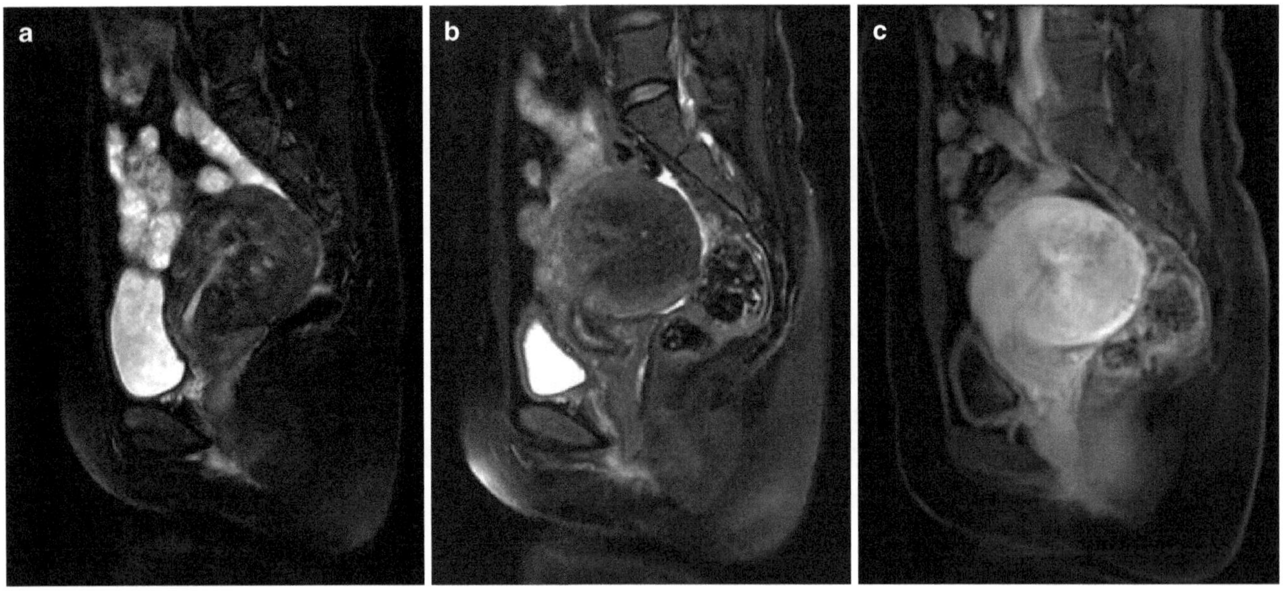

Fig. 5.12 MRI follow-up of adenomyoma at 3 months (**a**) and 5 months (**b**, **c**) after the second treatment. (**a**) T2WI_FS sagittal, (**b**) T2WI_FS sagittal, (**c**) T1WI_FS + C sagittal

T1WI follow-up showed only a small remaining non-perfusion necrotic area. However, the residual adenomyosis lesion in the surrounding uterine tissues significantly thickened and relapsed. Five months after the first treatment, the patient's dysmenorrhea recurred again. A second focused ultrasound ablation was performed, and a high ablation rate was achieved.

- The acoustic power was reduced during the repeat focused ultrasound ablation to avoid endometrial injury. The uterine volume was significantly reduced 3 months after the repeat ablation, and the uterine shape and size returned to almost normal. Five months later, the necrosis ablation area was completely absorbed and disappeared. The uterine wall was generally thick, and the endometrium was well repaired. Ongoing follow-up is needed to observe long-term efficacy.

5.1.5 Case 5

5.1.5.1 Case Description

The female patient was 43 years old and had dysmenorrhea with progressive exacerbation for more than 2 years. Transvaginal ultrasound (TVUS) showed uterine adenomyosis.

5.1.5.2 Pre-Treatment Assessment

MRI showed localized thickening of the anterior uterine wall of the uterus with low signals and scattered speckled hyperin-

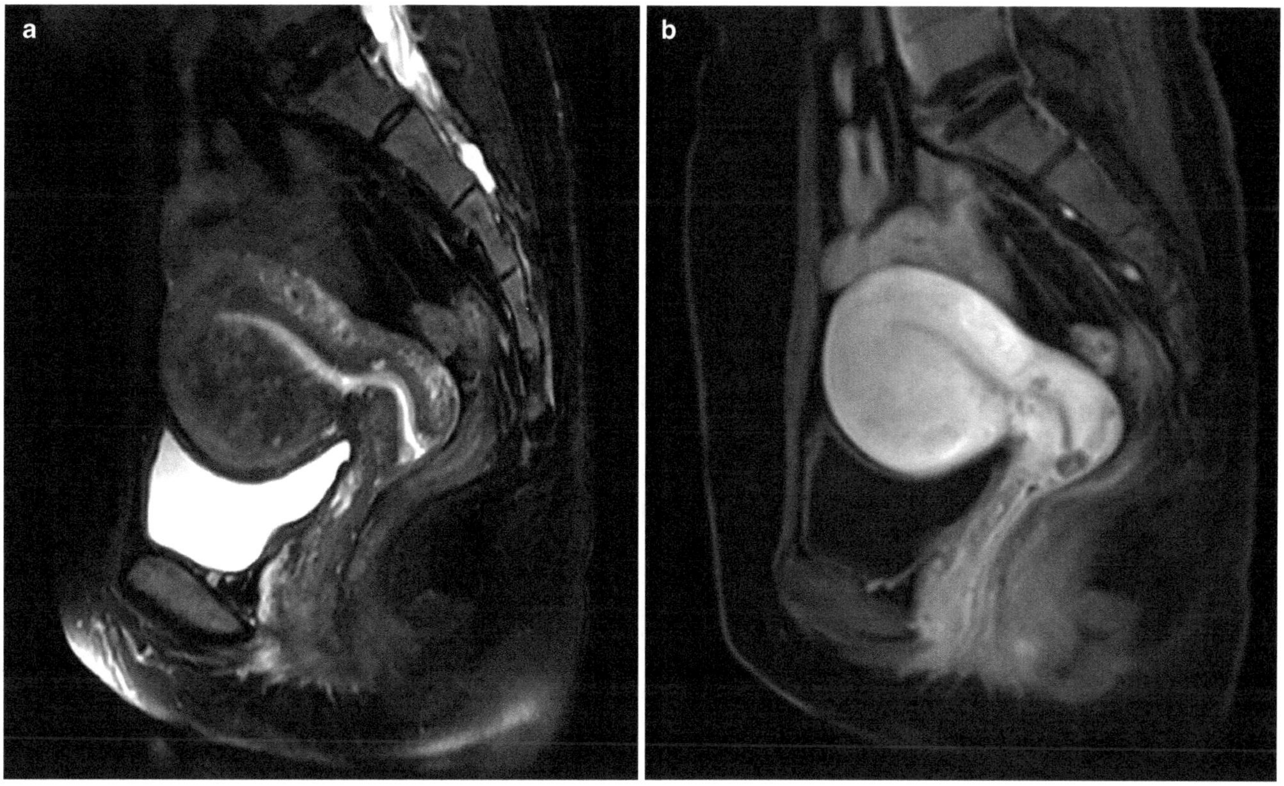

Fig. 5.13 Adenomyoma before treatment. (**a**) T2WI_FS sagittal, (**b**) T1WI_FS + C sagittal

tensity on T2WI (Fig.5.13a). The contrast-enhanced T1WI demonstrated that it had a moderate blood supply (Fig. 5.13b). The lesion located in the anterior wall of the anteverted uterus was closed to anterior abdominal wall; the focused ultrasound might achieve a good ablation effect due to its low intense signals on T2WI and the good acoustic pathway.

5.1.5.3 Treatment Techniques

1. **Focused ultrasound parameters.** Average acoustic power: 136 W, sonication time: 1359 s, duration of treatment: 111 mins, total energy: 220,190 J.
2. **Focused ultrasound ablation techniques.** Although the adenomyoma is localized, there is no clear boundary between the lesion and normal tissue unlike the uterine fibroid, and it originates from the endometrium. It is important to deploy the initial focal regions of focused ultrasound at least 10 mm away from the endometrial layer; meanwhile, once the grayscale changes occur, the focal regions move to the shallow layer of the lesion.

5.1.5.4 Post-Treatment Assessment

1. **MRI evaluation after treatment.** The signal intensity in the lesion area of the anterior wall significantly increased on T2WI (Fig. 5.14a). The contrast-enhanced T1WI showed that the non-perfused area covered almost all of the adenomyoma with some small breakthrough of the endometrium (Fig. 5.14b).
2. **MRI follow-up at 6 months after treatment.** The previous ablated area of the adenomyoma became significantly smaller with the intact endometrium line, and the anterior wall was thinner than that before and the volume of the uterus decreased (Fig. 5.15a, b).

5.1.5.5 Discussion

- For the patients with adenomyoma on the anterior wall of the anteverted uterus, a bladder of appropriate size could be filled by the degassed saline while the incident angle of focused ultrasound must be adjusted, which creates the axis of focused ultrasound parallel to the endometrial line, so as to make the endometrium not in the ultrasonic pathway as much as possible.
- Apart from improving the therapeutic strategy to reduce and avoid damage to the endometrium by ultrasound ablation, the medications also promote the intima repair after treatment.

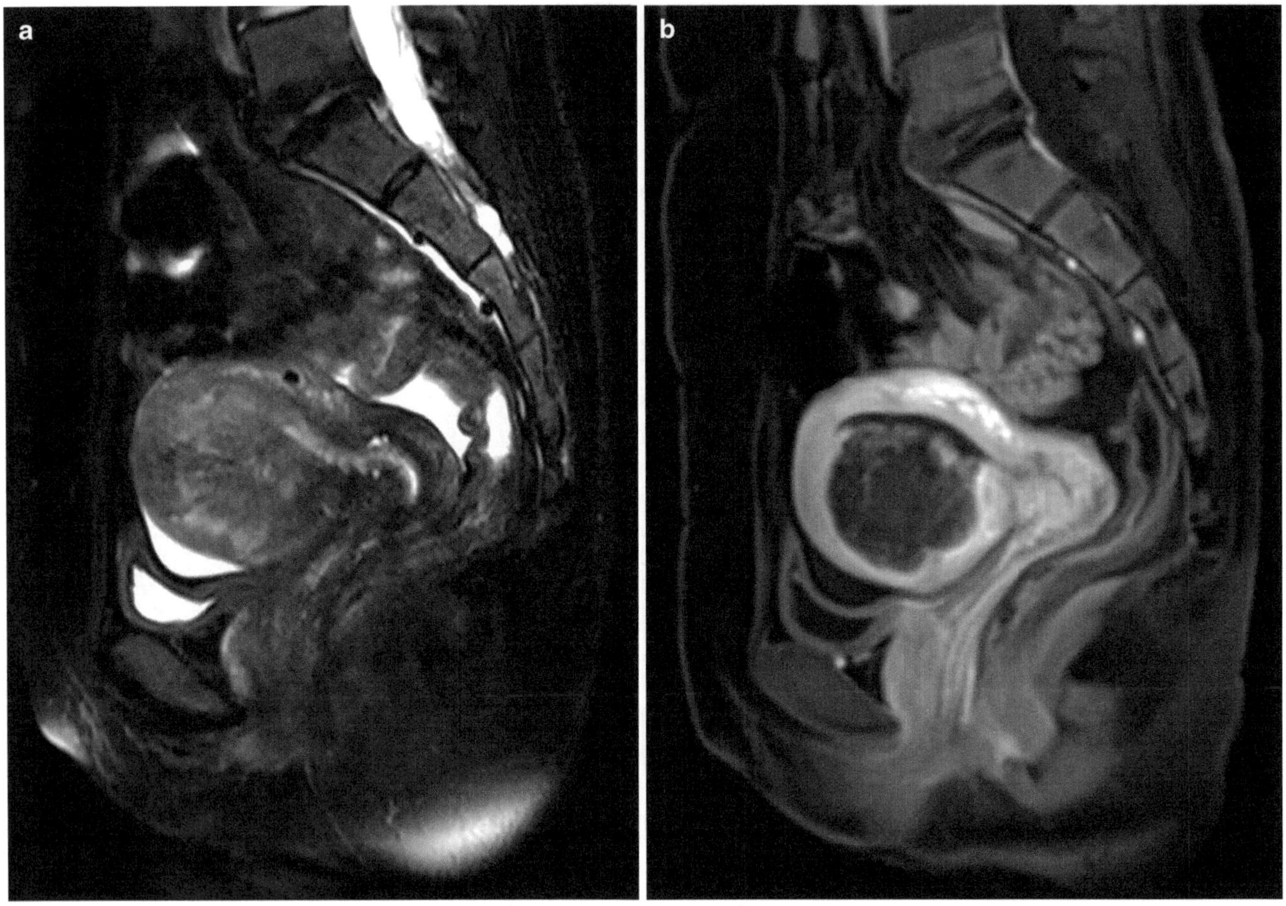

Fig. 5.14 MRI evaluation of adenomyoma after treatment. (**a**) T2WI_FS sagittal, (**b**) T1WI_FS + C sagittal

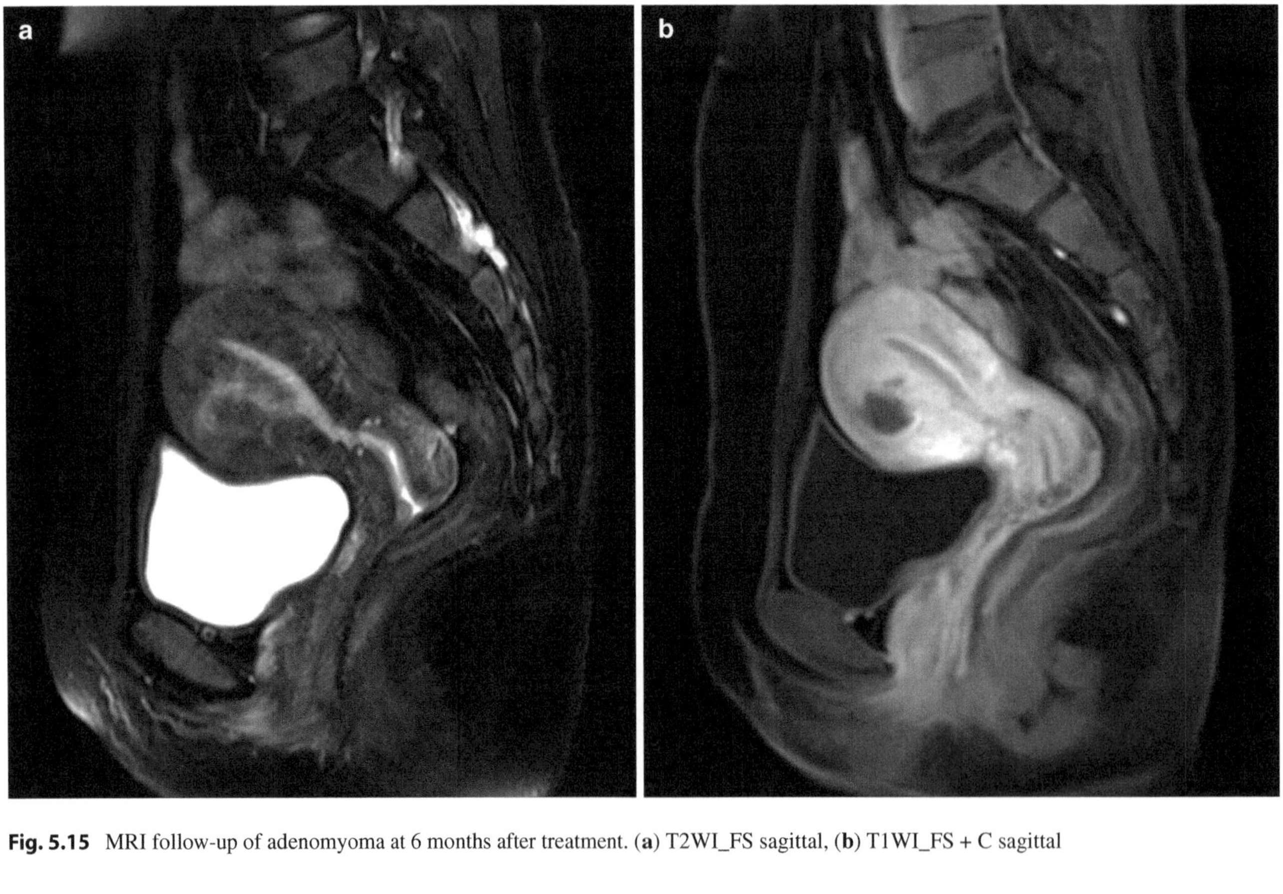

Fig. 5.15 MRI follow-up of adenomyoma at 6 months after treatment. (**a**) T2WI_FS sagittal, (**b**) T1WI_FS + C sagittal

5.2 Focused Ultrasound Ablation for Diffuse Adenomyosis

5.2.1 Case 1

5.2.1.1 Case Description

The female patient was 43 years old. She suffered from adenomyosis for many years. She complained of dysmenorrhea which gradually increased in severity for 1 year and was associated with increased menstrual blood flow. After focused ultrasound ablation treatment, the patient had a small amount of pink vaginal discharge, which was treated symptomatically and which had shown improvement. Subsequent follow-up visits showed that dysmenorrhea disappeared and the menstrual blood flow reduced.

5.2.1.2 Pre-Treatment Assessment

MRI showed adenomyosis lesions of the uterus. They had mixed hypo- and hyperintense signals on T2WI. The adenomyosis was diffusely located on the posterior wall and fundus of the uterus. There was a small fibroid with low intense signals at the anterior wall of the uterus near the bladder (Fig. 5.16a). The contrast-enhanced T1WI showed that the adenomyosis was heterogeneously enhanced, with an abundant blood supply (Fig. 5.16b). The fundus and the posterior wall of the uterus had a good acoustic pathway, and the expected effect of focused ultrasound ablation is good.

5.2.1.3 Treatment Techniques

1. **Focused ultrasound parameters.** Average acoustic power: 253 W, sonication time: 3274 s, duration of treatment: 150 mins, total energy: 825,800 J.
2. **Focused ultrasound ablation techniques.** Since adenomyosis did not have any anatomical boundary, it was necessary to use lower acoustic power irradiation so that the areas of focused ultrasound ablation could be easy to control.

5.2.1.4 Post-Treatment Assessment

MRI Evaluation after Treatment The muscle layer of the anterior abdominal wall had limited mild edema, and the signal intensity of the treated area, especially the fundus of the uterus, increased on T2WI. The contrast-enhanced T1WI showed that most of the ablation area showed non-perfusion. The endometrium at the uterine fundus was partially ablated, and the serosa of the posterior uterine wall was completely protected (Fig. 5.17).

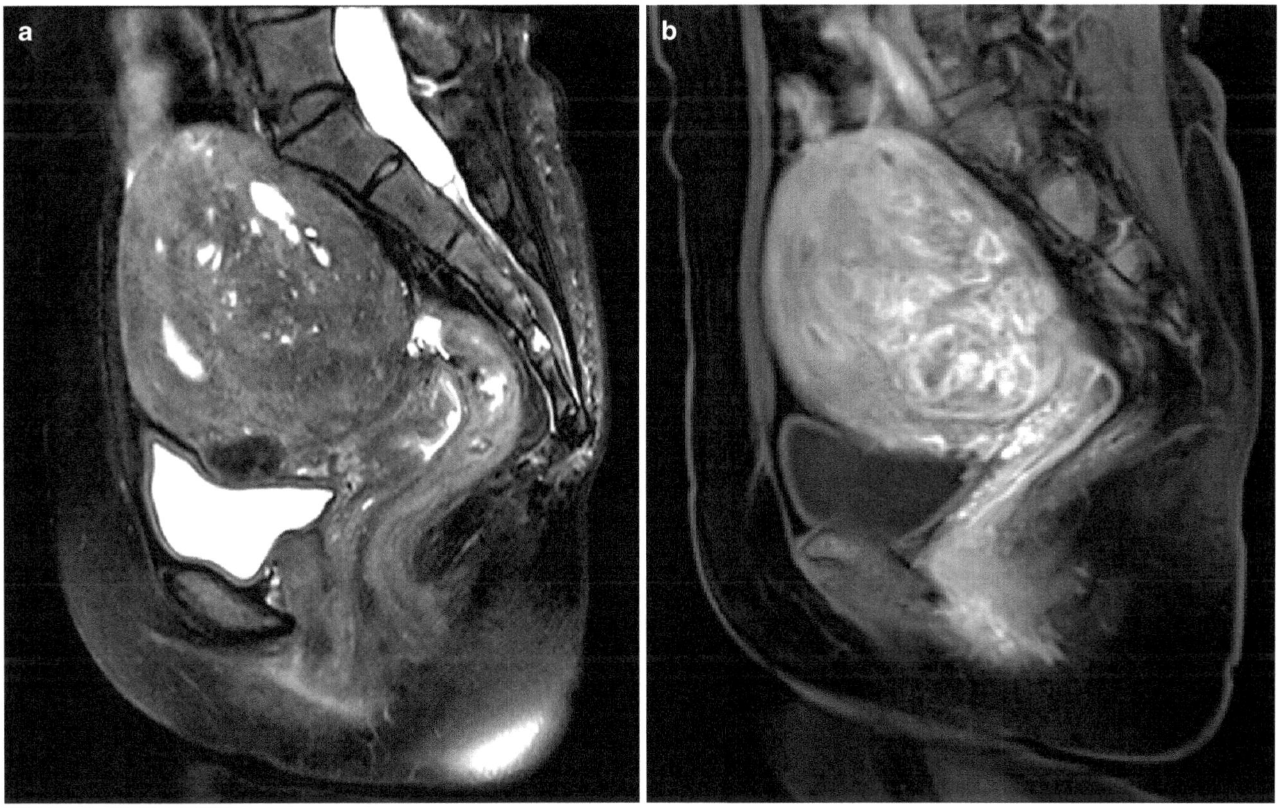

Fig. 5.16 Uterine adenomyosis before the treatment. (**a**) T2WI_FS sagittal, (**b**) T1WI_FS + C sagittal

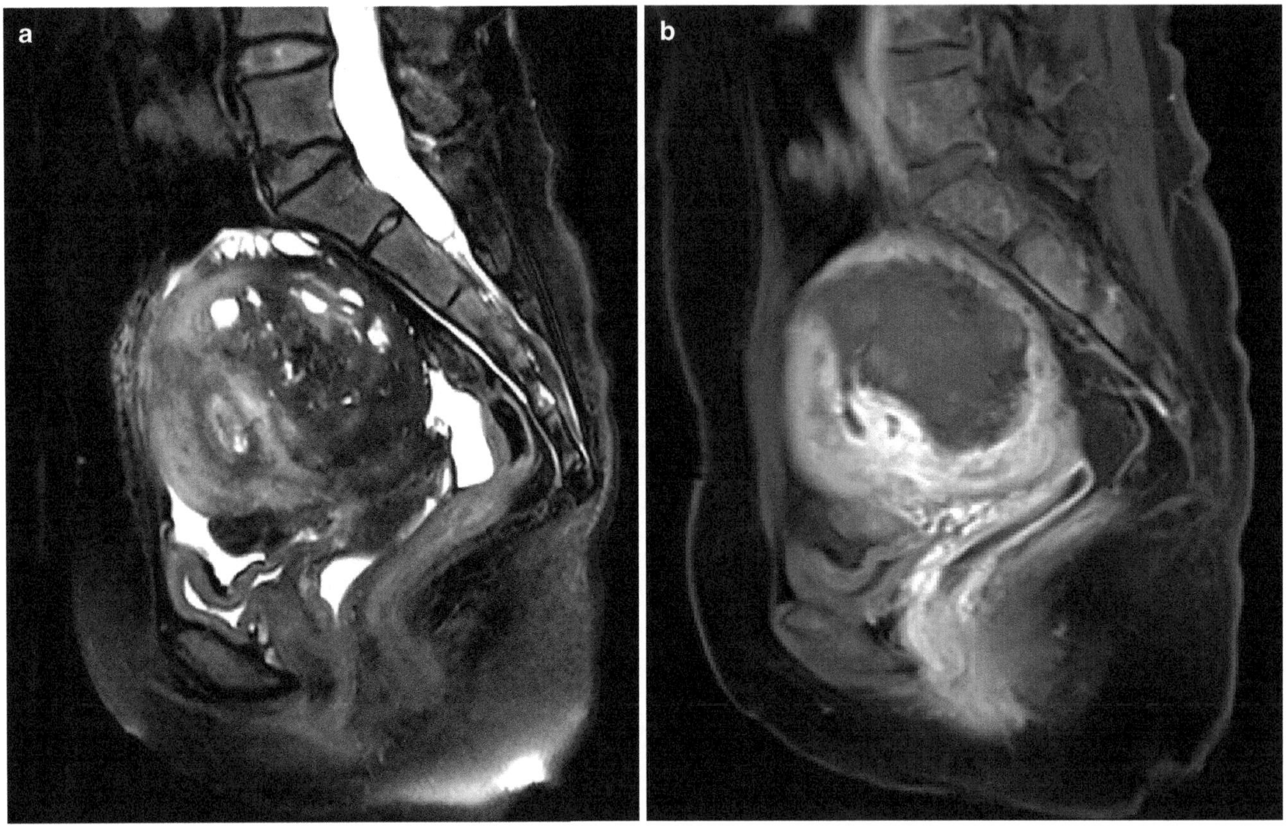

Fig. 5.17 MRI evaluation of uterine adenomyosis after treatment. (**a**) T2WI_FS sagittal, (**b**) T1WI_FS + C sagittal

5.2.1.5 Discussion

- Many adenomyosis were located at the posterior wall of the uterus. In adenomyosis treatment, focused ultrasound ablation can also thermally ablate the endometrium of uteirne fundus side partially, which was similar to radiofrequency or microwave endometrial ablation. Thus, it may reduce menstrual blood loss and improve the quality of life.

5.2.2 Case 2

5.2.2.1 Case Description

The female patient was 48 years old. She had heavy menstrual blood flow accompanied by dysmenorrhea and moderate anemia. The patient's menstrual blood flow had increased for 2 months after the focused ultrasound ablation treatment and then returned to normal, and her dysmenorrhea disappeared.

5.2.2.2 Pre-Treatment Assessment

MRI showed posterior adenomyosis showing a diffuse lesion with thickening of the posterior uterine wall. The lesion had hypointensity mixed with some spot-like signals on T2WI (Fig. 5.18a). The contrast-enhanced T1WI showed that the adenomyosis had a moderate blood supply (Fig. 5.18b, c). The entire uterus was enlarged with a spherical shape, and the acoustic pathway was good. It was predicted that the focused ultrasound ablation effect would be good.

5.2.2.3 Treatment Techniques

1. **Focused ultrasound parameters.** Average acoustic power: 260 W, sonication time: 1551 s, duration of treatment: 70 mins, total energy: 424,310 J.
2. **Focused ultrasound ablation techniques.** The anterior part of the adenomyosis was close to the endometrium, and the posterior was adjacent to the rectum and sacral spine. It should be noted that the focal region should be more than 15 mm away from the serosa of the uterus. In this case, the menstrual flow was heavy, and there was no fertility requirement, so some parts of the endometrium near the fundus of the uterus could be ablated.

5.2.2.4 Post-Treatment Assessment

MRI Evaluation after Treatment There was a small amount of slightly high signals in the lesion of the posterior uterine wall on T2WI (Fig. 5.19a). The contrast-enhanced T1WI showed that most adenomyosis was ablated (Fig. 5.19b, c). The non-perfusion area included the endometrium of the uterine body and fundus adjacent to the lesion, thus, reducing the endometrial tissue and subsequent menstrual flow.

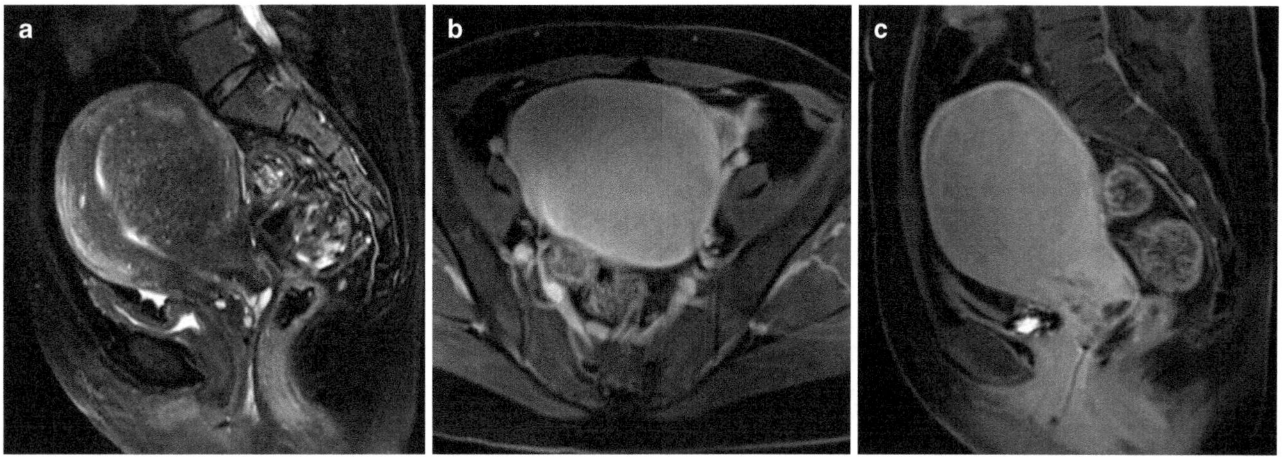

Fig. 5.18 Uterine adenomyosis before treatment. (**a**) T2WI_FS sagittal, (**b**) T1WI_FS + C axial, (**c**) T1WI_FS + C sagittal

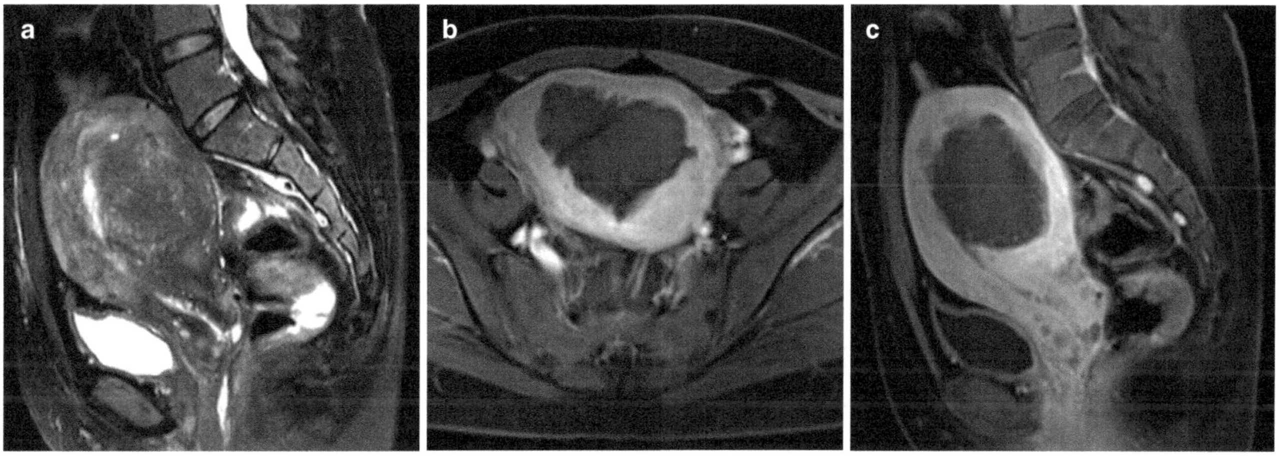

Fig. 5.19 MRI evaluation of uterine adenomyosis after treatment. (**a**) T2WI_FS sagittal, (**b**) T1WI_FS + C axial, (**c**) T1WI_FS + C sagittal

5.2.2.5 Discussion

- The boundary between diffuse adenomyosis and normal uterine tissue is unclear, and focused ultrasound ablation is a local thermal ablation for conformal treatment of the lesions.
- During the treatment of this case, the focused ultrasound ablation focus was more than 10 mm away from the endometrium. However, the heat diffusion can still cause coagulative necrosis to the adjacent endometrium, destroying the endometrial layer to reduce menstrual blood flow and improve anemia.

5.2.3 Case 3

5.2.3.1 Case Description

The female patient was 46 years old. She suffered from dysmenorrhea for 5–6 years, gradually worsening. In the past 2 months, her menstrual flow had increased and excessive and shortened menstrual periods, accompanied by severe anemia. Her follow-up after focused ultrasound ablation treatment showed that her menstrual blood flow was significantly decreased, and dysmenorrhea was significantly relieved.

5.2.3.2 Pre-Treatment Assessment

MRI showed anterior wall adenomyosis of the uterus, showing hypointensity with spot scattered high signals on T2WI (Fig. 5.20a). The contrast-enhanced T1WI showed that the adenomyosis had a poor blood supply, with no obvious boundary and small punctate hemorrhages scattered inside the lesion (Fig. 5.20b, c). The uterus was retroverted, and the bowels in front of the uterus had to be pushed away from the acoustic pathway by distending the bladder. The focused ultrasound ablation effect was predicted to be good.

5.2.3.3 Treatment Techniques

1. **Focused ultrasound parameters.** Average acoustic power: 250 W, sonication time: 1626 s, duration of treatment: 65 mins, total energy: 406,500 J.
2. **Focused ultrasound ablation techniques.** There is no obvious boundary between the anterior wall adenomyosis

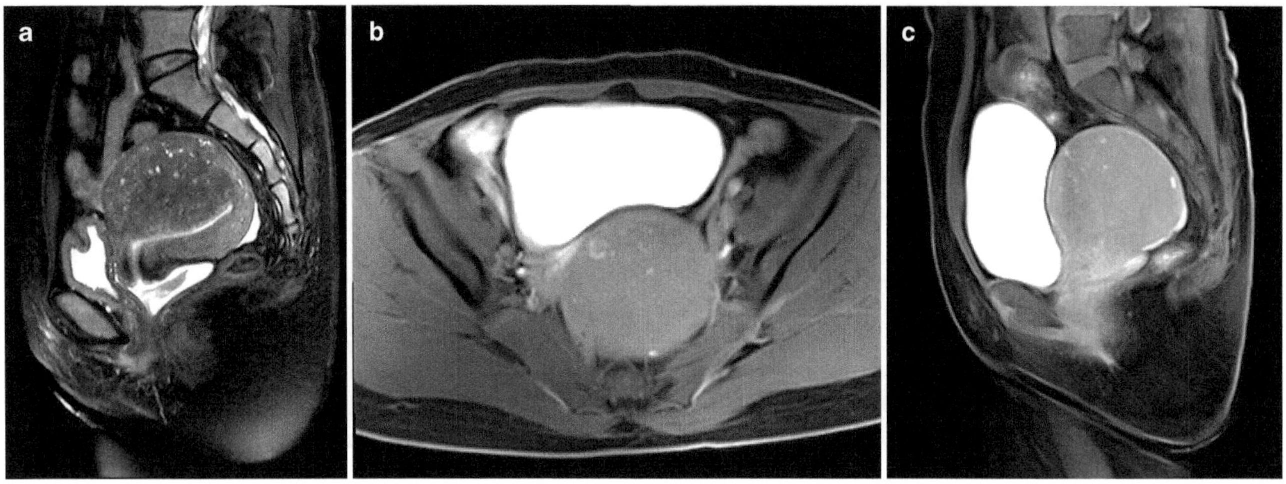

Fig. 5.20 Uterine adenomyosis before treatment. (**a**) T2WI_FS sagittal, (**b**) T1WI_FS + C axial, (**c**) T1WI_FS + C sagittal

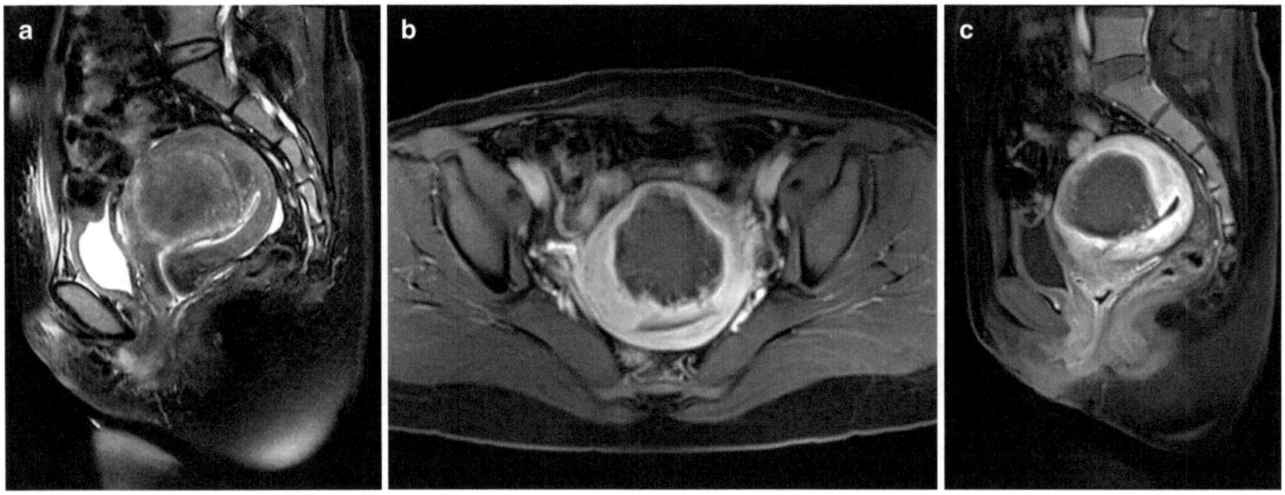

Fig. 5.21 MRI evaluation of uterine adenomyosis after treatment. (**a**) T2WI_FS sagittal, (**b**) T1WI_FS + C axial, (**c**) T1WI_FS + C sagittal

with the endometrium and surrounding tissues. It is not easy to control the ablation spread during treatment. In order to avoid the simultaneous breakthrough of the endometrium and serosal layer of the uterus, it is necessary to use low acoustic power and closely monitor the grayscale changes in the treatment area during treatment.

5.2.3.4 Post-Treatment Assessment

1. **MRI evaluation after treatment.** There was localized subcutaneous soft tissue and edema of the muscle layer in the anterior abdominal wall (Fig. 5.21a). The contrast-enhanced T1WI showed that most of the anterior uterine adenomyosis was ablated as a non-perfusion area (56 mm × 53 mm × 58 mm). The serosal layer was intact, and the endometrium had been partially ablated (Fig.5.21b, c).
2. **MRI follow-up at 3 months after treatment.** The volume of the uterus was reduced, the non-perfused area of the anterior uterine wall was significantly reduced (37 mm × 37 mm × 37 mm), and the endometrium was basically repaired and thickened (Fig. 5.22).

5.2.3.5 Discussion

- The endometrial injury, in this case, is caused by the heat diffusion from the ablation area, but it can be repaired in a short time.
- This is a typical case of adenomyosis after focused ultrasound ablation treatment, with improved clinical symptoms and reduced lesions.

5.2.4 Case 4

5.2.4.1 Case Description

The female patient was 51 years old. She had adenomyosis with severe dysmenorrhea, constipation, and urinary fre-

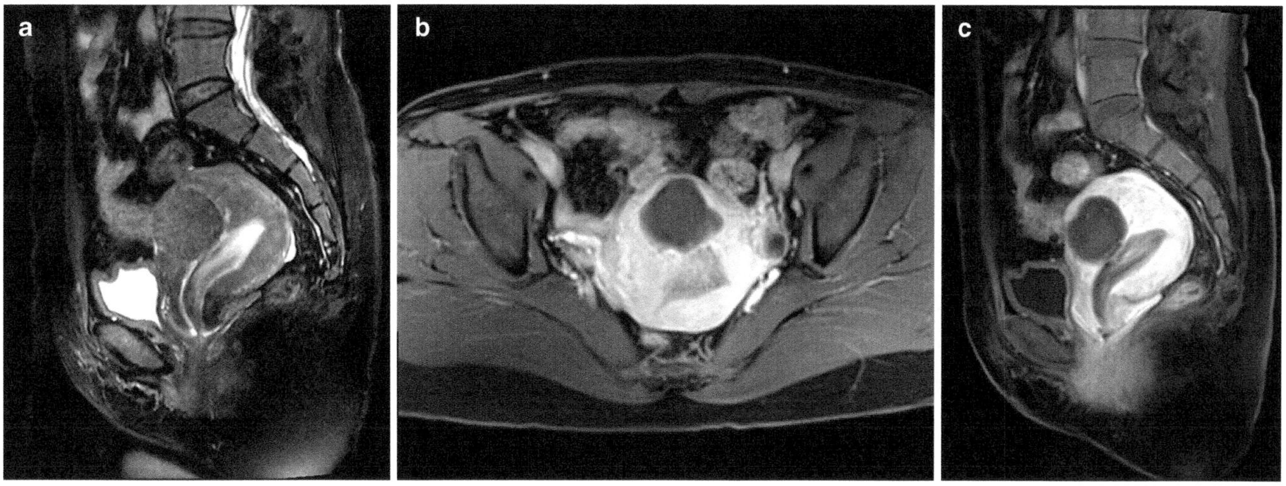

Fig. 5.22 Follow-up of uterine adenomyosis at 3 months after treatment. (**a**) T2WI_FS sagittal, (**b**) T1WI_FS + C axial, (**c**) T1WI_FS + C sagittal

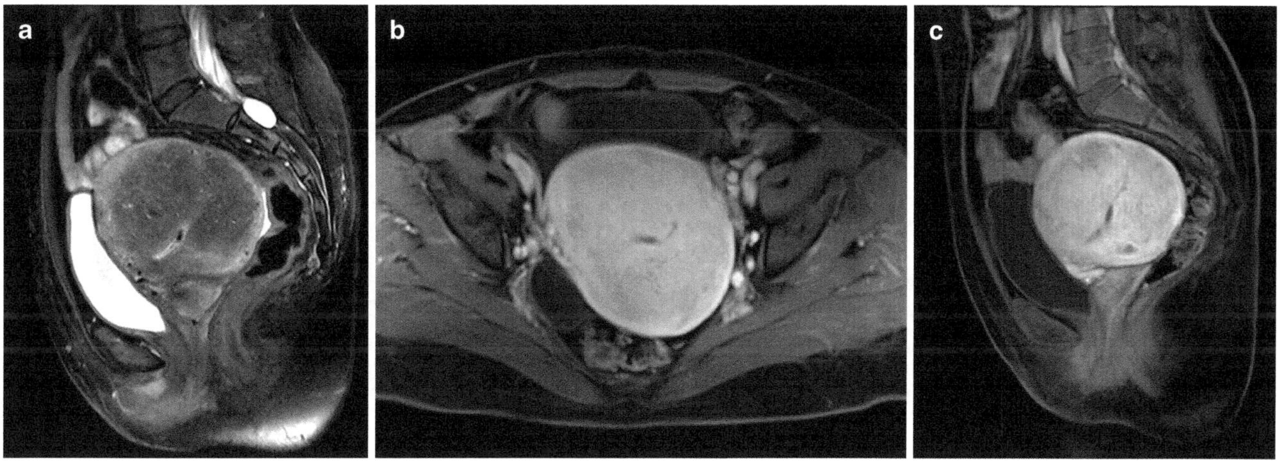

Fig. 5.23 Uterine adenomyosis before treatment. (**a**) T2WI_FS sagittal, (**b**) T1WI_FS + C axial, (**c**) T1WI_FS + C sagittal

quency for more than 3 years. Her symptoms did not improve after taking hormonal contraceptives and using intrauterine devices (Levonorgestrel Intrauterine system). Her menstrual period became prolonged in the past 2 months, with increased menstrual blood flow and moderate anemia. Her follow-up after focused ultrasound ablation treatment showed that the menstrual blood flow was significantly improved, and the dysmenorrhea disappeared.

5.2.4.2 Pre-Treatment Assessment

MRI showed diffuse adenomyosis, which had significantly thickened both the anterior and posterior walls of the uterus, showing low signals with scattered dot-shaped high signals on T2WI. The contraceptive device (Mirena) was visible in the uterine cavity. The shape of uterus was enlarged and spherical in shape. It compressed the bladder in front and rectum at the back (Fig. 5.23a). The contrast-enhanced T1WI showed that the adenomyosis was of moderate blood supply (Fig. 5.23b, c).

5.2.4.3 Treatment Techniques

1. **Focused ultrasound parameters.** Average acoustic power: 256 W, sonication time: 3200 s, duration of treatment: 135 mins, total energy: 820,400 J.
2. **Focused ultrasound ablation techniques.** Focused ultrasound ablation treatment for diffuse adenomyosis had a large ablation area. The endometria could be affected by heat diffusion. In the presence of a contraceptive device in the uterine cavity, the ultrasound focal region should avoid areas close to the endometrium.

5.2.4.4 Post-Treatment Assessment

MRI Evaluation after Treatment There is no edema in the anterior abdominal wall. The treated area of the uterine anterior and posterior walls showed heterogenous hyperintense signals on T2WI (Fig. 5.24a). The contrast-enhanced T1WI showed that most of the lesions of anterior and posterior walls were ablated without perfusion. The endometrium was

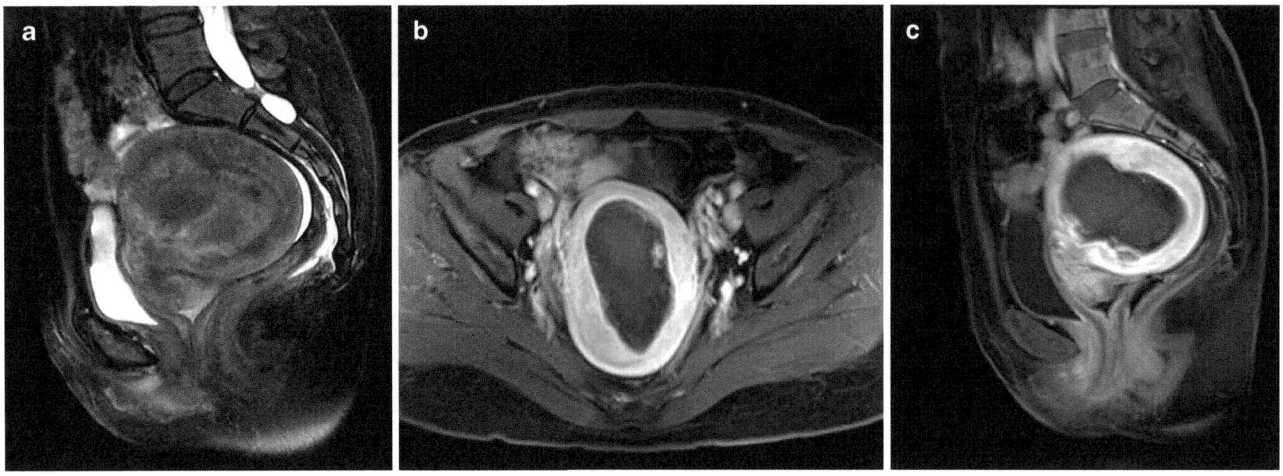

Fig. 5.24 MRI evaluation of uterine adenomyosis after treatment. (**a**) T2WI_FS sagittal, (**b**) T1WI_FS + C axial, (**c**) T1WI_FS + C sagittal

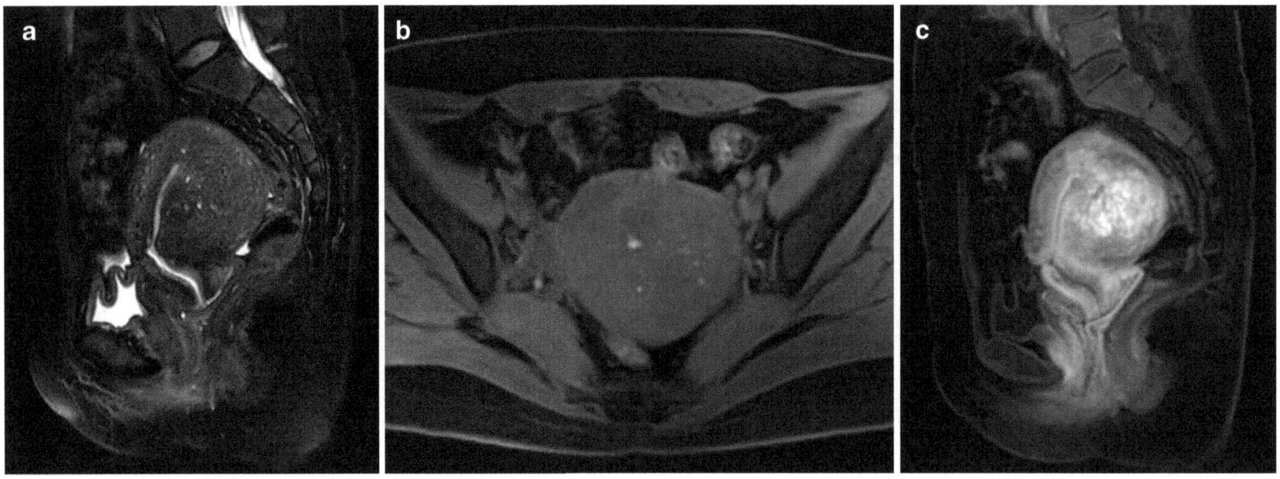

Fig. 5.25 Uterine adenomyosis before treatment. (**a**) T2WI_FS sagittal, (**b**) T1WI_FS axial, (**c**) T1WI_FS + C sagittal

ablated, but the outer layer of myometrium and serosal were completely protected (Fig. 5.24b, c).

5.2.4.5 Discussion

- Diffuse adenomyosis involves the entire uterine wall, and the increase in uterine volume would increase the corresponding endometrial area. Then treatment can ablate the adenomyosis and the endometrium together. The latter would achieve the therapeutic effect of endometrial ablation. The ultrasound treatment can be used for patients with adenomyosis who have no intention to become pregnant.

5.2.5 Case 5

5.2.5.1 Case Description

The female patient was 38 years old. She had dysmenorrhea and heavy menstrual blood flow. Follow-up for more than 1 year after focused ultrasound ablation treatment showed that her dysmenorrhea disappeared, and her menstrual blood flow decreased significantly.

5.2.5.2 Pre-Treatment Assessment

MRI showed diffuse adenomyosis in the posterior wall of the uterus without a clear boundary, and it compressed on the rectum at the back on T2WI (Fig. 5.25a). T1WI scan showed scattered bleeding spots in the lesion (Fig. 5.25b), and its contrast-enhanced T1WI showed that the adenomyosis was of an abundant blood supply (Fig. 5.25c). There were many bowels between the uterus and the anterior abdominal wall. Therefore, the procedure was somewhat difficult even if this posterior wall adenomyosis could be ablated.

5.2.5.3 Treatment Techniques

1. **Focused ultrasound parameters.** Average acoustic power: 244 W, sonication time: 2100 s, duration of treatment: 106 mins, total energy: 512,500 J.

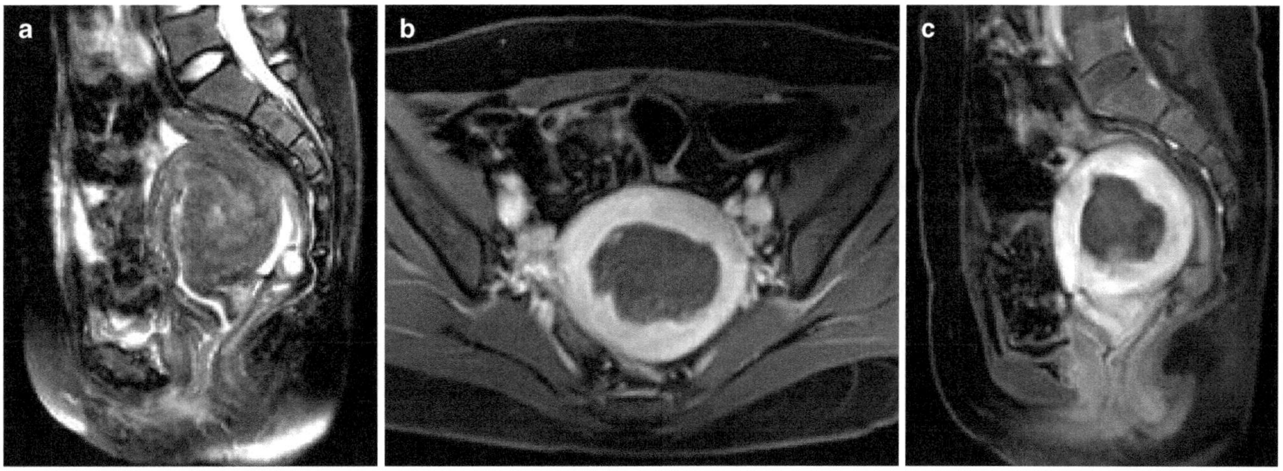

Fig. 5.26 MRI evaluation of uterine adenomyosis after treatment. (**a**) T2WI_FS sagittal, (**b**) T1WI_FS + C axial, (**c**) T1WI_FS + C sagittal

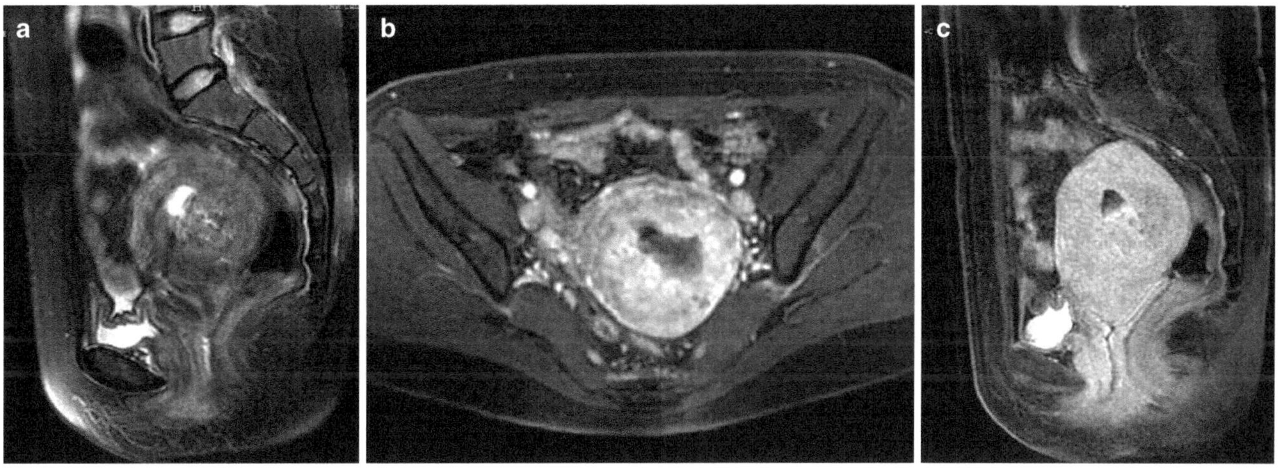

Fig. 5.27 MRI follow-up of adenomyosis at 14 months after treatment. (**a**) T2WI_FS sagittal, (**b**) T1WI_FS + C axial, (**c**) T1WI_FS + C sagittal

2. **Focused ultrasound ablation techniques.** The posterior adenomyosis of the uterus was diffused and adjacent to the rectum posteriorly. A lower acoustic power should be used during treatment. The ablation should be monitored by real-time ultrasound to prevent the breakthrough in the serosal layer of the posterior wall of the uterus.

5.2.5.4 Post-Treatment Assessment

- **MRI evaluation after treatment.** The muscular layer of the anterior abdominal wall was edematous. The thickened posterior wall with the adenomyosis showed increased T2WI signals (Fig. 5.26a). The contrast-enhanced T1WI showed that the adenomyosis had ablation without perfusion involving the adjacent endometrium. The posterior wall serosa and myometrial layer were completely protected and intact (Fig. 5.26b, c).
- **MRI follow-up at 14 months after treatment.** The size of the uterus was reduced, and the adenomyosis in the posterior wall was smaller. The ablation area without perfusion was significantly absorbed and reduced. The part of the ablated endometrium was repaired (Fig. 5.27).

5.2.5.5 Discussion

- After focused ultrasound ablation treatment, heat accumulation and diffusion affected the endometrium adjacent to the ultrasound focal area. This impaired part of the endometrium can be spontaneously repaired 14 months after treatment. Yet, this treatment should be more suitable for adenomyosis patients who have no fertility intention.

5.2.6 Case 6

5.2.6.1 Case Description

The female patient was 40 years old. She had dysmenorrhea, heavy menstrual blood flow, anal swelling, pain, and discomfort in the left lower limb, and mild anemia. Follow-up after focused ultrasound ablation treatment showed that the patient's menstrual blood flow was reduced, and her dysmenorrhea disappeared.

5.2.6.2 Pre-Treatment Assessment

MRI showed that the adenomyosis was mainly located on the posterior wall of the uterus, showing low signals with high spot intense signals on T1WI without a clear boundary (Fig. 5.28a). The contrast-enhanced T1WI showed that the adenomyosis lesion had a rich-moderate blood supply (Fig. 5.28b). It was predicted that focused ultrasound ablation could be feasible.

5.2.6.3 Treatment Techniques

1. **Focused ultrasound parameters.** Average acoustic power: 224 W, sonication time: 4041 s, duration of treatment: 153 mins, total energy: 905,640 J.
2. **Focused ultrasound ablation techniques.** The adenomyosis of the posterior uterine wall was adjacent to the lumbosacral spine, and it had no boundary. Therefore it would be advisable to use lower acoustic power for sonication. Pay attention to the patient's response during treatment to avoid damage to the sacral nerve plexus.

5.2.6.4 Post-Treatment Assessment

MRI Evaluation after Treatment There was no edema in the anterior abdominal wall, and the T2WI signal intensity in the center of the lesion significantly increased. The contrast-enhanced T1WI showed that the adenomyosis area of the posterior wall was partially ablated with non-perfusion areas. The posterior wall of the uterus and the adjacent serosa were protected. There were no lumbosacral injury signs (Fig. 5.29).

5.2.6.5 Discussion

- Although this patient had only partial ablation of the adenomyosis, her clinical symptoms improved significantly.
- The assessment of focused ultrasound ablation efficacy for adenomyosis differs from that of uterine fibroids. We often encountered adenomyosis with an NPV ratio of more than 90% after ultrasound ablation. Still, the symptoms of dysmenorrhea had not improved, and some patients had NPV ratios of less than 50%, but the symptoms of dysmenorrhea disappeared. Therefore, the effect of focused ultrasound ablation for adenomyosis mainly depends on improving clinical symptoms.

5.2.7 Case 7

5.2.7.1 Case Description

The female patient was 37 years old and had adenomyosis with dysmenorrhea, increased menstrual blood flow and a prolonged menstrual period for 10 years, and her dysmenorrhea has gradually worsened. After focused ultrasound abla-

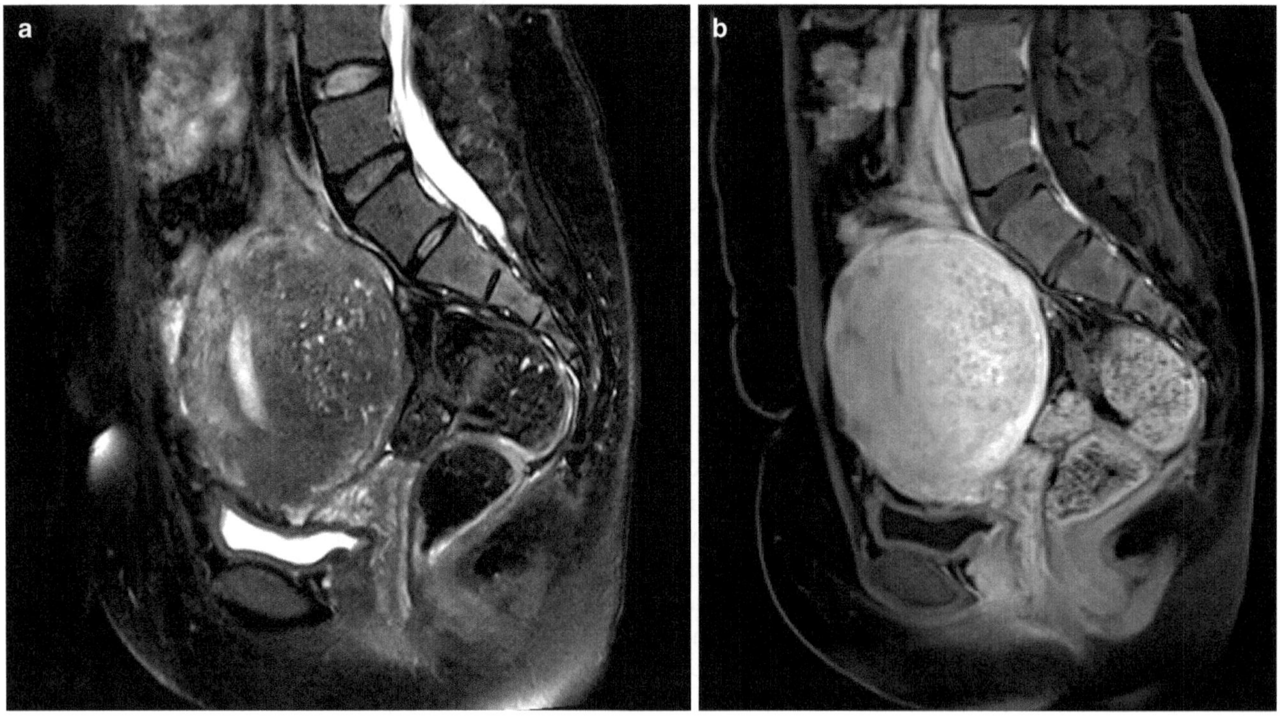

Fig. 5.28 Uterine adenomyosis before treatment. (**a**) T2WI_FS sagittal, (**b**) T1WI_FS + C sagittal

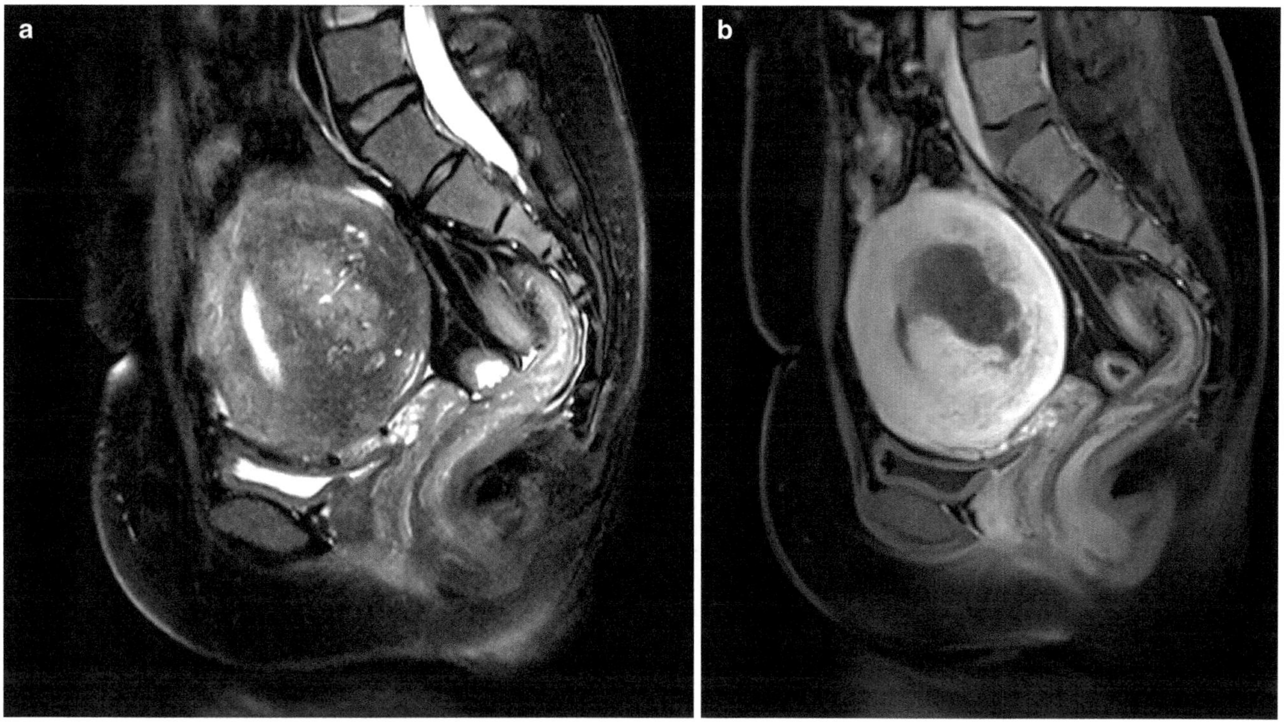

Fig. 5.29 MRI evaluation of uterine adenomyosis after treatment. (**a**) T2WI_FS sagittal, (**b**) T1WI_FS + C sagittal

tion treatment, the patient was administrated with three doses of GnRHa (Goserelin) at an interval of 28 days. Then LNG-IUS was inserted after MRI evaluation of uterus size. The patient's dysmenorrhea improved significantly, and menstrual flow had returned to normal.

5.2.7.2 Pre-Treatment Assessment

MRI demonstrated adenomyosis in the posterior wall and fundus of the uterus showing heterogeneously mixed high and low signals on T2WI. The anteverted uterus had enlarged and compressed on the bladder (Fig. 5.30a). The contrast-enhanced T1WI showed that the lesion had partially abundant blood supply without a clear boundary (Fig. 5.30b).

5.2.7.3 Treatment Techniques

1. **Focused ultrasound parameters.** Average acoustic power: 271 W, sonication time: 2600 s, duration of treatment: 131 mins, total energy: 704,650 J.
2. **Focused ultrasound ablation techniques.** The lesion was close to the lumbosacral vertebrae, and attention should be paid to avoid the focused ultrasound ablation area breaking through the serosa of the posterior uterine wall because the acoustic energy of the far-field was reflected by the lumbosacral bone surface, which made the thermal energy easily accumulated in post-focus. Therefore, the acoustic power need be reduced and the focal regions should be deployed at least 15 mm away from the posterior serosal layer.

5.2.7.4 Post-Treatment Assessment

1. **MRI evaluation after treatment.** There was locally moderate edema in the anterior abdominal wall, and the signal intensity of the treated area increased significantly on T2WI (Fig. 5.31a). The contrast-enhanced T1WI revealed that most of the lesion was ablated without perfusion, and the serosal layer and its adjacent myometrium of the posterior wall were protected and intact (Fig. 5.31b).
2. **MRI follow-up at 3 months after treatment.** The volume of the uterus decreased, and the ablation non-perfusion area was significantly reduced (Fig. 5.32a, b).

5.2.7.5 Discussion

- In this patient, the pain was severe during the ablation procedure since the treated lesion located at the posterior wall of the uterus was close to the lumbosacral bone, and ultrasound waves would stimulate the periosteum. The lower acoustic power was employed to prevent intolerable pain and improve patient compliance, apart from that the focal regions were set as far away from the lumbosacral vertebrae as possible.
- The combined treatment regimen of focused ultrasound ablation, GnRH-a, and LNG-LUS for adenomyosis had low long-term recurrence rates in dysmenorrhea and menorrhagia, and the focused ultrasound ablation combined with GnRH-a could make the uterine volume shrink significantly in the short period of time as in this case.

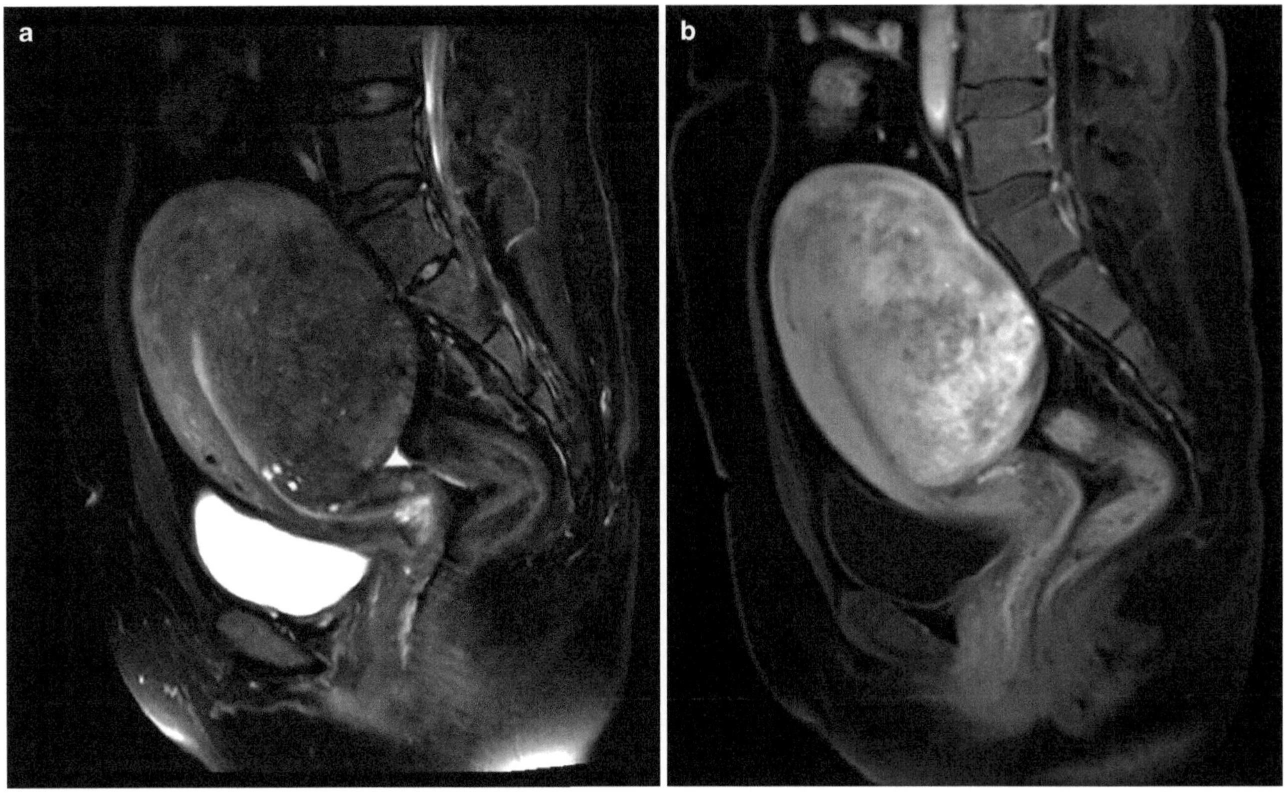

Fig. 5.30 Uterine adenomyosis before treatment. (**a**) T2WI_FS sagittal, (**b**) T1WI_FS + C sagittal

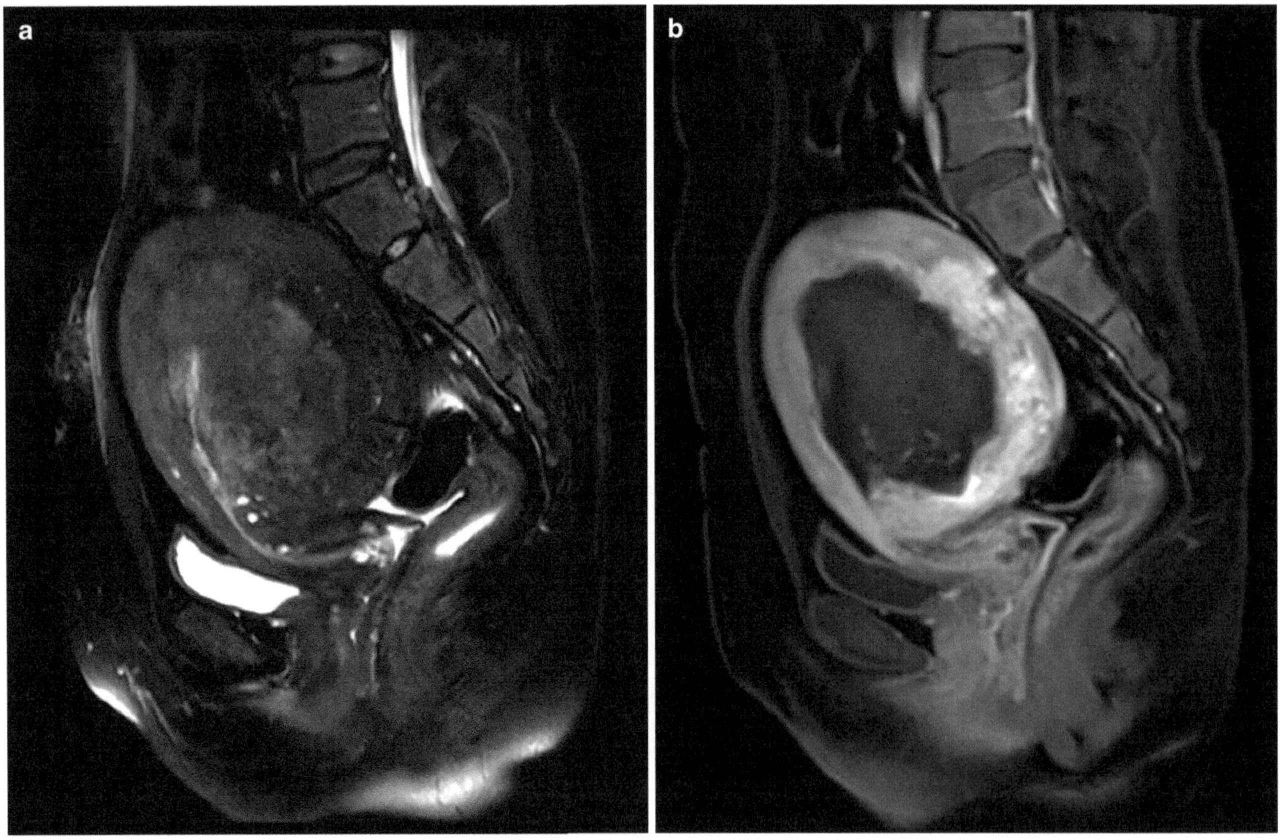

Fig. 5.31 MRI evaluation of uterine adenomyosis after treatment. (**a**) T2WI_FS sagittal, (**b**) T1WI_FS + C sagittal

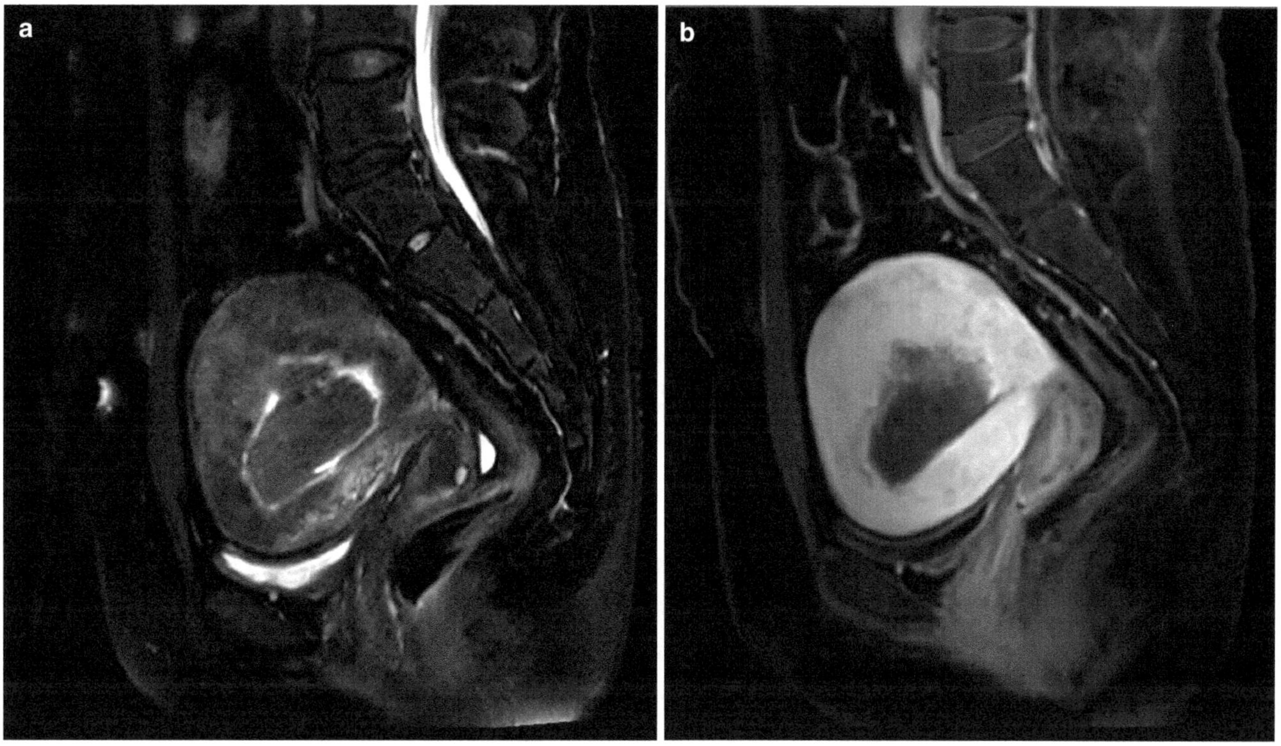

Fig. 5.32 MRI follow-up of adenomyosis at 3 months after treatment. (**a**) T2WI_FS sagittal, (**b**) T1WI_FS + C sagittal

5.2.8 Case 8

5.2.8.1 Case Description

The female patient was 39 years old with reproductive desire. She suffered from dysmenorrhea for more than 20 years, accompanied by lower abdominal soreness. The patient's dysmenorrhea disappeared after the focused ultrasound ablation treatment, and the menstrual blood flow remained relatively heavy. She became pregnant 5 months after ablation treatment and delivered a healthy baby girl by cesarean section.

5.2.8.2 Pre-Treatment Assessment

MRI showed diffuse adenomyosis of the posterior uterine wall with unclear boundaries. It showed mixed low signals with scattered speckled high signals on T2WI (Fig. 5.33a). The contrast-enhanced T1WI showed that the adenomyosis had an abundant blood supply (Fig. 5.33b, c). The acoustic pathway was clear, and focused ultrasound ablation was predicted to be feasible.

5.2.8.3 Treatment Techniques

1. **Focused ultrasound parameters.** Average acoustic power: 302 W, sonication time: 3000 s, duration of treatment: 131 mins, total energy: 905,750 J.
2. **Focused ultrasound ablation treatment technique** The blood supply of the adenomyosis was abundant. In this case, with a good acoustic pathway, higher acoustic power could be recommended. Pay close attention to the ablation areas during treatment, and avoid injury to the endometrium as much as possible.

5.2.8.4 Post-Treatment Assessment

MRI Evaluation after Treatment Local edema in the soft tissues of the anterior abdominal wall was seen, and the T2WI signal intensity in the adenomyosis had increased (Fig. 5.34a). The contrast-enhanced MRI showed that the central area of the posterior wall adenomyosis was ablated with no perfusion. The endometrium and the serosal layer of the uterus were completely protected and intact (Fig. 5.34b, c).

5.2.8.5 Discussion

- The ultrasound focal region should be ≥10 mm away from the endometrium for patients with fertility requirements. To avoid damage to the adjacent rectum and sacrococcyx, it must also be ≥15 mm away from the posterior edge of the uterus. In this case, most of the central area of the lesion was ablated, and the endometrium and serosal layer remained intact, which did not affect her to get subsequent pregnancy.

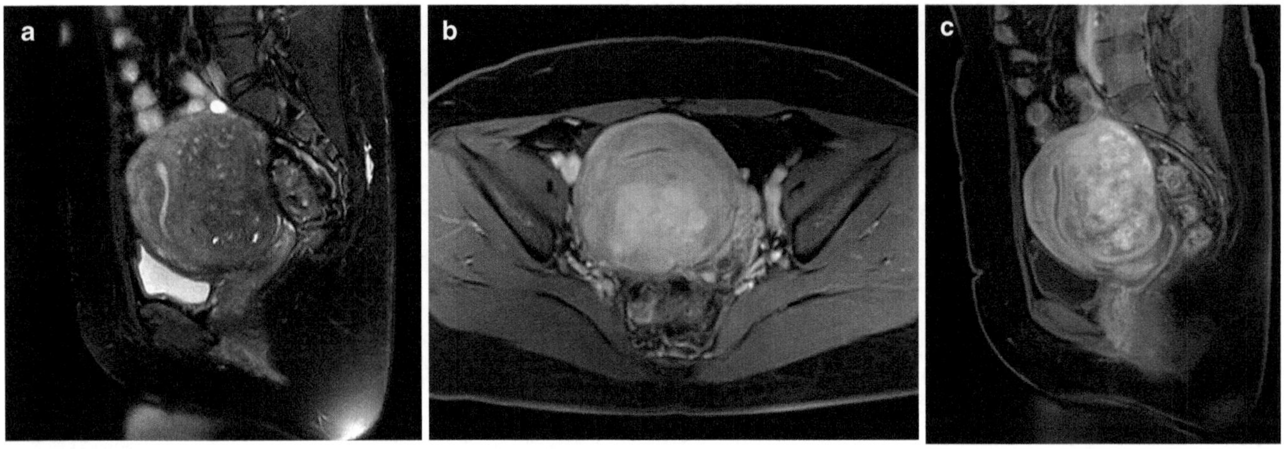

Fig. 5.33 Uterine adenomyosis before treatment. (**a**) T2WI_FS sagittal, (**b**) T1WI_FS + C axial, (**c**) T1WI_FS + C sagittal

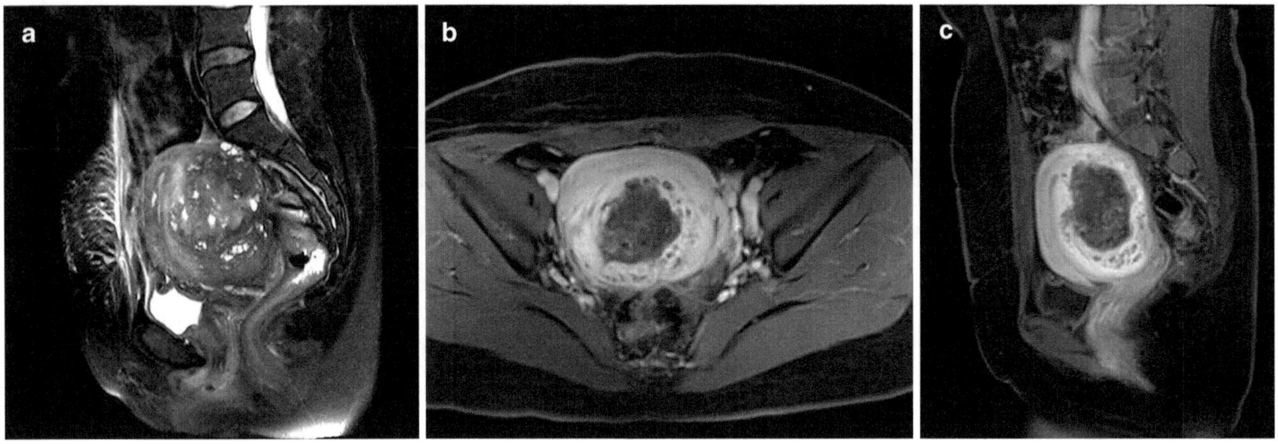

Fig. 5.34 MRI evaluation of uterine adenomyosis after treatment. (**a**) T2WI_FS sagittal, (**b**) T1WI_FS + C axial, (**c**) T1WI_FS + C sagittal

5.2.9 Case 9

5.2.9.1 Case Description

The female patient was 43 years old. She had dysmenorrhea and heavy menstrual blood flow. Long-term follow-up after focused ultrasound ablation treatment showed that the patient's menstrual blood flow decreased and his dysmenorrhea improved.

5.2.9.2 Pre-Treatment Assessment

MRI showed adenomyosis in the posterior wall of the uterus, showing low signals on T2WI. There were also scattered miliary hyperintense T2WI signals in the lesion. One small fibroid was seen on the anterior wall of the uterus, showing low signal on T2WI (Fig. 5.35a). According to the MRI T2WI signal characteristics, it was predicted that the lesions were feasible to ablate.

5.2.9.3 Treatment Techniques

1. **Focused ultrasound parameters.** Average acoustic power: 257 W, sonication time: 2200 s, duration of treatment: 136 mins, total energy: 564,860 J.
2. **Focused ultrasound ablation techniques.** Patients with heavy menstrual blood flow and no pregnancy plan could be treated by focused ultrasound ablation involving the endometrium of the fundus and the adenomyosis of the uterus. Small fibroids in the anterior wall of the uterus can be treated with focused ultrasound ablation simultaneously.

5.2.9.4 Post-Treatment Assessment

MRI Evaluation after Treatment The anterior abdominal wall was edematous, there was a small amount of fluid in the pouch of Douglas, and the signal of the posterior wall and fundal areas slightly increased on T2WI (Fig. 5.35b). The contrast-enhanced T1WI showed that these lesions of the

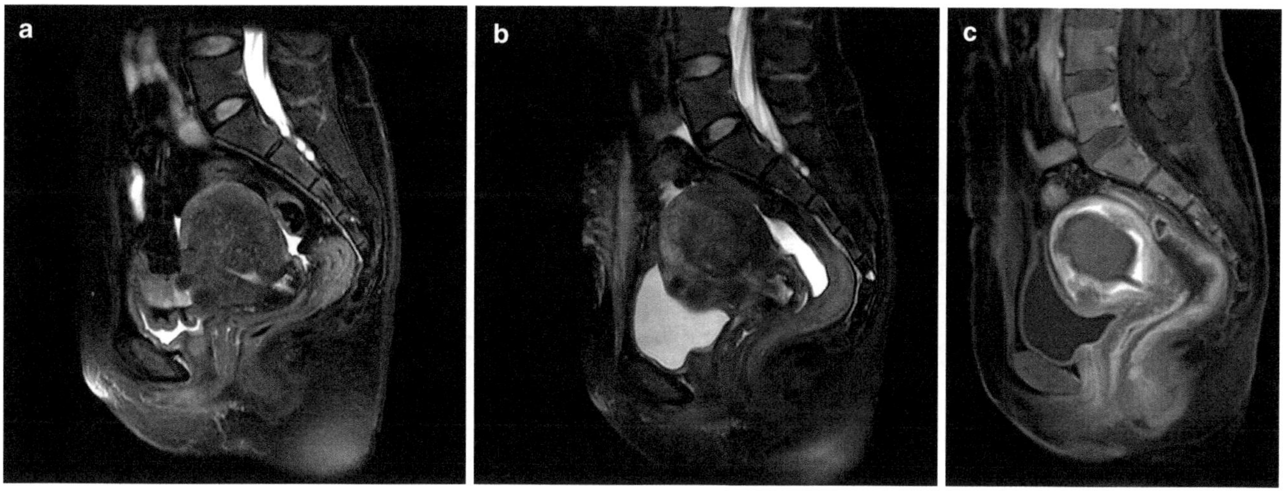

Fig. 5.35 MRI evaluation of uterine adenomyosis with uterine fibroids before treatment (**a**) and after treatment (**b**, **c**). (**a**) T2WI_FS sagittal, (**b**) T2WI_FS sagittal, (**c**) T1WI_FS + C sagittal

posterior uterine wall were almost completely ablated with no perfusion. The endometria of the fundus and posterior wall of the uterus were also ablated, but the posterior myometrium and serosal layer were preserved, and the small fibroid of the anterior wall was ablated (Fig. 5.35c).

5.2.9.5 Discussion

- This is a typical case of complete focused ultrasound ablation of adenomyosis, and it plays a role in reducing the endometrium.
- Focused ultrasound ablation in the treatment of adenomyosis sometimes involves the endometrium. The fundus of the uterine cavity is a blind end, so the ablation in this area does not need to consider the possibility of intrauterine adhesion.

5.2.10 Case 10

5.2.10.1 Case Description

The female patient was 38 years old. Her adenomyosis had progressively worsened in the past 2 years, with dysmenorrhea accompanied by increased menstrual blood flow. Follow-up after focused ultrasound ablation treatment showed that her dysmenorrhea and increased menstrual blood flow disappeared.

5.2.10.2 Pre-Treatment Assessment

MRI showed that adenomyosis had diffuse distributions on the posterior wall and fundus, resulting in obvious thickening of the posterior uterine wall. There were mixed high and low signals on T2WI (Fig. 5.36a). The contrast-enhanced T1WI showed that the lesion area without a clear boundary was homogeneously enhanced, with a moderate blood supply, and it had a good acoustic pathway (Fig. 5.36b, c). It was predicted that the focused ultrasound ablation would be feasible.

5.2.10.3 Treatment Techniques

1. **Focused ultrasound parameters.** Average acoustic power: 341 W, sonication time: 1440 s, duration of treatment: 110 mins, total energy: 490,700 J.
2. **Focused ultrasound ablation technique.** The uterus was anteverted. The adenomyosis was mainly located on the posterior wall of the uterus, closer to the sacrum. The ultrasound focal region should be more than 15 mm away from the serosa of the posterior uterine wall. Some lesions were adjacent to the endometrium, and care should be taken to keep a distance between the ablation focal region and the endometrium of at least 10 mm during treatment.

5.2.10.4 Post-Treatment Assessment

1. **MRI evaluation after treatment.** The muscle layer of the anterior abdominal wall was edematous, and a small amount of fluid was found in the pouch of Douglas (Fig. 5.37a). The contrast-enhanced T1WI showed that the adenomyosis was almost completely ablated with no perfusion. The endometria of the uterine fundus and posterior wall were partially ablated. The corresponding myometrial and serosal layers were well protected and intact (Fig. 5.37b, c).
2. **MRI follow-up at 20 months after treatment.** It showed that the size of the uterus had shrunk and gradually returned to its normal shape. Most of the necrotic tissue was discharged, and only some portion of the remaining necrotic tissue seemed to protrude into the uterine cavity (Fig. 5.38).
3. **MRI follow-up at 3 years after treatment.** It showed that the uterus had returned to its normal shape, no

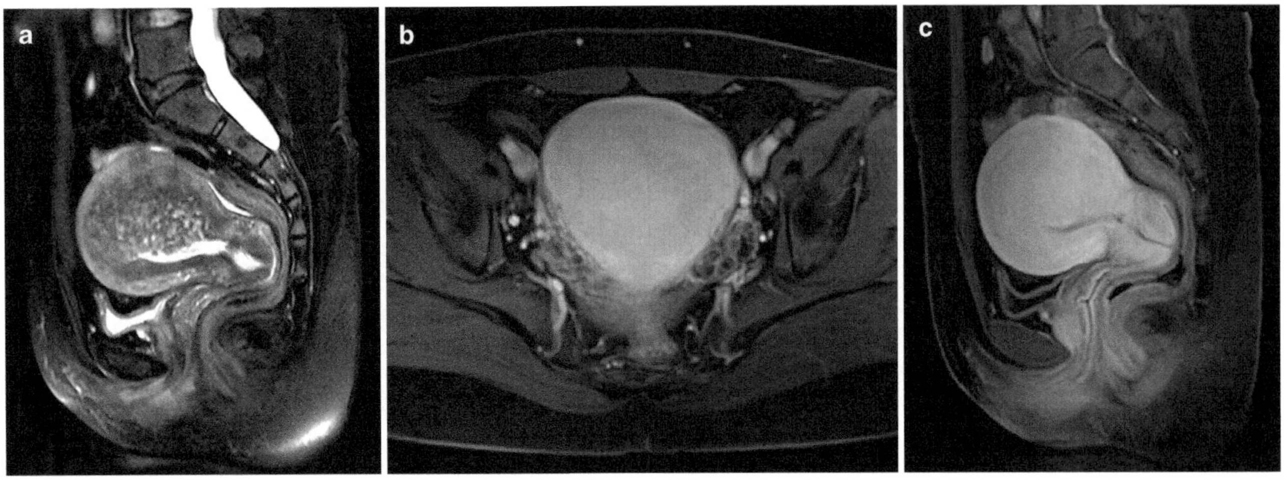

Fig. 5.36 Uterine adenomyosis before treatment. (**a**) T2WI_FS sagittal, (**b**) T1WI_FS + C axial, (**c**) T1WI_FS + C sagittal

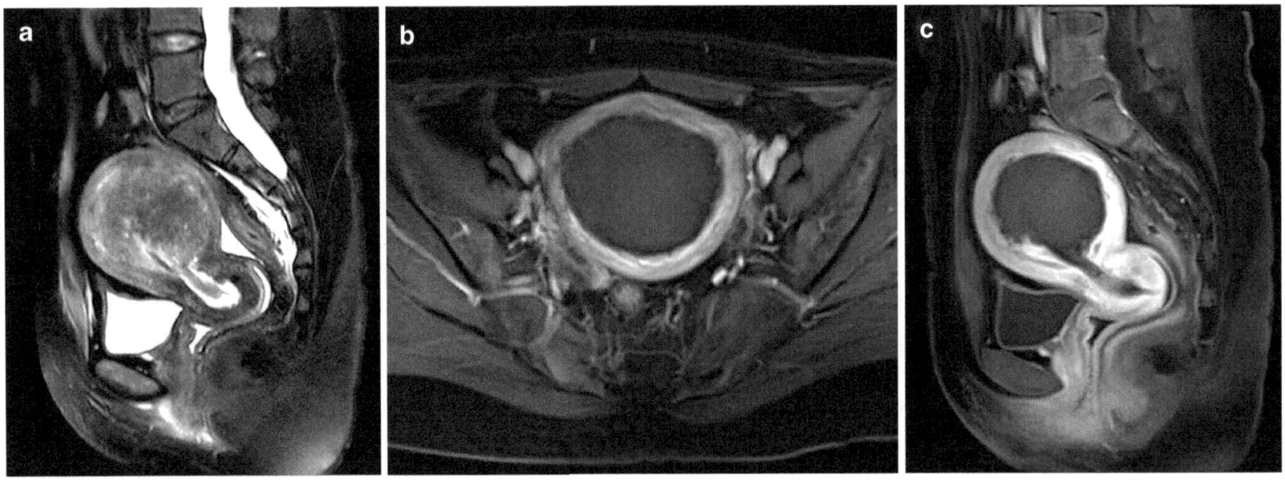

Fig. 5.37 MRI evaluation of uterine adenomyosis after treatment. (**a**) T2WI_FS sagittal, (**b**) T1WI_FS + C axial, (**c**) T1WI_FS + C sagittal

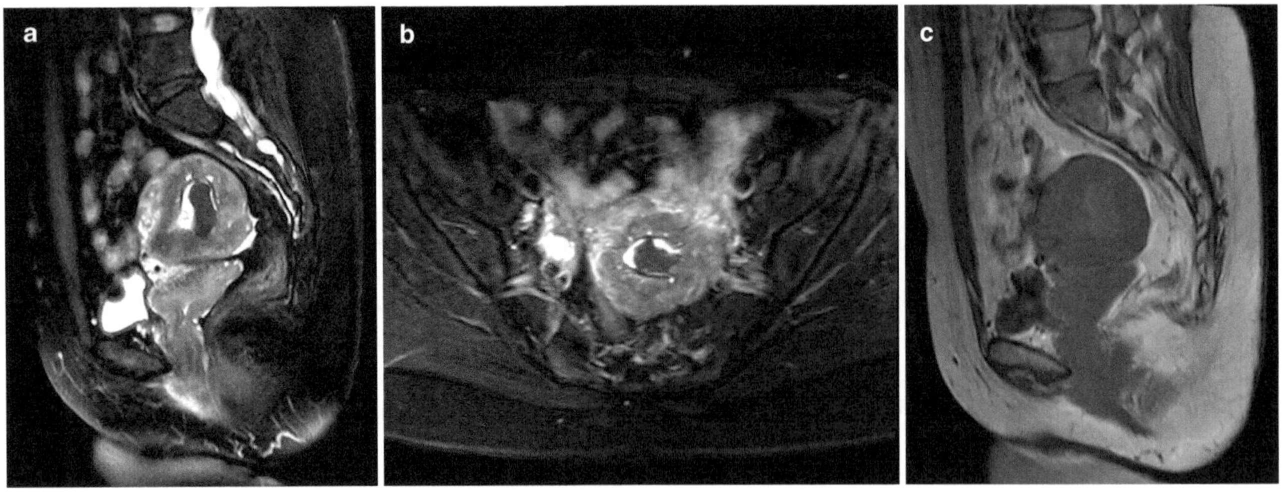

Fig. 5.38 MRI follow-up of uterine adenomyosis at 20 months after treatment. (**a**) T2WI_FS sagittal, (**b**) T2WI_FS axial, (**c**) T1WI sagittal

necrotic tissue was visible, and the endometrium had become normal (Fig. 5.39).

5.2.10.5 Discussion

- This is a typical case of adenomyosis cured by ultrasound ablation.
- The MRI examination showed that the uterus returned to its normal shape, and the part of the endometrium broken by heat diffusion of the ablation was repaired completely.

5.2.11 Case 11

5.2.11.1 Case Description

The female patient was 41 years old. She had dysmenorrhea for 7 years, progressive worsening with heavy menstrual blood flow, and severe anemia.

5.2.11.2 Pre-Treatment Assessment

MRI showed the adenomyosis was diffusely located on the posterior wall of the uterus. The junctional zone at the fundus and the body of the uterus were significantly enlarged. The adenomyosis showed homogeneous hyperintense signals on T2WI, with spotted hyperintense signals within the lesion on T1WI (Fig. 5.40a, b). The contrast-enhanced T1WI showed that the lesion was homogeneously enhanced and had an abundant blood supply (Fig. 5.40c). It was predicted that it would be difficult to perform focused ultrasound ablation treatment.

5.2.11.3 Treatment Techniques

1. **Focused ultrasound parameters.** Average acoustic power: 395 W, sonication time: 2403 s, duration of treatment: 165 mins, total energy: 948,650 J.
2. **Focused ultrasound ablation techniques.** The T2WI signals of the adenomyosis suggested that focused ultrasound ablation would be difficult. Therefore, when the ultrasound pathway was good and the ultrasound focal region was set to a certain distance ($\geq$ 15 mm) from the posterior edge of the uterus, a higher acoustic power was used for focused ultrasound ablation treatment.

5.2.11.4 Post-Treatment Assessment

1. **MRI evaluation after treatment.** The subcutaneous tissue and muscle layer of the anterior abdominal wall were edematous. The central portion of the adenomyosis showed circular T2WI high signals (Fig. 5.41a). The

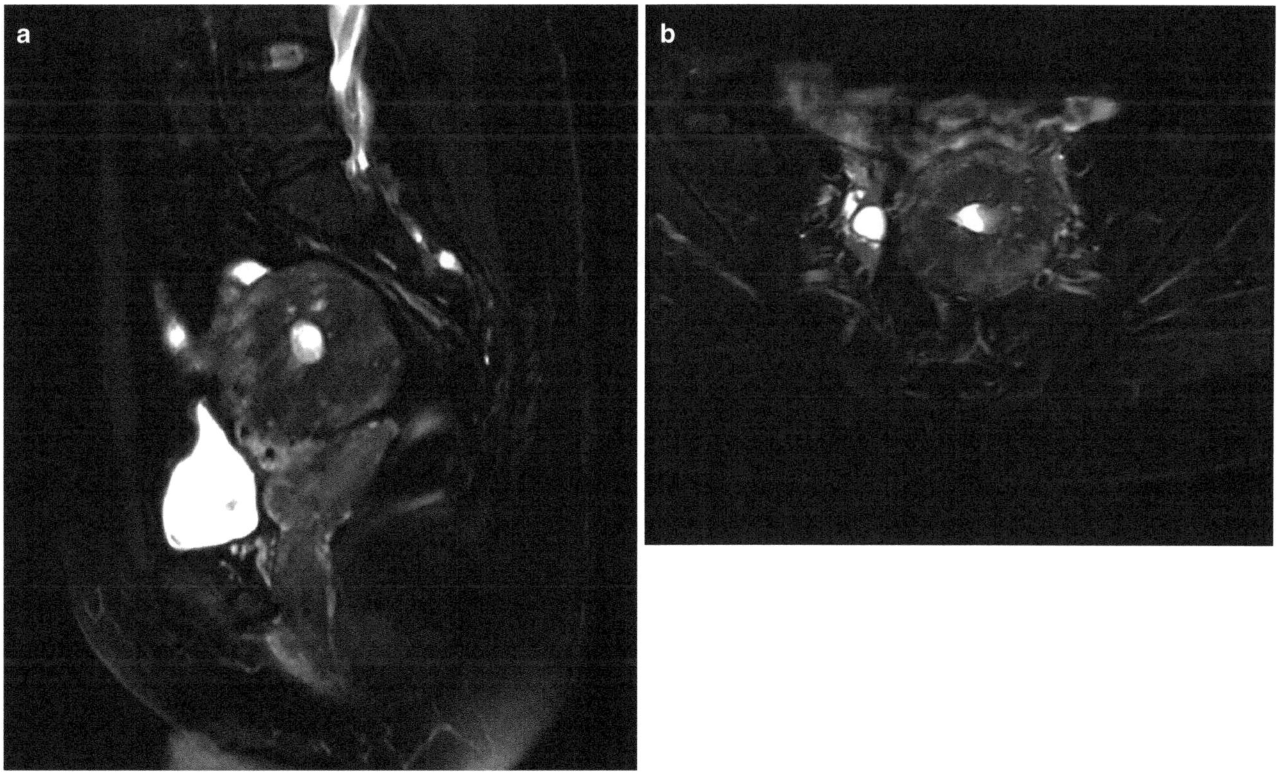

Fig. 5.39 MRI follow-up of uterine adenomyosis at 3 years after treatment. (**a**) T2WI_FS sagittal, (**b**) T2WI_FS axial

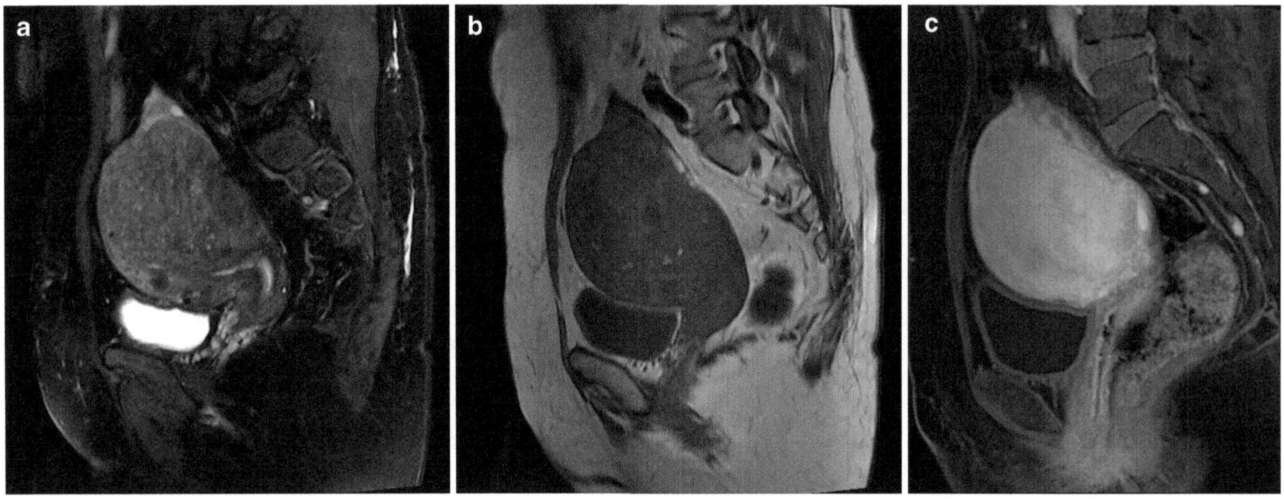

Fig. 5.40 Uterine adenomyosis before treatment. (**a**) T2WI_FS sagittal, (**b**) T1WI sagittal, (**c**) T1WI_FS + C sagittal

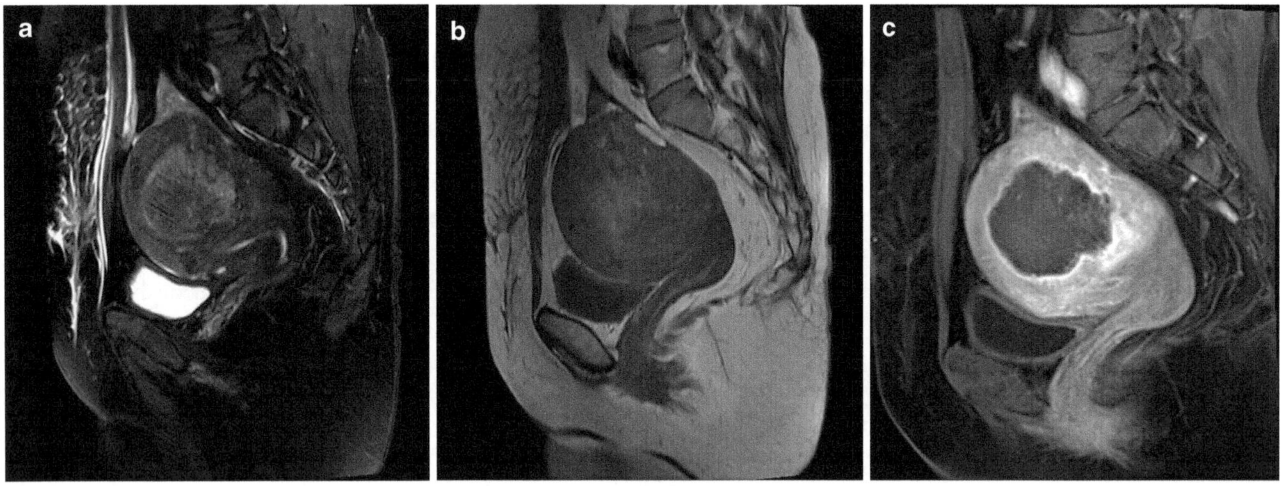

Fig. 5.41 MRI evaluation of uterine adenomyosis after treatment. (**a**) T2WI_FS sagittal, (**b**) T1WI sagittal, (**c**) T1WI_FS + C sagittal

contrast-enhanced T1WI showed that most of the ablation in the center of the lesion was non-perfused, and the surrounding lesions remained. The myometrial and serosal layers were well protected and intact (Fig. 5.41b, c).

2. **MRI follow-up at 21 months after treatment.** The edema of the anterior abdominal wall disappeared, the volume of the uterus was larger than that before, and the adenomyosis lesion area of the posterior wall was slightly enlarged. Scattered spots of T1WI high signals were seen, suggesting signs of recurrence (Fig. 5.42).

5.2.11.5 Discussion

- The purpose of treatment of adenomyosis is to improve clinical symptoms. Because the boundary between the lesion and the surroundings is unclear, it is safe to ablate as many adenomyosis as possible. It is generally believed that symptom improvement is related to the degree and extent of ablation.
- The ablation effect, in this case, was good. Still, the follow-up revealed that dysmenorrhea and heavy menstrual flow were not significantly improved, so the therapeutic strategy of focused ultrasound ablation for adenomyosis still needs to be further explored.
- Although there will be obvious edema of the soft tissues of the anterior abdominal wall after ultrasound ablation, this type of subcutaneous soft tissue edema can be gradually absorbed and disappear as long as the skin burns are avoided.

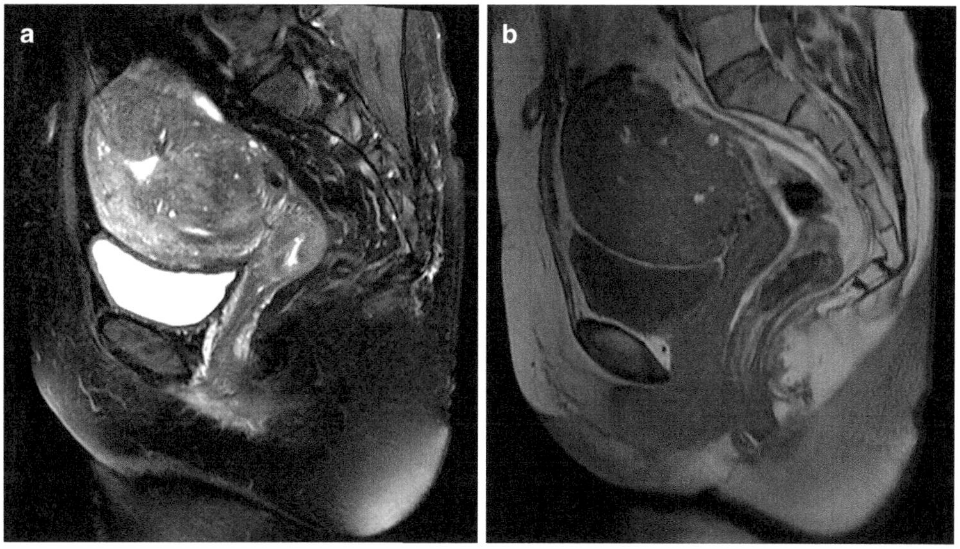

Fig. 5.42 MRI follow-up of uterine adenomyosis at 21 months after treatment. (**a**) T2WI_FS sagittal, (**b**) T1WI sagittal

Focused Ultrasound Ablation for Other Gynecological Related Diseases

6

Xiaogang Zhu, Yonghua Xu, Ming Xue, and Felix Wong

Abstract

Abdominal wall endometriosis, a rare extrapelvic disease, normally is related to obstetric or gynecologic surgery; however, focused ultrasound surgery may be an alternative with a lower incidence of adverse events. Contrast-enhanced ultrasonography and magnetic resonance imaging were used to assess and observe abdominal wall endometriosis before and after focused ultrasound ablation. The therapeutic techniques, focused ultrasound parameters, and treatment outcomes are revealed, and the treatment outcomes with follow-up are shown and discussed. Cesarean scar pregnancy, which is the gestational sac implanted in a cesarean section scar, has a high risk of severe hemorrhage and uterine perforation after curettage. The therapeutic strategies, focused ultrasound parameters, and treatment outcomes are revealed to ablate the lesion without or with subsequent curettage.

Keywords

MRI · Contrast-enhanced ultrasonography · High-intensity focused ultrasound · Ablation · Abdominal wall endometriosis · Cesarean scar pregnancy · Curettage

Since 1997, the first patient with a malignant bone tumor was successfully treated with extracorporeal high-intensity focused ultrasound (HIFU) in the world; the focused ultrasound ablation has been used to treat liver cancer, pancreatic cancer, breast cancer, renal cancer, and other malignant tumors. As the treatment technology of uterine fibroids and adenomyosis has become more and more mature, Focused ultrasound ablation surgery (FUAS) application in gynecology has exhibited greater advantages. In recent years, it has also attracted the attention of some experts and clinicians in the application of pregnancy-related diseases, such as abdominal endometriosis and cesarean scar pregnancy. This chapter describes the clinical application of focused ultrasound for treating abdominal endometriosis and cesarean section scar pregnancy.

6.1 Focused Ultrasound Ablation for Abdominal Wall Endometriosis

6.1.1 Case 1

6.1.1.1 Case Description

The female patient was 28 years old. She had periodic abdominal pain for more than 3 years. The abdominal pain started one year after a cesarean section, and it occurred during menstruation and was relieved after menstruation. A mass was found in the abdominal wall for 5 months. Because of the progressive abdominal wall pain, treatment was required.

6.1.1.2 Pre-Treatment Assessment

MRI sagittal scan showed mixed high and low signals on T2WI suggestive of abdominal wall endometriosis, with a range of about 39 mm ×31 mm × 13 mm, T1WI contrast-enhanced T1WI showed abundant blood supply of the lesion, and the arrow in the figure showed abdominal wall endometriosis lesions (Fig. 6.1).

6.1.1.3 Treatment Techniques

1. **Focused ultrasound parameters.** Average acoustic power: 125 W, sonication time: 381 s, duration of treatment: 76 min, total energy: 47,625 J.

X. Zhu · M. Xue (✉)
The Third Xiangya Hospital of Central South University, Changsha, China

Y. Xu
Zhongshan-Xuhui Hospital, Fudan University, Shanghai, China

F. Wong
The University of New South Wales, Sydney, NSW, Australia

Y. Xu et al. (eds.), *Surgical Techniques of Focused Ultrasound Ablation in Benign Uterine Diseases*,
https://doi.org/10.1007/978-981-19-7180-8_6

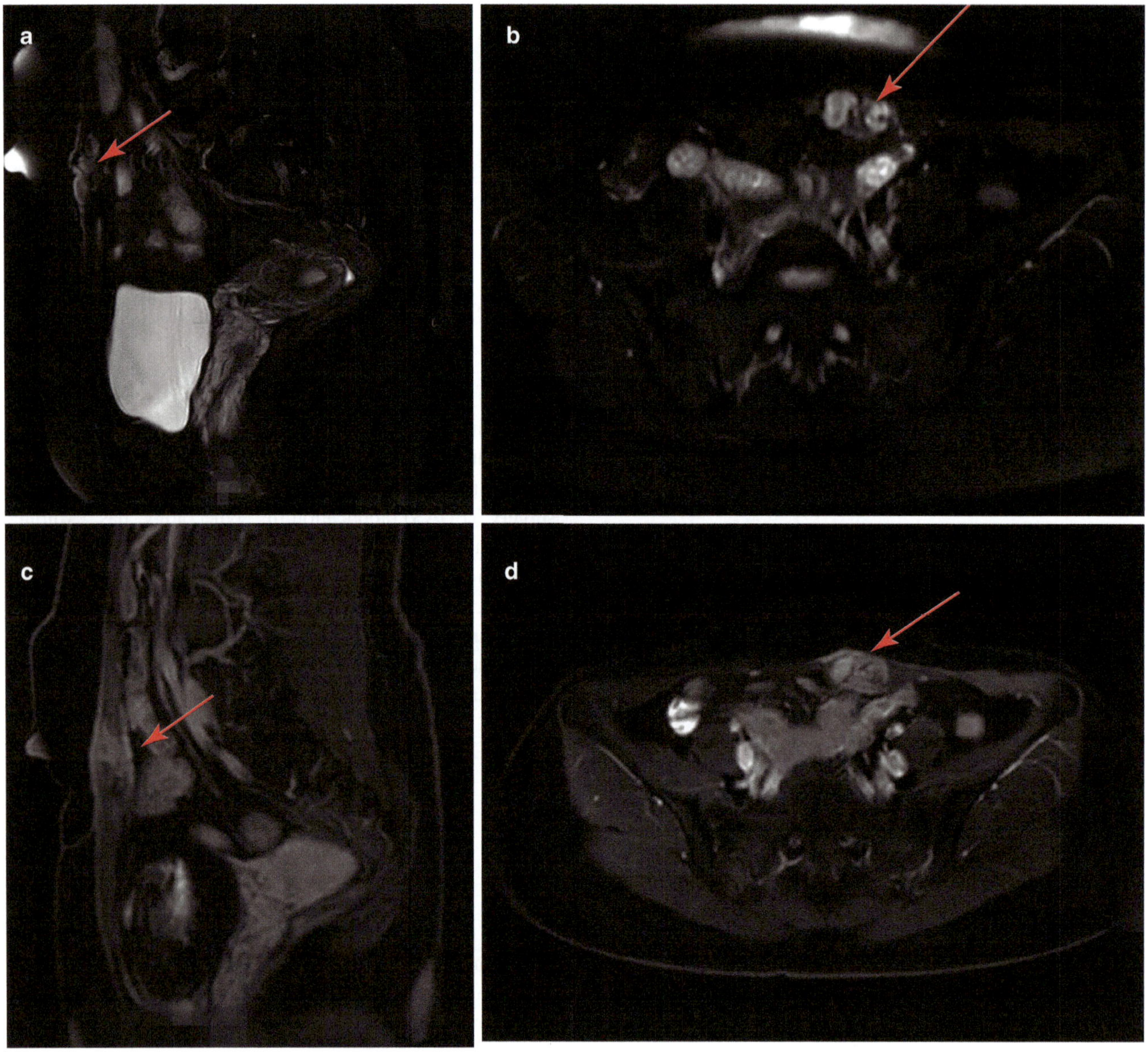

Fig. 6.1 Abdominal wall endometriosis before treatment. (**a**) T2WI_FS sagittal (the lesion reached the muscular layer), (**b**) T2WI_FS axial, (**c**) T1WI_FS +C sagittal, (**d**) T1WI_FS +C axial

2. **Focused ultrasound ablation techniques.** The ablation range was 0.5–1.0 cm around the lesion. For patients with abdominal wall thickness less than 3 cm, focused ultrasound ablation should be chosen carefully.

6.1.1.4 Post-Treatment Assessment

MRI follow-up at 5 months after treatment. After 5 months of treatment, the abdominal wall endometriosis lesions were significantly reduced and absorbed (1.2 m × 0.7 cm). The arrow in the figure showed the abdominal wall had reduced endometriosis lesions (Fig. 6.2).

6.1.1.5 Discussion

- The patient was a typical case of abdominal wall endometriosis and was unwilling to choose the traditional surgical treatment. After focused ultrasound ablation, the abdominal wall pain disappeared completely. Five months after the ablation treatment, MRI showed significantly reduced lesions.
- In this case, the lesion was deep and close to the parietal peritoneum, and the risk of focused ultrasound ablation was high. During the treatment, attention should be paid to distending the bladder and covering the lesion with the

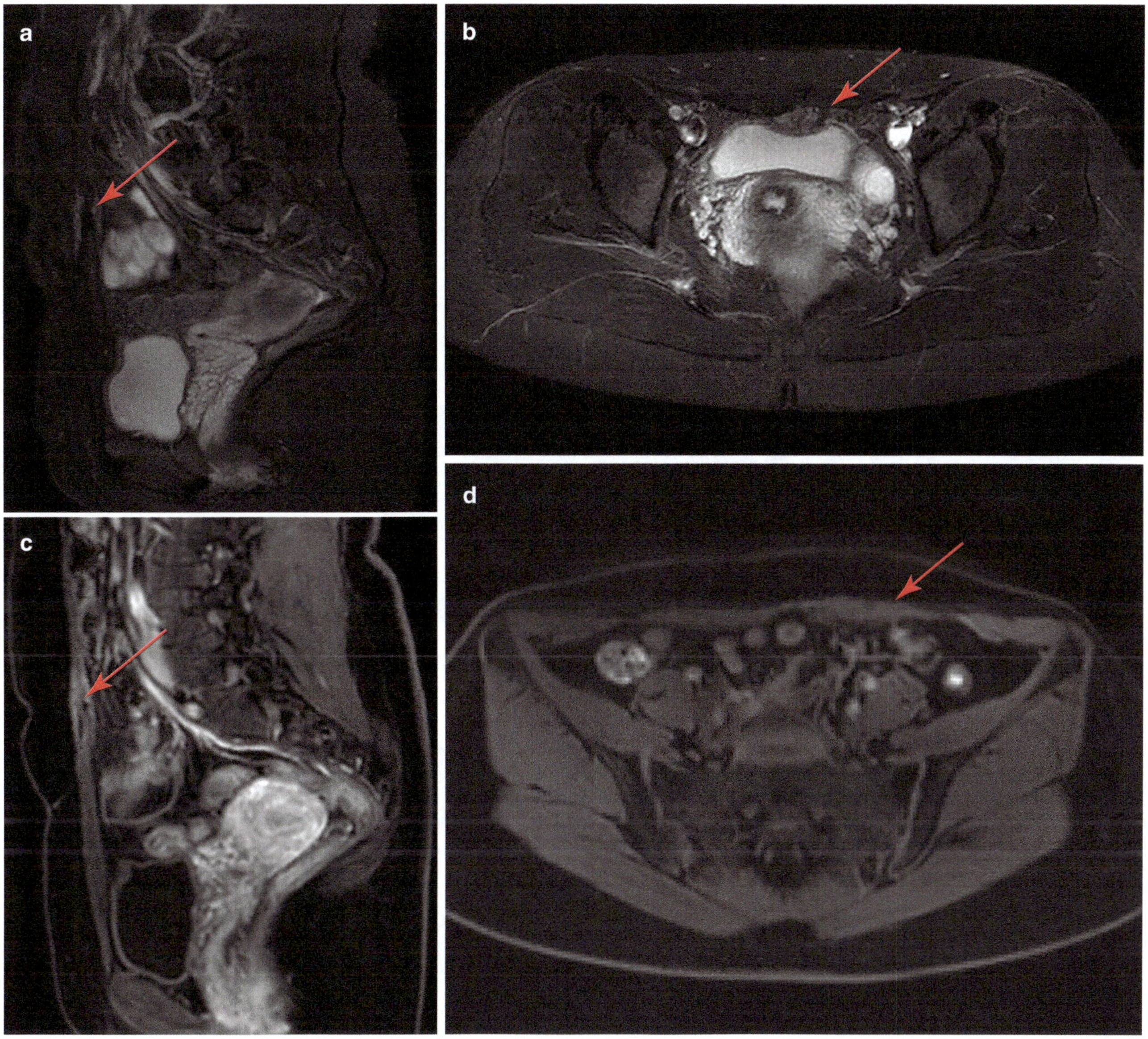

Fig. 6.2 MRI follow-up of abdominal wall endometriosis at 5 months after treatment. (**a**) T2WI_FS sagittal; (**b**) T2WI_FS axial; (**c**) T1WI_FS+C sagittal, (**d**) T1WI_FS+C axial

bladder to prevent intestinal tissue damage by ultrasound ablation. If there is a bladder behind the lesion, the focus point should be placed 1 cm away from the abdominal peritoneum and avoid urinary retention after treatment.

6.1.2 Case 2

6.1.2.1 Case Description

The female patient was 38 years old. She had menstrual abdominal pain for more than 2 years. After the focused ultrasound ablation treatment, abdominal pain was relieved.

6.1.2.2 Pre-Treatment Assessment

MRI sagittal scan showed abdominal wall endometriosis with mixed high and low signals on T2WI measuring 32 mm × 45 mm × 32 mm. Contrast-enhanced T1WI showed that the lesion had an abundant blood supply (Fig. 6.3). Color Doppler ultrasound showed blood perfusion in the lesion (Fig. 6.4a).

6.1.2.3 Treatment Techniques

1. **Focused ultrasound parameters.** Average acoustic power: 119 W, sonication time: 891 s, duration of treatment: 115 min, total energy: 106,030 J.

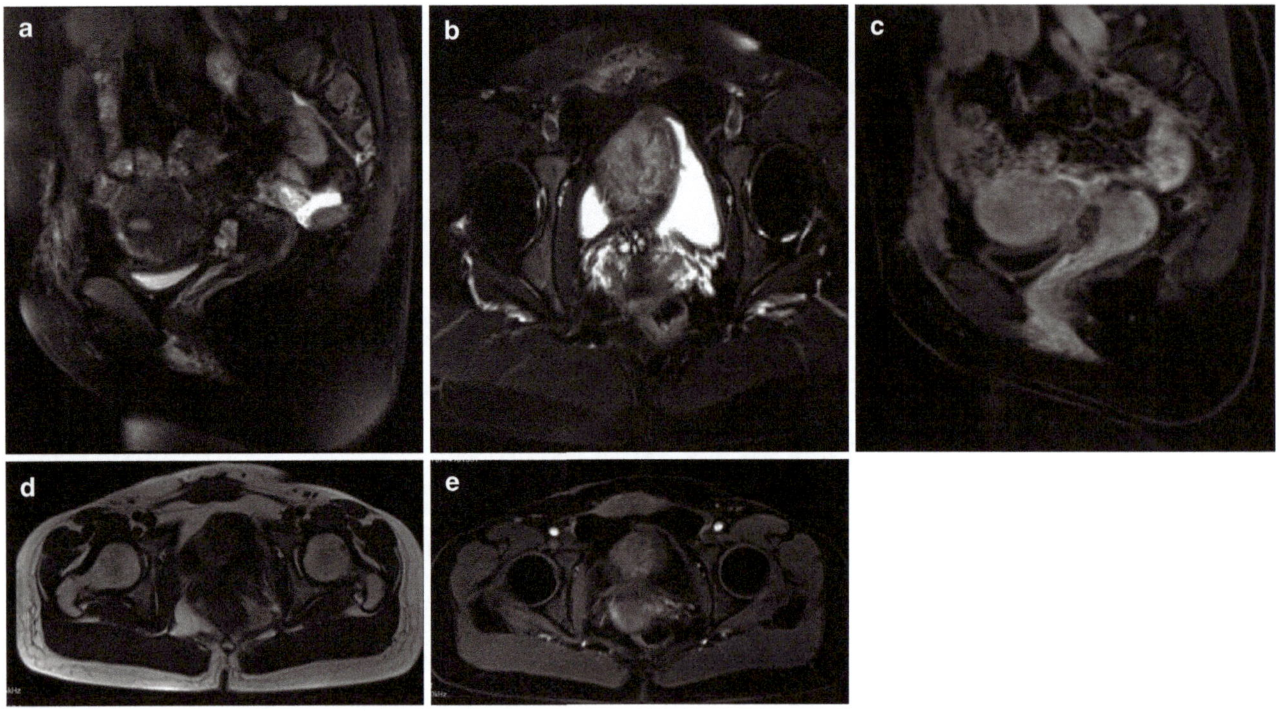

Fig. 6.3 Abdominal wall endometriosis before treatment. (**a**) T2WI_FS sagittal, (**b**) T2WI_FS axial, (**c**) T1WI_FS+C sagittal, (**d**) T1WI axial, (**e**) T1WI_FS+C axial

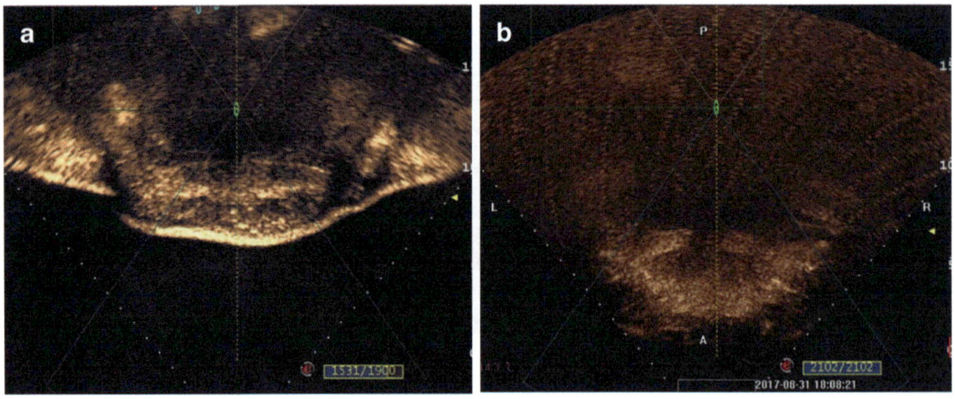

Fig. 6.4 Contrast-enhanced ultrasound of abdominal wall endometriosis. (**a**) There was blood perfusion in the endometriosis before treatment, (**b**) There was no blood perfusion in the endometriosis after treatment

2. **Focused ultrasound ablation techniques.** During the operation, the bladder was distended to the appropriate size to push the bowels away from behind the lesion to establish a safe acoustic pathway. Check the skin of the abdominal wall regularly to prevent skin scald or burn.

6.1.2.4 Post-Treatment Assessment

No obvious blood perfusion was found in the lesions by color Doppler ultrasound immediately after treatment (Fig. 6.4b).

6.1.2.5 Discussion

- This patient is a typical case of abdominal wall endometriosis. The lesion diameter is large (about 4.5 cm), so choosing the over-range ablation during the treatment would be better. It must be noted that the ablation is 0.5 cm outside the junction of the normal tissue and the lesion. To avoid the influence of abdominal wall movement on the treatment, we should pay attention to controlling the pain reaction of patients and inform them to cooperate with the ablation.

6.1.3 Case 3

6.1.3.1 Case Description

The female patient was 27 years old. She had periodic abdominal pain for more than 4 years and a mass at the abdominal wall for 2 years.

6.1.3.2 Pre-Treatment Assessment

Sagittal MRI scan showed abdominal wall endometriosis with mixed high and low signals on T2WI, measuring 34 mm × 58 mm × 16 mm. Contrast-enhanced T1WI revealed that the lesion had an abundant blood supply (Fig. 6.5). Color Doppler ultrasound showed blood perfusion in the lesion (Fig. 6.6a).

6.1.3.3 Treatment Techniques

1. **Focused ultrasound parameters.** Average acoustic power: 197 W, sonication time: 800 s, duration of treatment: 129 min, total energy: 157,600 J.
2. **Focused ultrasound ablation techniques.** The location of the lesion was low in the abdominal wall, and the uterus was behind it. The uterus could block the bowels to establish a safe acoustic pathway. The treatment can be carried out close to the deep layer of the lesion.

6.1.3.4 Post-Treatment Assessment

The lesion did not have obvious blood perfusion immediately after treatment (Fig. 6.6b). The abdominal wall pain was relieved after follow-up.

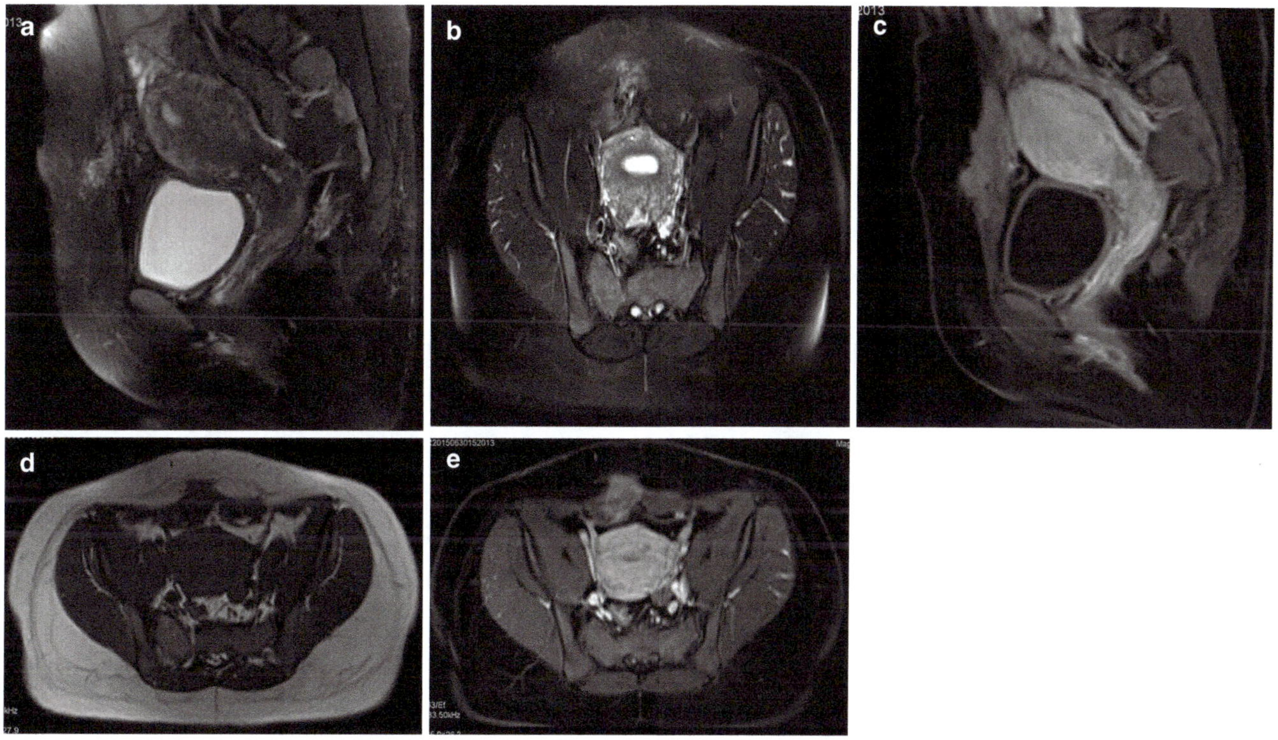

Fig. 6.5 Abdominal wall endometriosis before treatment. (**a**) T2WI_FS sagittal, (**b**) T2WI_FS axial, (**c**) T1WI_FS+C sagittal, (**d**) T1WI axial, (**e**) T1WI_FS+C axial

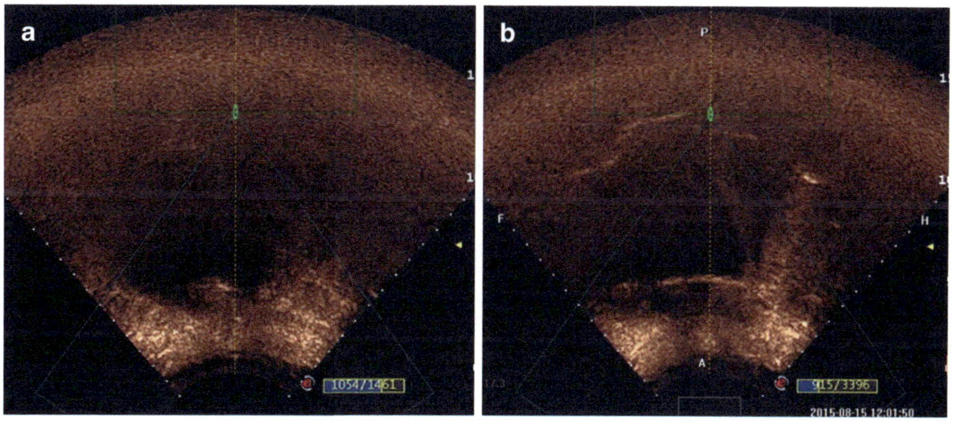

Fig. 6.6 Contrast-enhanced ultrasound of abdominal wall endometriosis. (**a**) Before treatment, there was blood perfusion in the lesions of abdominal wall endometriosis, (**b**) after treatment, there was no blood perfusion in the lesions of abdominal wall endometriosis

6.1.3.5 Discussion

- If patients have large lesions, use long treatment time and high power. Treatment should pay attention to the pain response of patients.
- It is suggested that the treatment intensity should be gradually increased from low to high power. The acoustic power should start to increase after the effect of sedation and analgesia is satisfied. The treatment intensity should be maintained at 1:3 (1s sonication: 3s cooling interval).

6.1.4 Case 4

6.1.4.1 Case Description

The female patient was 33 years old and had left sub-abdominal pain during the menstrual period for more than one year. A nodule (around 2 cm in diameter) could be subcutaneously palpated near but not at the original cesarean scar in the left lower abdomen and it became larger with time. Abdominal wall endometriosis was diagnosed to refer to focused ultrasound ablation treatment. Three months after ultrasound ablation, the pain disappeared, and the nodule became smaller.

6.1.4.2 Pre-Treatment Assessment

MRI T2WI showed mini-cystic hyperintensity mixed with slightly high signals within the lesion (20 mm × 28 mm × 35mm) involving the rectus abdominis (Fig. 6.7a, black arrow), and heterogeneous enhancement was observed on the contrast-enhanced T1WI before treatment (Fig. 6.7b, c).

The lesion was located at the deep musculus layer of left side from the cesarean section scar, which did not influence the near-field of focused ultrasound.

6.1.4.3 Treatment Techniques

1. **Focused ultrasound parameters.** Average acoustic power: 100 W, sonication time: 1100 s, duration of treatment: 45 min, total energy: 110,000 J.
2. **Focused ultrasound ablation techniques.** The strategy with low acoustic power and longer sonication time would be employed because of the lesions involving the

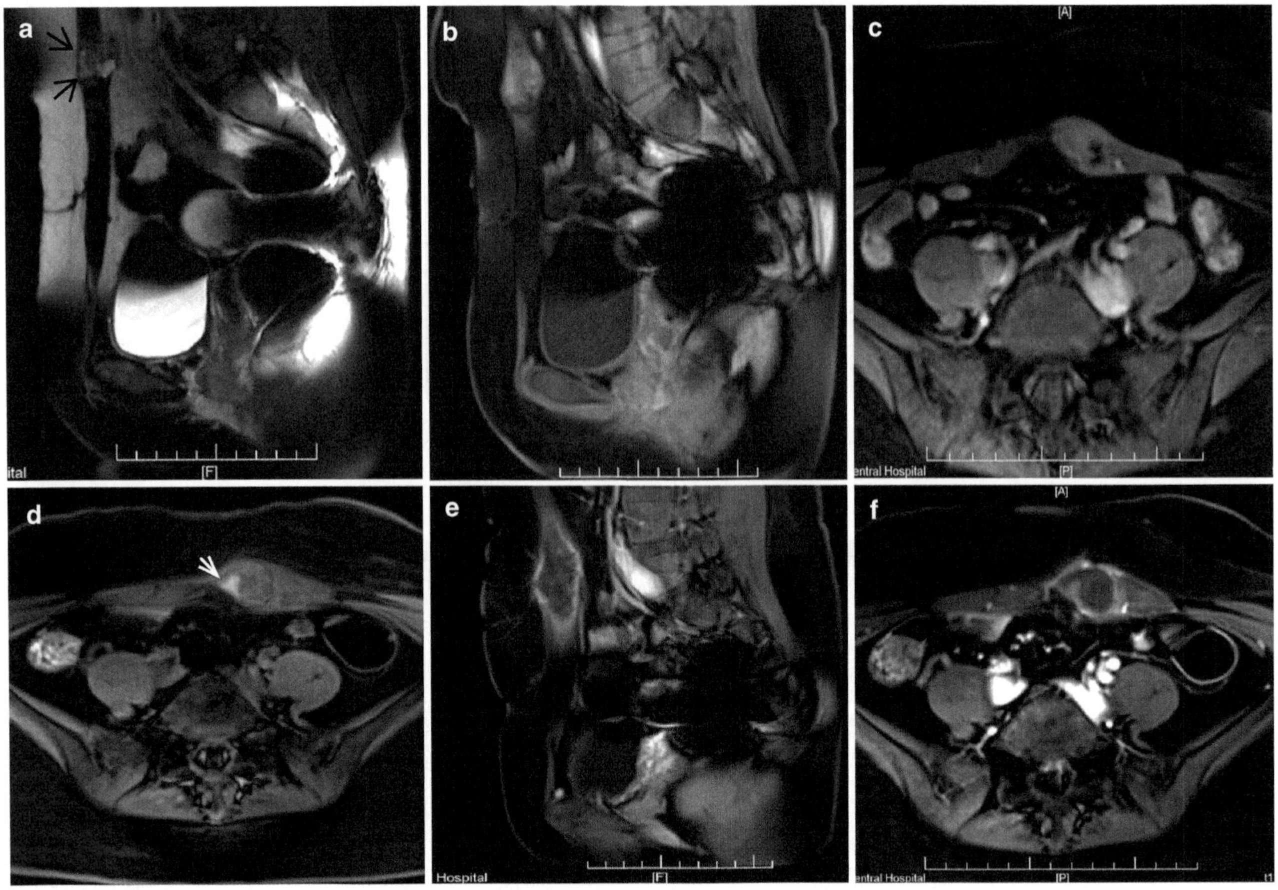

Fig. 6.7 Abdominal wall endometriosis before (**a–c**) and after treatment (**d–f**). (**a**) T2WI_FS sagittal, (**b**) T1WI_FS+C sagittal, (**c**) T1WI_FS+C axial, (**d**) T1WI_FS axial, (**e**) T1WI_ FS+C sagittal, (**f**) T1WI_FS+C axial

rectus abdominis. Each energy exposure lasted for 1 s and ceased for 2–3 s for cooling.

6.1.4.4 Post-Treatment Assessment

MRI evaluation after treatment: The treated lesion showed isointensity with a small portion of high signal (white arrow, tiny bleeding) on the T1WI image (Fig. 6.7d) and contrast-enhanced T1WI demonstrated the whole lesion of endometriosis was completely ablated within the swollen rectus abdominis (Fig. 6.7e, f).

6.1.4.5 Discussion

- This patient had an intrauterine metal device (IUD) that interfered with MR imaging, but it did not influence the display of abdominal wall endometriosis. So, there is no need for the patient to remove the IUD.
- Rarely the endometriosis lesion was not at cesarean incision, which is beneficial to ultrasound thermal ablation. Even so, the lower acoustic power still needs to be used.
- When the endometriosis lesion involves abdominal muscles, it is recommended to expand the scope of surgery resection to prevent recurrence appropriately, but the risk might increase. Under such circumstances, non-invasive focused ultrasound ablation would be an alternative therapy.

6.1.5 Case 5

6.1.5.1 Case Description

The female patient, 28 years old, had periodic abdominal pain for more than one year, which started one year after a cesarean section. The pain occurred during menstruation and became severe. A sub-abdominal mass (around 50 mm × 80 mm) was found in the cesarean scar over 1 year, and no medication was effective.

6.1.5.2 Pre-Treatment Assessment

MRI scan showed the endometriosis lesion of cystic hyperintensity mainly mixed with low signals in the muscle of the sub-abdominal wall on T2WI, measuring about 35 mm × 58 mm × 75 mm (Fig. 6.8a). Contrast-enhanced T1WI revealed that the lesion had a moderately homogenous enhancement (Fig. 6.8b).

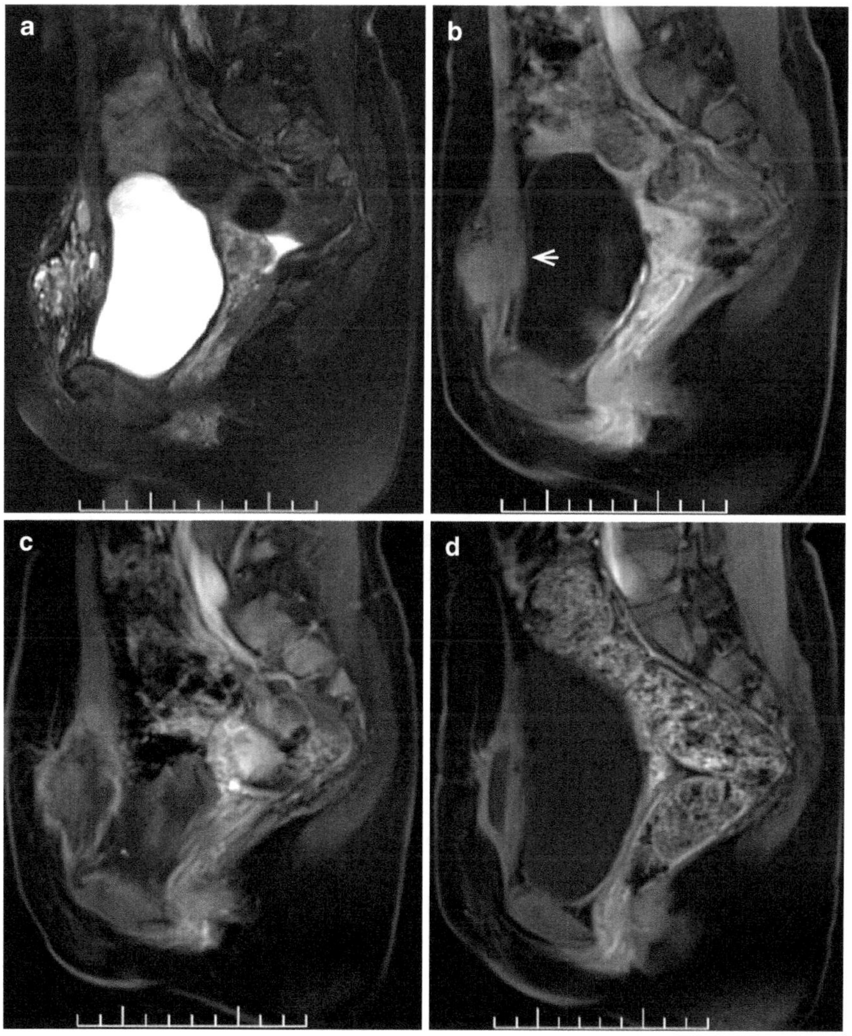

Fig. 6.8 MRI evaluation of abdominal wall endometriosis before and after FUAS. (**a**) T2WI_FS sagittal, (**b**) T1WI_FS+C sagittal before treatment, (**c**) T1WI_ FS+C sagittal 1 day after treatment, (**d**) T1WI_FS+C sagittal 3 months after treatment

6.1.5.3 Treatment Techniques

1. **Focused ultrasound parameters:** Average acoustic power: 89 W, sonication time: 3200 s, duration of treatment: 150 min, total energy: 284,800 J.
2. **Focused ultrasound ablation techniques:** The lesion was located in the sub-abdominal wall adjacent to small bowels. The bladder was to be distended to separate them, avoiding the thermal injury to bowels (Fig. 6.8b, white arrow) since the energy deposit in the far-field of sound focus should be considered.

6.1.5.4 Post-Treatment Assessment

MRI evaluation after treatment: The lesion was completely ablated with a larger range than the original one. The peripheral enhancement around the non-perfused area was observed (Fig. 6.8c).

MRI follow-up at 3 months after treatment. The treated lesion significantly decreased on the contrast-enhanced T1-weighted image without recurrence after focused ultrasound ablation, and the pseudoenhancement around the lesion disappeared (Fig. 6.8d).

6.1.5.5 Discussion

- The endometriosis was large in the abdominal muscle with fussy boundaries. It is difficult to completely remove the whole lesion by traditional surgery, and the probability of postoperative recurrence is high.
- The lesion invades the rectus abdominis, and the surgical resection of the lesion would cause muscle loss resulting in an abdominal incisional hernia.
- The fully distended bladder should be used to establish a safe acoustic pathway, avoiding the injury of the intestinal during the focused ultrasound ablation procedure because the lesion was located in the deeper layer of the abdominal wall.
- Focused ultrasound ablation treatment can preserve the integrity of the abdominal wall and avoid the complications and sequelae of surgical resection.

6.2 Focused Ultrasound Ablation for Cesarean Scar Pregnancy

6.2.1 Case 1

6.2.1.1 Case Description

The female patient was 25 years old. She was hospitalized for 13 days due to vaginal bleeding after a drug-induced abortion. B-ultrasound showed mixed echo mass and abundant blood flow signal in the previous cesarean incision of uterus. The risk of curettage was high, so focused ultrasound ablation was proposed. After focused ultrasound ablation, MRI follow-up showed no abnormal vaginal bleeding, and hCG decreased gradually.

6.2.1.2 Pre-Treatment Assessment

MRI sagittal scan showed the lesions of cesarean scar pregnancy with mixed high and low signals on T2WI, and the implanted scar was deep into the serosal layer of uterus (Fig. 6.9a, b). The lesion measured about 35 mm × 30 mm × 28 mm. Contrast-enhanced T1WI showed abundant blood supply (Fig. 6.9c, d)

6.2.1.3 Treatment Techniques

1. **Focused ultrasound parameters.** Average acoustic power: 400 W, sonication time: 1085 s, duration of time: 210 min, total energy: 434,000 J.
2. **Focused ultrasound ablation techniques.** During the treatment the pregnancy tissue should be ablated. The focused ultrasound ablation can ablate the blood vessels less than 2 mm in diameter, but it is unnecessary to ablate the large blood vessels around the lesions. After the pregnancy tissue is ablated, the blood vessels can atrophy by themselves. The focus point should be more than 1.0 cm away from the serosal layer during the treatment to avoid energy diffusion to the myometrium and bladder injury.

6.2.1.4 Post-Treatment Assessment

MRI follow-up at 3 months after treatment: After treatment, MRI showed no obvious pregnancy tissue in the cesarean scar, which was completely ablated and discharged (Fig. 6.10).

6.2.1.5 Discussion

- The lesion was implanted into the scar with abundant blood flow signals around. The curettage was prone to massive bleeding and uterine perforation, and the lesion was completely discharged after focused ultrasound ablation.

6.2.2 Case 2

6.2.2.1 Case Description

The female patient was 30 years old. She was hospitalized because of a small amount of vaginal bleeding for a day after having amenorrhea for 53 days. After focused ultrasound ablation, she had regular follow-ups, and her menstruation returned with no special symptoms.

6.2.2.2 Pre-Treatment Assessment

T2WI showed that the lower edge of the gestational sac of cesarean scar pregnancy was close to the scar, most of the gestational sac was in the uterine cavity, and the contrast-enhanced T1WI showed that the pregnancy tissue had an abundant blood supply (Fig. 6.11).

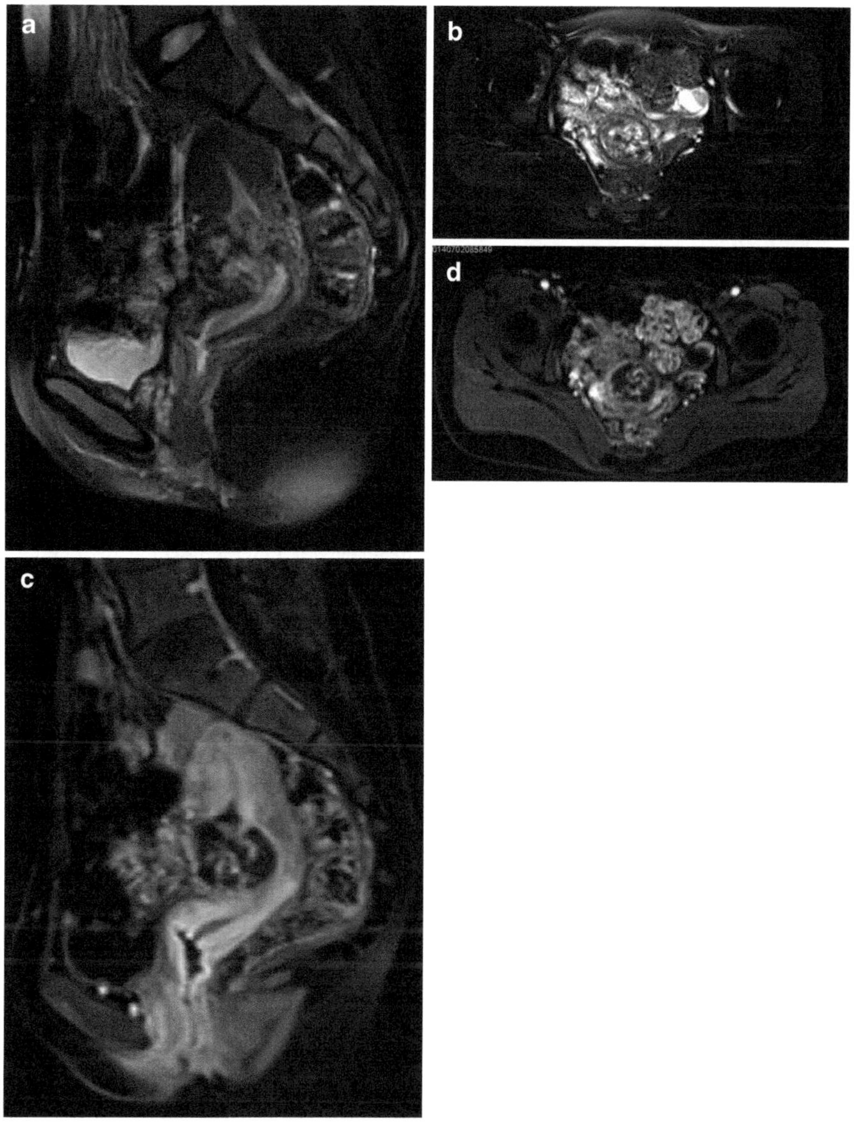

Fig. 6.9 Type III cesarean scar pregnancy before treatment. (**a**) T2WI_FS sagittal, (**b**) T2WI_FS axial, (**c**) T1WI_FS+C sagittal, (**d**) T1WI_FS+C axial

6.2.2.3 Treatment Techniques

1. **Focused ultrasound parameters:** Average acoustic power: 400 W, sonication time: 750 s, duration of time: 73 min, total energy: 300,000 J.
2. **Focused ultrasound ablation techniques:** High-intensity focused ultrasound (HIFU) was used to ablate the embryo and make the original heart tube beat disappear. The small blood vessels around the gestational sac, especially between the gestational sac and the anterior wall of the uterus, were destroyed. To avoid bladder injury, we should pay attention to keeping a distance from the serosal surface of the uterus.

6.2.2.4 Post-Treatment Assessment

- **Ultrasound imaging evaluation after treatment.** The contrast-enhanced ultrasound showed that the pulsation of the cardiac tube disappeared, and the blood perfusion around the gestational sac decreased significantly. The curettage was performed 2 days after the operation, and the curettage process was smooth with less blood loss.

6.2.2.5 Discussion

- The patient had an endophytic cesarean scar pregnancy. The lower edge was close to the scar. Most of the gestational sac was in the uterine cavity. There were abundant blood flow signals around it. Curettage was prone to massive bleeding. After focused ultrasound ablation, the curettage process and postoperative recovery were successful.

6.2.3 Case 3

6.2.3.1 Case Description

The female patient was 33 years old. She was hospitalized because of vaginal bleeding for 3 days after 47 days of amenor-

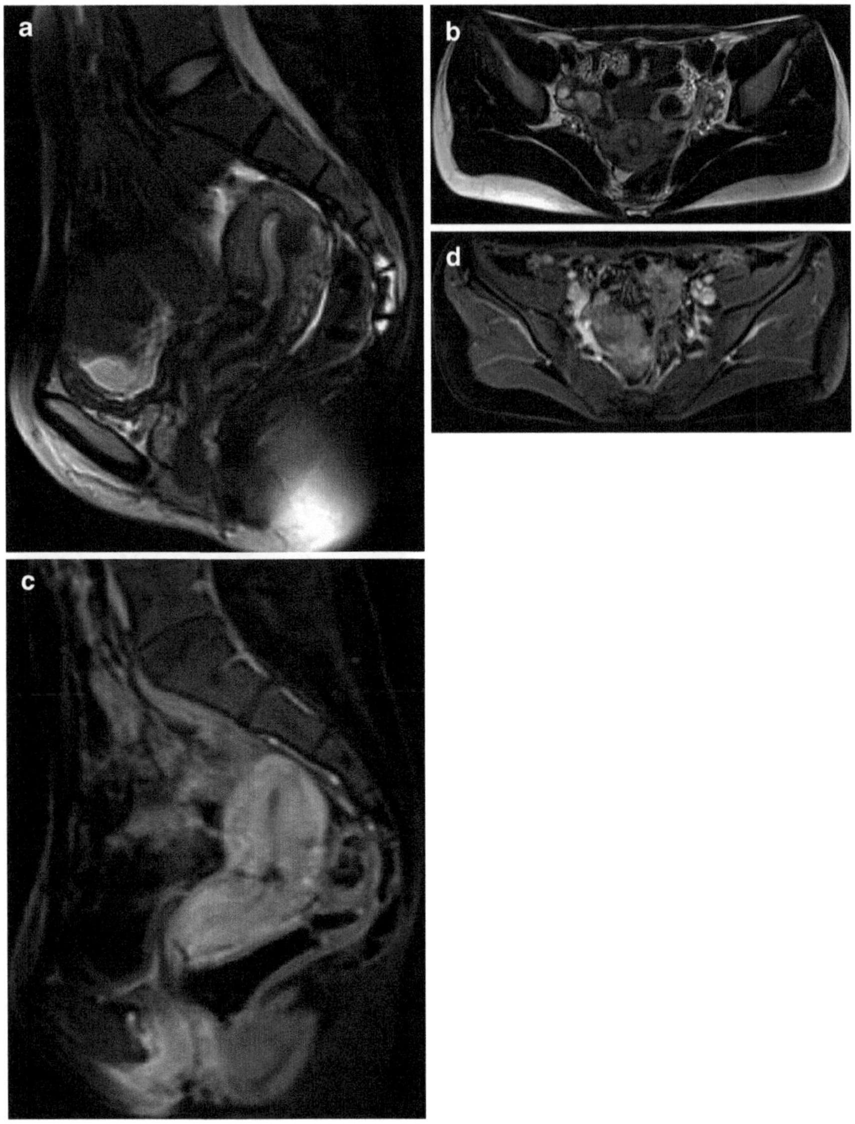

Fig. 6.10 MRI follow-up at 3 months after treatment. (**a**) T2WI_FS sagittal, (**b**) T2WI axial, (**c**) T1WI_FS+C sagittal, (**d**) T1WI_FS+C axial

rhea. After focused ultrasound ablation, there were no special symptoms, and menstruation was recovered after 25 days.

6.2.3.2 Pre-Treatment Assessment

MRI T2WI showed that the gestational sac of cesarean scar pregnancy was completely located in the scar, protruding the serous layer outwards. It was considered an exogenous scar pregnancy. The contrast-enhanced T1WI showed that the lesion had an abundant blood supply (Fig. 6.12).

6.2.3.3 Treatment Techniques

1. **Focused ultrasound parameters:** Average acoustic power: 400 W, sonication time: 500 s, duration of time: 74 min, total energy: 200,000 J.
2. **Focused ultrasound ablation techniques:** High-intensity focused ultrasound (HIFU) was used to ablate the embryo, and the fetal heart tube pulsation had disappeared. The blood flow of the cesarean scar should be treated according to the thickness of the myometrium. If its thickness is less than 5 mm, it should be treated carefully to avoid perforation of the uterus during curettage.

6.2.3.4 Post-Treatment Assessment

- After treatment, color Doppler ultrasound showed that the primitive heart tube pulsation disappeared. The curettage was performed 2 days after the ablation treatment, and the process of curettage was smooth with little blood loss.

6.2.3.5 Discussion

- The gestational sac was completely located in the cesarean section scar. The gestational sac protruded through the serosal layer with a thin myometrial layer (only 2 mm). The focused ultrasound ablation should only treat the original heart tube pulsation and avoid overtreatment damaging the muscle layer and leading to scar perforation during curettage.

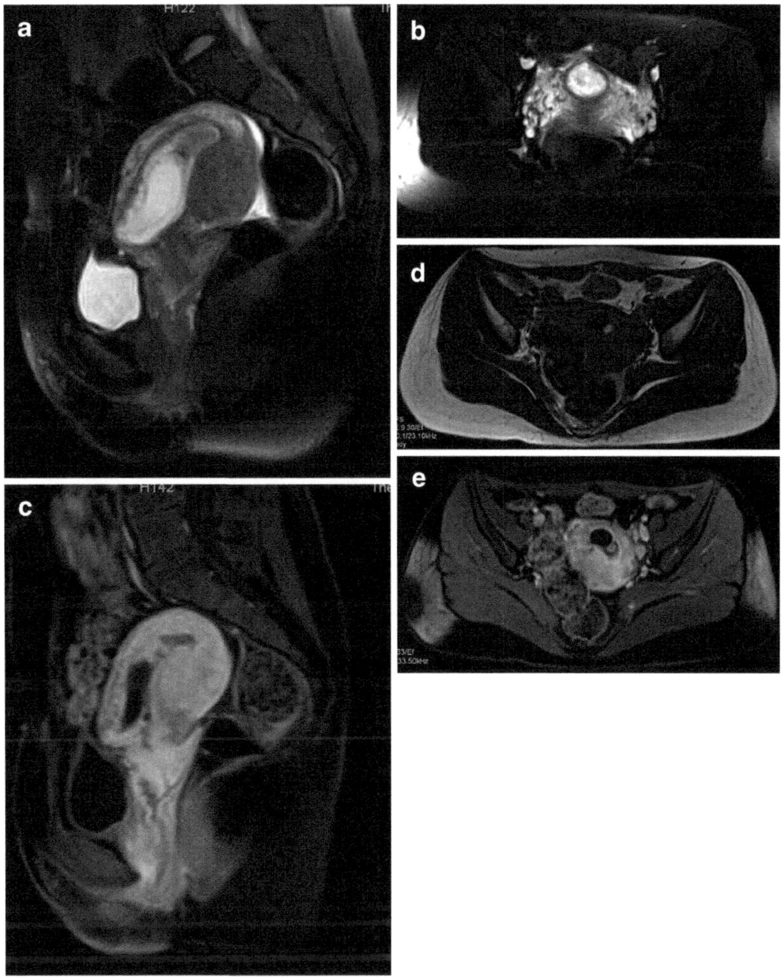

Fig. 6.11 Cesarean scar pregnancy (endogenous) before treatment. (**a**) T2WI_FS sagittal, (**b**) T2WI_FS axial, (**c**) T1WI_FS+C sagittal, (**d**) T1WI axial, (**e**) T1WI_FS+C axial

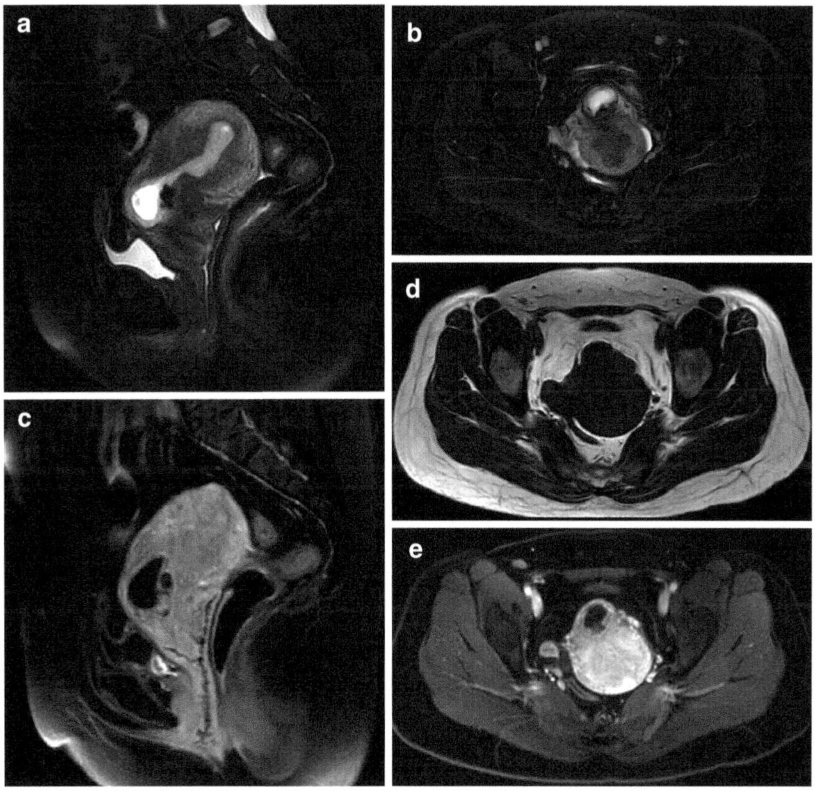

Fig. 6.12 Cesarean scar pregnancy (exogenous) before treatment. (**a**) T2WI_FS sagittal, (**b**) T2WI_FS axial, (**c**) T1WI_FS+C sagittal, (**d**) T1WI axial, (**e**) T1WI_FS+C axial

Complications and Management of Patients After Focused Ultrasound Ablation

7

Qian Chen, Felix Wong, and Yonghua Xu

Abstract

The adverse events and complications following the focused ultrasound ablation are classified and graded according to the Society of Interventional Radiology classification system for complications by outcome, and the incidences are mentioned. The real world of various complications and adverse events is revealed after the focused ultrasound ablation surgery, such as persistent low-grade fever, abdominal wall edema and pain, hematuria, urinary retention, abdominal wall injury and skin burn, discharged necrotic fibroid incarcerated at the cervix, intrauterine infection and adhesion, intestinal perforation, sacrococcygeal injury, nerve injury or irritation, and so on. The prevention measures and management strategies for them are recommended, and the outcomes and sequelae also are described.

Keywords

Adverse event · Complication · High-intensity focused ultrasound · Incidence · Classification · Management · Benign uterine disease

Post-treatment complications are the main issues with regard to all surgeries. As long as it is an iatrogenic operation, there is the possibility of complications, which is the last thing the doctors and the patients want to happen. Therefore, before focused ultrasound ablation surgery, the physicians should be familiar with the causes and prevention measures of various adverse events that may result from the ablation procedure, evaluating comprehensively the patient's condition and assessing the treatment risk in detail. The operating doctors must be well trained in the FUAS principle, therapeutic plans formulating, therapeutic processes, and fault management of the respective devices making corresponding measures and emergency plans. Thus, the occurrence of adverse events and complications would be minimized. This chapter introduces general complications (such as post-treatment fever, hematuria, abdominal pain, etc.) and specific complications related to focused ultrasound ablation.

7.1 Classification and Grading of Complications After Focused Ultrasound Ablation Treatment

Focused ultrasound ablation is a non-invasive treatment under real-time ultrasound or MR imaging guidance. In clinical practice, the complications related to focused ultrasound ablation are classified with reference to the Society of Interventional Radiology classification system and categorized using the definitions as follows [1]: 1. Minor Complications: A. No therapy, no consequence; B. Nominal therapy, no consequence including overnight admission for observation only. 2. Major Complications: C. Require therapy, minor hospitalization (<48 h); D. Require major therapy, unplanned increase in level of care, prolonged hospitalization (>48 h); E. Permanent adverse sequelae; F. Death. The sequence from A to F represents the complications from mild to severe.

The incidences of complications after the focused ultrasound ablation for the treatment of benign uterine diseases are different in each medical center based on the operators' learning curve for FUAS techniques and the accumulated volume of patient number. A retrospective review of the complications of 10,018 women treated with focused ultrasound ablation in 10 medical institutes between 2006 and 2013 showed that 10.6% (1062) of all patients pre-

Q. Chen
Hangzhou Integrative Medicine Hospital, Hangzhou, China

F. Wong
The University of New South Wales, Sydney, NSW, Australia

Y. Xu (✉)
Zhongshan-Xuhui Hospital, Fudan University, Shanghai, China

Y. Xu et al. (eds.), *Surgical Techniques of Focused Ultrasound Ablation in Benign Uterine Diseases*,
https://doi.org/10.1007/978-981-19-7180-8_7

sented with 1338 adverse events [2]. Among them, 1281 of these events were classified as class A, 45 as class B, 6 as Class C, and 6 as Class D. However, a recent multicenter study showed that the incidence of complications after focused ultrasound ablation of uterine fibroids was 0.18%, of which class A accounted for about 99.6%. The complications of classes C and D are very few, including the abdominal skin burn that required surgical removal of the necrotic tissue, numbness on the lower limbs or leg pain because of thermal injury to the sciatic nerve, and acute renal failure and intestinal perforation. There were no class E and class F complications. Herein, we will introduce the complications one by one according to chronological order and locations of their occurrence.

7.2 Post-Treatment Complications and Preventive Management

7.2.1 Case 1 Persistent Low-Grade Fever Caused by Necrotic Fibroid Infection

7.2.1.1 Case Description

The female patient was 42 years old. She had a uterine fibroid for 5 years, and the fibroid gradually increased in size, associated with heavy menstrual blood flow for two years.

7.2.1.2 Diagnosis and Treatment

Before treatment, the MRI scan showed a uterine fibroid located on the left uterine wall (Fig. 7.1a–c).

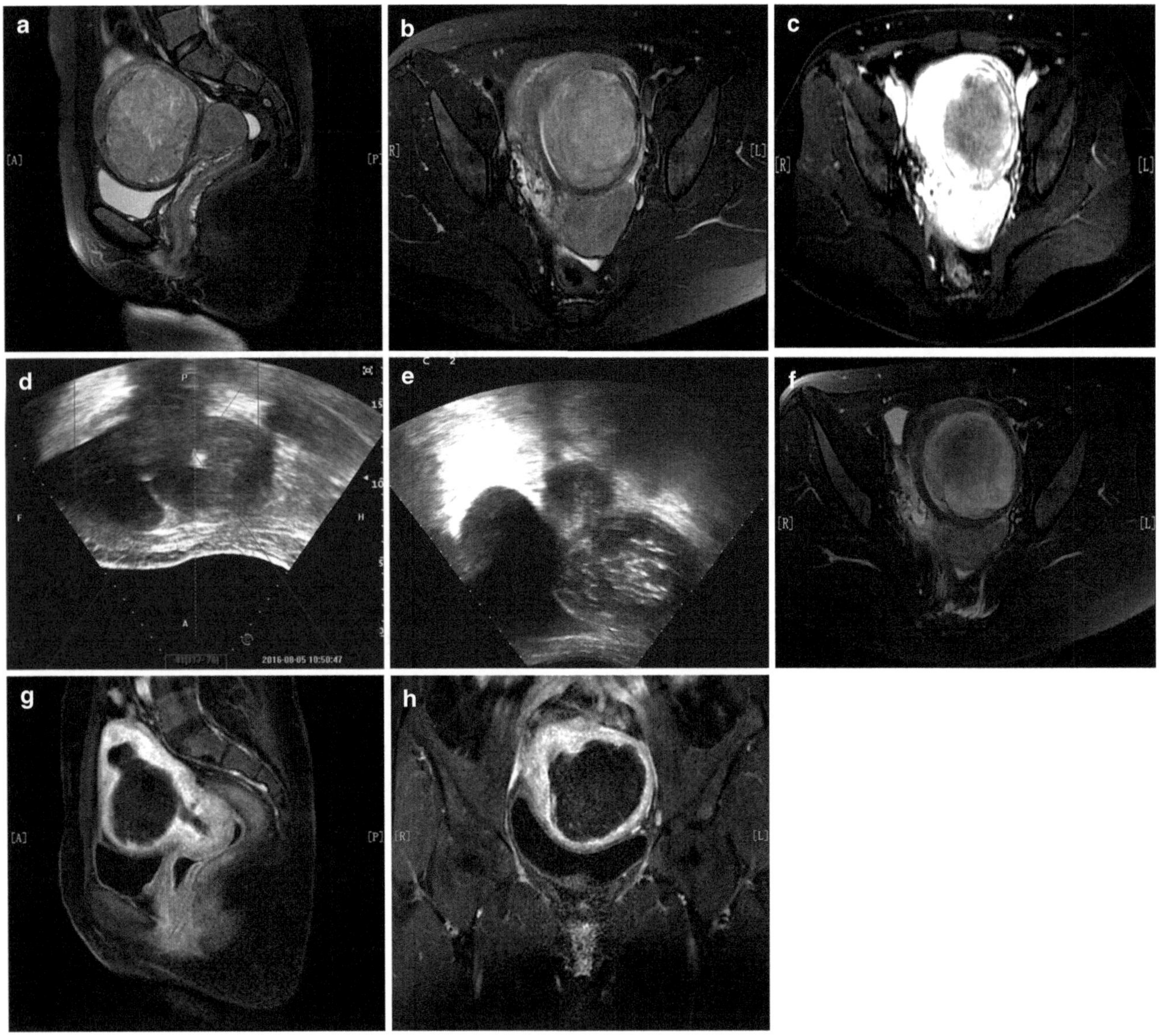

Fig. 7.1 Persistent low-grade fever after focused ultrasound ablation treatment. (**a**) T2WI_FS sagittal before treatment, (**b**) T2WI_FS axial before treatment, (**c**) T1WI_FS+C axial before treatment, (**d**) Ultrasound image during treatment, (**e**) Ultrasound image at the end of treatment, (**f**) T2WI_FS axial after treatment; (**g**) T1WI_FS+C sagittal after treatment, (**h**) T1WI_FS+C coronal after treatment

- After 50 s of sonication, the lesion had grayscale changes on ultrasound imaging (Fig. 7.1d). At the end of the treatment, ultrasonography showed a significantly enhanced echo of the entire fibroid (Fig. 7.1e).

7.2.1.3 Post-Treatment Assessment

1. **MRI evaluation after treatment:** The contrast-enhanced T1WI showed that the fibroid had 93% NPV with a breakthrough in the endometrium (Fig. 7.1f–h).
2. **Complications:** The patient had a light-yellow vaginal discharge and low-grade fever on the 10th day after treatment. These were relieved by symptomatic treatment. She had a persistent low-grade fever for three months, during which there was an intermittent vaginal discharge of rotten flesh-like tissues, and it took about five months to return to normal.

7.2.1.4 Discussion

- It was considered that the ablated fibroid is complicated by infection in this case, leading to the persistent low-grade fever. The vaginal discharge, the absorption of necrotic fibroid, and the repair of the endometrium had led to the return to normal.
- The incidence of fever in patients after focused ultrasound ablation treatment is 1.8%–2%. The etiology, mechanism, and treatment are as follows: (1) Acoustic energy absorption: During treatment, the patient's body temperature can rise, which is mostly transient, and no special treatment is required, but it is necessary to pay attention to supplementing saline and electrolytes; (2) there might be the absorption of heat or stress-related fever after treatment, which was mostly low-grade fever, lasting 1 to 3 days. No special treatment was required; (3) the infectious fever: there are corresponding tissue infections, and the body temperature can quickly return to normal after the infection is controlled by antibiotics.

7.2.2 Case 2 Abdominal Wall Edema After Focused Ultrasound Ablation Treatment

7.2.2.1 Case Description

The female patient was 42 years old. Ultrasound examination revealed uterine fibroids for 3 years, and the fibroid gradually increased in size with the heavy menstrual flow for a year. She had three previous abdominal operations.

7.2.2.2 Diagnosis and Treatment

- Before treatment, the physical examination showed a 13 cm longitudinal incision scar in the lower abdomen (Fig. 7.2a). The scar showed skin contracture at the scar, no redness, firm on touch, poor mobility, and decreased pain and temperature perception. MRI showed a submucosal fibroid on the anterior wall of the uterus (Fig. 7.2b, c). Sonography showed an obvious abdominal scar (Fig. 7.2d).
- The patient's skin became hot during the treatment. Ultrasound showed increased skin attenuation after treatment (Fig. 7.2e), and the abdominal wall skin was intact without redness and burns (Fig. 7.2f).

7.2.2.3 Post-Treatment Assessment

1. **MRI evaluation after treatment:** Sagittal T2-weighted imaging showed the subcutaneous tissue in the lower abdominal wall had flaky high intense signals, indicating edema (Fig. 7.2g); contrast-enhanced T1WI demonstrated inhomogeneous enhancement of these regions of the abdominal wall (Fig. 7.2h)
2. **Complications:** The patient developed pain in the abdominal wall, which disappeared after three days. She had no complaint for one-month follow-up.

7.2.2.4 Discussion

- The abdominal wall scar of this patient was obvious with significant ultrasound attenuation on sonography. During the procedure, the treatment speed should slow down, and the sonication should have enough cooling interval to ensure intact abdominal skin without injury.
- High-risk factors for abdominal wall injury include: a) the fat thickness of abdominal wall exceeding 5 cm; b) obvious surgical scars; c) fast and high energy delivery without regular breaks in focused ultrasound ablation treatment; d) using a large distending water balloon during ablation.
- The clinical manifestations of abdominal skin injury were edematous abdominal wall swelling with tenderness. A few patients may have redness associated with swelling; the ultrasound imaging showed increased skin attenuation, and MRI also showed edema of the abdominal wall.
- If the skin of the abdominal wall is intact, the subcutaneous soft tissue edema can be recovered in a short time after cooling management. Generally, there would be no sequelae.

7.2.3 Case 3 Abdominal Pain Caused by Peritoneal Injury During Treatment

7.2.3.1 Case Description

The female patient was 40 years old. She had abdominal pain during menstruation for ten years, and the pain got worse with increased menstrual blood flow for one year.

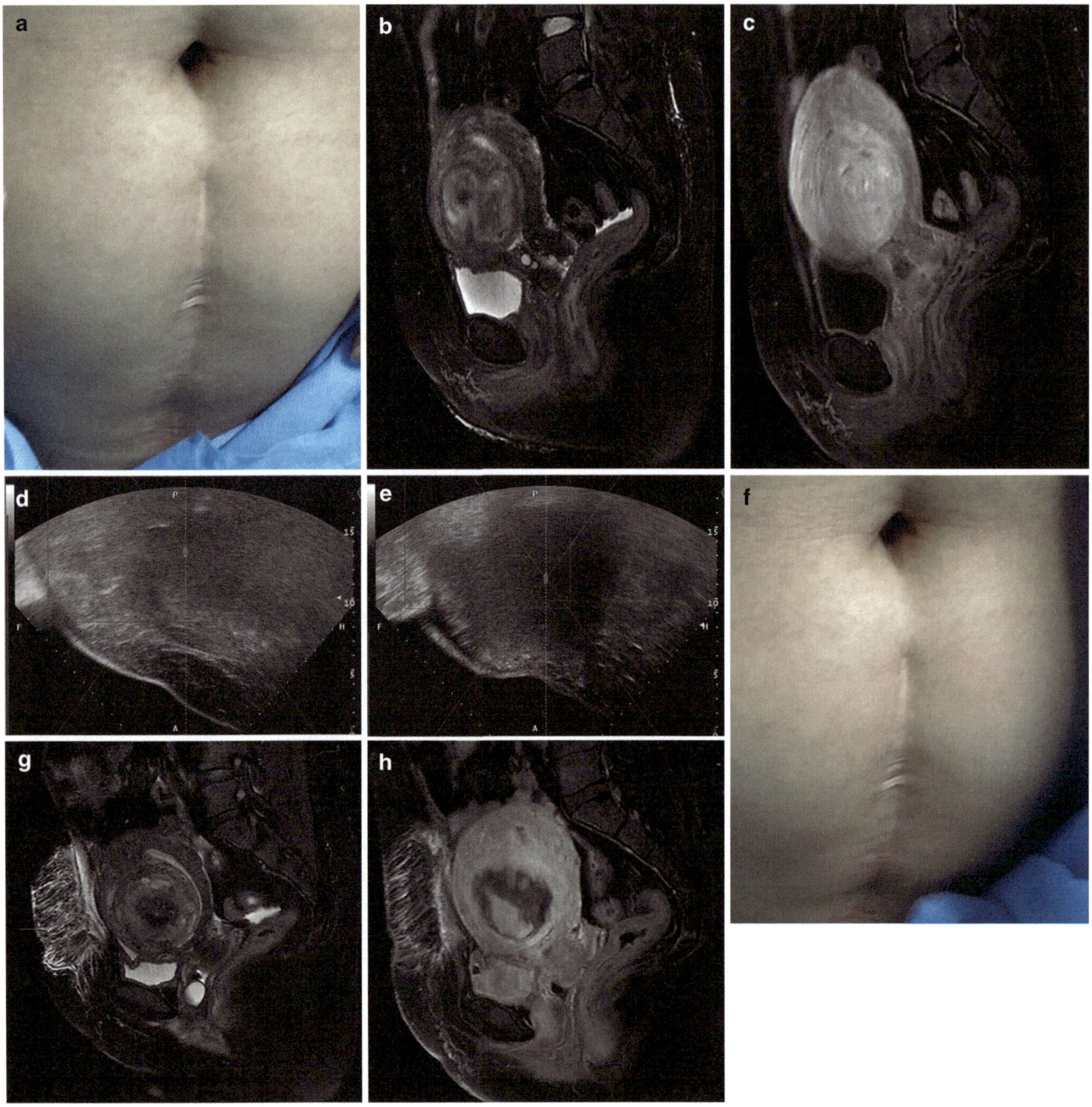

Fig. 7.2 Abdominal wall was edematous after focused ultrasound ablation treatment. (**a**) Abdominal wall before treatment, (**b**) T2WI_FS sagittal before treatment, (**c**) T1WI_FS+C sagittal before treatment, (**d**) Ultrasound image of the abdominal wall before treatment, (**e**) Ultrasound image of the abdominal wall after treatment, (**f**) Abdominal wall after treatment, (**g**) T2WI_FS sagittal after treatment, (**h**) T1WI_FS+C sagittal after treatment.

7.2.3.2 Diagnosis and Treatment

- Before treatment MRI revealed left-sided uterine adenomyosis (Fig. 7.3a–c), and the contrast-enhanced ultrasound showed a clear lesion area (Fig. 7.3d). After treatment, the contrast-enhanced ultrasound showed obvious attenuation, and the lesion became not well displayed (Fig. 7.3e).
- After focused ultrasound ablation treatment, MRI examination showed that the abdominal wall was edematous. The contrast-enhanced T1WI showed no perfused area with well-demarcated edges in the subcutaneous tissue of the lower abdominal wall, 83% of adenomyosis showed no perfusion area, and the uterine serosal layer had an obvious breakthrough (Fig. 7.3f–h).

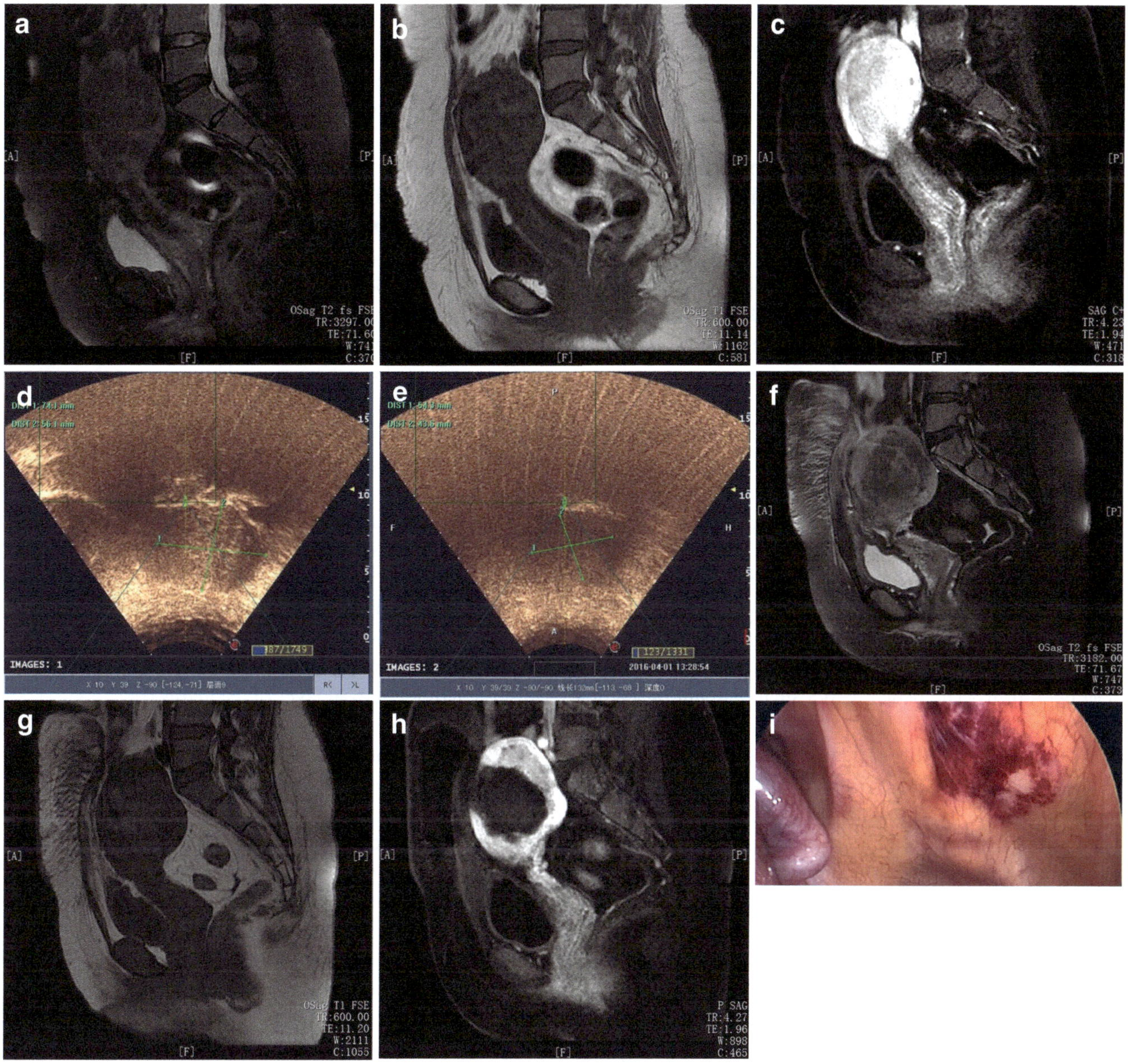

Fig. 7.3 Abdominal wall injury after focused ultrasound ablation treatment. (**a**) T2WI_FS sagittal before treatment, (**B**) T1WI sagittal before treatment, (**C**) T1WI_FS+C sagittal before treatment; (**d**) Contrast ultrasound with IV microbubble before treatment, (**e**) Contrast ultrasound after treatment, (**f**) T2WI_FS sagittal after treatment, (**g**) T1WI sagittal after treatment; (**h**) H. T1WI_FS+C sagittal after treatment; I. Laparoscopic finding at pelvic peritoneum after treatment.

- The patient had persistent post-operative pain in the lower abdomen. Due to acute appendicitis, the patient underwent laparoscopic surgery at a local hospital one month later. During laparoscopy, the abdominal wall was found to have a thermal peritoneal injury (Fig. 7.3i).

7.2.3.3 Discussion

- Peritoneal injury would occur in treating subserosal fibroids close to the abdominal wall using a large, high-tension water balloon, which affected the heat dissipation over the abdominal skin.
- Peritoneal injury may occur if a patient complains of persistent severe pain and sometimes sharp pain in the abdomen during focused ultrasound ablation, since the superficial sensory nerves innervate the peritoneum. The abdomen's appearance is generally normal on physical examination, and the abdomen is soft. Still, there may be mild tenderness and rebound tenderness, and there may be muscle stiffness.
- MRI can show edema in the peritoneal layer or non-perfusion areas, local reactive effusion, but no free gas under the diaphragm. Laparoscopy or open surgery can confirm the diagnosis.

- The peritoneum is an epithelial tissue that repairs quickly. The abdominal pain lasts for a short time after symptomatic treatment, with no sequelae.

– The pain, abdominal pain caused by the aseptic inflammation of the necrotic fibroid on the surrounding myometrium is generally continuous dull pain, lasting for several days or even weeks.

7.2.4 Case 4 Persistent Abdominal Pain Caused by Uterine Serosa Injury

7.2.4.1 Case Description

The female patient was 45 years old. Ultrasound examination revealed a fibroid, and it gradually enlarged over a period of 7 years. She felt lower abdominal discomfort for one year.

7.2.4.2 Diagnosis and Treatment

- MRI before treatment showed a fibroid at the anterior wall of the uterus (Fig. 7.4a–c).
- After 150 s of sonication, the ultrasound image showed grayscale changes in the fibroid (Fig. 7.4d)
- Postoperative MRI showed increased T2 signals of the anterior wall of uterine myometrium, and the abdominal wall was edematous. About 94% of the fibroid and its adjacent serosal layer showed non-perfusion areas (Fig. 7.4f–h). The patient had a small amount of vaginal bleeding after treatment.
- After treatment, the patient continued to have mild abdominal pain, and persistent abdominal pain worsened during the first menstrual period after treatment.

7.2.4.3 Discussion

- In this case, the focal regions of focused ultrasound were deployed at a shallow position in the fibroid during treatment. Therefore, the acoustic energy spread to the uterine serosal layer, resulting in its damage.
- Abdominal pains during and after focused ultrasound ablation treatment, except for the acute abdomen pain caused rarely by intestinal injury, generally have the following possibilities:

  – Uterine contraction pain caused by oxytocin is usually accompanied by increased blood pressure and heart rate. The abdominal pain can be significantly relieved after stopping oxytocin.
  – Abdominal pain is caused by acoustic energy stimulation of the endometrium during treatment. Pain is experienced when ultrasound energy is activated, but it is relieved when the sonication stopped.
  – The pain caused by the heated fibroid thermally stimulating the surrounding myometrium is more common in large fibroids. Postoperatively, the ice pad compression can relieve the pain.

7.2.5 Case 5 Hematuria After Focused Ultrasound Ablation

7.2.5.1 Case Description

The female patient was 32 years old. Ultrasound examination revealed a uterine fibroid for 3 years, and it gradually increased in size for one year.

7.2.5.2 Diagnosis and Treatment

- MRI before treatment demonstrated a fibroid at the anterior wall of the uterus (Fig. 7.5a–c).
- During the treatment, ultrasound monitoring showed obvious changes in the grayscale of the lesion (Fig. 7.5d). After treatment, the patient had gross hematuria.
- Postoperative MRI showed increased T2-weighted signals of the fibroid close to the bladder, and the contrast-enhanced T1WI showed no perfusion of the fibroid with the breakthrough of the serosal layer of the uterus (Fig. 7.5e–g).
- After treatment, the foley catheter was kept in situ, with the urine alkalized at the same time. The patient was advised to drink more water. The hematuria disappeared the next day.

7.2.5.3 Discussion

The common causes of hematuria after focused ultrasound ablation treatment are:

- Damage to the urethral mucosa during catheterization.
- During the treatment, gas bubbles in the bladder under the cavitation effect due to the ultrasound sonication will cause damage to the bladder mucosa.
- A fibroid adjacent to the bladder will receive heat energy during treatment. The heat may spread to the bladder wall causing thermal damage to the bladder.
- It might be due to misjudged operation or sudden changes in the patient's posture during treatment. Then the off-target ultrasound focus can directly damage the bladder mucosa.
- The patient has gross hematuria with urinary tract irritation or may be complicated by a urinary tract infection. Instruct the patient to drink more water, alkalize the urine, and use antibiotics if necessary. The hematuria usually disappears within 1–3 days.
- In this case, the patient developed hematuria after treatment. It is considered that the uterine serosa was damaged with thermal energy spread to the bladder wall.

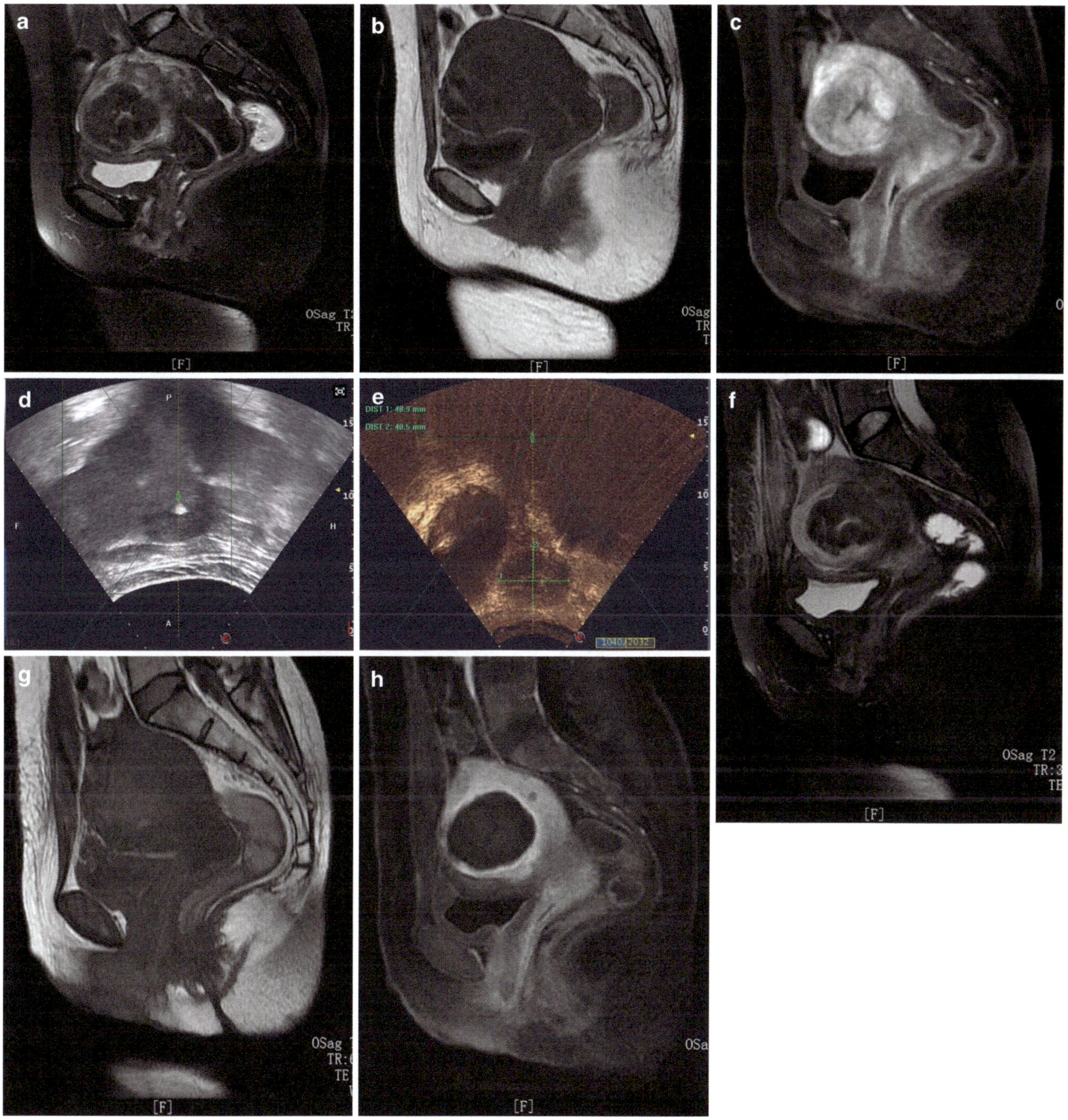

Fig. 7.4 Uterine serosal injury after focused ultrasound ablation treatment. (**a**) T2WI_FS sagittal before treatment, (**b**) T1WI sagittal before treatment, (**c**) T1WI_FS+C sagittal before treatment, (**d**) Real-time ultrasound image during treatment, (**e**) Contrast ultrasound image at the end of treatment, (**f**). T2WI_FS sagittal after treatment, (**g**) T1WI sagittal after treatment, (**h**) T1WI_FS+C sagittal after treatment

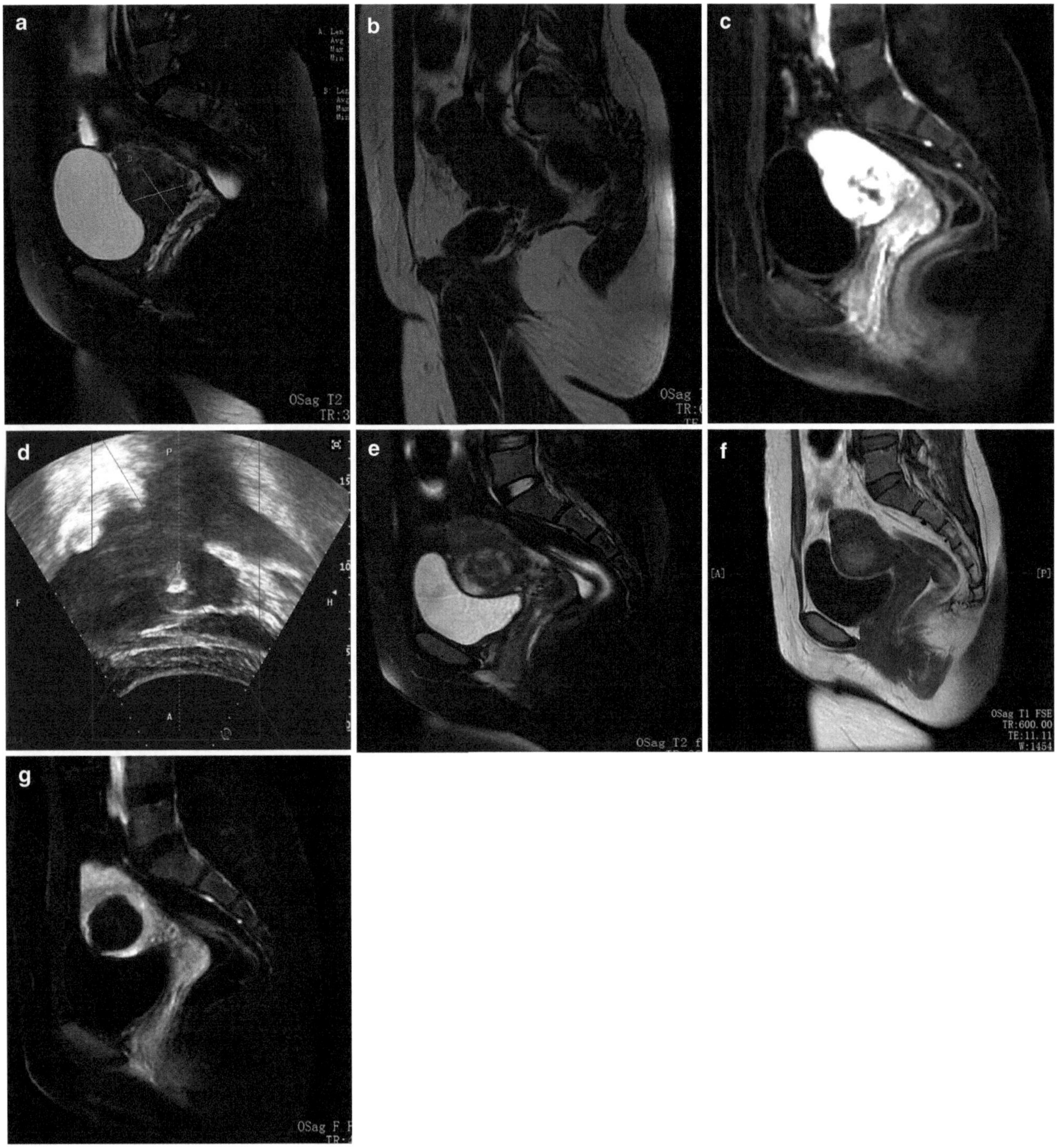

Fig. 7.5 The fibroid of anterior uterine wall is close to the bladder, and heat diffusion leads to hematuria. (**a**) T2WI_FS sagittal before treatment, (**b**) T1WI sagittal before treatment, (**c**) T1WI_FS+C sagittal before treatment, (**d**) Ultrasound image during treatment, (**e**) T2WI_FS sagittal after treatment, (**f**) T1WI sagittal after treatment, (**g**) T1WI_FS+C sagittal after treatment

7.2.6 Case 6 Acute Urinary Retention After Focused Ultrasound Ablation

7.2.6.1 Case Description

The female patient was 28 years old. Her ultrasound examination revealed a uterine fibroid for 3 years, and it gradually increased in size over a period of 1 year.

7.2.6.2 Diagnosis and Treatment

- Before treatment, MRI showed a fibroid at the posterior wall of the uterus (Fig. 7.6a, b). Ultrasound examination showed a normal bladder (Fig. 7.6c).
- The bladder was distended with 1200 mL of normal saline during the treatment, and the patient had abdominal distension and pain.

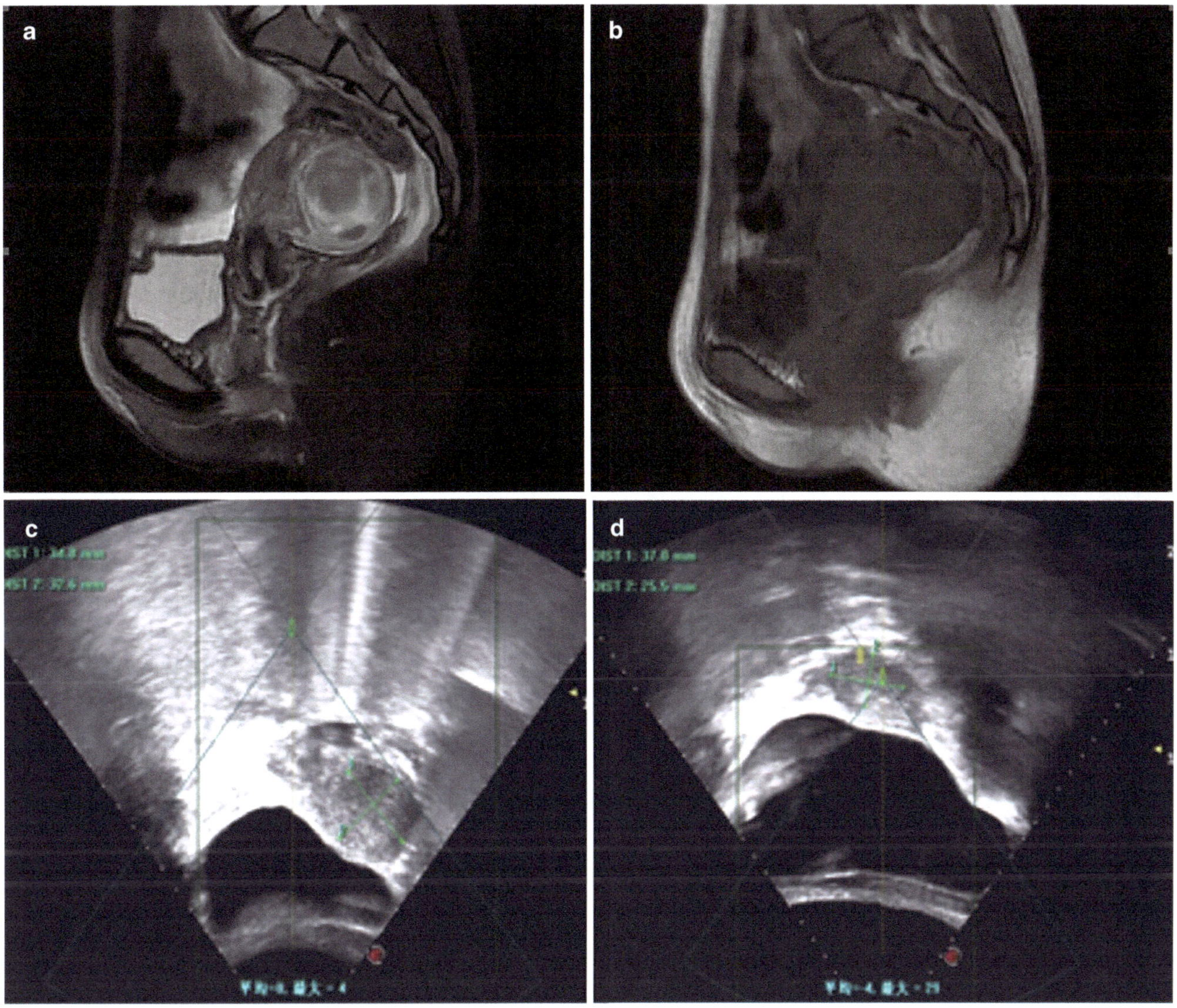

Fig. 7.6 Acute urinary retention after ultrasound ablation. (**a**) T2WI_FS sagittal before treatment, (**b**) T1WI sagittal before treatment, (**c**) Ultrasound examination showed normal bladder, (**d**) Ultrasound examination showed overfilling of the bladder

- Urinary retention occurred when the catheter was removed after the treatment (Fig. 7.6d). After the Foley catheter was reinserted and was regularly clamped and released, the bladder recovered its function back to normal after 2 days.

7.2.6.3 Discussion

- The patient had a retroverted uterus with a posterior fibroid. It is impossible to establish a safe acoustic pathway through the extracorporal water balloon, and we can choose the distended bladder to create a safe ultrasound pathway.
- After overfilling it during treatment, the bladder was extremely distended, which affected the smooth muscle's function and led to stress urinary incontinence.
- Urinary retention occurred after focused ultrasound ablation treatment. In addition, this patient may not be used to urinating lying in bed or alternatively due to using atropine and other drugs during treatment. However, the most common causes are the excessive infusion of normal saline into the bladder and over-distending it, leading to smooth muscle dysfunction.
- During the treatment, the bladder should not be overdistended too much; regularly reduce the saline in the bladder to release the pressure of the distended bladder; regularly relax and push the water balloon or the transducer head to avoid excessive pressing on the bladder for a long time. These measures can effectively prevent urinary retention after treatment.

- After treatment, urinary retention can quickly restore to normal without sequelae after re-catheterization and training bladder function. Sometimes, acupuncture and hot compress may be useful.

7.2.7 Case 7 Crush Injury of the Abdominal Wall

7.2.7.1 Case Description

The female patient was 38 years old. Ultrasound examination revealed uterine fibroids for 10 years, and the fibroids gradually increased in size with the prolonged menstrual periods for one year.

7.2.7.2 Diagnosis and Treatment

After focused ultrasound ablation, the patient found an "H" shaped erythematous lesion on the abdomen (Fig. 7.7). She complained of mild pain in the treatment area. She did not need any special treatment. The erythema disappeared, and the abdomen returned to normal after 3 days.

7.2.7.3 Discussion

- Abdominal wall crush injury is a soft tissue contusion. The reasons include (1) the treatment transducer head or ultrasound probe has pressed against the abdominal wall for a long time; (2) the skin of some patients is loose with less elasticity; (3)the treatment transducer head moves while it is firmly pressed against the skin, causing shearing of the subcutaneous tissue and breaking underlying subcutaneous blood vessels.
- Preventive measures for skin crush injury: (1) Do not press the skin with the treatment transducer head or diagnostic ultrasound probe too tightly or too long; (2) Regularly loose the skin to improve local microcirculation; (3) Keep the treatment transducer head separated from the skin when moving it.
- In this case, the treatment transducer head was probably touching the skin during treatment for a longer time, and the skin was squeezed, resulting in contusion injury.

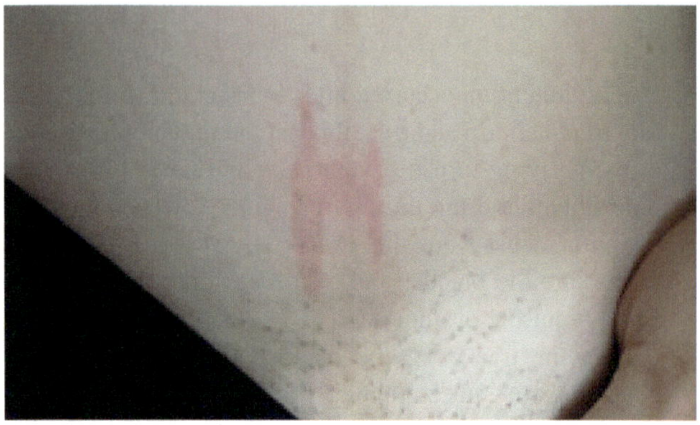

Fig. 7.7 Crush injury of abdominal skin
Immediately after the focused ultrasound ablation treatment, there is an "H" shaped indentation in the lower abdomen near the pubic symphysis, which is consistent with the shape of the ultrasound probe in the HIFU treatment system (Note: Photo courtesy of Huiyan LIU).

7.2.8 Case 8. One-Stage Debridement and Suture for Skin Burn

7.2.8.1 Case Description

The female patient was 29 years old. Her ultrasound examination revealed multiple fibroids for 3 years and dysmenorrhea for three months.

7.2.8.2 Diagnosis and Treatment

- MRI showed multiple uterine fibroids (Fig. 7.8a–c).
- During the treatment, the patient intermittently complained of hot skin. The intraoperative ultrasound monitoring showed that the fibroids were at the fundus of the uterus. The abdominal wall was pressed hard by the ultrasound probe to displace and show the fundal fibroids on sonography (Fig. 7.8d). After treatment, there was a blister of 2 cm in diameter on the skin (Fig. 7.8e).
- After treatment, the wound was debrided with one-stage suturing (Fig. 7.8f). The sutures were removed 10 days later. The wound healed well (Fig. 7.8g).

7.2.8.3 Discussion

- In this case, a large water balloon with high tension was used to push the abdominal wall, and the heat dissipation from the skin was limited. Thus, the skin was easily burned. The wound healed well after debridement of the skin burn area.
- Skin burn is the main complication of focused ultrasound ablation treatment; however, its incidence is very low. It is important to understand the causes of skin burns and focused ultrasound ablation principles for ensuring the safety of treatment.
- Due to the deposit of the focused ultrasound energy in the full-thickness abdominal wall, cooling intervals are needed to allow dissipation of the heat, which can avoid skin injuries.
- Scar tissue attenuates ultrasound significantly, and energy is easily deposited in the scar. The patient feels a dull ache without sharp pain in the scar area, which is a high-risk factor for skin injury. Before treatment, it is particularly important to know how to distinguish between normal and scarred skin by ultrasound examination.

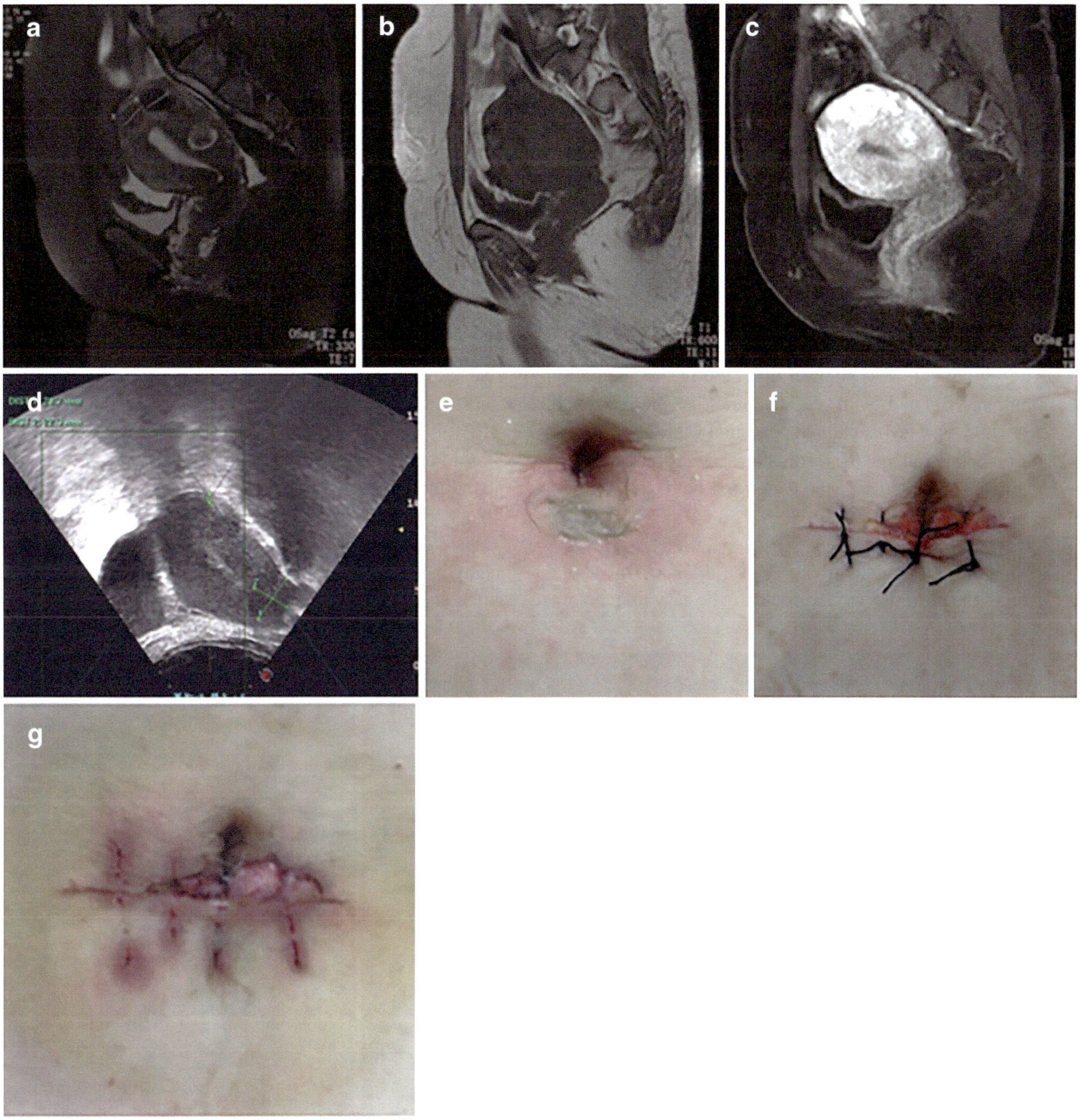

Fig. 7.8 One-stage debridement of II° skin burn (Note: Photo courtesy of Xiaofeng GU). (**a**) T2WI_FS sagittal before treatment, (**b**) T1WI sagittal before treatment, (**c**) T1WI_FS+C sagittal before treatment, (**d**) Ultrasound image during treatment, (**e**) Skin blister immediately after treatment, (**f**) Skin of one-stage surgical debridement and suture, (**g**) Skin after suture removal

7.2.9 Case 9 Continuous Vaginal Discharge After Treatment

7.2.9.1 Case Description

The female patient was 28 years old. She experienced menstrual pain for 5 years, gradually worsening for one year.

7.2.9.2 Diagnosis and Treatment

- MRI showed an adenomyoma at the posterior wall of the uterus before treatment (Fig. 7.9a–c).
- During the treatment, the patient complained of pain in the sacral coccyx, and there was no skin and nerve injury after the treatment.
- After treatment, MRI showed that 78% of the adenomyoma was ablated with the endometrial breakthrough (Fig. 7.9d–f). The patient had persistent vaginal discharge after the ablation, but the dysmenorrhea was relieved. The vaginal discharge disappeared after 6 months.

7.2.9.3 Discussion

- In this case, the adenomyoma had a thickness of about 4 cm of the posterior wall. It could not be easy to maintain a safe distance between the acoustic focus and the endometrium during treatment (safe distance >10 mm). Thus it may lead to endometrial damage.
- The sonication time may be too long during the treatment. After the treatment, the MRI showed that the posterior endometrial lining was broken through, and the ablated coagulated lesion directly communicated with the uterine cavity. Aseptic inflammation continued to stimulate the endometrium, resulting in persistent vaginal discharge.
- Vaginal drainage after focused ultrasound ablation treatment is generally divided into acute and chronic vaginal discharge.
- Causes of acute vaginal discharge: (1) some necrotic tissues of submucosal fibroids are discharged per vagina after ablation; (2) the diffusion of heat from the ablated fibroid or the aseptic inflammation of the necrotic fibroid irritating continually the endometrium; (3) endometrial injury leading the continuous inflammatory exudation.
- Causes for chronic vaginal discharge: (1) incomplete discharge of necrotic fibroid or unhealed wounds formed after shedding of submucous fibroid; (2) the necrotic

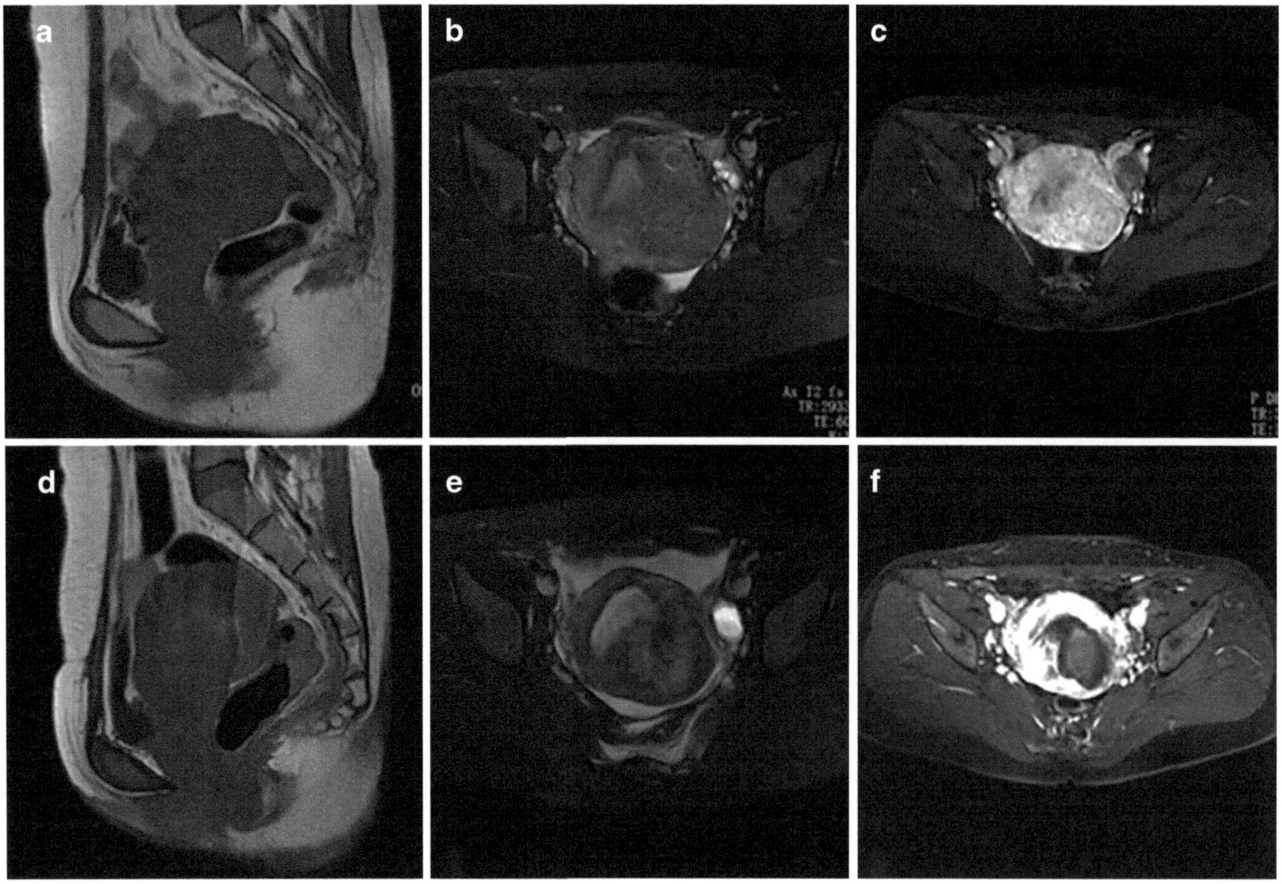

Fig. 7.9 Continuous vaginal discharge after focused ultrasound ablation treatment. (**a**) T1WI sagittal before treatment, (**b**) T2WI_FS axial before treatment, (**c**) T1WI_FS+C axial before treatment, (**d**) T1WI sagittal after treatment, (**e**) T1WI axial after treatment, (**f**) T1WI_FS+C axial after treatment

fibroid stimulating continually the endometrium; (3) the formation of a sinus in the endometrial layer.

- Continuous vaginal bleeding after treatment can seriously affect a patient's quality of life, and it takes a long time to recover.

7.2.10 Case 10 The Discharged Necrotic Fibroids Incarcerated at the Cervix

7.2.10.1 Case Description

The female patient was 28 years old. Ultrasound examination revealed a submucous fibroid for 3 years, and she had increased menstrual blood flow for 6 months.

7.2.10.2 Diagnosis and Treatment

- During the focused ultrasound ablation treatment, ultrasound monitoring showed the grayscale in the fibroid was significantly enhanced and spread (Fig. 7.10a).
- After treatment, MRI showed that the fibroid was completely ablated (Fig. 7.10b–d). Vaginal bleeding occurred. Two weeks later, the patient had a sudden abdominal pain. The gynecological examination found that the treated fibroid was discharged and incarcerated in the cervix, and then the intact fibroid was taken out (Fig. 7.10e). The bleeding volume was about 30 mL.

7.2.10.3 Discussion

- The fibroid in this case is a type I submucosal fibroid. After treatment, the MRI showed complete ablation of the fibroid. The fibroid eventually fell off and was incarcerated at the cervix, which stimulated uterine contractions and caused abdominal pain.
- The delivery of fibroid through the cervix may require surgical removal or be aborted spontaneously. Antibiotics can be used to prevent infection after the removal. The patient recovered well after treatment, and follow-up showed that she had no discomfort.

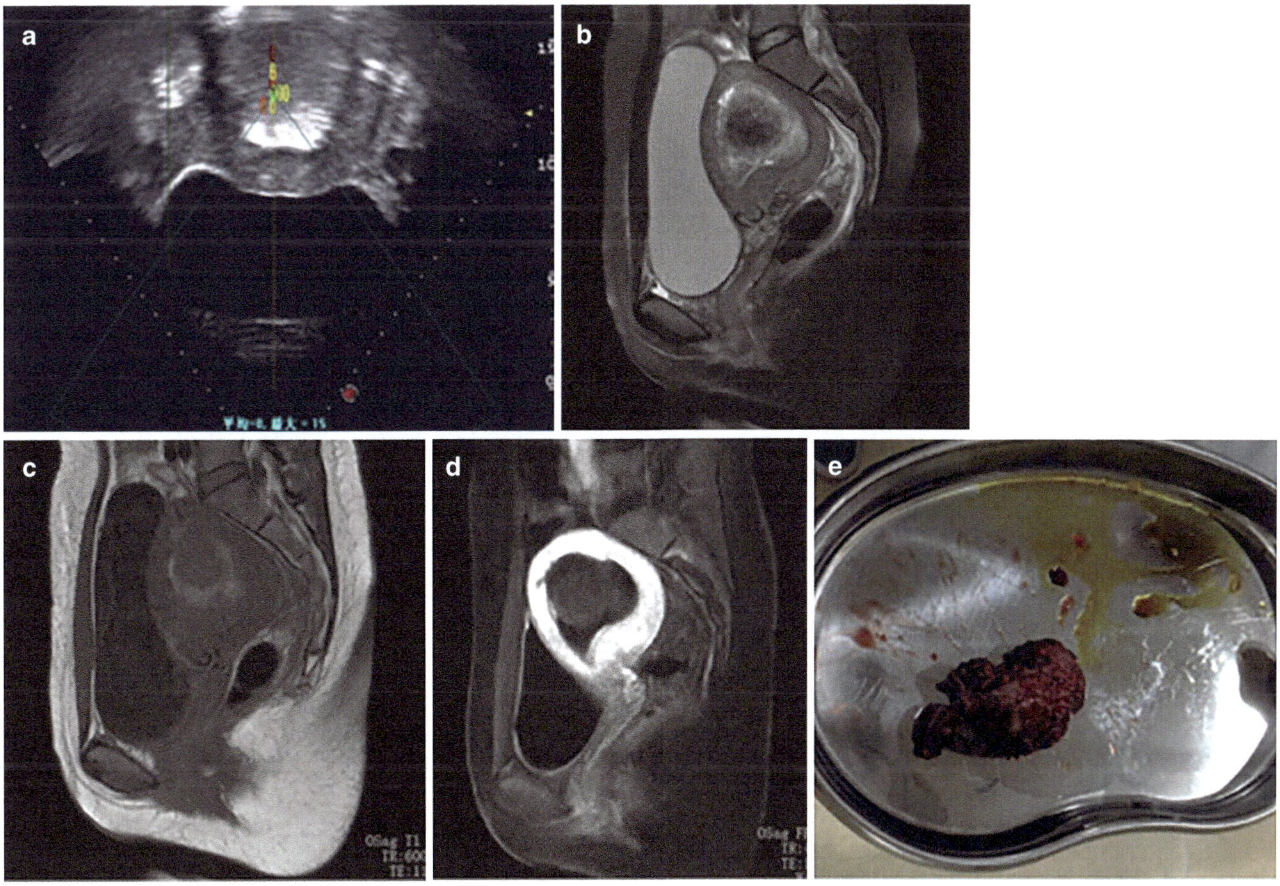

Fig. 7.10 After treatment, the necrotic fibroids were discharged and incarcerated at the cervix (Note: Photo courtesy of Dr. Yuzhen Zhou). (**a**) Ultrasound image during treatment, (**b**) T2WI_FS sagittal after treatment, (**c**) T1WI sagittal after treatment, (**d**) T1WI_FS+C sagittal after treatment, (**e**) Fibroid removed

7.2.11 Case 11 Continuous Discharge of Necrotic Tissue After Focused Ultrasound Ablation

7.2.11.1 Case Description

The female patient was 42 years old. She had abdominal pain during menstruation for 5 years, and it worsened for one year.

7.2.11.2 Diagnosis and Treatment

- MRI showed adenomyosis at the posterior wall of the uterus (Fig. 7.11a–c). After focused ultrasound ablation treatment, MRI demonstrated a large ablation area in the treated adenomyosis with a non-perfused volume of more than 93% on contrast-enhanced T1WI, and a breakthrough in the endometrium. There was a small amount of pelvic effusion on T2WI (Fig. 7.11d–f).

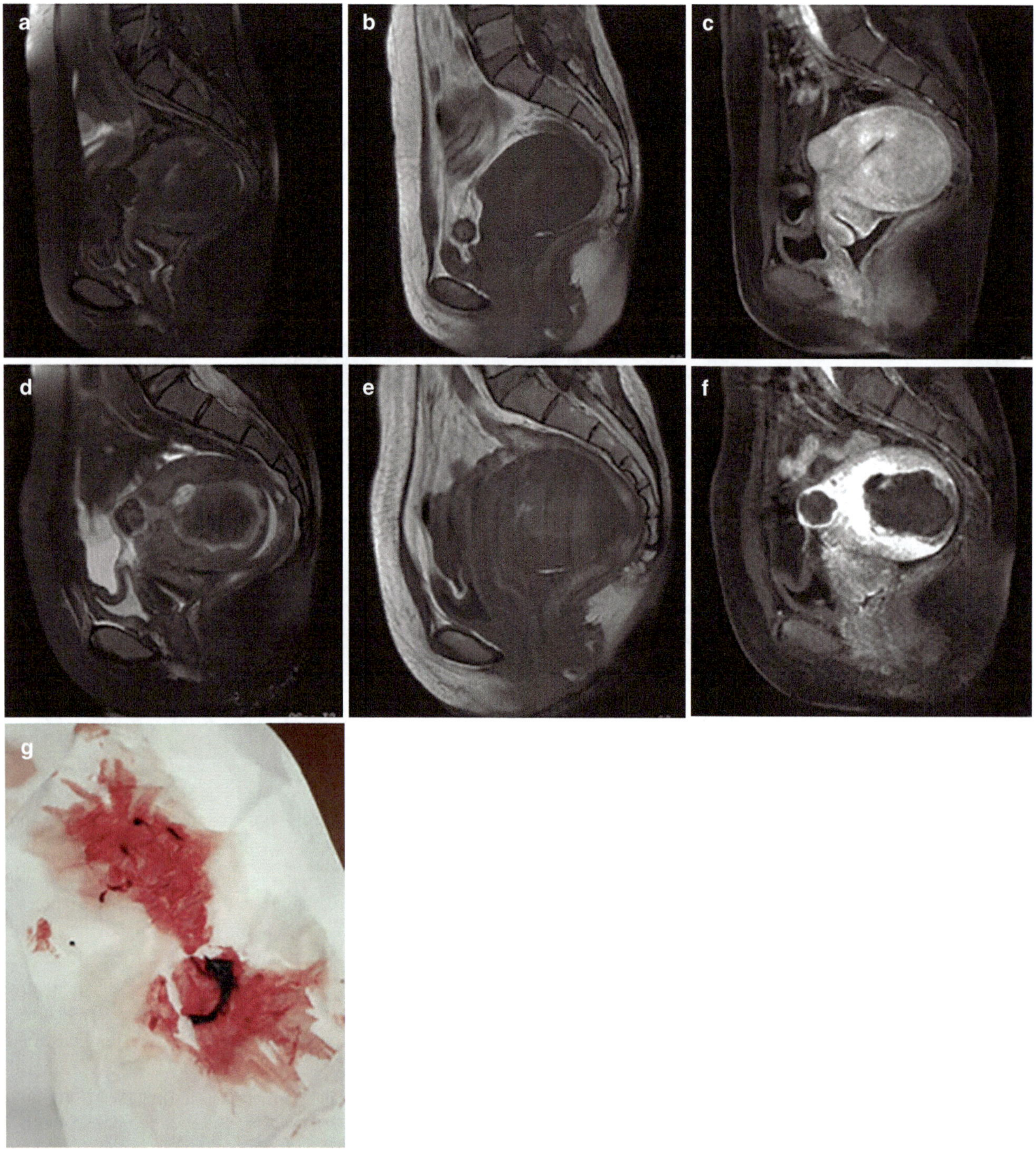

Fig. 7.11 The necrotic tissue continued to be discharged after the treatment. (**a**) T2WI_FS sagittal before treatment, (**b**) T1WI sagittal before treatment, (**c**) T1WI_FS+C sagittal before treatment, (**d**) T2WI_FS sagittal after treatment, (**e**) T1WI sagittal after treatment, (**f**) T1WI_FS+C sagittal after treatment, (**g**) Intermittent discharge of dark brown objects

- After the treatment, the patient had intermittent abdominal pain with continuous discharge of black blood clots (Fig. 7.11g) or tofu-like tissues, and returned to normal after the second menstruation.

7.2.11.3 Discussion

- After treatment, this patient experienced continuous vaginal discharge of necrotic tissue, considering that the adenomyosis lesion communicated with the uterine cavity after the endometrial breakthrough. After the tissue necrosis and liquefaction, it continues to be discharged through the endometrial gap. With the expulsion and absorption of necrotic lesions and the repair of the endometrial layer, it would eventually return to normal.

7.2.12 Case 12 Intrauterine Adhesions After Focused Ultrasound Ablation

7.2.12.1 Case Description

The female patient was 43 years old. Her ultrasound examination revealed uterine fibroids for 5 years, and she had increased menstrual flow for 1 year.

7.2.12.2 Diagnosis and Treatment

- MRI showed a posterior submucosal fibroid before treatment (Fig. 7.12a–c). Intraoperative ultrasound showed a breakthrough of the endometrium during the ablation procedure (Fig. 7.12d).
- After treatment, MRI showed that 95% of the uterine fibroid and a small portion of the anterior wall had no perfusion area with a small amount of fluid in the uterine cavity, suggestive of a breakthrough in the endometrium and an injury to the anterior wall of the uterus (Fig. 7.12e–g). A light yellow vaginal discharge was associated with decreased menstrual blood flow and occasional dysmenorrhea. Hysteroscopy was performed 5 months after the treatment and showed adhesions in the uterine cavity (Fig. 7.12h), and the adhesions were resected under hysteroscopic vision (Fig. 7.12i).
- Three months after hysteroscopy, her menstruation returned to normal, with no abnormal vaginal bleeding or other symptoms.

7.2.12.3 Discussion

- In this case, the ultrasound echo of the anterior wall showed increased echogenicity near the endometrium during the treatment, indicating that the overlying endometrium might have been injured. Postoperative MRI showed a breakthrough at the anterior and posterior endometrium of uterus.
- During the repair of the endometrium, adhesions occur over the injured area of the anterior and posterior uterine walls, which leads to intrauterine adhesions.
- Common causes of intrauterine adhesions after treatment include (1) focused ultrasound ablation of submucosal fibroids and adenomyosis can damage the endometrium; (2) intrauterine infection after treatment. The clinical presentations of intrauterine adhesions are abnormal menstruation, secondary reduced menstrual blood flow, and period pain. Hysteroscopy can help to separate the intrauterine adhesions.

7.2.13 Case 13 Intestinal Perforation After Focused Ultrasound Ablation

7.2.13.1 Case Description

The female patient was 47 years old. Ultrasound examination revealed uterine fibroids for one year, accompanied by increased menstrual flow for 6 months.

7.2.13.2 Diagnosis and Treatment

- MRI showed two submucosal fibroids before treatment (Fig. 7.13a–c).
- During focused ultrasound ablation treatment, ultrasound monitoring at the 50 s of sonication showed that the lesion had mass grayscale changes and spread well (Fig. 7.13d).
- MRI evaluation on the second day after treatment showed a large ablation area of fibroids that had a breakthrough in the anterior serosa on contrast-enhanced T1WI, and a small amount of fluid in the pelvic cavity on T2WI (Fig. 7.13e–g).
- One week after treatment, the patient suddenly developed severe abdominal pain, and free air under the diaphragm was seen in the erect position of the abdominal X-ray (Fig. 7.13h). An emergency laparotomy was performed, and perforation of the small intestine was found near the uterus (Fig. 7.13i). She underwent a repair of the intestinal perforation and recovered after the surgical treatment.

7.2.13.3 Discussion

- In this case, the mass grayscale change spread to the anterior uterine serosa during treatment, and a breakthrough in the serosal layer could be seen in MRI after treatment. It is considered that heat diffusion has caused thermal damage to the intestine. Five days later, the necrosis area of the intestinal tract ruptured, resulting in an intestinal perforation.
- For those who have a history of surgery, it is considered that there may be adhesions in the bowels, the grayscale change spread out of the serosal layer during the treatment, and a breakthrough in the serosal layer diagnosed by MRI are the high-risk factors for intestinal injury.
- Intestinal injury is a rare and serious complication of focused ultrasound ablation surgery. Patients usually develop abdominal pain and fever from immediately after

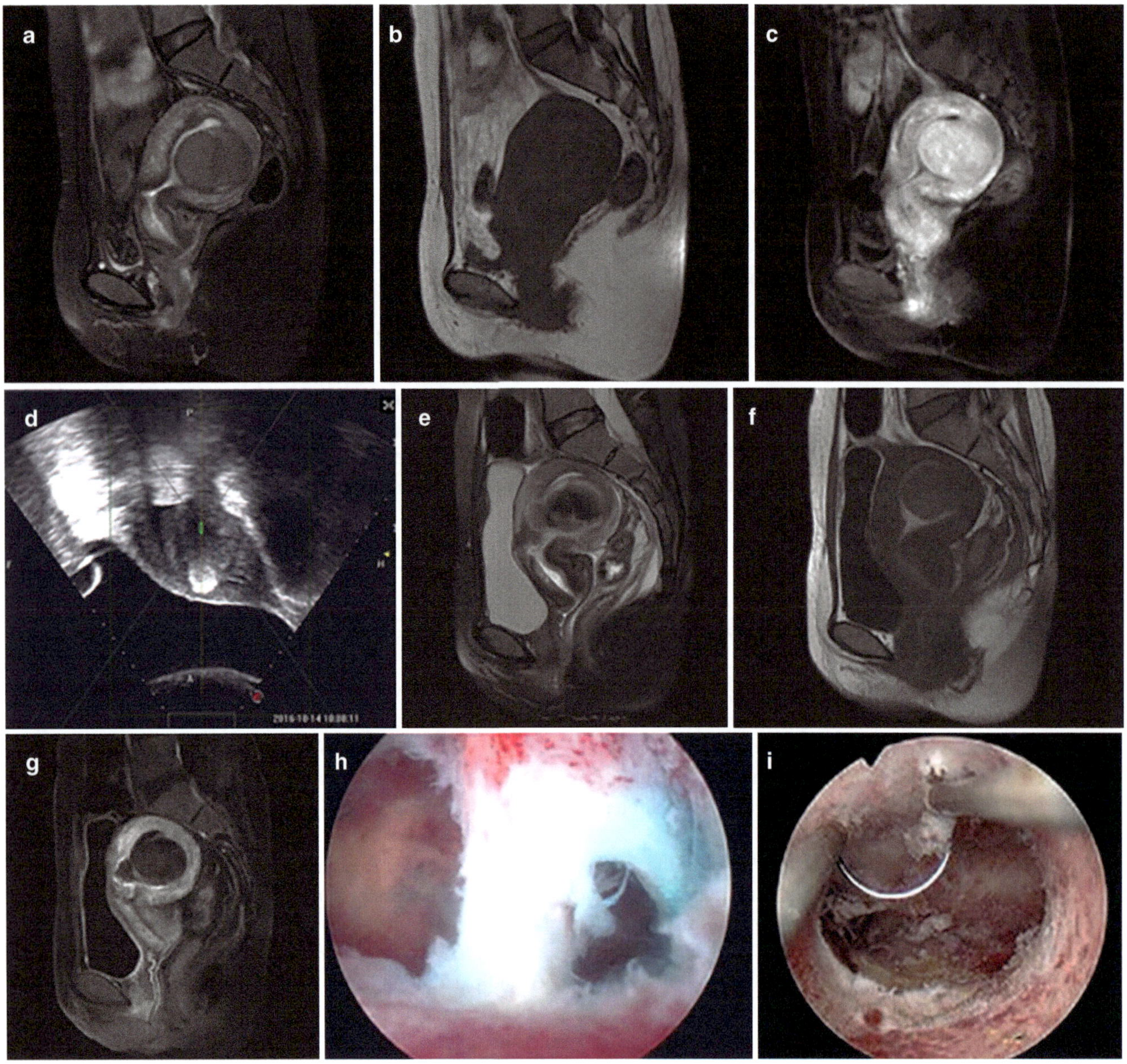

Fig. 7.12 Uterine adhesions after focused ultrasound ablation treatment. (**a**) T2WI_FS sagittal before treatment, (**b**) T1WI sagittal before treatment, (**c**) T1WI_FS+C sagittal before treatment, (**d**) Ultrasound image during treatment, (**e**) T2WI_FS sagittal after treatment, (**f**) T1WI sagittal after treatment, (**g**) T1WI_FS+C sagittal after treatment, (**h**) Hysteroscopy after treatment showed intrauterine adhesions, (**i**) Hysteroscopy showed removal of adhesions

treatment to 1 week after treatment, and the signs of peritonitis can be found on physical examination. The treatment of intestinal injury is mainly surgical therapy.

7.2.14 Case 14 Sacrococcygeal Injury Caused by Focused Ultrasound Ablation

7.2.14.1 Case Description

The female patient was 40 years old. Her ultrasound examination revealed uterine fibroids for 5 years, with enlarging fibroids and heavy menstrual blood flow for one year.

7.2.14.2 Diagnosis and Treatment

- Before treatment, MRI showed a fibroid at the anterior wall of the uterus (Fig. 7.14a–c).
- During focused ultrasound ablation treatment, the sacrococcygeal pain was severe, and sonography showed ultrasound echo changes could be seen in the coccyx (Fig. 7.14d). On the second day after treatment, MRI demonstrated a large ablation area of fibroids with a non-perfused volume ratio of 93% and enhancement along the anterior wall of the upper rectum adjacent to the uterus on the contrast-enhanced T1WI, and a small amount of fluid in the pelvic cavity and the increased signal intensity in

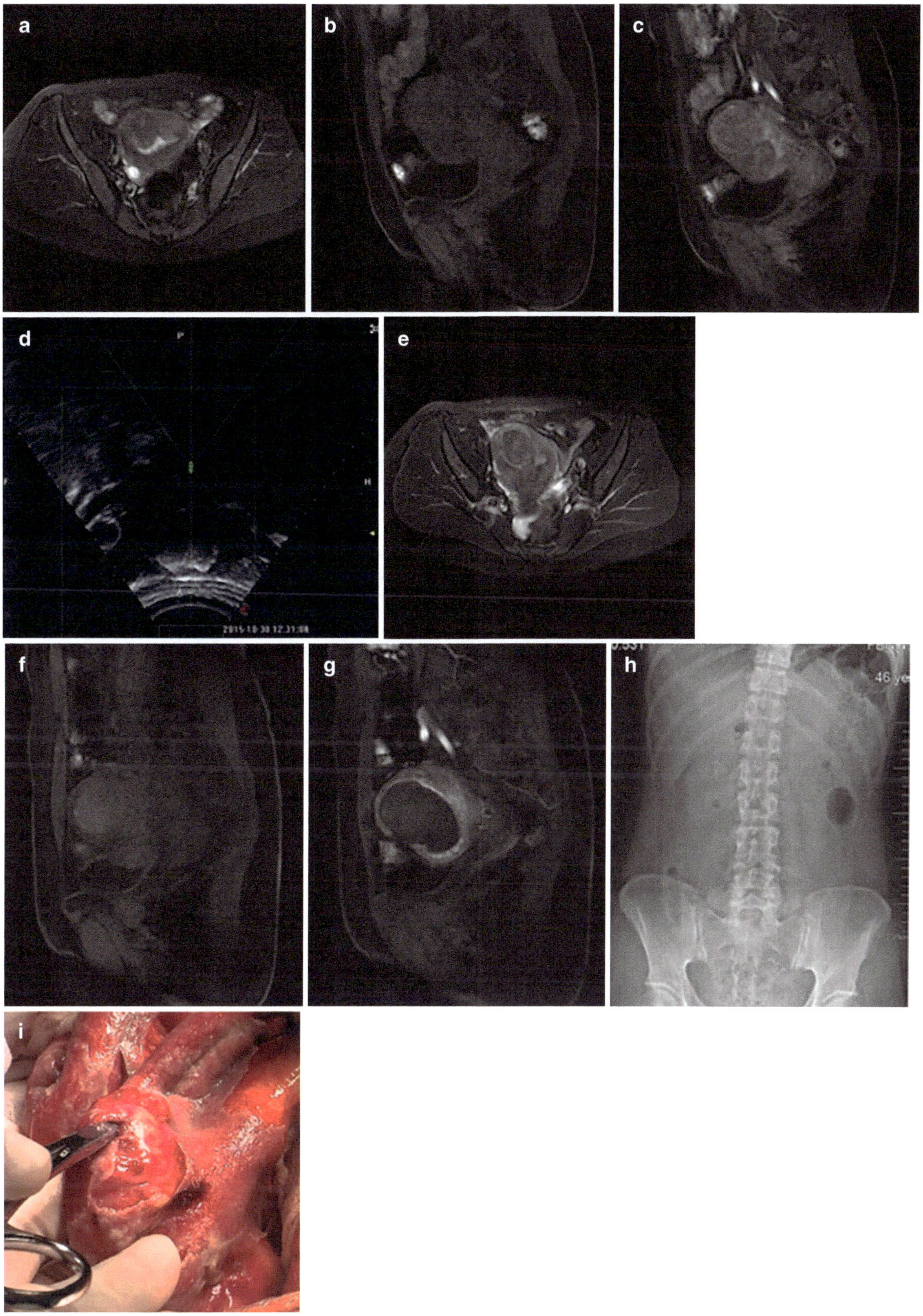

Fig. 7.13 Intestinal perforation after focused ultrasound ablation therapy. (**a**) T2WI_FS sagittal before treatment, (**b**) T1WI sagittal before treatment, (**c**)T1WI_FS+C sagittal before treatment, (**d**) Ultrasound image during treatment, (**e**) T2WI_FS sagittal after treatment, (**f**) T1WI sagittal after treatment, (**g**) T1WI_FS+C sagittal after treatment, (**h**) Abdominal radiograph at 8 days after treatment, (**i**) Laparotomy at 9 days after focused ultrasound ablation treatment

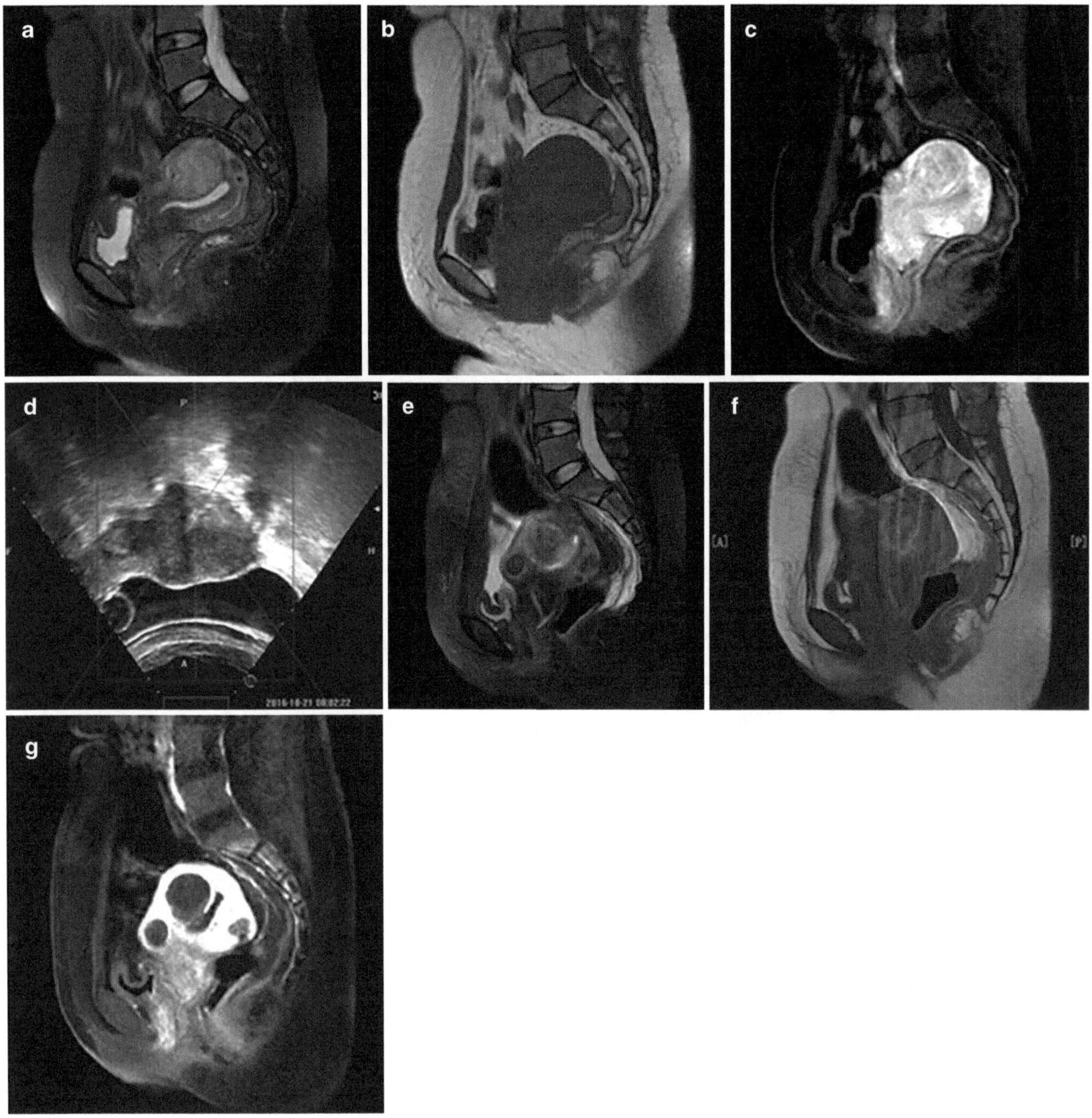

Fig. 7.14 Sacrococcygeal injury after ultrasound ablation. (**a**) T2WI_FS sagittal before treatment, (**b**) T1WI sagittal before treatment, (**c**) T1WI_FS+C sagittal before treatment, (**d**) Ultrasound image during treatment, (**e**) T2WI_FS sagittal after treatment, (**f**) T1WI sagittal after treatment, (**g**) T1WI_FS+C sagittal after treatment

the posterior fascia and sacrococcygeal bone on T2WI (Fig. 7.14e–g).
- Persistent sacrococcygeal pain occurred after treatment, especially aggravated after exercise. Sacrococcygeal pain disappeared after 2 months of symptomatic treatment.

7.2.14.3 Discussion
- In this case, the large distended bladder pushed the uterus posteriorly to the back during treatment, and the focused ablation area was closer to the sacrococcyx. And the treatment time was probably longer, which could cause more energy to be absorbed by the sacrococcyx and suffered the sacrococcygeal injury.
- Sacrococcygeal injury usually presents as sacrococcygeal pain without affecting the body's movement or activities. Symptomatic treatment is sufficient, and it also can be cured by itself.

7.2.15 Case 15 Nerve Damage Caused by Focused Ultrasound Ablation

7.2.15.1 Case Description
The female patient was 42 years old. Her ultrasound examination revealed a uterine fibroid for 5 years, and it gradually increased in size with lower abdominal distension and pain for one year.

7.2.15.2 Diagnosis and Treatment
- Before treatment, MRI showed a fibroid in the right wall of the uterus (Fig. 7.15a, b). Before treatment, ultrasound positioning showed the posterior part of the fibroid close to the pelvic nerves and blood vessels (Fig. 7.15c).
- During the treatment, the patient intermittently complained of pain in the right calf, and immediately after the treatment, the patient did not complain of any special discomfort.
- After the treatment, the fascia around the neurovascular plexus was edematous at the right pelvic posterior wall (Fig. 7.15d), and the NPV ratio of the fibroid was around 91% on contrast-enhanced MR imaging (Fig. 7.15e). However, the patient experienced persistent pain in the right leg. Symptomatic treatment was given to relieve the pain, the muscle strength of the right foot decreased, and there was edema after exercise (Fig. 7.15f). The edema subsided after resting in the supine position.
- Six months later, a follow-up showed that the muscle strength of the right foot returned to normal, and the right foot still had slight edematous.

7.2.15.3 Discussion
- In this case, there is a nerve behind the fibroid, and the backfield energy of focused ultrasound directly stimulates the nerve during the treatment, so radiating pain to the calf occurred during the treatment.
- When the nerve was injured, neuro-sensitivity symptoms like leg pain and muscle weakness appeared. After symptomatic treatments such as inhibition of inflammation and pain relief, which would promote nerve regeneration, the pain disappeared after the nerve recovered from injury.

7.2.16 Case 16 Necrotic Fibroid with Aseptic Inflammation Causing Nerve Irritation

7.2.16.1 Case Description
The female patient was 32 years old. Her ultrasound examination revealed a uterine fibroid for 2 years, and the fibroid gradually increased in size, causing anal discomfort for one year.

7.2.16.2 Diagnosis and Treatment
- MRI showed a fibroid on the posterior wall of the uterus before treatment (Fig. 7.16a–c), and the patient did not complain of discomfort during treatment.
- After the treatment, the contrast-enhanced T1WI showed 96% NPV of the posterior fibroid (Fig. 7.16d–f). On the third day, the patient developed a persistent pain in his left leg. After symptomatic treatment, the pain was gradually relieved and disappeared after 1 week.

7.2.16.3 Discussion
- In this case, the fibroid was close to the sacrum. After the ablation treatment, the aseptic inflammation from the necrotic fibroid stimulated the pelvic nerve plexus lying in the front and sides of the sacrum, causing leg pain. The aseptic inflammation subsided after anti-inflammatory treatment, and the nerve irritation disappeared.
- The causes for nerve damage include (1) the nerve tissue absorbing the heat energy at ultrasound backfield; (2) aseptic inflammation of the necrotic fibroid affecting the above nerve plexus; (3) the heat spreading to the nerves during prolonged treatment.
- The cause of leg pain is sometimes due to ultrasound irradiation, and then the patient will have radiating pain during treatment. In the early stage, the treatment mainly uses anti-inflammatory drugs to reduce inflammation and edema. If the patient has no radiating pain during the treatment, the

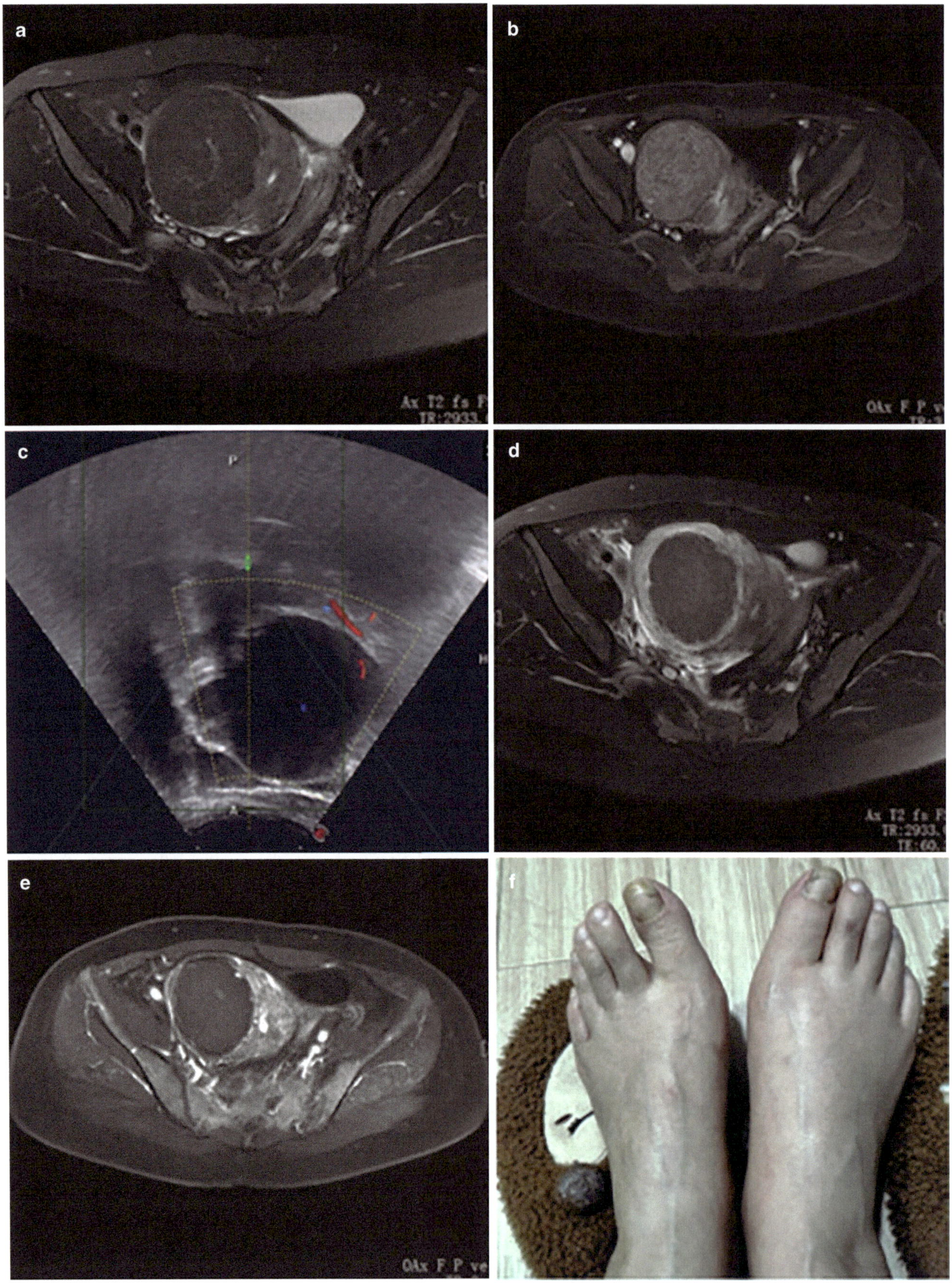

Fig. 7.15 Focused ultrasound ablation resulting in nerve injury. (**a**) T2WI_FS axial before treatment, (**b**) T1WI_FS+C axial before treatment, (**c**) Ultrasound image during treatment, (**d**) T2WI_FS axial after treatment, (**e**) T1WI_FS+C axial after treatment, (**f**) There is still edematous in the right foot at 1 month after treatment

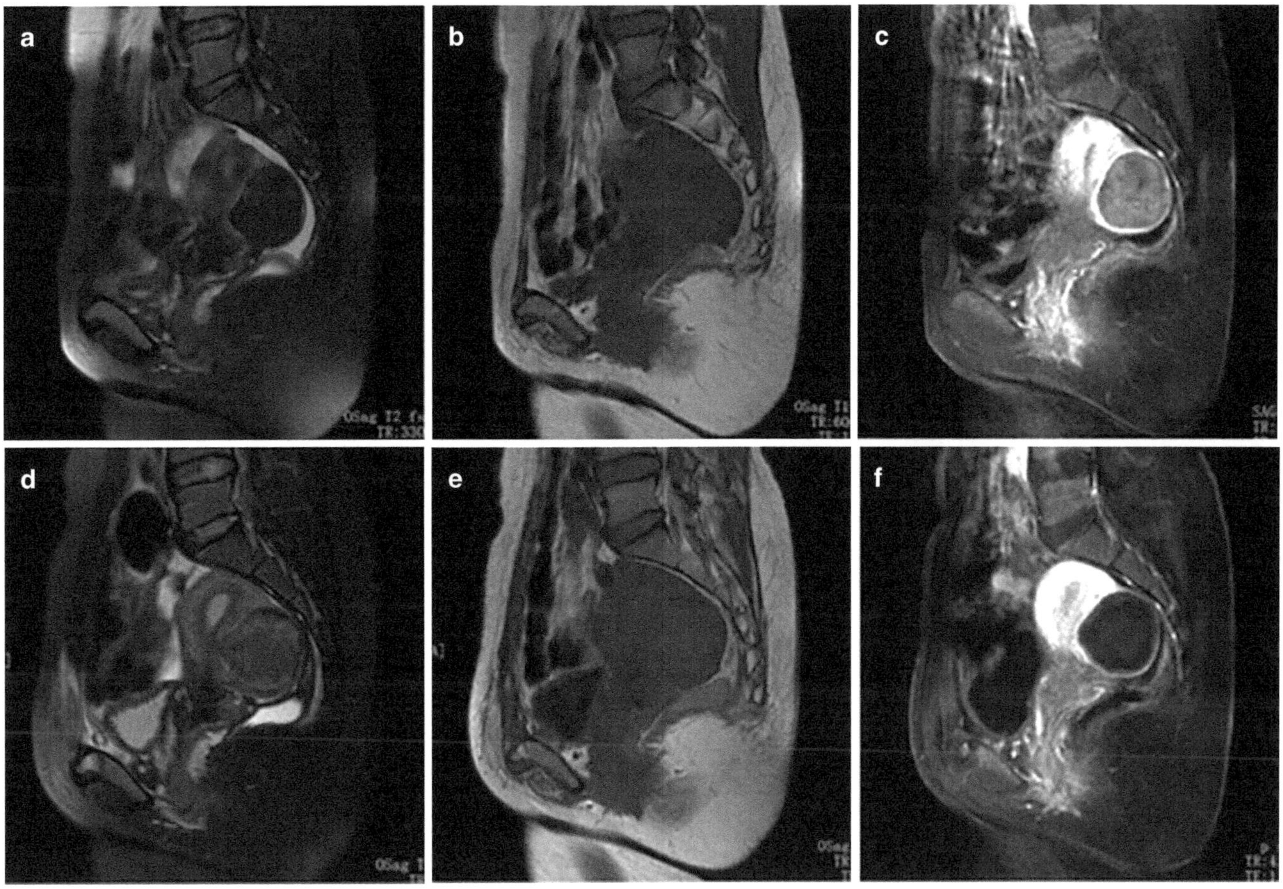

Fig. 7.16 Necrotic fibroid stimulated the sacral plexus after focused ultrasound ablation treatment. (**a**) T2WI_FS sagittal before treatment, (**b**) T1WI sagittal before treatment, (**c**) T1WI_FS+C sagittal before treatment, (**d**) T2WI_FS sagittal after treatment, (**e**) T1WI sagittal after treatment, (**f**) T1WI_FS+C sagittal after treatment

cause could be the nerve stimulation from the necrotic fibroids, and the patient will show continuous aggravating nerve pain after treatment. Treatment with anti-inflammatory and symptomatic treatment is sufficient.

- Prevention of nerve damage: After treatment, the patient rests in the prone position for 2 hours, which can avoid thermal nerve injury from the diffusion of residual heat of the necrotic fibroid, causing injury to the sacral plexus.

References

1. Sacks D, McClenny TE, Cardella JF, Lewis C. Society of interventional radiology clinical practice guidelines. J Vasc Interv Radiol. 2003;14:S199–202.
2. Zhang L, Zhang W, Orsi F, et al. Ultrasound-guided high intensity focused ultrasound for treating gynaecological diseases: a review of safety and efficacy. Int J Hyperthermia. 2015;31(3):280–4.

GPSR Compliance

The European Union's (EU) General Product Safety Regulation (GPSR) is a set of rules that requires consumer products to be safe and our obligations to ensure this.

If you have any concerns about our products, you can contact us on ProductSafety@springernature.com

In case Publisher is established outside the EU, the EU authorized representative is:

Springer Nature Customer Service Center GmbH
Europaplatz 3
69115 Heidelberg, Germany

Batch number: 10731524

Printed by Printforce, the Netherlands